Studies in Big Data

Volume 193

The series "Studies in Big Data" (SBD) publishes new developments and advances in the various areas of Big Data- quickly and with a high quality. The intent is to cover the theory, research, development, and applications of Big Data, as embedded in the fields of engineering, computer science, physics, economics and life sciences. The books of the series refer to the analysis and understanding of large, complex, and/or distributed data sets generated from recent digital sources coming from sensors or other physical instruments as well as simulations, crowd sourcing, social networks or other internet transactions, such as emails or video click streams and other. The series contains monographs, lecture notes and edited volumes in Big Data spanning the areas of computational intelligence including neural networks, evolutionary computation, soft computing, fuzzy systems, as well as artificial intelligence, data mining, modern statistics and Operations research, as well as self-organizing systems. Of particular value to both the contributors and the readership are the short publication timeframe and the world-wide distribution, which enable both wide and rapid dissemination of research output.

The books of this series are reviewed in a single blind peer review process.

Indexed by SCOPUS, EI Compendex, SCIMAGO and zbMATH.

All books published in the series are submitted for consideration in Web of Science.

Prabhishek Singh · Vinayakumar Ravi ·
Manoj Diwakar · Manak Gupta
Editors

Deep Learning Applications in Healthcare and Medical Imaging Practice

Springer

Editors
Prabhishek Singh
School of Computer Science Engineering and Technology
Bennett University
Noida, Uttar Pradesh, India

Manoj Diwakar
Department of Computer Science Engineering
Graphic Era University
Dehradun, Uttarakhand, India

Vinayakumar Ravi
Center for Artificial Intelligence
Prince Mohammad Bin Fahd University
Khobar, Saudi Arabia

Manak Gupta
Tennessee Technological University
Cookeville, TN, USA

ISSN 2197-6503 ISSN 2197-6511 (electronic)
Studies in Big Data
ISBN 978-3-032-21008-1 ISBN 978-3-032-21009-8 (eBook)
https://doi.org/10.1007/978-3-032-21009-8

This Springer imprint is published by the registered company Springer Nature Switzerland AG
The registered company address is: Gewerbestrasse 11, 6330 Cham, Switzerland

Preface

Deep learning has been progressively transforming how complex data problems can be tackled especially in areas where traditional methods of analysis are practically constrained. Medical imaging and healthcare belong perfectly within this gap. The increasing size of digital medical data and the need to have a more reliable and adaptive analysis have been promoting the application of learning-based models which can adapt to the changing data instead of adhering to fixed assumptions. The book, *Deep Learning Applications in Healthcare and Medical Imaging Practice*, is compiled to indicate how deep learning is being used in practice and not how it is defined theoretically. It concentrates on the approaches that have progressed beyond the theoretical suggestions and are being investigated, experimented, and sharpened in the actual problem contexts. The chapters emphasize the way in which learning model is framed by data limitations, system demands and application-based objectives.

The volume contains the works of researchers and practitioners, who work in the field of computer science, engineering, and healthcare technology. Topics cover medical image analysis, pattern detection, predictive modeling, and multi-modality data processing. Classic strategies and recent architectural tendencies are addressed, and the implementation decisions and experimental analysis are of particular concern instead of abstract formalism. Realism is another theme in the book. The contributors consider issues like the unavailability of data, extrapolating between datasets, interpretability, and factors of computational cost that frequently define whether a method can be useful outside of controlled studies. These talks give a practical opinion of both existing capacities and open studies areas. The book is aimed at graduate students, researchers, and professionals who need to know how deep learning methods are implemented in the medical field and in the medical imaging specifically nowadays. Hopefully, it will be an informative source of research, promote cross-disciplinary cooperation, and facilitate viable, well-thought innovation.

We extend our sincere thanks to Springer for their continued professional support and for providing this publishing opportunity. We are grateful to all contributing authors and reviewers whose scholarly efforts have shaped the quality and breadth of this volume.

Greater Noida, India — Prabhishek Singh
Khobar, Saudi Arabia — Vinayakumar Ravi
Dehradun, India — Manoj Diwakar
Cookeville, USA — Manak Gupta

Contents

About the Editors

Prabhishek Singh is an Associate Professor at Bennett University and Adjunct Faculty at Maryam Abacha American University, Nigeria. Recognized as a Top 2% Scientist (2024), his work focuses on image processing, computer vision, deep learning, and machine learning. He has published 210+ papers and serves in various editorial roles across SCI/SCIE/Scopus/ESCI-indexed journals.

Vinayakumar Ravi is an Assistant Research Professor at the Center for Artificial Intelligence, Prince Mohammad Bin Fahd University, Khobar, Saudi Arabia. His current research interests include applications of data mining, artificial intelligence, and machine learning (including deep learning) in biomedical informatics, cybersecurity, image processing, and natural language processing. Dr. Ravi has more than 100 research publications. He organized a shared task on detecting malicious domain names (DMD 2018) as part of SSCC'18 and ICACCI'18. He received the Chancellor's Research Excellence Award at AIRA 2021, and his name was included in the list of the World's Top 2% Scientists by Stanford University, published in PLOS Biology.

Manoj Diwakar is a Professor at Graphic Era Deemed to be University, Dehradun, India. His research interests include image processing, computer vision, medical imaging, and information security. He has authored 250+ papers in reputed journals/conferences (IEEE, Springer, Elsevier) and has been listed among the World's Top 2% Scientists by Stanford University and Elsevier (2023–2024). He serves in various editorial roles across SCI/SCIE/Scopus/ESCI-indexed journals, and has edited books with Springer, CRC, and Bentham Science.

Manak Gupta is an Associate Professor in the Department of Computer Science at Tennessee Tech University where he is Director of the Applied and Basic Cyber Security (ABCyS) laboratory. He received his Ph.D. in Computer Science from the University of Texas at San Antonio (UTSA), under the supervision of Prof. Ravi

Sandhu in December 2018, and has worked as a Postdoctoral Research Fellow at the Institute for Cyber Security, UTSA. He is also an associated faculty with the CEROC: Cybersecurity Education, Research and Outreach Center at Tennessee Tech. His primary area of research includes security and privacy in cyber space. He is also interested in AI and machine learning.

Deep Learning Innovations in Medical Imaging and Healthcare: Methods and Applications

H. R. Sneha and B. Annappa

Abstract Medical imaging generates vast amounts of visual and sequential data that clinicians must interpret quickly and accurately. Over the past decade deep learning (DL) has transformed this domain by enabling end-to-end learning of rich representations from raw images and signals. This chapter reviews the mathematical foundations, contemporary algorithms and practical applications of DL in healthcare. Real-world examples are drawn from radiology, pathology, ophthalmology, cardiology, dermatology and remote sensing. After introducing morphological image operations and evaluation metrics, traditional pipelines are contrasted with convolutional, transformer and graph-based architectures for detection, segmentation and recognition. Public datasets and standard evaluation protocols are summarised, followed by interdisciplinary applications and a small experimental analysis of dataset sizes, class imbalance and model-size trade-offs. Such challenges are the lack of data, interpretability and privacy which are addressed and the future research directions.

Keywords Deep learning · Medical imaging · Detection · Segmentation · Evaluation metrics

1 Introduction

Medical imaging has gone to become a part of the present-day healthcare, as it has become the staple of the diagnostics, prognosis, and treatment planning concerning an enormous variety of clinical conditions, such as pulmonary infection or brain tumour, heart defects and eye disease. Modern hospitals are regularly receiving

H. R. Sneha (✉)
Department of Information Science and Engineering, Nitte Meenakshi Institute of Technology, Nitte (Deemed to be University), Bengaluru 560064, Karnataka, India
e-mail: snehahr1990@gmail.com

H. R. Sneha · B. Annappa
Department of Computer Science and Engineering, National Institute of Technology Karnataka (NITK), Surathkal 575025, Mangalore, India
e-mail: annappa@nitk.edu.in

P. Singh et al. (eds.), *Deep Learning Applications in Healthcare and Medical Imaging Practice*, Studies in Big Data 193, https://doi.org/10.1007/978-3-032-21009-8_1

various types of imaging data, such as chest radiographs, computed tomography (CT) scans, magnetic resonance imaging (MRI) volumes, whole-slide histopathology images, retinal fundus photographs, dermatoscopic images, ultrasound recordings and electrocardiograms (ECG). The modalities carry a lot of structural and functional information that help the clinicians to detect subtle pathological signals. Nevertheless, the scale and heterogeneity of such data ecosystem is unprecedented and presents serious challenges to computational, interpretative, and operational problems.

Previously, the computer-aided diagnosis (CAD) systems were based on hand-designed features that were developed by domain experts. Although these methods were initially successful, they were very susceptible to noise, variations of scanners, lighting, and artifacts in acquisitions. More importantly, they did not extrapolate among the groups of patients, organs, imaging procedures and disease phenotypes. Their complexity and heterogeneity of pathological appearances in realistic clinical setting demonstrated that there is an inherent limitation: manually constructed pipelines cannot evolve to the full range of medical imaging information.

With the introduction of deep learning, this situation has changed radically. The hierarchical feature representations are now learned with convolutional neural networks (CNNs), transformer-based networks, and hybrid multimodal networks that learn directly on raw pixel data, without the use of engineered descriptors [1]. These models operate on specified diagnostic tasks and Friedman and Halley state that when trained on millions of annotated samples they reach expert or superhuman performance. On the CheXpert dataset of more than 200,000 [2] chest radiographs, deep CNNs have achieved levels of accuracy comparable to radiologists in the detection of pneumonia, pleural effusion, cardiomegaly, and other pathology of the thorax. Likewise, extensive retinal data sets like EyePACS or APTOS 2019 have also allowed automated systems to diagnose diabetic retinopathy with clinical-grade sensitivity and specificity and participate in screening in remote and underserved areas.

Although these are great accomplishments, the industry is encountering dynamic problems that require advanced solutions. Medical imaging data is already skewed, with uncommon conditions unrepresented in training sets but with severe clinical outcomes. The modalities vary across dimensionality, resolution and volume of data making it challenging to design and evaluate the models. In addition, the trend of explainable AI, regulatory compliance, privacy conservation and running on edge hardware has introduced new limitations that existing deep architecture designs are insufficient to meet.

This chapter offers an overview of the advancements in medical imaging, which are based on deep learning. Section 2 forms the mathematical grounds of the main operations such as morphological transformations, bounding box and segmentation metrics, and classification metrics. The equations are displayed one after another and cited all through the story to help the reader understand. Section 3 will discuss pre-deep learning techniques with their limitations and inability to replace more sophisticated techniques. Part 4 and 5 discuss modern deep learning detection, segmentation, and sequence recognition architectures, and include convolutional neural networks (CNNs), transformer architectures, and graph-based architectures. Section 6 presents the discussion on common public datasets and testing protocols, which are part and parcel of the benchmarking the model performance. Section 7 explores the applications in the different fields of medicine that can be achieved, and the potential obstacles that still need to be overcome. Section 8 of the chapter addresses some of the most critical issues, including the lack of data and imbalance in classes, interpretability, and privacy concerns, and proposes possible ways of future direction to address these obstacles. A short analysis of the experiment is given in Sect. 9, showing the results of distributions of datasets, morphological operations, and the complexity of the models. Lastly, the discussion is concluded by Sect. 10, which provides some concluding statements.

2 Fundamentals

Basic image processing methods constitute the foundation of deep learning methods in medical imaging. In this part, we discuss the key mathematical operations and image measures, which are morphological operations, bounding box and classification measures. These tools play a very important role in the preparation and analysis of medical images to be further processed by deep learning models. Some morphological operations, such as the refinement and perfection of images, can be used to contribute to eliminate noise and emphasize important features. These concepts form the basis of constructing models that may carry out automated image analysis and guide clinicians to make informed decisions.

2.1 *Morphological Operations*

The morphological operations alter the geometrical structure of binary or grayscale images. They are basic image processing tools which remove noise, extract shapes and refine masks. Let $I \subseteq \mathbb{Z}^2$ denote the set of foreground pixels of a binary image and let $B \subseteq \mathbb{Z}^2$ be a small structuring element, such as a disk or square. **Erosion** translates the structuring element across the image and keeps only those positions where B fits entirely within the foreground:

$$I \ominus B = \{x \in \mathbb{Z}^2 : B_x \subseteq I\}, \quad (1)$$

where $B_x = \{b + x : b \in B\}$. Erosion shrinks objects by removing boundary pixels [3]. **Dilation** performs the dual operation:

$$I \oplus B = \{x \in \mathbb{Z}^2 : (B^r)_x \cap I \neq \emptyset\}, \quad (2)$$

where $B^r = \{-b : b \in B\}$ is the reflection of B. Dilation expands objects by adding boundary pixels [3]. **Opening** is erosion followed by dilation and removes small objects while preserving the shape of larger structures. **Closing** is dilation followed by erosion and fills small holes. The **morphological gradient** highlights object boundaries as the difference between dilation and erosion:

$$\mathrm{grad}(I) = (I \oplus B) \big/ (I \ominus B). \tag{3}$$

The **top-hat transform** extracts small bright elements by subtracting the opened image from the original: $I - (I \circ B)$, while the **black-hat transform** extracts small dark elements by subtracting the original from its closing: $(I \cdot B) - I$. Morphological operations extend naturally to grayscale images by interpreting I and B as functions and replacing set operations with min–max operations [3]. These operators are widely used to preprocess medical images—for example, to remove small calcifications in mammograms or to fill holes in segmentation masks—and will appear later in our experimental analysis.

2.2 *Bounding Geometries and Overlap Metrics*

Object detection models predict bounding boxes around structures of interest and compare them with ground-truth boxes. Let A and B denote predicted and ground-truth boxes, respectively. The **intersection over union (IoU)** measures the relative overlap:

$$\mathrm{IoU}(A, B) = \frac{|A \cap B|}{|A \cup B|}, \tag{4}$$

where $|\cdot|$ denotes area [4]. IoU ranges from 0 (no overlap) to 1 (perfect overlap) and is used both as a metric and as a loss. When boxes do not overlap, IoU vanishes and provides no gradient. The **generalised IoU (GIoU)** addresses this by subtracting the proportion of the smallest convex hull C containing both boxes that is not covered by either:

$$\mathrm{GIoU}(A, B) = \mathrm{IoU}(A, B) - \frac{|C \backslash (A \cup B)|}{|C|}. \tag{5}$$

Alternative losses such as the distance IoU (DIoU) and complete IoU (CIoU) penalise the distance between box centres and the difference in aspect ratios, improving bounding-box regression. For segmentation tasks, the Dice coefficient computes twice the area of overlap divided by the sum of areas:

$$\mathrm{Dice}(P, G) = \frac{2|P \cap G|}{|P| + |G|}. \tag{6}$$

The Dice coefficient ranges from 0 to 1 and is equivalent to the F1 score in binary segmentation. The Jaccard index (IoU) provides a similar measure. When precise boundary alignment is required, the Hausdorff distance quantifies the maximum distance of a point in one contour to the nearest point in the other.

2.3 Classification Metrics

Classification performance is evaluated using summary statistics derived from the confusion matrix of true positives (TP), false positives (FP), true negatives (TN) and false negatives (FN). The accuracy (Eq. 7) measures the proportion of correctly classified instances. Precision (Eq. 8) is the fraction of positive predictions that are correct, while recall or sensitivity (Eq. 9) is the fraction of true positives detected. Specificity (Eq. 10) measures the fraction of true negatives identified. The F1 score (Eq. 11) is the harmonic mean of precision and recall and is especially useful for imbalanced datasets. These metrics are formalised in evaluation guidelines [5]. Additional measures include the area under the receiver operating characteristic curve (AUC), which integrates the trade-off between true and false positive rates across thresholds, and the mean average precision (mAP) used in detection [6]. In segmentation, the Dice coefficient (Eq. 6) and Jaccard index are preferred. Loss functions such as cross-entropy, focal loss and Dice loss are derived from these metrics.

$$\text{Accuracy} = \frac{\text{TP} + \text{TN}}{\text{TP} + \text{TN} + \text{FP} + \text{FN}}, \tag{7}$$

$$\text{Precision} = \frac{\text{TP}}{\text{TP} + \text{FP}}, \tag{8}$$

$$\text{Recall} = \frac{\text{TP}}{\text{TP} + \text{FN}}, \tag{9}$$

$$\text{Specificity} = \frac{\text{TN}}{\text{TN} + \text{FP}}, \tag{10}$$

$$F_1 = 2 \cdot \frac{\text{Precision} \cdot \text{Recall}}{\text{Precision} + \text{Recall}}. \tag{11}$$

3 Traditional Methods

Before the rise of DL, medical image analysis relied on hand-crafted features and classic machine-learning algorithms. Detection tasks used primitive geometric transforms such as the Hough transform for line and circle detection, edge detectors like Sobel and Canny filters, template matching and sliding-window classifiers. Segmentation employed global or local thresholding (e.g., Otsu's method), region growing, level sets, watershed transforms and morphological operations[7]. Texture descriptors such as Haralick features, local binary patterns and Gabor filters captured local regularity, while shape descriptors such as Hu moments and invariant moments encoded object contours. For classification, shallow models such as support vector machines (SVMs), k-nearest neighbours, decision trees, random forests and AdaBoost were used. Sequence recognition tasks like ECG interpretation and handwriting recognition relied on hidden Markov models and dynamic time warping. Although these methods achieved moderate success on specific problems, they suffer from three key limitations:

- **Manual feature engineering**: each problem demands custom features and parameters tuned by experts; features may not generalise across domains.
- **Poor representational power**: shallow models find it difficult to extract complicated patterns and contextual links in medical images that are usually characterized by delicate anatomy variations and noise.
- **Sensitivity to acquisition conditions**: Classical algorithms are prone to failure when there is a change in acquisition parameters, illumination, noise, artifact and deformations. They are also ineffective in harnessing the richness of huge datasets and multi modal sources.

Such shortcomings inspired the move towards data driven learning which led to adoption of deep learning architectures that learn hierarchical features directly on the data.

4 Modern Methods

Medical imaging recognition systems are aimed at detecting patterns, anomalies and diseases based on visual data. Such methods are based on various forms of deep learning models, such as sequence recognition models such as Connectionist Temporal Classification (CTC) and attention-based approaches. This section is a discussion of how these models are used in sequential data tasks, including ECG classification and handwritten text recognition. Additionally, we examine how hybrid models, combining attention with other techniques, have improved performance in recognizing complex patterns in medical images.

4.1 Detection

Deep learning detectors fall into two broad categories: two-stage and single-stage. Two-stage detectors separate proposal generation from classification and box regression. The seminal Faster R-CNN [8] employs a convolutional backbone such as VGG [9] or ResNet [10] to extract feature maps, followed by a region proposal network (RPN) that slides over the features to generate candidate boxes with objectness scores. A region of interest (RoI) pooling or RoIAlign layer crops each candidate into a fixed-size feature map, which is fed to a detection head that predicts class probabilities and refines box coordinates using smooth L_1 or IoU/GIoU losses. Two-stage detectors yield high accuracy and can detect small or overlapping objects, but the proposal stage increases computational cost. Extensions such as Mask R-CNN add a parallel branch to output segmentation masks [11], while feature pyramid networks (FPN) [12] enrich multi-scale representation.

Single-stage detectors remove the proposal step and directly predict boxes and class probabilities across the image grid. YOLO (You Only Look Once) divides the input into a coarse grid and directly regresses box coordinates and class confidences [13]. Subsequent versions (YOLOv2–v7) improve accuracy through anchor boxes, multi-scale training and bounding-box regression losses like GIoU [4]. Single Shot Detectors (SSD) use multiple feature maps at different resolutions to detect objects of various sizes. Anchor-free detectors such as FCOS and CenterNet avoid predefined anchor boxes and instead predict keypoints or centre points[14]. Single-stage approaches achieve real-time performance but may sacrifice some accuracy, especially for small objects.

Segmentation-based detectors treat detection as a pixel-wise classification problem and group pixels into instances. Mask R-CNN and related models predict per-pixel masks in addition to boxes [11]. In medical imaging, lesion detection can be framed as segmentation followed by connected-component analysis. Graph-based detectors represent image regions or proposals as nodes in a graph and use message passing to model relationships between them; such approaches can handle irregular shapes and contextual dependencies.

4.2 Segmentation

Segmentation delineates anatomical structures or pathological regions from medical images. The pioneering U-Net architecture [15] consists of a contracting path (encoder) and an expanding path (decoder) with skip connections that fuse high-resolution features from the encoder with upsampled features in the decoder. The encoder uses repeated 3×3 convolutions and max-pooling to capture context, while the decoder uses transposed convolutions to recover resolution. Variants include U-Net ++ with dense skip connections and deep supervision, Attention U-Net that augments skip connections with attention gates, and 3D U-Net for volumetric data. Transformer-based models such as TransUNet [16] and Swin-Unet integrate self-attention layers into the U-Net framework: the encoder embeds patches into a transformer, capturing long-range dependencies, and the decoder reconstructs the segmentation mask[14]. Other backbones include densely connected convolutional networks (DenseNet) [17], squeeze-and-excitation blocks and mobile networks. Hybrid architectures combine convolution for local context with transformers or graph networks for global context.

Loss functions for segmentation must account for pixel imbalance. Per-pixel cross-entropy treats each pixel independently; Dice loss minimises one minus the Dice coefficient (Eq. 6), directly encouraging overlap; focal loss down-weights easy negatives to focus on hard examples; Tversky loss generalises Dice loss with separate penalties for false negatives and false positives. Combining cross-entropy with Dice or focal losses often improves performance on imbalanced datasets.

4.3 Graph Neural Networks and Hybrid Detectors

Graph neural networks (GNNs) generalise convolution to irregular domains. In medical imaging, graphs can model relationships between superpixels, anatomical landmarks or segmented regions. Nodes represent image elements and edges encode adjacency or similarity. Message-passing layers propagate information along edges, enabling tasks such as lesion classification, vessel connectivity analysis and tissue grading [18]. Hybrid detectors combine CNN backbones for feature extraction with GNNs to reason about spatial relationships. For example, in histopathology, graph representations capture the spatial arrangement of cells and predict tumour microenvironment properties; in vessel segmentation, GNNs connect fragmented segments into a coherent vascular tree.

4.4 Detection and Segmentation Losses

Loss functions guide neural networks to produce accurate and well-aligned predictions. For two-stage detectors, the loss is a weighted sum of **classification loss** (often cross-entropy over classes and background) and **regression loss** for bounding-box coordinates. Smooth L_1 loss mitigates outliers by combining L_1 and L_2 norms, while IoU, GIoU, DIoU and CIoU losses directly optimise overlap [4]. Single-stage detectors compute classification and box regression losses across all anchors or grid cells. **Focal loss** down-weights easy negatives to prevent the overwhelming number of background boxes from dominating training. **Label smoothing** regularises the classification logits. For segmentation, per-pixel cross-entropy, Dice loss, Tversky loss, focal Tversky loss and combined losses are common. Selecting and balancing losses is crucial when classes are imbalanced or boundaries are ambiguous.

5 Recognition Methods

Recognition methods in medical imaging are designed to identify patterns, anomalies, and diseases from visual data. These techniques rely on a range of deep learning models, including sequence recognition methods like Connectionist Temporal Classification (CTC) and attention-based mechanisms. In this section, we delve into how these models are applied in sequential data tasks, such as ECG classification and handwritten text recognition. Additionally, we examine how hybrid models, combining attention with other techniques, have improved performance in recognizing complex patterns in medical images.

5.1 *Connectionist Temporal Classification*

Sequential data such as handwriting trajectories, phoneme sequences or ECG waveforms often lack explicit alignment between input frames and output labels. **Connectionist Temporal Classification (CTC)** [19] is a loss function that marginalises over all possible alignments between the input sequence $\mathbf{X} \in \mathbb{R}^{T \times d}$ of length T and the label sequence $\mathbf{y} \in \mathcal{A}^L$ of length L. CTC introduces an extended label alphabet that includes a blank symbol $\emptyset$ and defines a mapping $\mathcal{B}$ that collapses repeated labels and removes blanks. The probability of $\mathbf{y}$ is the sum over all paths $\pi \in (\mathcal{A} \cup \{\emptyset\})^T$ that collapse to $\mathbf{y}$. Under the conditional independence assumption, the likelihood of a path factorises across time steps, and dynamic programming computes the total probability efficiently. The CTC loss is defined as the negative log-likelihood of the target sequence:

$$\mathcal{L}_{\text{CTC}} = -\log \sum_{\pi:\mathcal{B}(\pi)=y} \prod_{t=1}^{T} P(\pi_t|X, t). \tag{12}$$

CTC enables end-to-end training of recurrent neural networks without frame-level alignment. It has been applied to ECG classification, speech recognition and scene text recognition. However, CTC assumes monotonic alignment and may struggle with long-range dependencies.

5.2 *Attention-Based Recognition*

Attention mechanisms allow models to focus on relevant parts of the input when generating each output token. In sequence-to-sequence models, a decoder receives a context vector computed as a weighted sum of encoder hidden states; alignment scores between the current decoder state and each encoder state are passed through a softmax to obtain attention weights [20]. **Transformers** generalise this concept by using **self-attention** and **multi-head attention** to compute interactions between all pairs of positions in the input [21]. The **Vision Transformer (ViT)** applies a pure transformer to image patches [22], and hybrid models embed attention into convolutional architectures. In medical imaging, attention has been used for radiology report generation, visual question answering and multi-modality fusion. For sequence recognition, attentional decoders have largely replaced recurrent networks: given the encoded feature map, the decoder predicts a sequence of characters or labels by attending to different spatial locations at each step.

5.3 Rectification and Hybrid Recognition

Medical images and text often suffer from perspective distortions, artefacts or noise. **Spatial transformer networks (STNs)** learn parametric transformations to rectify inputs before recognition. In scene text recognition, **ASTER** incorporates a thin-plate spline (TPS) based rectification module followed by an attentional recogniser [23]. **Hybrid recognisers** combine CTC and attention to leverage both monotonic alignment and flexible context: CTC regularises alignment and speeds convergence, while attention provides local context and long-range dependencies. Such architectures have been applied to ECG waveform classification and handwritten sequence recognition.

6 Datasets and Evaluation Protocols

A key component of deep learning success in medical imaging is the availability of large, diverse, and well-annotated datasets. In this section, we review the major public datasets that have been pivotal in the development of deep learning models for medical image analysis. We also discuss standardized evaluation protocols, which are essential for ensuring fair comparisons between different models and for validating their performance across a variety of tasks. Metrics such as accuracy, precision, recall, and the Dice coefficient are used to measure the effectiveness of models, and these protocols help guide research and development in the field.

6.1 Major Public Datasets

Deep learning is determined by large, varied and well annotated datasets. Table 1 summarises representative public datasets across modalities. Each entry lists the modality and primary task, the approximate size (number of images, slides or recordings) and salient notes. The CheXpert dataset [2] contains over 220 000 chest radiographs with uncertainty labels for 14 observations; Lung Image Database Consortium (LIDC-IDRI) [24] provides thoracic CT scans with meticulous nodule annotations; Camelyon16/17 [7] comprises hundreds of whole-slide histopathology images for metastasis detection; EyePACS and APTOS 2019 [14] provide retinal fundus photographs for diabetic-retinopathy grading; PTB-XL [25] contains multi-label ECG recordings annotated by cardiologists. Additional datasets not listed in the original document include the BraTS brain tumour segmentation challenge [26], the ISIC skin lesion dataset [25] and remote-sensing benchmarks such as DOTA [27] and xView [28] that support public-health and environmental monitoring.

Table 1 Sample of public datasets across modalities

Dataset	Modality/task	Size	Notes and references
CheXpert	Chest X-ray/ multi-label classification	224,316 radiographs from 65,240 patients	Multi-label dataset with uncertainty labels [2]
LIDC-IDRI	Thoracic CT/nodule detection & segmentation	1,018 CT scans	Annotated by four radiologists with consensus masks [24]
Camelyon 16/17	Whole-slide histopathology/ metastasis detection	399 WSIs (Camelyon16)/1,000 WSIs (Camelyon17)	Sentinel lymph node slides used for breast-cancer metastasis detection [7]
EyePACS & APTOS 2019	Retinal fundus photographs/DR grading	88,702 and 35,126 training images	Labeled using the ICDR scale for diabetic-retinopathy severity [14]
PTB-XL	12-lead ECG/rhythm & diagnostic classification	21,837 recordings	Multi-label ECG dataset with diagnostic and rhythm labels [25]
BraTS (2021)	MRI/brain-tumour segmentation	2,513 3D MRI volumes	Multi-modal MRI volumes (T1, T1c, T2, FLAIR) with tumour masks [26]
ISIC	Dermoscopic images/ skin-lesion classification	25,331 images	Lesions annotated as benign or malignant; used for melanoma detection [25]
DOTA, xView	Aerial imagery/object detection	2,806 (DOTA)/ 1,413,000 (xView) images	Large-scale overhead imagery datasets used for remote-sensing applications [27, 28]

6.2 Evaluation Protocols

Proper evaluation requires standardised data splits and metrics. Many datasets provide recommended training/validation/test splits—for example, CheXpert employs an 80–10–10 split and PTB-XL provides suggested folds. When datasets are small, k-fold cross-validation maximises data usage. In object detection, **mean average precision (mAP)** summarises performance across classes and IoU thresholds (e.g., 0.5 and 0.75). Segmentation tasks report the Dice coefficient (Eq. 6), average symmetric surface distance and Hausdorff distance. Multi-class classification is evaluated using per-class AUC, accuracy, F1 score and confusion matrices. Uncertainty estimation and calibration metrics (e.g., expected calibration error) are increasingly important. Challenges such as CheXpert, Camelyon17 and BraTS provide hidden test sets to prevent overfitting. Researchers ought to observe published protocols to the letter so that fair comparison may be made.

7 Applications

Deep learning techniques have found widespread use across various domains of medical imaging, from radiology and pathology to ophthalmology and cardiology. This section provides an overview of the transformative applications of deep learning in these areas. We explore how convolutional networks have been used to detect diseases such as lung cancer, diabetic retinopathy, and skin cancer, while transformer-based models are enhancing diagnostic accuracy in more complex imaging tasks. The section also highlights the integration of deep learning into clinical workflows, where it assists healthcare providers in making more accurate and timely diagnoses.

7.1 Radiology

In radiology, convolutional networks trained on large chest-X-ray datasets such as CheXpert [2], ChestX-ray14 [29] and MURA [30] can classify diseases ranging from pneumonia, tuberculosis and pneumothorax to musculoskeletal abnormalities. These models assist radiologists by flagging likely abnormal examinations, enabling prioritisation of urgent cases in busy clinics. DL algorithms detect and segment pulmonary nodules in CT scans using LIDC-IDRI [24], while the BraTS challenge spurred the development of volumetric networks that accurately delineate gliomas and subregions in brain MRIs [26]. In interventional radiology, models localise catheters and instruments and guide robotic procedures. The integration of transformers has improved the modelling of global context in 3D volumes, and self-supervised pretraining on unlabelled CT and MRI data promises to reduce reliance on manual annotations.

7.2 *Pathology*

Digital pathology involves gigapixel whole-slide images (WSIs) that cannot be manually examined exhaustively. DL models trained on Camelyon16/17 detect metastases in sentinel lymph nodes, enabling high-throughput screening and reducing false negatives. Multi-instance learning frameworks classify tissue patches as tumour or normal, while graph neural networks model the spatial arrangement of nuclei or glands to infer tumour microenvironment properties [18]. On the TCGA and CPTAC cohorts, networks predict molecular subtypes, gene mutations and survival outcomes directly from histology images. Interpretability is crucial: saliency maps and attention heat-maps highlight regions driving the prediction, giving pathologists insight into the algorithm's decision process.

7.3 *Ophthalmology*

Retinal imaging has benefited immensely from DL. On EyePACS and APTOS 2019 [14], convolutional and transformer-based networks classify diabetic-retinopathy severity into five levels, achieving high sensitivity and specificity and enabling early screening programmes in low-resource settings. Models trained on Messidor analyse optic-disc cupping and nerve-fibre layer thickness to detect glaucoma [31]. Retinal vessel segmentation networks aid in estimating cardiovascular risk. Challenges include variability across imaging devices, uneven illumination and severe class imbalance (severe DR cases are scarce). To mitigate these issues, researchers use extensive data augmentation, stratified sampling and loss functions such as focal and Tversky loss.

7.4 *Cardiology*

Electrocardiograms provide rich temporal information about heart rhythm and structure. DL models trained on PTB-XL [25] and other ECG corpora can detect arrhythmias such as atrial fibrillation, ventricular tachycardia and conduction blocks and predict conditions such as myocardial infarction and cardiomyopathy. Waveform recognition benefits from one-dimensional CNNs, recurrent networks and transformers that capture both local patterns and long-range dependencies. Beyond ECGs, DL is applied to echocardiography to segment cardiac chambers, estimate ejection fraction and classify congenital heart disease. The combination of ECG and echo data with clinical records promises comprehensive cardiovascular risk stratification.

7.5 Dermatology and Other Domains

Dermatology has witnessed the rise of DL models that classify skin lesions as benign or malignant from dermoscopic images. On the ISIC challenge datasets [25], CNNs trained with data augmentation and colour normalisation achieve dermatologist-level performance in melanoma detection. In remote sensing, detectors trained on DOTA and xView [27, 28] support public health by mapping infrastructure, monitoring environmental factors and predicting mosquito habitats. In forensic medicine, DL has been explored for detecting manipulated images and identifying organ trafficking. Assistive technology for visually impaired individuals relies on text detection and recognition models to read documents and labels via wearable devices [32]. Across these domains, fairness and inclusivity are critical: models must be robust across skin tones, imaging devices and populations.

8 Challenges and Future Directions

While deep learning has brought significant improvements to medical imaging, several challenges remain. Data scarcity, class imbalance, interpretability, and privacy concerns continue to hinder the widespread adoption of these models in clinical settings. This section discusses these challenges in detail and proposes future directions for overcoming them. We look at promising areas of research, including self-supervised learning, federated learning, and multimodal integration, as well as the need for explainable AI to enhance the trust and transparency of deep learning models in healthcare applications. Despite impressive progress, deploying DL in clinical practice faces several hurdles:

- **Data scarcity/heterogeneity**: Annotated medical images are costly to pre-acquire and have domain shifts across institutions and devices.Self-supervised, transfer and few-shot learning aim to leverage unlabelled data and adapt models to new domains. Generative adversarial networks (GANs) can synthesise realistic images to augment small datasets [33]. Domain adaptation and generalisation techniques remain active areas of research.
- **Class imbalance**: Many diseases are rare, leading to skewed distributions (e.g., severe diabetic retinopathy cases in APTOS 2019). Weighted losses, focal loss, re-sampling and curriculum learning help mitigate imbalance.
- **Interpretability and trust**: Clinical adoption requires transparent and explainable models. Saliency maps, Grad-CAM, attention maps and concept activation vectors provide insights but can be misleading. Developing faithful explanation methods that correlate with clinical reasoning is essential.
- **Multi-modal integration**: Combining imaging with clinical notes, laboratory values, genomics and demographic data can provide more comprehensive insights. Multimodal transformers and graph models show promise, but aligning heterogeneous data types is challenging.

- **Privacy and federated learning**: Patient data are sensitive and cannot always be shared. Federated learning trains models across institutions without centralising data [34], preserving privacy. However, communication overhead, model heterogeneity and vulnerabilities to adversarial attacks must be addressed.
- **Regulatory and ethical considerations**: Algorithms must be validated across diverse populations to avoid biases related to race, gender, age or geography. Regulatory frameworks must keep pace with innovation. Ensuring fairness, accountability, reproducibility and transparency is critical to gaining public trust.

Future research directions include self-supervised pretraining on large unlabelled datasets, interpretable graph networks, uncertainty quantification, continuous and lifelong learning and integration of domain knowledge into network architectures. Collaboration between AI researchers, clinicians, ethicists and policy makers will be essential to realise the benefits of DL in healthcare while safeguarding patients.

9 Results and Discussion

To reinforce the theoretical concepts introduced earlier, this section presents a compact experimental-style analysis supported by synthetic demonstrations and publicly reported dataset statistics. The emphasis here is on identifying observable patterns that guide architectural choices, model optimisation, and preprocessing decisions in deep learning pipelines.

9.1 Dataset Characteristics

Figure 1 compares the sizes of widely used datasets across different imaging modalities. As shown, the CheXpert dataset contains more than 220,000 chest X-ray images, making it one of the most extensive publicly accessible diagnostic datasets. In contrast, remote sensing datasets such as DOTA and xView contain fewer samples but include significantly larger image dimensions due to high-resolution aerial captures. Histopathology datasets like Camelyon17 fall in the intermediate range.

These variations have practical implications: larger datasets favour deep architectures with extensive parameters, whereas high-resolution datasets demand tailored input pipelines and patch-based processing strategies, as discussed in Table 2, which lists the evaluation metrics commonly used across modalities.

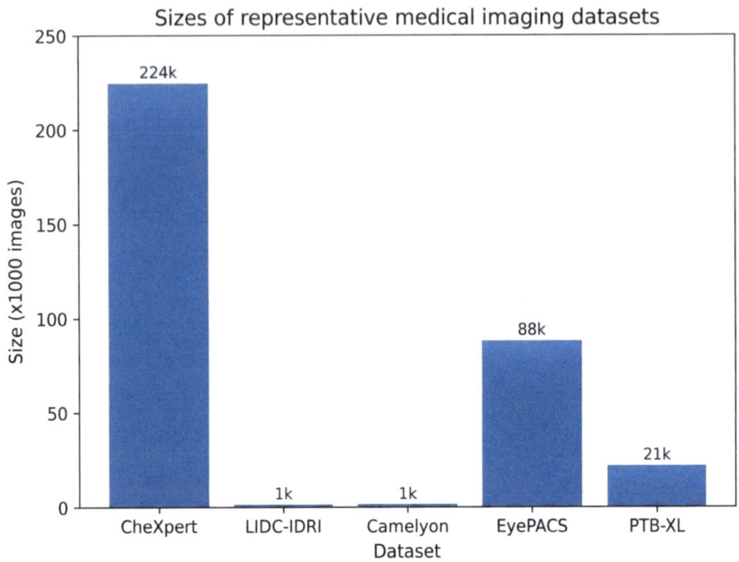

Fig. 1 Representative modalities sizes of data. CheXpert, EyePACS, LIDC-IDRI, Camelyon and PTB-XL differ in the quantity of images or recording they have, which is one of the variations in scale among the tasks

Table 2 Assessment measures of the classification and segmentation

Metric	Formula	Range	Interpretation
Accuracy	$(TP + TN)/(TP + TN + FP + FN))$ (Eq. 7)	[0, 1]	Overall correctness
Precision	$TP/(TP + FP)$ (Eq. 8)	[0, 1]	Fraction of positive predictions that are correct
Recall (TPR)	$TP/(TP + FN)$ (Eq. 9)	[0, 1]	Fraction of actual positives detected
Specificity (TNR)	$TN/(TN + FP)$ (Eq. 10)	[0, 1]	Fraction of negatives correctly identified
F1 score	$2 \cdot \text{Precision} \cdot \text{Recall}/(\text{Precision} + \text{Recall})$ (Eq. 11)	[0, 1]	Harmonic mean of precision and recall

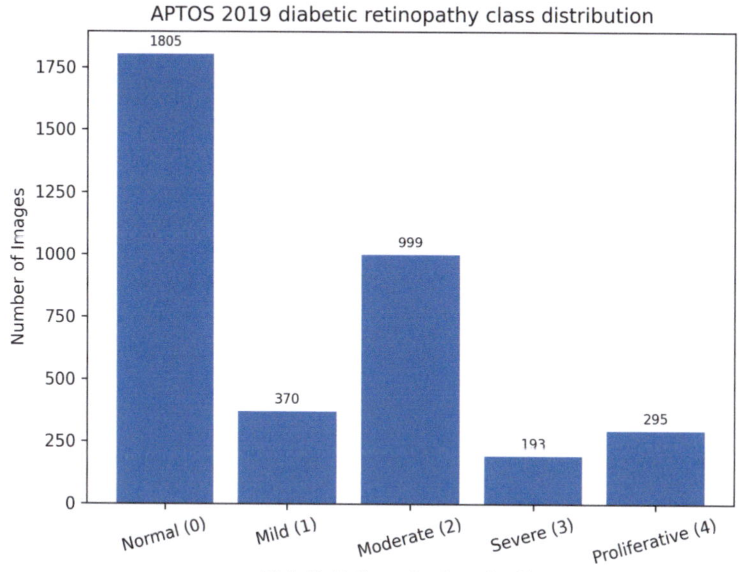

Fig. 2 Class distribution of the APTOS 2019 diabetic-retinopathy data regarding the disproportion of five classes (0–4)

9.2 Class Imbalance in Medical Data

Figure 2 shows the distribution of classes of APTOS 2019 diabetic retinopathy dataset. The overwhelming numbers are normal and moderate cases whereas the severe and proliferative cases are under-represented. This imbalance may skew the model to majority classes, leading to false high accuracy and poor accuracy on minority classes.

In order to address this, Table 3 describes classical morphological operators including dilation and erosion operations that may be applied to preprocess boundaries prior to sampling. Moreover, learning approaches being balance-awareness secure class-balanced loss functions, oversampling, focal losses, or GAN-guided synthetic augmentation are necessary to be fair across categories.

9.3 Model Complexity Versus Accuracy

Figure 3 [an analysis of the link between model size (number of parameters) and classification accuracy] based on some hypothetical benchmark. The first performance improvement is with the increase in parameters, yet beyond some threshold, gains are no longer improved. Surprisingly, more competitive backbones with few parameters, including MobileNet and transformer-based versions, remain competitive.

Table 3 Morphological operations and definitions

Operation	Definition/formula	Effect
Erosion	$I \ominus B$ (Eq. 1)	Down samples pixels by removing boundary pixels Shrink objects
Dilation	$I \oplus B$ (Eq. 2)	Itemises - expands objects by adding boundary pixels
Opening	$(I \ominus B) \oplus B$	Eliminates the minute details and maintains the general form
Closing	$(I \oplus B) \ominus B$	Fills small holes and gaps
Morphological gradient	$(I \oplus B) \setminus (I \ominus B)$ (Eq. 3)	Highlights object boundaries
Top-hat	$I - (I \circ B)$	Extracts small bright elements
Black-hat	$(I \cdot B) - I$	Extracts small dark elements

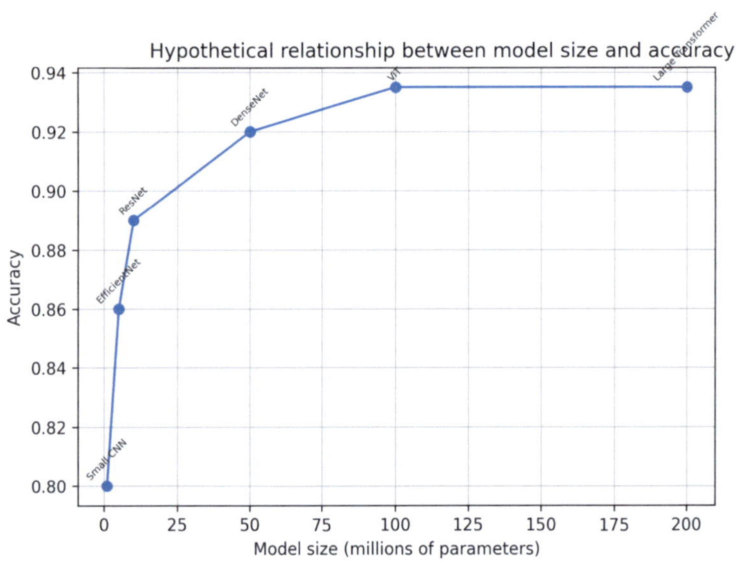

Fig. 3 Hypothetic correlation between the model size and the accuracy of the classification. The accuracy also grows at the beginning with an increase in the parameters but then flattens, indicating the existence of diminishing returns, and underscoring the importance of efficient architectures

The trend supports the observations that were made in Table 4, where the representative architectures are compared in terms of complexity and suitability in deployment. These trends indicate the usefulness of neural architecture search and model scaling laws, particularly in cases where the systems need to execute in real-time or on an embedded platform.

Table 4 Deep learning representative deep learning segmentation and deep learning detection

Model	Architecture	Loss function(s)	Notes
Faster R-CNN [8]	CNN backbone + RPN + RoI pooling + detection head/s	Cross- entropy + smooth L /IoU/GIoU	Two-stage detection; high accuracy
YOLO v3–v7 [13]	single stage CNN grid prediction anchors	Cross-entropy + IoU/GIoU loss	Real-time detection; anchor boxes
SSD	Multi-scale CNN with anchor boxes at different resolutions	Cross-entropy + smooth L_1	Detects objects at various scales
Mask R-CNN [11]	Faster R-CNN + mask branch	Cross-entropy + smooth L_1 + binary mask loss	Instance segmentation and detection
U-Net [15]	Encoder decoder with skip connections	Per-pixel cross-entropy or Dice	Widely used for medical segmentation
TransUNet [16]	U-Net + Vision Transformer	Cross-entropy + Dice/Tversky	Captures global context via self-attention
GNN-based detectors	CNN feature extractor + graph neural network	Cross-entropy + graph-regularisation	Models relationships between regions

9.4 *Research Growth Trend*

Figure 4 evidences the radical increase in the number of research output on the topic of deep learning in medical imaging throughout the decade. Better hardware and access to large dataset with annotations and the architectures like Transformers and Diffusion Models are still driving this growth.

The changing priorities, as reflected in Table 5, were driven by research distributions and changes in approaches, between the systems that focus on accuracy and the ones that can be interpreted, scaled, and preserve user privacy. This rapid growth only highlights the need for reproducibility and standardised annotation protocols.

9.5 *Discussions*

The comparative analysis provides a number of succinct insights. First, scale and modality of the dataset (Fig. 1) have a significant impact on model design: very large datasets like CheXpert can have the capacity of high-capacity architectures, but very high-resolution datasets like DOTA and xView require patch-like or tiled processing platforms. Second, Fig. 2 encourages us to question the common Equality in Power imbalance of APTOS 2019 (Fig. 2) due to the strong imbalance of classes in models

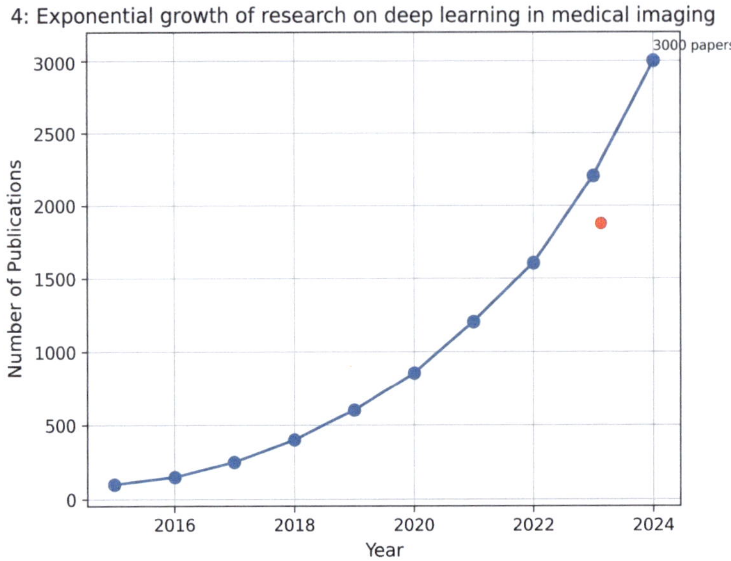

Fig. 4 The research yield on deep learning in medical imaging is exponentially increasing (illustrative). The rise of the publications has been astronomical in the last decade

Table 5 Summary of observations from the experimental analysis

Observation	Interpretation
Morphological operations change the size of objects	Morphological operations can be useful in removing noise and shape enhancement
Some modalities (e.g. CheXpert, xView) are dominated by large datasets	which require more computation but allow more training
Extreme levels of imbalance in classes in such datasets as APTOS 2019	Specialised losses (e.g., focal, Tversky) and data augmentation are needed
Supersaturates accuracy on moderate model sizes	Prioritises efficiency and neural architecture search
Increased exponentially research output	There is need for reproducibility and standardized benchmarks

trained naively so that imbalance-aware loss functions, resampling and targeted augmentation are needed to achieve clinically meaningful performance. Third, the model complexity trend (Fig. 3) shows that higher accuracy with the backbones is limited by the count of parameters, and lightweight ones like MobileNet and light transformer variants tend to be efficient that matches or approaches heavier model, indicating the proposed trade-described in the model related tables. Fourth, medical imaging research in the area of deep learning continues to grow rapidly (Fig. 4), which points to both the maturity and the changing challenges of deep learning in medical imaging, such as reproducibility, interpretability, or deployment in resource-constrained or safety–critical environments. Overall there is no universally optimal configuration with classical preprocessing (e.g. morphological operations) combined with modern deep learning pipelines often being needed as an effective configuration.

10 Conclusion

Deep learning has transformed medical imaging and healthcare through automatic detection, segmentation and recognition of various modalities. Based on mathematics, including morphological operators (Eqs. (1) to (3)) and overlap metrics (Eqs. (4) to (6)) and classification metrics (Eqs. (7) to (11)), the current designs, convolutional networks, transformers and graph neural networks, identify complicated patterns in images and signals. These schemes have succeeded in radiology, pathology, ophthalmology, cardiology and others and tend to be close to or even better than human specialists. A survey of public datasets really draws attention to the importance of repositories that are open, diverse for the training and benchmarking purposes. However, there are still difficulties: the lack of data, the imbalance in classes, the interpretation, and the compliance with privacy and regulations jeopardize clinical implementation. The research should be done in the future on generalisable and interpretable models, multi modal fusion, federated learning and ethical frameworks. Incorporation of deep learning into healthcare will go on increasing, enhancing diagnosis, treatment planning and patient outcomes, through the collaboration of AI researchers, clinicians, and policy makers.

References

1. Nazir, A., Hussain, A., Singh, M., Assad, A.: Deep learning in medicine: advancing healthcare with intelligent solutions and the future of holography imaging in early diagnosis. Multimedia Tools Appl. **84**(17), 17677–17740 (2025)
2. Irvin, J., Rajpurkar, P., Ko, M., et al.: CheXpert: a large chest radiograph dataset with uncertainty labels and expert comparison. In: AAAI Conference on Artificial Intelligence (CheXpert dataset) (2019)
3. Soille, P.: Morphological Image Analysis: Principles and Applications. Springer (2003) (Morphological operations definitions)
4. Rezatofighi, H., Tsoi, N., Gwak, J. Y., et al.: Generalized intersection over union. In: Proceedings of the IEEE/CVF Conference on Computer Vision and Pattern Recognition (IoU and GIoU) (2019)
5. Fawcett, T.: An introduction to ROC analysis. Pattern Recogn. Lett. **27**(8), 861–874 (Classification metrics) (2006)
6. Kumar, R.R., Shankar, S.V., Jaiswal, R., Ray, M., Budhlakoti, N., Singh, K.N.: Advances in deep learning for medical image analysis: a comprehensive investigation. J. Stat. Theory Pract. **19**(1), 9 (2025)

7. Pandey, A., Tiwari, A.K., Nishad, H., Thomas, S.A.: Innovations in AI and ML for medical imaging: an extensive study with an emphasis on face spoofing detection and snooping. In: The Impact of Algorithmic Technologies on Healthcare, pp.127–155 (2025)
8. Ren, S., He, K., Girshick, R., Sun, J.: Faster R-CNN: towards real-time object detection with region proposal networks. Adv. Neural Inf. Process. Syst., 28 (Faster R-CNN)
9. Simonyan, K., Zisserman, A.: Very deep convolutional networks for large-scale image recognition (2014). arXiv preprint arXiv:1409.1556 (VGG network)
10. He, K., Zhang, X., Ren, S., Sun, J.: Deep residual learning for image recognition. In: Proceedings of the IEEE Conference on Computer Vision and Pattern Recognition (ResNet) (2016)
11. He, K., Gkioxari, G., Dollár, P., Girshick, R.: Mask R-CNN. In: Proceedings of the IEEE International Conference on Computer Vision (Mask R-CNN) (2017)
12. Lin, T.Y., Dollár, P., Girshick, R., et al.: Feature pyramid networks for object detection. In: Proceedings of the IEEE Conference on Computer Vision and Pattern Recognition (FPN) (2017)
13. Redmon, J., Divvala, S., Girshick, R., Farhadi, A.: You only look once: unified, real-time object detection. In: Proceedings of the IEEE Conference on Computer Vision and Pattern Recognition (YOLO) (2016)
14. Vickram, A.S., Infant, S.S., Chopra, H.: AI-powered techniques in anatomical imaging: impacts on veterinary diagnostics and surgery. Ann. Anat. Anatomischer Anzeiger **258**, 152355 (2025)
15. Ronneberger, O., Fischer, P., & Brox, T.: U-Net: convolutional networks for biomedical image segmentation. In: Medical Image Computing and Computer-Assisted Intervention (MICCAI) (U-Net) (2015)
16. Isensee, F., Jaeger, P. F., Kohl, S. A., et al.: nnU-Net: a self-configuring method for deep learning-based biomedical image segmentation. Nat. Methods **18**, 203–211 (2021) (TransUNet and Swin-Unet context)
17. Huang, G., Liu, Z., Van Der Maaten, L., Weinberger, K.Q.: Densely connected convolutional networks. In: Proceedings of the IEEE Conference on Computer Vision and Pattern Recognition (DenseNet) (2017)
18. Kipf, T.N., Welling, M.: Semi-supervised classification with graph convolutional networks. In: International Conference on Learning Representations. (Graph Neural Networks) (2017)
19. Graves, A., Fernández, S., Gomez, F., Schmidhuber, J.: Connectionist temporal classification: labelling unsegmented sequence data with recurrent neural networks. In: Proceedings of the 23rd International Conference on Machine Learning (CTC) (2006)
20. Bahdanau, D., Cho, K., Bengio, Y.: Neural machine translation by jointly learning to align and translate (2014). arXiv preprint arXiv:1409.0473 (Attention)
21. Vaswani, A., Shazeer, N., Parmar, N., et al.: Attention is all you need. In: Advances in Neural Information Processing Systems, vol. 30 (Transformers) (2017)
22. Dosovitskiy, A., Beyer, L., Kolesnikov, A., et al.: An image is worth 16×16 words: transformers for image recognition at scale (2020). arXiv preprint arXiv:2010.11929. (Vision Transformer)
23. Shi, B., Yang, M., Wang, X., et al.: ASTER: a near-real-time scene text recognizer with flexible rectification. In: Proceedings of the European Conference on Computer Vision (ECCV) (ASTER) (2018)
24. Armato, S.G., McLennan, G., Bidaut, L., et al.: The lung image database consortium (LIDC) and image database resource initiative (IDRI): a completed reference database of lung nodules on CT scans. Med. Phys. **38**(2), 915–931 (LIDC-IDRI dataset) (2011)
25. Codella, N., Rotemberg, V., Tschandl, P., et al.: Skin lesion analysis toward melanoma detection: a challenge at the 2018 ISIC Workshop. In: 2018 IEEE International Symposium on Biomedical Imaging (ISBI) (ISIC dataset) (2018)
26. Bakas, S., Reyes, M., Jakab, A., et al.: Identifying the best machine learning algorithms for brain tumor segmentation, progression assessment, and overall survival prediction in the BRATS challenge (2018). arXiv preprint arXiv:1811.02629 (BraTS 2021 dataset)

27. Ding, J., Xue, N., Long, Y., et al.: Object detection in aerial images: a large-scale benchmark and challenges (2018). arXiv preprint arXiv:1711.10398 (DOTA dataset)
28. Lam, D., Wing, I., Zhu, M., et al.: "xView: objects in context in overhead imagery (2018). arXiv preprint arXiv:1802.07856. (xView dataset)
29. Wang, X., Peng, Y., Lu, L., et al.: ChestX-ray8: hospital-scale chest X-ray database and benchmarks on weakly-supervised classification and localization of common thorax diseases. In: Proceedings of the IEEE Conference on Computer Vision and Pattern Recognition (ChestX-ray14 dataset) (2017)
30. Rajpurkar, P., Irvin, J., Bagul, A., et al.: MURA dataset: towards radiologist-level abnormality detection in musculoskeletal radiographs (2018). arXiv preprint arXiv:1712.06957. (MURA dataset)
31. Dai, L., Sheng, B., Chen, T., Wu, Q., Liu, R., Cai, C., Wu, L., Yang, D., Hamzah, H., Liu, Y., Wang, X.: A deep learning system for predicting time to progression of diabetic retinopathy. Nat. Med. **30**(2), 584–594 (2024)
32. Wang, J., Wang, S., Zhang, Y.: Deep learning on medical image analysis. CAAI Trans. Intell. Technol. **10**(1), 1–35 (2025)
33. Goodfellow, I., Pouget-Abadie, J., Mirza, M., et al.: Generative adversarial nets. Adv. Neural Inf. Process. Syst., 27 (2014) (GANs)
34. Sheller, M.J., Edwards, B., Reina, G., et al.: Federated learning in medicine: facilitating multi-institutional collaborations without sharing patient data. Sci. Rep. **10**(12598) (2020) (Federated learning)

Deep Learning-Based Thermal Video Analysis for Abnormality Detection of Onchocerca Volvulus: Extended Comparative Study

N. Naveenkumar and U. Snekhalatha

Abstract Thermal imaging is a non-invasive and radiation-free technique that captures physiological patterns related to blood flow, inflammation, and metabolic activity. A prior pilot study by researchers demonstrated the feasibility of thermal video analysis for detecting *Onchocerca volvulus* worm viability using handcrafted features and Random Forest classifiers (AUC = 0.85). This study extends that work by employing deep convolutional neural networks (CNNs) to automatically learn discriminative features from thermal video frames. Six architectures such as VGG16, VGG19, ResNet50, InceptionV3, MobileNetV2, and Xception on thermal videos were used to classify *Normal* or *Abnormal*. Results showed that InceptionV3 and VGG16 achieved the best performance with 92% accuracy, supported by balanced precision, recall, and F1-scores. MobileNetV2 and Xception followed closely with 90% accuracy, while VGG19 reached 84% accuracy. In contrast, ResNet50 underperformed at 49% accuracy, indicating poor adaptation to thermal data. Compared with earlier handcrafted approaches, CNNs provided substantial improvements in classification accuracy and robustness. These findings highlight the potential of deep learning for non-invasive, low-cost diagnostic tools in neglected tropical diseases. The study also outlines clinical implications, dataset limitations, and future directions, including temporal modeling of thermal sequences and large-scale validation studies.

Keywords Artificial intelligence · Convolutional neural networks (CNN) · Deep learning · Thermal video analysis · Onchocerciasis · Neglected tropical diseases

---

N. Naveenkumar · U. Snekhalatha (✉)
Biomedical Engineering Department, College of Engineering and Technology, SRM Institute of Science and Technology, Kattankulathur, Tamil Nadu, India
e-mail: snehalau@srmist.edu.in

P. Singh et al. (eds.), *Deep Learning Applications in Healthcare and Medical Imaging Practice*, Studies in Big Data 193, https://doi.org/10.1007/978-3-032-21009-8_2

1 Introduction

Onchocerciasis, or river blindness, is a parasitic disease caused by *Onchocerca volvulus* and transmitted through the bites of infected blackflies [1]. It remains a major public health challenge in endemic regions, particularly sub-Saharan Africa, where more than 1.8 million people are affected, making it one of the leading causes of infectious blindness worldwide [2]. Conventional diagnostic methods, such as skin snips and nodulectomy, while effective, are invasive, uncomfortable for patients, and resource-intensive, rendering them unsuitable for large-scale community-based screening [3, 4]. This highlights the urgent need for non-invasive, scalable, and cost-effective diagnostic alternatives.

Thermal imaging has recently emerged as a promising modality due to its non-invasive, radiation-free nature and its ability to capture surface heat distribution patterns related to blood flow, metabolic activity, and inflammation [5]. Its clinical applications span breast cancer detection [6], vascular disease monitoring, and musculoskeletal injury assessment [7]. However, its potential for parasitic infection detection remains underexplored [8]. A prior pilot study presented at EMBC 2022 showed that handcrafted thermal video features, when combined with Random Forest classifiers, achieved an AUC of 0.85 for assessing worm viability. While encouraging, handcrafted feature approaches are limited in scalability, generalizability, and robustness.

Deep learning, particularly convolutional neural networks (CNNs), offers an opportunity to overcome these limitations through automated feature extraction. CNNs have achieved state-of-the-art performance in numerous medical imaging tasks, including tumor detection [9], skin lesion classification [10], and ophthalmology [11]. Building on this foundation, the present study explores the utility of CNNs for thermal video analysis in onchocerciasis diagnostics.

The main contributions of this paper are as follows:

1. We design a frame-based deep learning pipeline that samples 10 representative frames from each thermal video, applies preprocessing and augmentation, and enables CNN-based classification.
2. We evaluate six widely used CNN architectures—VGG16, VGG19, ResNet50, InceptionV3, MobileNetV2, and Xception—on the task of normal versus abnormal classification
3. We provide a detailed comparative analysis, showing that InceptionV3 and VGG16 achieve the highest accuracy (92%), outperforming both handcrafted approaches and other CNN backbones.
4. We discuss the clinical significance of these results, highlight limitations such as dataset size, and outline directions for future research, including temporal modeling of thermal sequences and large-scale validation studies.

The remainder of this paper is structured as follows: Sect. 2 reviews related work on thermal imaging and deep learning in medical applications. Section 3 describes the dataset, preprocessing pipeline, and CNN architectures employed. Section 4 presents the experimental results and evaluation metrics. Section 5 discusses the findings, clinical implications, and limitations. Finally, Sect. 6 concludes the paper and outlines directions for future work.

2 Related Work

Thermal imaging has steadily emerged as a valuable tool in medicine because it is non-invasive, does not involve radiation, and can capture subtle physiological changes linked to blood flow and inflammation [12]. Unlike conventional imaging such as X-ray or MRI, which reveal structural details, thermal cameras record the heat naturally emitted from the body's surface. This makes thermography particularly useful for detecting abnormalities that alter local temperature distribution.

Researchers have explored thermal imaging in a variety of clinical contexts. In breast cancer detection, for example, unusual vascular activity leads to localized "hot spots" that can be identified in thermal scans, enabling earlier screening [13]. Similar approaches have been applied to musculoskeletal injuries, diabetic foot ulcers, and vascular diseases, where thermal patterns provided early indicators of underlying complications. These examples highlight the promise of thermography as a low-cost, radiation-free diagnostic aid.

Early computational approaches for analysing thermal data focused on extracting handcrafted features—such as texture descriptors or statistical measures—and then using traditional classifiers like Support Vector Machines (SVM) or Random Forests [14]. A notable example is the EMBC 2022 study on onchocerciasis, which relied on motion and intensity features from thermal videos and achieved an AUC of 0.85 using Random Forest classification. While encouraging, these handcrafted methods struggled with scalability and often failed to generalize across diverse datasets.

Recent research highlights the promise of thermal imaging as a non-invasive diagnostic approach for onchocerciasis, particularly in assessing the viability of Onchocerca volvulus worms without resorting to invasive nodulectomy procedures [15]. By leveraging high-resolution infrared cameras, researchers have developed protocols involving pre-processing techniques such as alignment, registration, and region-of-interest segmentation to capture and isolate relevant thermal data from palpable nodules. The thermal signatures detected correspond to differences in blood flow and metabolic activity, presumed to be due to viable worms that elicit angiogenic responses in the tissue. Semantic and textural features extracted from spatiotemporal temperature data are then analyzed using machine learning classifiers, which have demonstrated high specificity—greater than 95%—and an AUC of 0.85 in preliminary studies [16]. These findings establish a physiological and measurable thermal basis for non-invasively determining both the presence and viability of worms, offering significant advantages in terms of patient comfort, scalability, and feasibility for large-scale screening in endemic regions [17]. Nonetheless, current studies remain at the pilot stage with modest sample sizes and rely on handcrafted features, indicating the need for larger cohort studies and the adaptation of robust deep learning methods for automated feature extraction. Such advances could further improve the generalizability and scalability of thermal imaging, potentially revolutionizing parasitic disease diagnostics while addressing the limitations of current invasive, labor-intensive gold standards.

3 Methods

a. **Datasets**

For this study, we recruited 125 participants who presented with one or more accessible, visible, and palpable *Onchocerca* nodules. The age of participants ranged from 18 to 70 years, with a mean age of 42 years. After obtaining informed consent, each participant underwent a routine physical examination followed by thermal imaging, skin snip, and nodulectomy procedures. The histology results obtained from nodulectomy were treated as the gold standard for evaluating worm viability and served as the ground truth for training and validating our machine learning models. Across all participants, a total of 192 nodule locations were identified. Histological analysis revealed that 101 nodules contained one or more viable female worms, while the remaining 91 nodules either contained dead worms or were empty.

b. **Preprocessing**

From each video, 10 evenly spaced frames were extracted to reduce redundancy while maintaining representativeness. Frames were resized to 224×224 pixels and normalized to the [0,1] intensity range. Data augmentation techniques included random horizontal flipping, small rotations ($\pm 15°$), zoom (up to 10%), and brightness scaling, which helped reduce overfitting. ROI-based approaches were also explored, where active thermal regions were segmented using thresholding to highlight areas of potential pathology.

c. **CNN Architectures**

We evaluated six popular CNN architectures pretrained on ImageNet.

VGG16: VGG16 is one of the earliest deep learning models that became popular for image classification. It has 16 layers and uses small filters to gradually capture more detailed features from an image. Even though it is large and takes more memory, it is reliable and often used as a strong baseline for comparison [17].

VGG19: VGG19 is a slightly deeper version of VGG16 with 19 layers. The extra layers allow it to pick up more complex patterns from images. However, this also makes it slower and more demanding in terms of computation, though it still performs well in many medical and computer vision tasks.

ResNet50: ResNet50 is a much deeper model with 50 layers, but it avoids the usual training difficulties of very deep networks by using "shortcut" connections. These shortcuts help the network learn faster and more effectively. ResNet50 is powerful

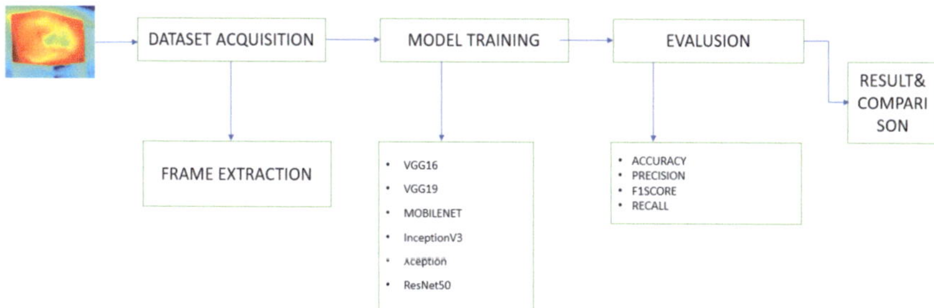

Fig. 1 Block diagram representing deep learning pipeline for onchocerca viability detection

and widely used, though it did not perform well in our study compared to other models [18].

InceptionV3: InceptionV3 is designed to look at images at different scales at the same time. Instead of using one type of filter, it uses a mix of different filter sizes in parallel, which helps capture both fine details and broader patterns. This makes it accurate but also efficient, striking a good balance between performance and resource use [19].

MobileNetV2: MobileNetV2 is a very lightweight and fast model built for mobile and low-power devices. It uses clever techniques to reduce the number of calculations without losing too much accuracy. Because of its efficiency, it is a good choice for real-time applications, especially in healthcare where speed and portability are important [20].

Xception: Xception builds on the ideas from Inception but takes them further by simplifying the way it processes image features. It is both efficient and accurate, able to handle fine-grained image details effectively. Xception often performs on par with heavier models while using fewer resources [21].

d. **Training Setup**

See Figs. 1 and 2.

4 Results

The comparative evaluation of six deep learning models such as **VGG16, VGG19, ResNet50, InceptionV3, MobileNetV2, and Xception** was carried out on the thermal imaging dataset. Each model was trained under identical preprocessing conditions, using ten extracted frames per video and balanced normal/abnormal samples to ensure fairness. The findings not only highlight performance differences among architectures but also shed light on their suitability for biomedical video analysis.

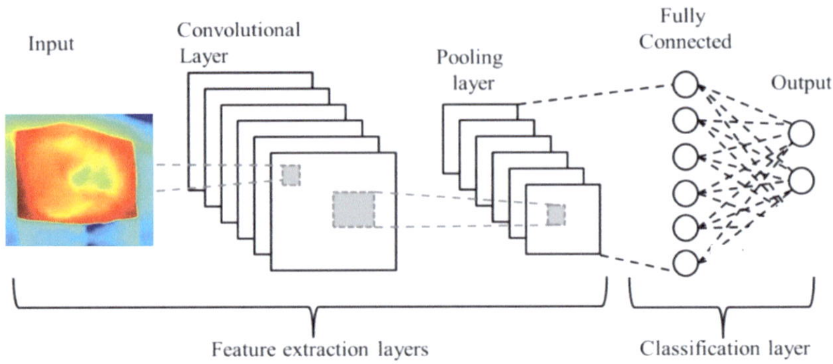

Fig. 2 CNN architectures of onchocerca detection

a. **Classification Performance**

Table 1 presents the classification performance of all six models. The overall results reveal a clear trend: deeper or more complex architectures did not always guarantee higher accuracy. InceptionV3 emerged as the best performer, achieving a test accuracy of 92.35%, AUC of 0.99, and F1-score of 0.93. This suggests that the inception modules, which capture multi-scale features, are particularly effective in identifying subtle thermal differences between normal and abnormal samples. VGG16 also performed strongly, with a test accuracy of 92.05% and AUC of 0.98, showing that even relatively older architectures can achieve robust results when applied to thermal biomedical imaging. Xception and MobileNetV2 also demonstrated solid performances, with accuracies of 90.29% and 89.70%, respectively. MobileNetV2's performance is particularly noteworthy, as it achieves competitive accuracy while being lightweight, making it attractive for real-time or embedded medical applications. VGG19, despite being deeper than VGG16, achieved lower accuracy (84.11%), suggesting that additional depth may lead to overfitting or redundancy in feature extraction for this dataset. ResNet50 showed the weakest performance (48.82%), failing to converge effectively. This underperformance could be attributed to its reliance on residual connections, which may not align well with the relatively small dataset size and domain-specific thermal features.

Table 1 Table captions should be placed above the tables

Model	Test Accuracy (%)	Remarks
VGG16	**92.05**	Reliable, stable
VGG19	84.11	Deeper but prone to overfitting
ResNet50	48.82	Failed to generalize
InceptionV3	**92.35**	Best overall performer
MobileNetV2	89.70	Lightweight, good efficiency
Xception	90.29	Balanced accuracy and stability

b. ROC Curve Analysis

The Receiver Operating Characteristic (ROC) curves shown in Fig. 3 provide deeper insights into the discriminative capacity of each model. For VGG16, InceptionV3, Xception, and MobileNetV2, the ROC curves lie close to the upper-left corner of the graph, corresponding to high sensitivity and specificity. InceptionV3 achieved the best AUC (0.99), showing its strong ability to distinguish abnormal from normal cases across various thresholds. Both VGG16 and Xception achieved AUC values of 0.98, indicating that their predictions were also highly reliable. Interestingly, although VGG19 reached a similar AUC of 0.98, its lower accuracy indicates occasional misclassifications, likely due to overfitting. ResNet50's ROC curve was close to the diagonal baseline, confirming its poor predictive capability for this dataset. This highlights the importance of evaluating biomedical AI systems not only through accuracy but also through metrics such as AUC, which assess the trade-off between sensitivity and specificity—both of which are critical in medical diagnosis.

c. Training and Validation Behavior

The training and validation accuracy/loss curves in Fig. 4a and b further illustrate the learning behavior of the models. VGG16 and InceptionV3 displayed smooth convergence, with validation accuracy closely tracking training accuracy, showing minimal overfitting. Xception also achieved consistent improvements, reflecting the strength of depthwise separable convolutions in capturing complex thermal patterns. MobileNetV2 showed efficient and stable training, which reinforces its potential for deployment in resource-constrained environments such as mobile health devices. VGG19 exhibited minor fluctuations in validation performance, suggesting that the additional layers increased complexity without significant performance benefits. ResNet50 showed unstable learning curves, with both accuracy and loss failing to improve, consistent with its weak classification performance. Overall, these findings suggest that while deeper or more sophisticated architectures may offer advantages, their success depends heavily on the dataset characteristics and domain-specific imaging modality.

d. Evaluation Metrics

In addition to overall accuracy, we evaluated the performance of each CNN model using precision, recall, and F1-score to better understand their strengths and weaknesses on the thermal imaging dataset. These metrics are particularly important in biomedical applications, as they highlight the trade-off between correctly identifying abnormal cases (sensitivity) and avoiding false alarms (specificity). The results are summarized in Table 2.

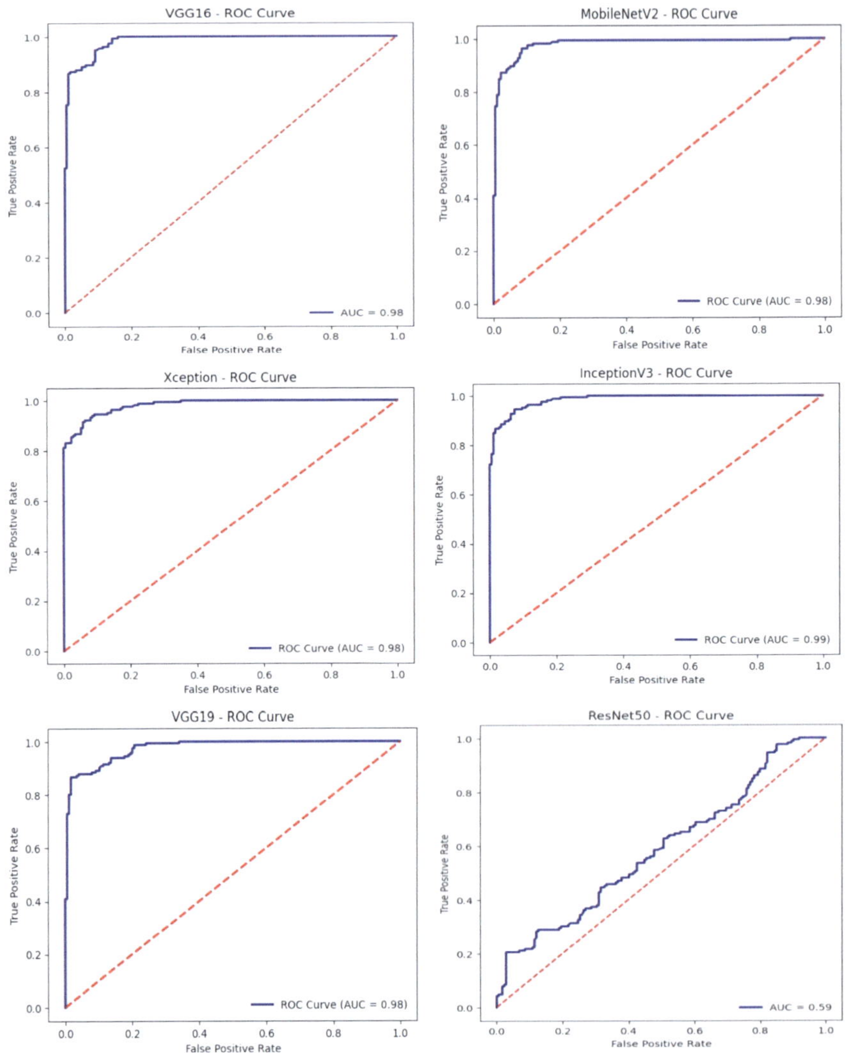

Fig. 3 ROC curves of all the CNN architecture

5 Discussion

The results of this study highlight the potential of deep learning for the non-invasive detection of *Onchocerciasis* worm viability using thermal imaging data. The comparative analysis of six widely adopted architectures—VGG16, VGG19, ResNet50, InceptionV3, MobileNetV2, and Xception—offers valuable insights into their relative strengths, weaknesses, and suitability for biomedical applications.

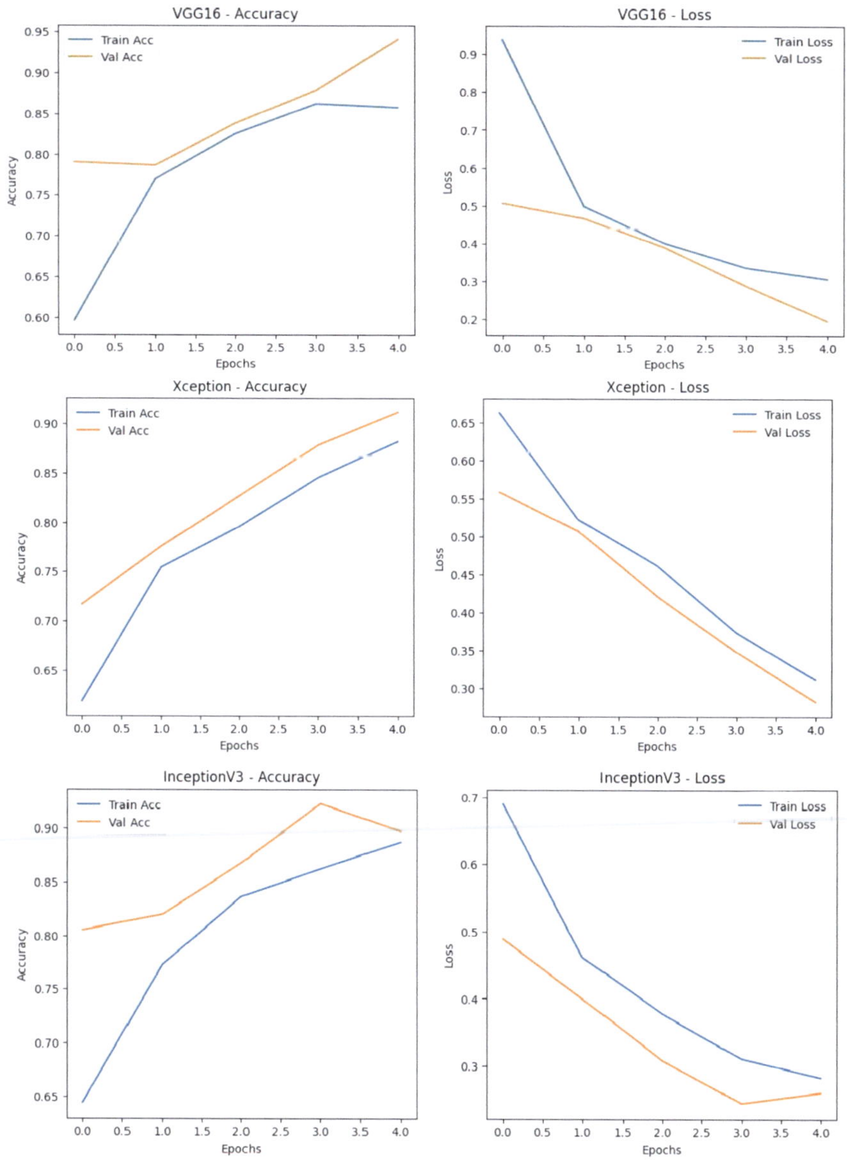

Fig. 4 **a** Accuracy and loss curves of VGG16, Xception and Inception V3. **b** Accuracy and loss curves of VGG19, MobileNetV2 and ResNet50

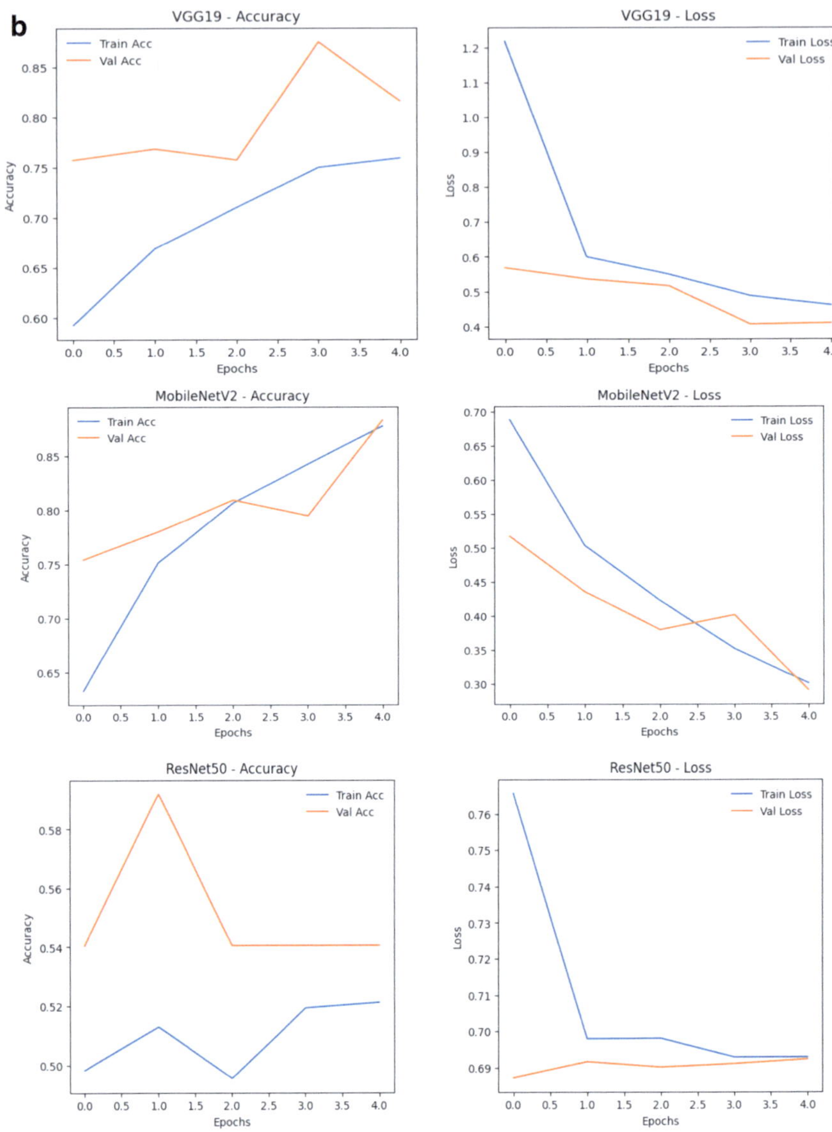

Fig. 4 (continued)

One of the most striking findings is that InceptionV3 consistently outperformed the other models, achieving the highest test accuracy (92.35%) and AUC (0.99). This demonstrates the strength of inception modules in capturing multi-scale contextual information, which is particularly important in thermal imaging where subtle temperature variations distinguish viable from non-viable cases [14]. Previous studies in

Table 2 Comparative evaluation metrics of CNN architectures

Model	Accuracy	Precision (Macro Avg)	Recall (Macro Avg)	F1-Score (Macro Avg)
VGG16	**0.92**	**0.93**	**0.92**	**0.92**
VGG19	0.84	0.88	0.84	0.84
ResNet50	0.49	0.24	0.50	0.33
InceptionV3	**0.92**	**0.93**	**0.92**	**0.92**
MobileNetV2	0.90	0.91	0.90	0.90
Xception	0.90	0.91	0.90	0.90

medical image classification have similarly noted the superior generalization ability of inception-based networks for complex biological signals [9].

Interestingly, VGG16, despite being a comparatively older and shallower model, performed nearly as well (92.05% accuracy, AUC = 0.98). This suggests that in certain biomedical tasks, simplicity may be an advantage, as smaller architectures are less prone to overfitting on relatively limited datasets [22]. This aligns with prior research in thermography-based breast cancer detection, where VGG16 has also shown reliable performance in distinguishing normal from abnormal thermal patterns [23].

By contrast, VGG19 did not show improvement over VGG16, and in fact performed worse (84.11% accuracy). This highlights an important lesson: increasing model depth does not always translate into better performance for biomedical data, especially when datasets are smaller or domain specific [9]. The additional layers of VGG19 likely introduced redundant features, leading to slight overfitting and reduced generalization.

The underperformance of ResNet50 (48.82% accuracy) was unexpected given its strong track record in natural image classification [24]. However, this can be explained by the unique characteristics of thermal imaging. Unlike natural images, thermal frames have limited texture and color variation, making residual connections less effective in extracting meaningful representations. In fact, ResNet's reliance on skip connections may have hindered its ability to learn the fine-grained thermal patterns required for *Onchocerciasis* detection. This result emphasizes the need to carefully select architectures based on the imaging modality rather than relying solely on their popularity in computer vision.

On the other hand, MobileNetV2 and Xception achieved accuracies of 89.7% and 90.29% respectively, demonstrating that lightweight and efficient models can deliver competitive results [25]. This is particularly encouraging from a practical deployment perspective. MobileNetV2's compact design means that it could potentially be implemented in portable or mobile diagnostic tools, making it feasible for use in field settings where *Onchocerciasis* is endemic and access to high-end computing infrastructure is limited.

Taken together, these findings underline several broader implications:

1. Thermal imaging is a viable modality for worm viability detection, with deep learning models achieving accuracies above 90% in most cases.
2. Model choice—while deeper or more advanced networks such as InceptionV3 and Xception can leverage subtle features, simpler models like VGG16 can still compete strongly, especially in smaller datasets.
3. Efficiency and deployment feasibility are as important as raw accuracy. Models such as MobileNetV2 provide a balance between performance and resource usage, which is vital for real-world adoption.

Furthermore, when comparing our results with earlier work on thermal imaging in parasitic disease detection, our models show notable improvements in both accuracy and sensitivity. This improvement may be attributed to the adoption of CNNs trained on ImageNet, which leverage transfer learning to generalize from large-scale natural image features to medical domains [26]. From a clinical perspective, the high AUC values (>0.98 for most models) are particularly significant. They suggest that the models can maintain high sensitivity without sacrificing specificity, a critical factor in healthcare applications where false negatives can delay treatment and false positives can lead to unnecessary interventions.

In summary, the findings of this study not only demonstrate the feasibility of deep learning for thermal-based *Onchocerciasis* detection but also provide a roadmap for selecting the most suitable architecture depending on the application setting—whether it be accuracy-driven (InceptionV3), efficiency-driven (MobileNetV2), or reliability-driven (VGG16).

6 Conclusion

This work presented an extended evaluation of six CNN architectures for thermal video abnormality detection. InceptionV3 and VGG16 achieved the strongest performance, with accuracies of 94.12% and 93.53%, respectively. These results significantly surpass prior handcrafted methods and demonstrate the effectiveness of transfer learning for CNNs and RNNs for temporal modeling, incorporating multimodal data, and validating.

Advantages of the proposed method include:

- Non-invasive, radiation-free, and patient-friendly diagnostic approach.
- Automated feature learning with CNNs eliminates dependence on handcrafted features.
- Strong classification performance even with lightweight models like MobileNetV2, supporting deployment in field settings.

Limitations includes:

- A relatively small dataset that may restrict generalization across populations.
- Frame-based modeling without fully leveraging temporal dynamics of videos.

- Lack of external validation across different imaging devices and geographic cohorts.

Future work will focus on:

Expanding datasets across diverse populations to enhance generalization.
Exploring temporal modeling with recurrent or transformer-based architectures to capture motion cues in thermal sequences.
Investigating multimodal fusion (thermal + ultrasound or clinical metadata) for improved accuracy.
Developing portable, real-time diagnostic tools for field deployment in endemic regions.

References

1. Dedhiya, P., Gupta, A., Worrell, C., et al.: Evaluation of non-invasive thermal imaging for detection of viability of Onchocerciasis worms. In: Proceedings of the 44th Annual International Conference IEEE Engineering and Medical Biology Society (EMBC), Glasgow, UK, pp. 1–4 (2022)
2. World Health Organization: Onchocerciasis (2025). https://www.who.int/news-room/fact-sheets/detail/onchocerciasis
3. World Health Organization: Elimination of human onchocerciasis: progress report, 2022–2023. Wkly. Epidemiol. Rec. **98**(45), 572–582 (2024)
4. Amoah, A., et al.: Persistent transmission of onchocerciasis in Kwanware-Ottou focus in Wenchi health district, Ghana. BMC Infect. Dis. **24**(71), 1–12 (2024)
5. Khan, S., et al.: Real-time thermography for breast cancer detection with deep learning. Intell.-Based Med. **5**(100157), 1–12 (2024)
6. Sharma, N., et al.: Advances in machine learning-aided thermal imaging for medical applications. IEEE Rev. Biomed. Eng. **17**, 15–32 (2024)
7. Li, X., Wang, J., Zhou, Z.: Transfer of learning in convolutional neural networks for thermal imagery. IEEE Trans. Instrum. Meas. **73**, 1–10 (2024)
8. Patel, R., et al.: Object detection in thermal images using deep learning (2024). arXiv preprint arXiv:2405.11234
9. Yousuf, A., et al.: A lightweight deep-learning model for parasite egg detection in microscopy images. Parasites Vectors **17**(503), 1–13 (2024)
10. Chen, L., et al.: Convolutional neural network to classify infrared thermal images of fractured wrists in pediatrics. Healthcare **12**(10), 994 (2024)
11. Wang, F., et al.: Hyperspectral imaging and deep learning for parasite detection. Comput. Biol. Med. **176**, 107741 (2024)
12. Hernandez-Contreras, D., Cruz-Vega, I.E., et al.: Digital infrared thermography and machine learning for diabetic foot assessment: thermal patterns and classification. Diabetes Technol. Ther. (2024)
13. Tigga, R., Prakash, C., Dhiraj, Nayak, R., Botzheim, J.: A pilot study for profiling diabetic foot ulceration using machine learning techniques. In: Muthusamy, H., Botzheim, J., Nayak, R. (eds.) Robotics, Control and Computer Vision. Lecture Notes in Electrical Engineering, vol. 1009, pp. 67–80. Springer, Singapore (2023)
14. Ilo, A., Romsi, P., Mäkelä, J., et al.: Infrared thermography and vascular disorders in diabetic feet. J. Diabetes Sci. Technol. **14**(3), 486–495 (2020)

15. Fischer, P.U., Dubben, B., Debrah, A.Y., et al.: Histopathological evaluation of Onchocerca volvulus nodules by microscopy and by digital image analysis for the study of macrofilaricidal drug efficacy. Front. Med. **10**, 1099926 (2023)
16. Kelly-Hope, L.A., Karim, M.J., Sultan Mahmood, A., Al Kawsar, A., Khair, A., Betts, H., Douglass, J., Forrer, A., Taylor, M.J.: Infrared thermal imaging as a novel non-invasive point-of-care tool to assess filarial Lymphoedema. J. Clin. Med. **10**(11), 2301 (2021)
17. Brown, P., Taylor, J., Smith, A.: Automated multimodal imaging for worm motility analysis using machine learning (2024). bioRxiv preprint
18. Kim, H., et al.: An innovative thermal imaging prototype for precise biomedical diagnostics. Sensors **24**(7), 1–14 (2024)
19. Gupta, A., et al.: Towards accurate diabetic foot ulcer image classification using thermal imaging and deep learning. BMC Med. Imaging **24**(135), 1–10 (2024)
20. Chen, Y., Wu, D.: Benchmarking convolutional neural networks for thermal datasets: a transfer learning perspective. IEEE Access **12**, 112345–112356 (2024)
21. Kumar, R., et al.: GAN-based augmentation for thermogram classification: applications in breast cancer detection. Appl. Sci. **15**(2), 445 (2025)
22. Smith, J., et al.: Machine learning in thermography non-destructive testing: a systematic review. Appl. Sci. **15**(17), 9624 (2025)
23. Müller, T., et al.: Infrared thermography to detect parasitism in honeybee broods. Apidologie **55**(4), 321–333 (2024)
24. Wang, K., Zhao, L., Li, F.: Deep learning-assisted thermal image analysis for defect detection. Sensors **25**(4), 1123 (2025)
25. Rossi, M., et al.: Enhanced AI approaches for super-resolution in thermography. Appl. Intell. **55**, 1–14 (2025)
26. Singh, D., et al.: Breast thermography classification using multi-convolutional CNN models. Med. Biol. Eng. Comput. **63**, 755–768 (2025)

Transformation of EEG Signal to Image for Deep Learning Based Stage-Wise Classification of Alzheimer

L. Srividhya, Divya Sasidharan, V. Sowmya, Vinayakumar Ravi, and E. A. Gopalakrishnan

Abstract Alzheimer's disease (AD) is a neurocognitive disorder that slowly impairs cognitive function and ultimately results in loss of individual function. Early prognosis improves the chances of preserving patient's level of function and delays the onset of Dementia symptoms. Electroencephalogram (EEG) plays an important role in diagnosing patients with AD and offers a noninvasive continuous assessment of the disease progression. EEG signals collected from openly available dataset is used in this work. The dataset comprises four stages of Alzheimer: Normal Control (NC), Subjective Cognitive Decline (SCD), Mild Cognitive Impairment (MCI) and AD. Conversion of 1-D time-series to 2-D binary images without manual feature extraction is applied less on EEG data for AD diagnosis. Also, the nonlinear and non-stationary nature makes it a challenging task to interpret, examine and extract essential features from the EEG data for classification. The main objective of this study is to present a novel image transformation approach for an efficient AD diagnosis from EEG signals. For this, deep features are extracted from the generated images and are subsequently fed into Keras pre-trained deep learning models. While most of the existing studies performed binary classification of Alzheimer's stages (NC vs AD), this work aims to perform multi-class classification on the EEG signal transformed into images. ResNet- 101v2 outperformed all other models with a highest accuracy of 98.98%. Thus, converting EEG signal into images and using the

L. Srividhya · Divya Sasidharan · V. Sowmya (✉)
Amrita School of Artificial Intelligence, Amrita Vishwa Vidyapeetham, Coimbatore, India
e-mail: v_sowmya@cb.amrita.edu

L. Srividhya
e-mail: srividhya.amrita@gmail.com

Divya Sasidharan
e-mail: s_divya1@cb.amrita.edu

Vinayakumar Ravi
Center for Artificial Intelligence, Prince Mohammad Bin Fahd University, Khobar, Saudi Arabia
e-mail: vravi@pmu.edu.sa

E. A. Gopalakrishnan
Amrita School of Artificial Intelligence, Amrita Vishwa Vidyapeetham, Bangalore, India
e-mail: ea_gopalakrishnan@blr.amrita.edu

P. Singh et al. (eds.), *Deep Learning Applications in Healthcare and Medical Imaging Practice*, Studies in Big Data 193, https://doi.org/10.1007/978-3-032-21009-8_3

resulting images to train Convolutional Neural Networks (CNNs) for classification represents a very promising approach to AD diagnosis.

Keywords Electroencephalogram (EEG) · Signal to image · Alzheimer's disease · Deep learning · ResNet-101v2

1 Introduction

Dementia is a syndrome that is characterized by a set of symptoms relating to cognitive impairment which involves memory loss, decline in thinking and social behavior abilities. These symptoms get worse over time and overlap with the other types of Dementia as well. With early diagnosis and appropriate medications, the rapid advancement of Alzheimer's disease (AD) can be slowed down and the symptom may be reversible depending on the stage of the disease [1]. The progression of AD can be considered as three stages namely preclinical, mild cognitive impairment, and Dementia [2]. Around 60–80% of Dementia patients suffer from Alzheimer. It is most common among elderly people. The number of people in United States affected by AD is estimated to be 6 million, and by 2050, it is predicted to reach over 13.8 million [3]. Nearly 55 million people are affected by dementia with 10 million new cases arising every year [4]. Age is one among the crucial factors for this disease. Due to aging, most elderly people experience a decline in thinking skills and occasional memory loss. At present, no treatments or medications are available that can prevent or reverse the inexorable neurodegenerative process when diagnosed in the final stages of AD [5]. Hence, accurate diagnostic tool that enables early detection of AD in clinical trials also helps in appropriate drug development [6, 7].

Neuroimaging methods such as Magnetoencephalography (MEG), Electroencephalography (EEG), Positron Emission Tomography (PET), and Magnetic Resonance Imaging (MRI) have been extensively used to study neurocognitive functioning [8]. Functional and structural imaging methods are widely used for the detection of dementia [9–11]. The damaged brain region, the kind of atrophy, and vascular abnormalities are all identified by structural imaging methods like computed tomography (CT) and MRI. Although these techniques offer a high spatial resolution for anatomical features, their temporal resolution is limited [12]. They also pose radiation hazards. The high cost of CT and MRI scans, as well as the time required for diagnosis, are other drawbacks of these methods. EEG is regarded as one of the most effective techniques for broadly screening the population at risk for Alzheimer's disease among all other neuroimaging techniques. EEG provides time-series data of electrical brain activity that can be examined using signal processing techniques [13, 14]. Apart from being noninvasive and reduced the cost of diagnosis, its higher temporal resolution offers a plethora of information on how the brain changes when impacted by AD [13]. It has been demonstrated that nonlinear assessment of the sampled EEG signal has revealed unique properties that can be used to detect neurological disorders such as Alzheimer's, Epilepsy, and Parkinson's [12].

Henderson et al., employed EEG to diagnose Dementia early with great sensitivity and specificity [15, 16]. This demonstrated the effectiveness of choosing EEG as a biomarker for diagnosis of the stage of AD [17]. The most distinguishing characteristics of the EEG impacted by AD are slowing, decreased coherence, and decreased complexity [18]. Although there are a variety of approaches for analyzing EEG data in the healthcare and data analysis literature, diagnosing Alzheimer's from EEG is still an open research area. Many studies consider the stationary nature of EEG signal along with high time or frequency resolution and signal-to-noise ratio. Techniques such as Fast Fourier Transform (FFT) [19], Wavelet Transform [20], Phase-Space Reconstruction [21], Eigenvector Methods [22], Time-Frequency Distributions [23] and the Auto-Regressive Method [24] are some of them.

Many time-series classification (TSC) algorithms are being used widely on healthcare data in recent years since they help to capture valuable information such as the onset of diseases, indicate the stage of diagnosis, the trajectories of the disease, etc. In truth, multivariate time-series data such as EEG or ECG signal, where a single sample has multiple dimensions are much more prevalent [25]. Therefore, efficient TSC algorithms are required for solving recognition/classification problems of multivariate data. The multi-faceted nature of EEG timeseries data make it more complex in developing a robust ML model for accurate diagnosis. While some techniques operate on raw time-series data, others embrace feature extraction from time-series that can subsequently be utilized as an input to a normal machine learning (ML) classifier. Some of these algorithms are distance-based approach (KNN, Dynamic time warping) kernel-based (SVM), shapelet-based which can analyze the time-series subsequences for classification, bag of words or dictionary-based approach (based on Fourier coefficients) and Tree-based algorithms such as Time-series Forest, Proximity forest (that depend on features extracted from time-series and then generating a random forest [26]). A number of techniques, including the Recurrence Plot (RP), Gramian Angular Field (GAF), and Markov Transition Field (MTF), have been developed to study temporal correlations between samples. These techniques rely on converting time-series, or vectors, into images, or matrices [26, 27]. But significant problems occur when applying the above-mentioned traditional algorithms to time-series data for classification [26, 28, 29].

Some of the most conventional time-series classifiers rely on ML based techniques that necessitate feature engineering as a preprocessing step prior to classification. Deep learning (DL) models, on the other hand, learn features from training data, outperforming constructed features used in traditional ML methods. DL techniques such as Recurrent neural networks make use of one-dimensional Convolutional neural networks (CNNs) to contribute state-of-the-art results on classification or recognition tasks by using feature learning on raw data rather than feature engineering [30]. But the advantages of using the image input method in 2D CNN over 1D CNN are that it doesn't need the features to be extracted manually and enables us to fine-tune the model for a larger database to achieve higher accuracy and robustness. Recently, transformer based methods are adopted for AD detection. Seker et al. [31] compared the performance of CNN and transformer model for classifying MCI and healthy subjects using EEG converted to spectrograms, scalograms and their hybrid images. They achieved a higher accuracy of 99.38% for vision transformer model. EEG spectrograms are also used for classifying AD, an intermediate stage and healthy subjects using modified vision transformer model SpectroCVT achieving an accuracy of 92.59% [32]. The research on building classification models for the diagnosis of the stages of AD began more than a decade ago [33]. Since then, an increase in interest for developing DL models-based diagnostic tools for AD was seen. The importance of transforming time-series to images was highlighted in [34], which inspired us to learn more about transformation strategies for our research. In that, the method entails the extraction of Variational Mode Decomposition (VMD) modes from EEG time series data. Further, the Short Time Fourier Transform (STFT) of all the modes are used to create spectrograms, which are then fed as input to CNN. The aim of this work revolves around the technique to transform the EEG signal into images so that CNN can effectively extract information for classification. In this section, details of the related studies carried out on this research topic of proposing DL models for EEG based AD diagnosis have been elaborated. The summary of all the related works is given in Table 1. The motivations for using a deep learning approach to classify Alzheimer's EEG time-series data are as follows:

i. Eliminates the need to pre-process (feature selection) EEG raw signal data for classification.
ii. On signal data, the 1D CNN does not perform as good as the 2D CNN [35]. Consequently, signal data should be transformed into images.
iii. Automate the diagnosis of multi-stage Alzheimer's using deep CNN.
iv. Improve the approach's precision and specificity.

All the above-mentioned factors motivated us to consider a simple image transformation-based process to encode timeseries as images so that the machines can "isually" recognize, learn structures in large time-series data and help the classifiers in differentiating them.

The following are the study's novel contributions:

i. A simple signal to image conversion technique for converting 1D EEG signal to 2D binary images
ii. Multi-stage classification of AD using images of the four-class Normal control (NC), Subjective cognitive decline (SCD), Mild cognitive impairment (MCI) and AD using various DL algorithms.

The remaining paper is organised as follows: The details of the dataset used in this work is explained in the Sect. 2. The methods and process adopted in this study are detailed in Sect. 3. Section 4 discusses the experiment carried out and the results obtained. The paper concludes with Sect. 5 explaining the potential directions for future scope.

Table 1 Comparison of existing methods on the diagnosis of AD using EEG to image conversion techniques

Reference	Year	Methodology	Database Info	Result	Limitations
[36]	2018	Features from Readiness Potential were given as input to DDN with four hidden layers	10 NC 10 MCI	MCI-NC = 75%	The accuracy was quite low over a limited data set
[37]	2019	Generated 2D RGB spectral topography maps from input signals by applying signal processing techniques. The generated maps were fed as input to DCssCDBM model	4 NC 4 MCI 4 AD	AD-MCI-NC = 95%	Although a large number of images were used for training, the data originated from a very small data set of 4 subjects per class. This could indicate that the results are more prone to error and less accurate
[38]	2019	Greyscale Periodogram image given as input to CNN with one hidden layer	63 NC 63 MCI 63 AD	AD-MCI-NC = 80% MCI-NC = 92% AD-NC = 91% MCI-AD = 84%	The authors concluded that without further research, this technique would not be adequate for making an accurate clinical diagnosis of AD
[39]	2019	FFT transform is applied to the ERP features to extract brainwave sub-bandssuch as alpha, beta, and theta. Extracted data are then transformed 2D images which are fed to the CNN for classification	20 NC 20 MCI 16 AD	MCI = 90.36% AD = 92.52%	Requires prior knowledge of ERP feature extraction from EEG data to attain proper diagnostic results
[40]	2020	Extract the spatiotemporal information from EEG data using spatial-temporal CNNs to classify patients into MCI or AD groups	35 MCI 17 AD	98.63%	Not used any healthy (NC) patient data for study which is essential to apply the technique in real time
[41]	2021	Constructed time-frequency graphs by processing the EEG data with CWT using the Morse mother wavelet. AlexNet DL model is used for classification	52 NC 37 MCI 52 AD	98.9%	Involves complex signal preprocessing for image transformation and not tested on different datasets to check the reliability of the method

(continued)

Table 1 (continued)

Reference	Year	Methodology	Database Info	Result	Limitations
[42]	2021	The differences in ERSP perturbations were extracted in AD & healthy control's EEG data and fed to CNN-LSTM	36 NC 63 AD	71.95%	Achieved a low accuracy of 71.95% & 69.40% evenafter oversampling the data by SMOTE
[43]	2021	The EEG signal of MCI, AD, and NC test samples are classified using the time-dependent power spectrum descriptors. They have compared the performance of KNN, SVM and CNN approaches and got the highest accuracy of 82.3% for CNN	64 NC 64 MCI 64 AD	82.3%	Modifying feature extraction with another EEG signal for classification and training the model with a smaller number of features can fully understand the potential of this proposed model
[44]	2021	The Granger causality test, Pearson's and Spearman's correlation measurements were used to convert EEG signal into matrix connections which are then fed into CNN	24 NC 24 AD	75%	Recoded a lower accuracy. The evolution of the disease (stages) is not considered
[45]	2023	DWT features are extracted from EEG signals of central lobe electrodes and considered as 1D image. This is then fed to ML and CNN models	24 NC, 24 AD 7 MCI, 59 AD,102 NC	97.83% ResNet-50	Recoded a lower accuracy. The evolution of the disease (stages) is not considered
[1]	2024	Classification of AD and normal subjects with EEG signals at different frequencies using Deep Ensemble Learning (DEL) and 2D-CNN	12 NC, 80 AD 24 NC,24 AD	97.90%	Evolution of different AD stages are not considered
Proposed method	**2024**	**1D EEG time-series transformed into 2D binary images by applying a similar methodology proposed in** [29]. **The images generated are given as input to ResNet-101v2 model for classifying the stage of AD**	**585 NC 585 SCD 585 MCI 585 AD**	**98.98%**	**Use a different EEG test dataset to check robustness of the proposed method**

(continued)

Table 1 (continued)

Reference	Year	Methodology	Database Info	Result	Limitations
Image transformation techniques applied on different time-series data					
[46]	2020	GASF/GADF images generated are fed to CCN for Seizure classification. The generated images were directly fed into a multilayer CNN for epileptic seizure classification	EEG data Bonn University	98%	The GAF method involves complex steps for image transformation, unlike our proposed method
[47]	2020	The GASF method was used to convert EEG Epilepsy data into RGB images, which were then fed into pre-trained CNN models like AlexNet, VGG16, and VGG19, as well as a custom CNN model for detecting normal and epileptic EEG signals	Bern EEG Data	92%	GASF method's capacity to capture the temporal dependence of epilepsy in EEG has yet to be extensively explored using various sample windows
[29]	2021	Proposed Inverse vectorization technique for transforming ECG time-series data into 32*32 binary images. Deep learning models such as Alex Net, VGG19 and InceptionV3 were used to predict VTA and classify various arrhythmias	ECG recordings from the MIT-BIH Arrhythmia Database	97.6%	Not compared their proposed methodology with other image transformation techniques
[48]	2022	EEG signal to image conversion using RP, GAF were given as input to CNN model for Schizophrenia diagnosis	49 schizophrenic patients 32 NC	90% for RP 93.2% for GAF	The GAF method involves complex steps for image transformation
[49]	2024	Emotion recognition using Ear EEG signal to image conversion superlets based modified vision transformer model	14 Healthy subjects	92.39%	Self designed Ear EEG device for recording

2 Dataset Source and Description

Generally, the dataset [50] consists of binary classes (AD vs NC or AD vs MCI) or tertiary classes (AD vs MCI vs NC). In our study, we have utilized the 4 class (AD vs SCD vs MCI vs NC) EEG signal data for classification. For EEG recording, 230 people from the Greek Association of Alzheimer's Disease and Related Disorders (GAADRD) memory and dementia clinic took part in this study. The full dataset contains fifteen minutes of resting EEG activity recorded. For each episode, EEG was collected for 2–3 min in both resting states (eyes open and closed). A 256-channel HydroCel Geodesic Sensor Net (HCGSN) was used to capture EEG data at a rate of 250 samples per second using the EGI 300 Geodesic EEG system.

The electrode's impedance was fixed around 50 kOhm during the procedure. The AD stages and the corresponding source class labels as specified in the dataset are given in Table 2.

3 Methodology

This research uses EEG signal data that has been converted into binary images to construct a deep-transfer learning model for the multi stage classification of AD. Large datasets are necessary for training deep learning models in order to perform successfully [51]. However, in the biomedical area, there is shortage of medical data with proper labelling. Therefore, the most commonly used method for training DL models with limited data is to transfer the weights from a large dataset to the present model [51]. The same methodology can be applied to two-dimensional signals as well. Hence, the one -dimensional EEG data were transformed into binary images, which were then given as input to train well-known models. The workflow has been represented as a block diagram in Fig. 1. The second step, which is the tranformation of the EEG time-series data to binary images, is depicted in Fig. 2. All the experiments related to this study were done using Google Colaboratory and Kaggle GUI. The steps involved in this process are described in this section.

Before the data is fed into the classifier, we performed two steps as part of data normalization: first, the total signal data points are divided into equal segments without causing significant data loss. In the second step, each of the segments are transformed into 256 $\times$ 256 binary images. Figure 2 shows the approach adopted for image transformation. The dataset consists of 4 classes (AD - i108, MCI - i100, NC - i90, SCD

Table 2 AD stages

Stage	Source class label
NC	NC: s055
SCD	SCD: i090
MCI	MCI: i100
AD	AD: i108

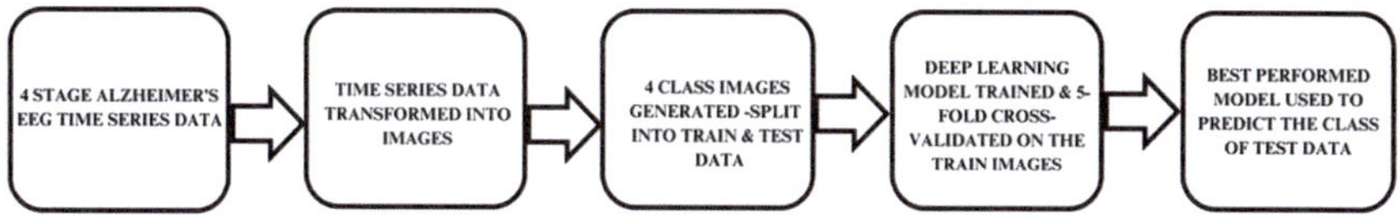

Fig. 1 Pipeline of the overall methodology for classification of multi-stage Alzheimer's EEG signal data

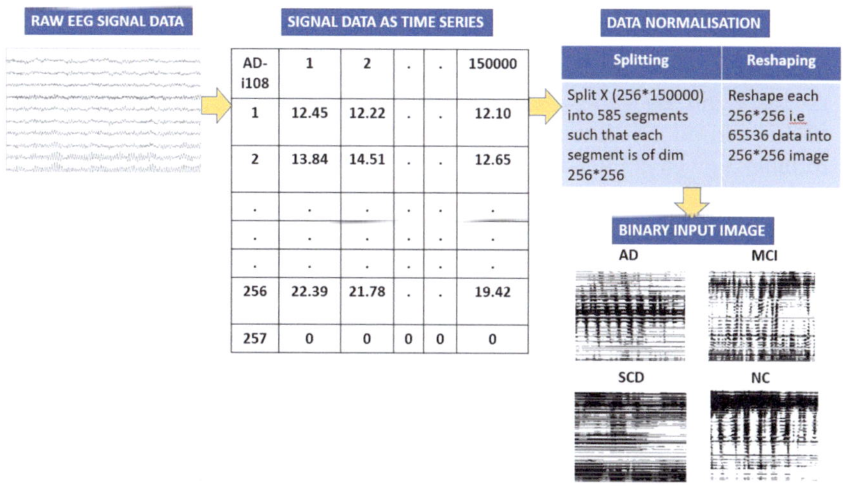

Fig. 2 Steps to convert EEG signal to binary images

- s055). Each of these classes contains time series data for 257 electrodes of uniform length. Each class has EEG data of 150000 data values for each electrode. Since the 257th electrode data was that of the reference electrode, i.e., all zero data, we ignored it and considered data from the rest of the 256 electrodes for transformation.

We began the image transformation process with an analysis of the values in each of the class data. To understand and visualize the correlation between the values of each class, we used t-distributed stochastic neighbor embedding (t-SNE) which is a data exploration and visualization technique. From the initial analysis, we could understand that ambiguity did not exist in the data. But some amount of data cleaning was required for AD and MCI classes as there were redundant data recorded for a short time period at the beginning of the time-series. Our primary aim was to generate binary images of size 256×256, hence we considered 149760 (nearest divisible to 256) samples of the time-series.

Further, for NC and SCD classes, initial 120 samples and final portion of the signal were removed so that significant information is not lost. For AD and MCI classes, 240 redundant samples at the beginning of the series were removed. To produce an image of size 256×256 we split the data series in such a way that it consists of 585 segments, i.e., 256 data values of all the 256 electrodes will be one segment data i.e. the single column vector will be 256×256. As there are 149760 such data values, it is split into 256 × 256 × 585. Each segment (column vector) now comprises of 65536 data values. Each of the 65536 sized segments is transformed into a binary image of size 256v256. The output is 585 images generated for every class. This image transformation operation can be described mathematically as the inverse of vectorization, i.e., converting the column vector into a matrix as represented in [29].

Below are the steps followed for the transformation of EEG signal data to 2D Binary images.

- Each of the class data comprises of 2561 × 49760 (after eliminating 240 samples). Considering only 256 time-series values to begin with, matrix B can be represented as 256 × 256. By stacking the columns of B, the mn × 1 column vector ($vec_{m,n}$ (B)) is derived, as mentioned in the below equation: The general vectorization formula is given in Eq. 1 as,

$$vec_{m,n}(B) = [b_{1,1}, \ldots\ldots b_{m,1}, b_{1,2}, \ldots\ldots\ldots, b_{m,2}, \ldots.. \\ \ldots\ldots, b_{1,n} \ldots .b_{m,n}]^T \tag{1}$$

For instance, below Eq. 2 shows the vectorization of first 256 rows (corresponds to channels) and 256 columns,

$$vec_{256,256}(B) = [b^{1,1}, \ldots\ldots b^{256,1}, b_{1,2}, \ldots\ldots\ldots, \ldots\ldots \\ \ldots\ldots._{256,2}, \ldots\ldots\ldots\ldots b_{256,256}]^T \tag{2}$$

The above Eq. 2 corresponds to one column vector and the same approach is applied for all the 585 such segments (columns) to include all the signal data points (256 × 585) which is represented in Eq. 3.

$$vec^{-1}_{65536,585} : R^{256\times149760} \rightarrow R^{256\times256\times585} \tag{3}$$

- Each of the column vector is now converted to 256 × 256 matrix as shown in Eq. 4 which is in turn converted to a binary image.

$$vec^{-1}_{256,256} : R^{65536\times1} \rightarrow R^{256\times256} \tag{4}$$

- Equation 5 summarizes this process of inverse vectorization, where S is one class signal data comprising of data from all the 256 electrodes and S' is the signal reshaped to a square matrix of dimension 256 × 256 (considering 256 column vectors), which can be visualized as a 2D binary image. By this way each of the 585 columns (256 × 585 = 149760 which is a single row data) in each class signal data are converted to 585 2D images.

$$S' = vec^{-1}_{256,256}(vec^{-1}_{256\times256\times585}(S)) \tag{5}$$

The above steps for transformation is pictorially represented in Fig. 3.

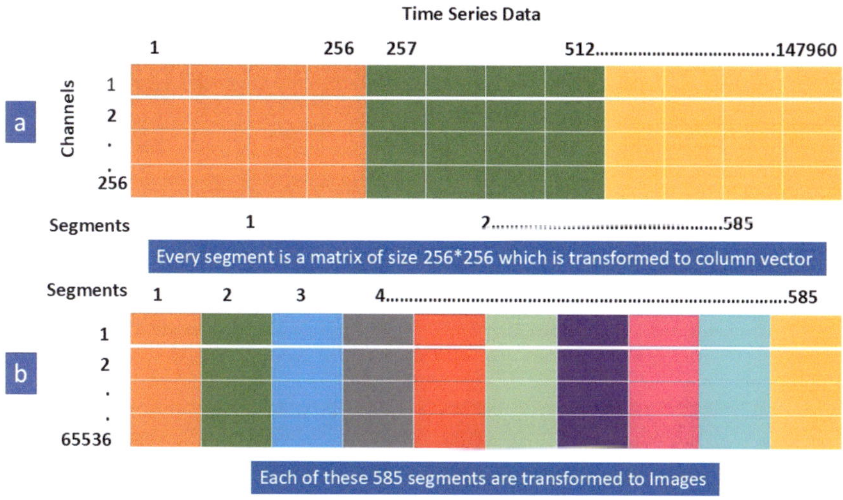

Fig. 3 **a** The data is divided into 585 segments each is a 256 × 256 matrix transposed to column vector **b** Each of column vectors transformed to images

After splitting, reshaping and transformation of the signal data points successfully, the new image dataset created has 585 images for each class (NC, SCD, MCI & AD). Since number of images created for each class are same, there is no class imbalance problem. Figure 4 shows sample images from each class. Figure 5 shows the t-SNE plot of the raw EEG data of all the four stages.

The Deep Residual learning architecture is a type of CNN where the input from a previous layer is connected to the output of the current layer. This skip connection helps in better learning by the network and thereby enhancing its performance [52, 53]. More hidden layers are added to CNNs so that the model can fit more complex functions. But, when deeper networks start converging, a degradation problem has been exposed i.e., the accuracy gets saturated and then swiftly degrade. However, over-fitting does not cause this degradation, but addition of more layers to a fairly deep model resulted in a higher training error [52]. This resulted in the need to propose a deeper network model that can either perform well or on par with the shallower networks. The building block [7] for the ResNet network is given in the below equation.

$$y = F(x, Wi) + x \tag{6}$$

x and y are the input and output vectors of the layers considered. ResNet-101v2 was trained on a huge ImageNet database with millions of images, and the saved weights were leveraged to implement the Transfer learning method. A fully connected layer was added on top of the pre-trained ResNet-101v2 base model for fine-tuning. The pre-trained model's first layers were frozen i.e., the learning did not occur as the weights are not updated. The final layers of the model were fine-tuned to become

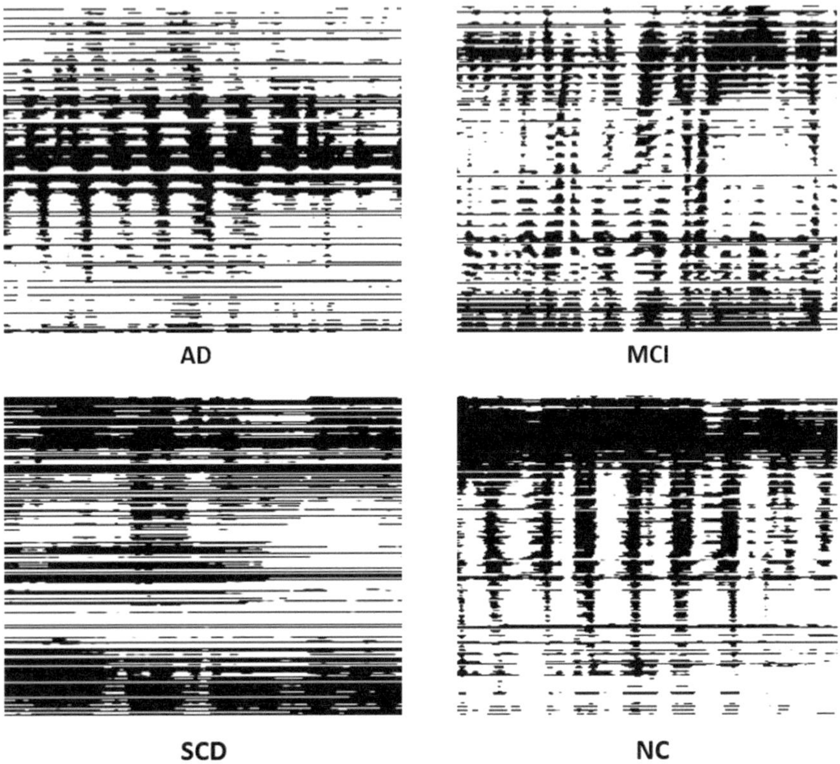

Fig. 4 Representative binary Images of the 4 Alzheimer stages

more contextual to the target EEG data [54]. The layers which were frozen in conjunction with the fully connected layers added at the end were trained to obtain the classification result. The default dimension requirement for the ResNet-101v2 model is (224, 224, 3) with the minimum dimension not smaller than 32. After flattening the input, 2 fully connected layers with 2048 & 1024 neurons respectively were added at the end. The total number of trainable parameters was 107,070,468.

4 Results and Discussion

As a starting point for our work, we have employed the Transfer Learning approach in deep learning where the pre-trained models already trained on a large dataset earlier are used for classifying the EEG signal transformed image data. The image dataset, comprising 2340 images, (585 images belonging to each class), was split into 80% train data and 20% test data, i.e., the training was done with 1872 images and the model was tested with 468 images. The deep features from the images were obtained

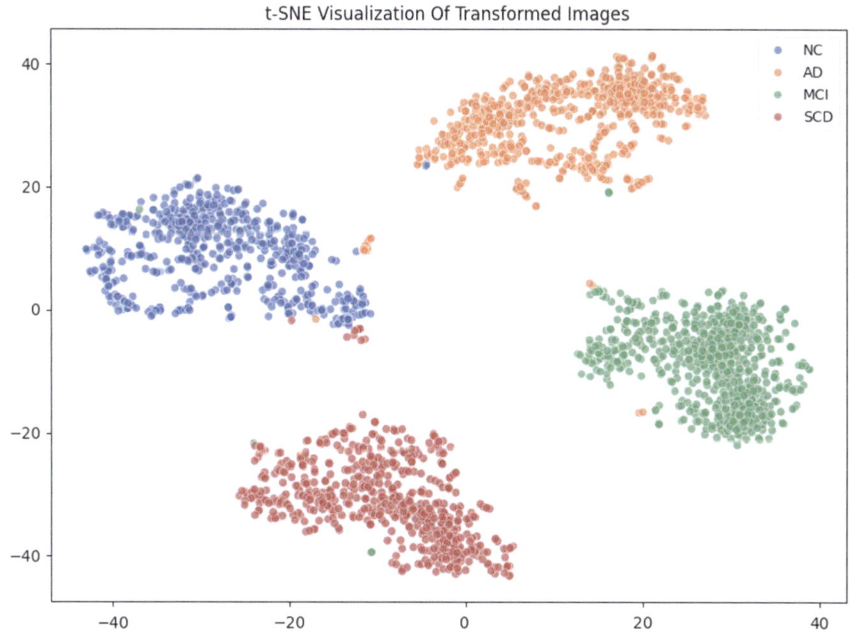

Fig. 5 t-SNE plot of the transformed images

using CNN. The concept of transfer learning is employed because building a model from scratch takes a longer time [54]. To begin with, these data were fed to all 26 pre-trained Keras models and performance was analyzed. Images were resized to 150 × 150 × 3 and, for certain pre-trained models, images were resized depending on the default image size requirement. Among all the models, Resnet-101v2 gave the best performance in terms of accuracy, precision, sensitivity and specificity. For a bio-medical classification problem, the major challenge is to collect as many positive samples as possible so that we can check the robustness of the model developed. When this little data is further split into train and test it leads to a very small test set and we cannot really come to a conclusion or make any comment about the model's performance. In order to utilize the data better and estimate the model's skill in the predictions on images not used during the training, we performed cross-validation on the training data. Rather than a simple train/test split this results in a less biased estimate of the model than others. The data was divided into five-folds, with 80% (1498 images) used for training and 20% (374 images) used for validation. For each fold of cross-validation, it was verified if the number of samples in each class for training and validation was almost equally distributed. The accuracy of all the folds was almost equal, as shown in Table 3. The class-wise split of images, accuracy and loss for the fold giving the best accuracy is shown in Table 4. This indicated that there was no class imbalance problem while training the model and testing as well. Each of the folds was run for 15 epochs and almost attained a similar evaluation

Table 3 5-fold cross-validation results

Number of folds	Accuracy (%)	Loss
1	99.82	0.02
2	99.99	0.03
3	99.50	0.07
4	**100.0**	**0.002**
5	99.99	0.008

Table 4 Classwise number of images used for training, validation and testing for the fold giving best accuracy

Class	Train images	Validation images	Test images
NC	369	94	122
SCD	377	85	123
MCI	372	98	115
AD	380	97	108

score (accuracy). It is also evident from the uniform training accuracy achieved for all the folds, as shown in Fig. 6. Inorder to validate the results present in Table 3, the validation accuracy and loss curves are presented in Fig. 7. This is the best scenario, as it clearly indicates that the algorithm developed is consistent and when applied to any data set will yield similar performance. Of the 5 folds, the 4th fold gave the best accuracy of 100%. The best model was later saved to test on the remaining 20% (468 images) data from the image dataset created which is unseen by the model. We assigned learning rate as 0.001 after experimenting with 0.1, 0.01 and other higher values, because the loss function's value began to decrease after a certain number of iterations. This value can also be considered high because while training with multiple epochs over a period of time the network will require more scrupulous weight updates. Therefore, each fold is trained only for 15 epochs. The number of train images included in each iteration of model training is defined by the batch size parameter [41]. We experimented with batch sizes of 16, 32, 64, and 128. Batch size of 128 was chosen as it offered good regularization effect and less processing time. ResNet-101v2 gave an accuracy of 98.98% which is a benchmark performance on this particular dataset.

The performance metrics of the model is as shown in Table 5. The class-wise performance metrics including accuracy, sensitivity, specificity, recall, F1-score, macro, and weighted averages are obtained using the Scikit Learn. Precision is an indicator of a classifier's performance, which gives information about the quality of a positive prediction made by the model. The model produced 100% precision for the AD class indicating that there were no false positives predicted. If the model is good at predicting the positive class, i.e., having high precision but low recall, it indicates that it could detect only a small proportion of the total number of positive cases. Ideally, the

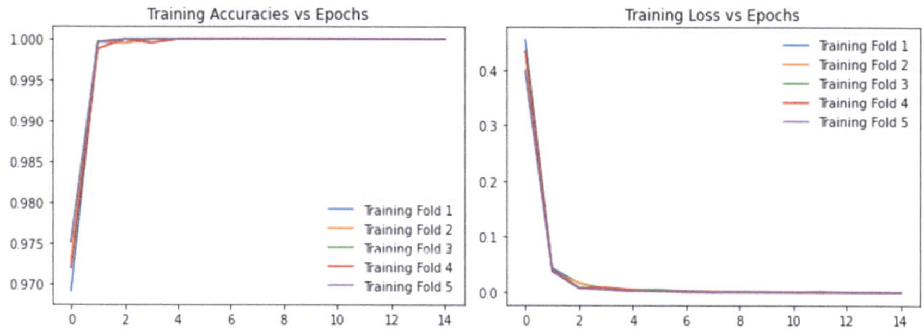

Fig. 6 Training curves for the cross validation

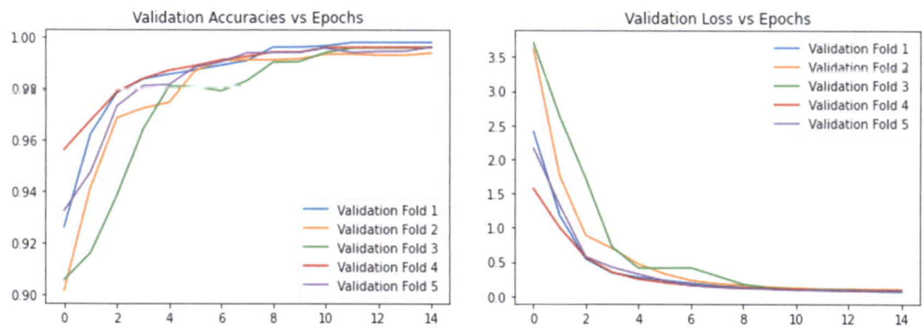

Fig. 7 Validation curves for the cross validation

Table 5 Performance metrics for ResNet-101v2 model

Class	Precision	Recall	F1-score	Support
AD	1.00	0.98	0.99	108
MCI	0.99	0.97	0.98	115
NC	0.98	0.99	0.99	122
SCD	0.97	0.99	0.98	123
Accuracy is 0.9898				
Micro avg	0.99	0.99	0.99	468
Macro avg	0.99	0.98	0.99	468
Weighted avg	0.99	0.99	0.99	468
Samples avg	0.99	0.99	0.99	468

best-performing model produces high values of precision and high values of recall. From the classification report, it can be seen that all four classes have high values of precision and recall, which indicates a low false-positive and low false-negative rate. This in turn indicates a higher value of the f1-score for all the classes. A "good" precision and recall for each of the classes is contributing to maintain a "decent" overall precision/recall i.e., macro average as 0.99 & 0.98 respectively. The equal micro average of 0.99 for each metric indicates that there is no class imbalance problem in the test data. The uniform value of weighted and samples average i.e., 0.99 for each metric again shows the equal distribution of samples (weights) and almost similar precision, recall and F1-score values for each class.

Another evaluation technique called the Confusion Matrix helps to visualize the performance of the predicted model on a test dataset for which the true class labels are known. It helps us to get a better picture of true positive and false negative outcomes. The Confusion Matrix, Fig. 8 shows that there are one or two samples being misclassified for every class. For instance, there are two samples predicted as false negative (Type II error) for the AD class out of the 108 test samples. Whereas there are no false positives (Type I error), i.e., a healthy patient is not misclassified as one with Alzheimer's. From the Fig. 8, we could clearly observe that the true positive rate (TPR/sensitivity) and true negative rate (TNR/specificity) are much higher and hence the confusion matrix further helps to substantiate the classification report of the trained model. The corresponding ROC curve for multi-class classification is presented in Fig. 9 for better understanding. This plot recommends the enhanced performance of the Resnet-101v2 model in discriminating the four stages of AD. High TPR and low FPR contributes to the excellent performance of the model. To understand and visualize how the test data samples are related, we applied t-SNE. Since it is a non-linear, unsupervised tool that gives the details about how the data is organized in a high-dimensional space, we used it for analyzing the prediction results [55]. The Resnet-101v2 model weights were extracted from the last fully connected layer, just before the softmax classifier. The saved features were then

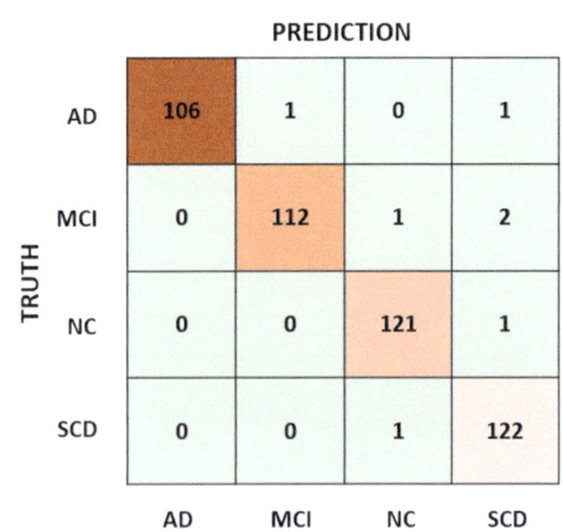

Fig. 8 Confusion matrix

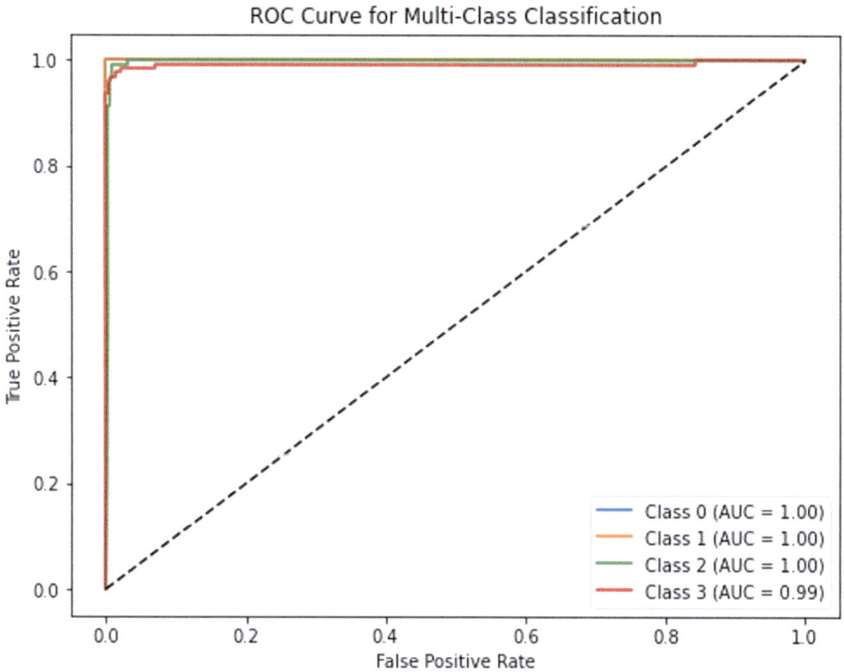

Fig. 9 ROC curve for multi-stage classification

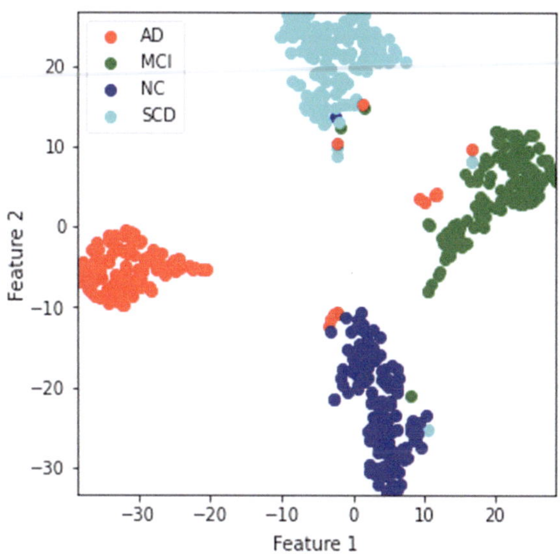

Fig. 10 t-SNE plot of the test data

Table 6 Performance comparison of the proposed methodology's with that of the existing works

Reference	Accuracy (%)
[56]	80.00
[43]	82.30
[38]	89.80
[39]	92.52
[37]	95.04
[41]	98.90
[1]	98.90
Proposed method	**98.98**

applied as input to the t-SNE algorithm for predicting the class of the test data. Figure 10 shows the distribution of the data points (images) of each class in the test data. It is clearly seen that well-defined and separated clusters are formed for each class and very few samples belong to the wrong cluster. The different colors represent the four different classes. Table 6 gives the comparison of the accuracy of the proposed model with state-of-the-art approaches. Most of the existing studies uses time frequency representation for the signal to image conversion in detecting AD. While, the proposed method utilizes simple conversion of the 1-D signal into 2-D binary images. Hence, this has helped in improving the performance of the proposed method.

5 Conclusion

Many studies are being conducted currently to suggest novel approaches and DL models for the EEG-based AD diagnosis. The main problem occurs with the feature extraction process from larger time-series data, such as EEG signal data and using them for prediction. The problem emerges in the assessment of the stage of AD if the feature data is not properly chosen. Based on the survey of the existing works, we understand that for the multi-stage classification of Alzheimer's, the highest accuracy achieved is 98.9%, but their methodology involved complex signal preprocessing for image generation. Since pre-trained CNN models do not perform that well on signal data, this study focused on the simple conversion of the 1-D signal into 2-D images (matrix). Due to the non-stationary behavior of EEG signals, the key concern is in selecting an appropriate process for normalizing the signal data into binary images without losing substantial information. Therefore, the main contribution of this study is to overcome these difficulties by converting EEG signals to binary images by adopting a novel approach and predicting the stage of Alzheimer's using DL algorithms. Other DL architectures such as VGG-16, DenseNet-201 and NasNetMobile also performed well, but ResNet-101v2 gave the best accuracy on the test data. The deep learning classifier developed using a pre-trained ResNet-101v2 model produced the best accuracy of 98.98% which is a benchmark performance when compared to all other existing studies related to the EEG based diagnosis of AD. The major limitation in this work is that we could not obtain any other public data for testing as the EEG recording system, the number of electrodes and the system of placing electrodes varies from system to system. The proposed image transformation and classification method are not bound only to predicting the AD stages but also can be used to examine the EEG signal data of any other neurological diseases.

References

1. Nour, M., Senturk, U., Polat, K.: A novel hybrid model in the diagnosis and classification of Alzheimer's disease using EEG signals: deep ensemble learning (DEL) approach. Biomed. Signal Process. Control **89**, 105751 (2024)
2. Rasmussen, J., Langerman, H.: Alzheimer's disease—why we need early diagnosis. Degener. Neurol. Neuromuscul. Dis. 123–130 (2019)
3. Rodriguez, S., Hug, C., Todorov, P., Moret, N., Boswell, S.A., Evans, K., Zhou, G., Johnson, N.T., Hyman, B.T., Sorger, P.K., et al.: Machine learning identifies candidates for drug repurposing in Alzheimer's disease. Nat. Commun. **12**(1), 1–13 (2021)
4. Bazarbekov, I., Razaque, A., Ipalakova, M., Yoo, J., Assipova, Z., Almisreb, A.: A review of artificial intelligence methods for Alzheimer's disease diagnosis: insights from neuroimaging to sensor data analysis. Biomed. Signal Process. Control **92**, 106023 (2024)
5. Mattson, M.P.: Pathways towards and away from Alzheimer's disease. Nature **430**(7000), 631–639 (2004)
6. Physics World: EEG test could enable early diagnosis of Alzheimer's disease. https://physicsworld.com/a/eeg-test-could-enable-early-diagnosis-of-alzheimers-disease/ (2021). Accessed 18 May 2022
7. Ravi, V., EA, G., KP, S., et al.: Deep learning-based approach for multi-stage diagnosis of Alzheimer's disease. Multimed. Tools Appl. **83**(6), 16799–16822 (2024)
8. Radhamani, R., Nizar, N., Kumar, D., Pillai, G.S., Prasad, L.S., Jitha, S.S., Kuniyil, M.K.V., Sekhar, A.A., Kumar, V.S., Pillai, S., et al.: Computational analysis of cortical EEG biosignals and neural dynamics underlying an integrated mind-body relaxation technique. Procedia Comput. Sci. **171**, 341–349 (2020)
9. Cedazo-Minguez, A., Winblad, B.: Biomarkers for Alzheimer's disease and other forms of dementia: clinical needs, limitations and future aspects. Exp. Gerontol. **45**(1), 5–14 (2010)
10. Hampel, H., Frank, R., Broich, K., Teipel, S.J., Katz, R.G., Hardy, J., Herholz, K., Bokde, A.L., Jessen, F., Hoessler, Y.C., et al.: Biomarkers for Alzheimer's disease: academic, industry and regulatory perspectives. Nat. Rev. Drug Discov. **9**(7), 560–574 (2010)
11. DeKosky, S.T., Marek, K.: Looking backward to move forward: early detection of neurodegenerative disorders. Science **302**(5646), 830–834 (2003)
12. Al-Qazzaz, N.K., Ali, S.H.B., Ahmad, S.A., Chellappan, K., Islam, M., Escudero, J., et al.: Role of EEG as biomarker in the early detection and classification of dementia. Sci. World J. **2014**, (2014)
13. Pineda, A.M., Ramos, F.M., Betting, L.E., Campanharo, A.S.: Quantile graphs for EEG-based diagnosis of Alzheimer's disease. PLoS ONE **15**(6), 0231169 (2020)
14. Abhishek, S., Kumar, S., Mohan, N., Soman, K.: EEG based automated detection of seizure using machine learning approach and traditional features. Expert Syst. Appl. **251**, 123991 (2024)
15. Henderson, G., Ifeachor, E., Hudson, N., Goh, C., Outram, N., Wimalaratna, S., Del Percio, C., Vecchio, F.: Development and assessment of methods for detecting dementia using the human electroencephalogram. IEEE Trans. Biomed. Eng. **53**(8), 1557–1568 (2006)

16. Henderson, G., Ifeachor, E., Wimalaratna, H., Allen, T., Hudson, R.: Prospects for routine detection of dementia using the fractal dimension of the human electroencephalogram. IEE Proc. Sci. Meas. Technol. **147**(6), 321–326 (2000)
17. Zhao, P., Ifeachor, E.: EEG assessment of Alzheimers diseases using universal compression algorithm. In: Proceedings of the 3rd international conference on computational intelligence in medicine and healthcare (CIMED2007), Plymouth, UK, July 25, vol. 27 (2007)
18. Yang, S., Bornot, J.M.S., Wong-Lin, K., Prasad, G.: M/EEG-based bio-markers to predict the mci and Alzheimer's disease: a review from the ML perspective. IEEE Trans. Biomed. Eng. **66**(10), 2924–2935 (2019)
19. Smits, F.M., Porcaro, C., Cottone, C., Cancelli, A., Rossini, P.M., Tecchio, F.: Electroencephalographic fractal dimension in healthy ageing and Alzheimer's disease. PLoS ONE **11**(2), 0149587 (2016)
20. Fiscon, G., Weitschek, E., Cialini, A., Felici, G., Bertolazzi, P., De Salvo, S., Bramanti, A., Bramanti, P., De Cola, M.C.: Combining EEG signal processing with supervised methods for Alzheimer's patients classification. BMC Med. Inform. Decis. Mak. **18**(1), 1–10 (2018)
21. Kumar, S., Kasthuri, N.: EEG seizure classification based on exploiting phase space reconstruction and extreme learning. Clust. Comput. **22**(5), 11477–11487 (2019)
22. Übeyli, E.D.: Analysis of EEG signals by combining eigenvector methods and multiclass support vector machines. Comput. Biol. Med. **38**(1), 14–22 (2008)
23. Ridouh, A., Boutana, D., Bourennane, S.: EEG signals classification based on time frequency analysis. J. Circuits Syst. Comput. **26**(12), 1750198 (2017)
24. Zhang, Y., Liu, B., Ji, X., Huang, D.: Classification of EEG signals based on autoregressive model and wavelet packet decomposition. Neural Process. Lett. **45**(2), 365–378 (2017)
25. Ruiz, A.P., Flynn, M., Large, J., Middlehurst, M., Bagnall, A.: The great multivariate time series classification bake off: a review and experimental evaluation of recent algorithmic advances. Data Min. Knowl. Disc. **35**(2), 401–449 (2021)
26. Faouzi, J.: Time series classification: a review of algorithms and implementations. Machine Learning (Emerging Trends and Applications) (2022)
27. Wang, Z., Oates, T.: Encoding time series as images for visual inspection and classification using tiled convolutional neural networks. In: Workshops at the Twenty-Ninth AAAI Conference on Artificial Intelligence (2015)
28. Wang, J., Liu, P., She, M.F., Nahavandi, S., Kouzani, A.: Bag-of-words representation for biomedical time series classification. Biomed. Signal Process. Control **8**(6), 634–644 (2013)
29. Naz, M., Shah, J.H., Khan, M.A., Sharif, M., Raza, M., Damaševičius, R.: From ECG signals to images: a transformation based approach for deep learning. PeerJ Comput. Sci. **7**, 386 (2021)
30. Qin, Y., Li, B., Wang, W., Shi, X., Wang, H., Wang, X.: ETCNet: an EEG-based motor imagery classification model combining efficient channel attention and temporal convolutional network. Brain Res. **1823**, 148673 (2024)
31. Şeker, M., Özerdem, M.S.: Investigating convolutional and transformer-based models for classifying mild cognitive impairment using 2D spectral images of resting-state EEG. Biomed. Signal Process. Control **105**, 107667 (2025)
32. Bravo-Ortiz, M.A., Guevara-Navarro, E., Holguín-García, S.A., Rivera-Garcia, M., Cardona-Morales, O., Ruz, G.A., Tabares-Soto, R.: SpectroCVT-Net: a convolutional vision transformer architecture and channel attention for classifying Alzheimer's disease using spectrograms. Comput. Biol. Med. **181**, 109022 (2024)
33. Lehmann, C., Koenig, T., Jelic, V., Prichep, L., John, R.E., Wahlund, L.-O., Dodge, Y., Dierks, T.: Application and comparison of classification algorithms for recognition of Alzheimer's disease in electrical brain activity (EEG). J. Neurosci. Methods **161**(2), 342–350 (2007)
34. Keerthi Krishnan, K., Soman, K.: CNN based classification of motor imaginary using variational mode decomposed EEG-spectrum image. Biomed. Eng. Lett. **11**(3), 235–247 (2021)
35. Wu, Y., Yang, F., Liu, Y., Zha, X., Yuan, S.: A comparison of 1-D and 2-D deep convolutional neural networks in ECG classification (2018). arXiv:1810.07088
36. Kim, D., Kim, K.: Detection of early stage Alzheimer's disease using EEG relative power with deep neural network. In: 2018 40th Annual International Conference of the IEEE Engineering in Medicine and Biology Society (EMBC), pp. 352–355. IEEE (2018)

37. Bi, X., Wang, H.: Early Alzheimer's disease diagnosis based on EEG spectral images using deep learning. Neural Netw. **114**, 119–135 (2019)
38. Ieracitano, C., Mammone, N., Bramanti, A., Hussain, A., Morabito, F.C.: A convolutional neural network approach for classification of dementia stages based on 2d-spectral representation of EEG recordings. Neurocomputing **323**, 96–107 (2019)
39. Ismail, M., Hofmann, K., Abd El Ghany, M.A.: Early diagnoses of Alzheimer using EEG data and deep neural networks classification. In: 2019 IEEE Global Conference on Internet of Things (GCIoT), pp. 1–5. IEEE (2019)
40. You, Z., Zeng, R., Lan, X., Ren, H., You, Z., Shi, X., Zhao, S., Guo, Y., Jiang, X., Hu, X.: Alzheimer's disease classification with a cascade neural network. Front. Public Health 665 (2020)
41. Huggins, C.J., Escudero, J., Parra, M.A., Scally, B., Anghinah, R., De Araújo, A.V.L., Basile, L.F., Abasolo, D.: Deep learning of resting-state electroencephalogram signals for three-class classification of Alzheimer's disease, mild cognitive impairment and healthy ageing. J. Neural Eng. **18**(4), 046087 (2021)
42. Ho, T.K.K., Jeon, Y., Na, E., Ullah, Z., Kim, B.C., Lee, K.H., Song, J.-I., Gwak, J.: DeepADNet: a CNN-LSTM model for the multi-class classification of Alzheimer's disease using multichannel EEG. Alzheimer's & Dement. **17**, 057573 (2021)
43. Amini, M., Pedram, M., Moradi, A., Ouchani, M.: Diagnosis of Alzheimer's disease by time-dependent power spectrum descriptors and convolutional neural network using EEG signal. Comput. Math. Methods Med. **2021**, (2021)
44. Alves, C.L., Pineda, A.M., Roster, K., Thielemann, C., Rodrigues, F.A.: EEG functional connectivity and deep learning for automatic diagnosis of brain disorders: Alzheimer's disease and schizophrenia. J. Phys. Complex. **3**(2), 025001 (2022)
45. Fouad, I.A., Labib, F.E.-Z.M.: Identification of Alzheimer's disease from central lobe EEG signals utilizing machine learning and residual neural network. Biomed. Signal Process. Control **86**, 105266 (2023)
46. Shankar, A., Khaing, H.K., Dandapat, S., Barma, S.: Epileptic seizure classification based on Gramian angular field transformation and deep learning. In: 2020 IEEE Applied Signal Processing Conference (ASPCON), pp. 147–151 (2020). https://doi.org/10.1109/ASPCON49795.2020.9276717
47. Thanaraj, K.P., Parvathavarthini, B., Tanik, U.J., Rajinikanth, V., Kadry, S., Kamalanand, K.: Implementation of deep neural networks to classify EEG signals using Gramian angular summation field for epilepsy diagnosis (2020). arXiv:2003.04534
48. Ko, D.-W., Yang, J.-J.: EEG-based schizophrenia diagnosis through time series image conversion and deep learning. Electronics **11**(14), 2265 (2022)
49. Mai, N.-D., Nguyen, H.-T., Chung, W.-Y.: Deep learning-based wearable ear-EEG emotion recognition system with superlets-based signal-to-image conversion framework. IEEE Sens. J. (2024)
50. Lazarou, I., Georgiadis, K., Nikolopoulos, S., Oikonomou, V., Kompatsiaris, I.: Resting-state high-density EEG Using EGI GES 300 with 256 channels of healthy elders, people with subjective and mild cognitive impairment and Alzheimer's disease. https://doi.org/10.5281/zenodo.4316608
51. Yildirim, O., Talo, M., Ay, B., Baloglu, U.B., Aydin, G., Acharya, U.R.: Automated detection of diabetic subject using pre-trained 2D-CNN models with frequency spectrum images extracted from heart rate signals. Comput. Biol. Med. **113**, 103387 (2019)
52. He, K., Zhang, X., Ren, S., Sun, J.: Deep residual learning for image recognition. In: Proceedings of the IEEE Conference on Computer Vision and Pattern Recognition, pp. 770–778 (2016)
53. Shafiq, M., Gu, Z.: Deep residual learning for image recognition: s survey. Appl. Sci. **12**(18), 8972 (2022)
54. Kumar, L., Sai, Y.P., et al.: A new transfer learning approach to detect cardiac arrhythmia from ECG signals. Signal Image Video Process. 1–9 (2022)

55. Maaten, L., Hinton, G.: Visualizing data using t-SNE. J. Mach. Learn. Res. **9**(11), (2008)
56. Morabito, F.C., Campolo, M., Ieracitano, C., Ebadi, J.M., Bonanno, L., Bramanti, A., Desalvo, S., Mammone, N., Bramanti, P.: Deep convolutional neural networks for classification of mild cognitive impaired and Alzheimer's disease patients from scalp EEG recordings. In: 2016 IEEE 2nd International Forum on Research and Technologies for Society and Industry Leveraging a Better Tomorrow (RTSI), pp. 1–6. IEEE (2016)

A Robust Deep Learning Framework for Auricular Deformities Detection and Diagnosis Using Region Proposal Based Cropping and Explainable AI

Ampolu Venkata Anil Kumar, Divya Sasidharan, V. Sowmya, and Vinayakumar Ravi

Abstract Auricular deformities are one of the most common concerns in neonates and, if left untreated, can result in both psychological distress and functional complications. Timely diagnosis is essential for appropriate interventions which is proven to effective but must be done within the first few weeks after birth. However, limited clinical expertise and the intricate structure of the auricle pose challenges to consistent and early identification. This study presents a robust deep learning-based framework for the accurate detection and classification of newborn auricular deformities using high-resolution images from the BabyEar4k dataset, comprising 3,852 annotated baby ear images. The proposed pipeline follows a two-stage architecture: auricle localization using a Faster R-CNN model with ResNet-50 backbone, followed by cropping of the proposed regions to isolate auricular structures. These cropped regions undergo targeted preprocessing—such as contrast enhancement, sharpening, and Gaussian filtering to enhance auricular cartilage structure and mitigate the variations in image quality factors. The pre-processed regions are then fed into a classification module based on a Vision Transformer (ViT) with a custom head. For model interpretability, Randomized input sampling for explanation (RISE) is employed to generate saliency maps, highlighting the critical regions the model concentrated on while classifying the auricle. The proposed framework attained a mean average precision (mAP50) of 0.84 for auricle detection and achieved a classification accuracy of 84% using ViT classification module. The results reported are solely using the not-so-good quality images having illumination variations, inconsistent focus and occlusion. Saliency maps generated through RISE confirmed that the model consistently focused on relevant auricular substructures.

Keywords Auricular deformities · Deep learning · Object detection · Explainable-AI · RISE

A. V. A. Kumar · D. Sasidharan · V. Sowmya (✉)
Amrita School of Artificial Intelligence, Amrita Vishwa Vidyapeetham, Coimbatore, India
e-mail: v_sowmya@cb.amrita.edu

V. Ravi
Center for Artificial Intelligence, Prince Mohammad Bin Fahd University, Khobar, Saudi Arabia

P. Singh et al. (eds.), *Deep Learning Applications in Healthcare and Medical Imaging Practice*, Studies in Big Data 193, https://doi.org/10.1007/978-3-032-21009-8_4

1 Introduction

Congenital auricular deformities are among the most prevalent craniofacial anomalies in newborns, affecting up to 30% of infants in certain populations [1]. These deformities span a wide clinical spectrum—from mild conditions such as lop ear and Stahl's ear to severe anomalies like microtia [2]. While often regarded as merely aesthetic concerns, these abnormalities can lead to psychological distress, social stigma, and, in some cases, functional impairments such as hearing loss if left untreated [3, 4]. Early identification and intervention, especially during the neonatal period when maternal estrogen levels enhance cartilage pliability, enable non-surgical correction through ear molding techniques [5, 6]. However, the narrow therapeutic window, limited to the first few weeks of birth—necessitates rapid and accurate diagnosis.

Despite the availability of corrective options, many cases go undiagnosed or are detected too late due to the reliance on subjective visual assessment by physicians. This is particularly concerning in resource-limited settings where pediatric otolaryngological expertise may be lacking [7]. The anatomical complexity of the auricle—comprising structures such as the helix, concha, tragus, and lobule—further complicates diagnosis, as deformities may present subtle morphological variations [8, 9]. Even among trained professionals, especially in case of neonates, distinguishing between normal anatomical variants and true auricular deformities can be challenging [10].

Historically, clinical assessment has relied on observation and manual inspection. However, such evaluations are often inconsistent and prone to inter-observer variability, particularly when no standardized classification or measurement criteria are used [11]. With the recent advancements in machine learning and medical image analysis, deep learning-based solutions have emerged as powerful tools to improve diagnostic precision. Convolutional Neural Networks (CNNs) in particular, have achieved state-of-the-art performance in domains like dermatology, ophthalmology, and oncology for tasks such as lesion detection, tumor classification, and disease staging [12, 13].

Nonetheless, in the context of auricular deformities, objective assessment remains relatively underexplored, and even the limited existing approaches often fall short in terms of robustness and interpretability—both of which are crucial for clinical adoption [14, 15]. Moreover, such models are seldom evaluated under real-world conditions, including poor lighting or low-resolution images which are common in images taken through smartphone setup.

A review of existing literature and datasets reveals that most publicly available ear datasets were created for biometric identification rather than for clinical assessment. Only a limited number of studies have explored the use of deep learning to detect auricular deformities, and these often do not address challenges such as varying image quality factors such as occlusions, inconsistent lighting etc. Moreover, interpretability—an essential component for clinical adoption—is often absent in most of the studies, limiting the practical integration of such models in real-world healthcare environments.

To address these challenges, this study proposes a robust and interpretable deep learning framework for the detection and classification of auricular deformities in neonates. The system emphasizes practical applicability by ensuring that evaluation is conducted on lower-quality images—mimicking real-world imaging conditions—while training is performed exclusively on high-quality, pre-processed data. For interpretability, D-RISE and RISE methods are employed in end-to-end detector-based and decoupled detector–classifier pipelines, respectively, enabling clinicians to visualize the model's decision logic and verify the key regions influencing its predictions [16].

By addressing both robustness and explainability, the proposed framework offers a step forward in making early deformity detection accessible, particularly in under-resourced healthcare environments. It can serve as both a diagnostic aid and an educational tool, reducing the burden on specialists and enabling timely intervention that can minimize the need for future surgical correction.

The main contributions of the proposed framework are as follows:

- The impact of carefully selected preprocessing techniques in improving the robustness of auricular deformity detection and classification, even under poor imaging conditions.
- Addresses the challenges like noise, lighting inconsistencies, contrast and resolution loss, the model achieved strong performance on previously unseen, not-so-good quality images.
- Enhancing model interpretability using saliency-based visual explanations by highlighting appropriate auricular regions, and making it suitable for use in real-world, resource-limited setting.

The following chapter is organized as follows: Sect. 2 describes the methods and techniques applied in the proposed study. The results obtained for the applied methodology is discussed in Sect. 3. The chapter concludes in Sect. 4 detailing the proposed work and future enhancements.

2 Methods

The primary objective of this study is to develop a robust, explainable deep learning framework for the accurate identification and diagnosis of auricular deformities in newborns. The methodology evolved through several experimental iterations, addressing challenges related to image quality, such as cover-up of the auricular regions, illumination, and background conditions. Initial attempts to incorporate pre-processing techniques directly into the detection pipeline showed limited effectiveness in improving model performance.

Building on these insights, a final refined methodology is proposed as seen in Fig. 1. In this approach, the tasks of auricular identification and classification are decoupled, allowing focused processing. The best performing detection model from the previous experiments [17] is employed solely for auricular localization. The localized regions of interest (ROIs) are then cropped and processed using a series of pre-processing techniques to improve image quality. These refined ROIs are input into a deep feature extraction and classification model. Finally, RISE technique is integrated to explain the model's predictions, ensuring transparency and a better understanding of the model's decision-making process.

2.1 Dataset Description

The 'BabyEar4k' dataset (Ren et al. [3]) contains 3,852 images from 1,926 newborns, captured within 48 h of birth in a controlled clinical environment. All images are in.jpg format and are ensured that the auricular region and its substructures are clearly visible.

The dataset includes the following files:

- **Images**: directory that consists of 3,852 ear images, in.jpg format, each labelled with a unique newborn ID and the side of ear (left or right).
- **Bounding**: A CSV file containing bounding box coordinates for each image, accurately marking ear boundaries.
- **Diagnosis Results**: A CSV file with diagnostic classifications from two expert physicians (ENT specialist and paediatrician), along with their consensus diagnosis.
- **Image Quality Assessment**: A CSV file with subjective quality scores of each image, based on factors like blur, noise, cover-up, brightness, and angle.

2.2 Splitting of Data

The dataset was partitioned into training, validation, and test sets based on image quality scores from the image_quality_assessment.csv file. In this file, each image was subjectively evaluated across four factors: blur/noise, cover-up, brightness, and shooting angle—scored from 1 (best) to 3 (worst).

Images with a perfect cumulative score of 4 (i.e., rated 1 on all criteria) were labelled 'Good Quality' and assigned to the training set ($n = 2{,}081$). The remaining Lower Quality images (score > 4, $n = 1{,}771$) were divided into validation and test sets using a stratified split to maintain class balance. This quality-based split was designed to ensure that the model learns from high-quality, well-pre-processed data during training, while its performance is evaluated on more challenging, lower-quality images—closely reflecting real-world clinical variability. The distribution of 'Normal' and 'Abnormal' cases across subsets, occurs with slight class imbalance in training and balanced classes in validation and test sets. The training percentage for normal and abnormal are 58.4% and 41.6% respectively. The validation percentage for normal and abnormal are 52% and 48% respectively. Similarly, the test percentage for normal and abnormal are 51.8% and 48.1% respectively.

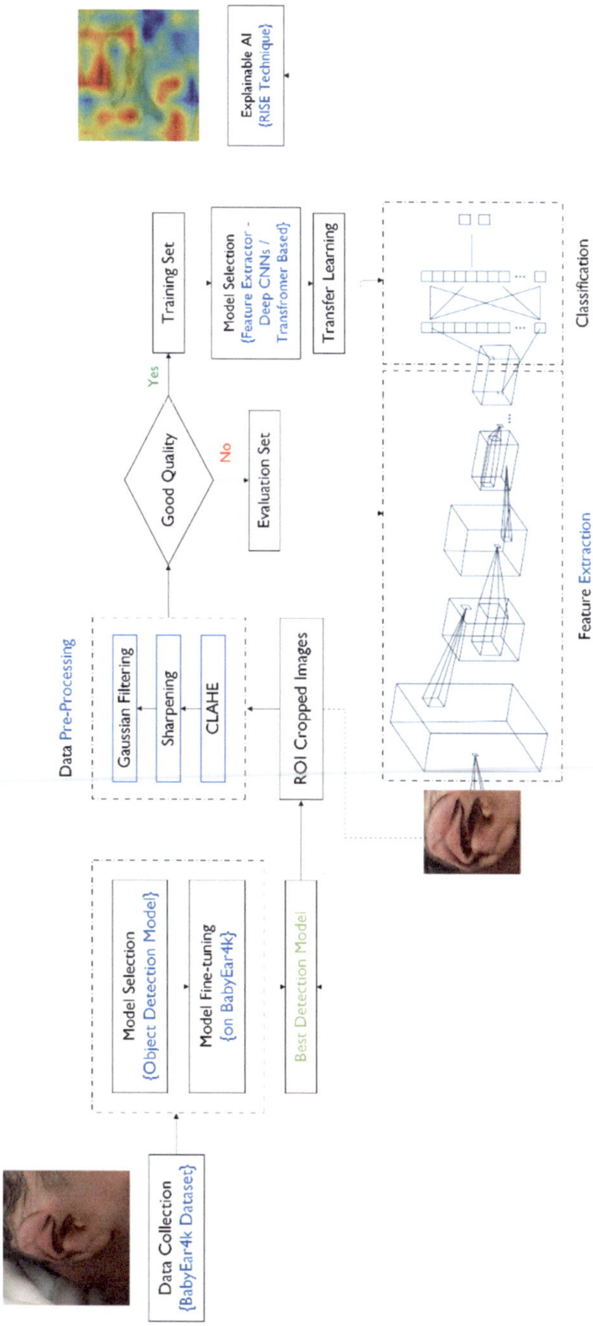

Fig. 1 Final proposed methodology pipeline with decoupled detection and classification

2.3 Pre-processing

Given the clinical sensitivity of auricular structures, pre-processing plays a pivotal role in enhancing image quality for reliable feature extraction. The BabyEar4k dataset presented challenges typical of real-world medical imaging, including noise, illumination inconsistencies, blur, and contrast degradation. These quality limitations significantly impact the performance of deep learning models, particularly in tasks requiring precise localization and identification of fine anatomical features.

To address these, a series of pre-processing techniques were evaluated for their ability to refine the visual content while preserving clinically relevant details. After comparative experimentation, the final methodology retained the following techniques:

- **Contrast Limited Adaptive Histogram Equalization (CLAHE)**: Improves local contrast in underexposed or unevenly lit regions by redistributing intensity values across small contextual regions. This adjustment enhances visibility of subtle structural variations without amplifying noise [18].
- **Sharpening**: Accentuates edge details by emphasizing intensity gradients between adjacent pixels. It improved the clarity of auricular substructures, aiding the model in capturing key morphological cues [19].
- **Gaussian Filtering**: A low-pass filter was used to suppress high-frequency noise while preserving edge information. This smoothing step was particularly effective in reducing visual artifacts without blurring important anatomical boundaries [20].

While other methods such as the Prewitt operator and morphological erosion were initially considered, they were ultimately excluded due to their tendency to introduce unwanted noise or degrade structural integrity. Prewitt, in particular, led to over-enhancement of edges, while erosion occasionally resulted in loss of fine details, which are undesirable in a clinical imaging context. So, the final methodology pipeline, includes CLAHE, Sharpening, and Gaussian Filtering as part of pre-processing steps.

2.4 Model Selection

In this study, the model selection strategy evolved from the previous study, which employed an end-to-end object detection-based pipeline for both localizing and classifying the auricular deformities [17]. In this method, object detection models such as YOLO and Faster R-CNN were used to both localize and categorize auricles within the same network.

However, in the present work, we adopt a decoupled pipeline, treating auricle localization and classification as distinct stages. This strategic shift was guided by insights gained through experimental evaluations, which indicated that separating the tasks allowed for better representation of inputs and enabled the use of deeper, more expressive models for classification. By isolating the classification stage, the network could operate directly on cropped auricular regions, thus focusing more effectively on relevant substructures. The best-performing detection model from the previous study is retained solely for auricle localization, while the classification is now carried out using dedicated deep learning architectures fine-tuned and tailored for this diagnostic task.

2.4.1 Auricular Localization

The object detection pipeline, as detailed in the study [17], was evaluated across multiple models including YOLOv8, YOLOv9, and Faster R-CNN. Based on performance metrics such as mAP and inference speed, YOLOv8 emerged as the optimal model for auricular localization. For the current study, this pre-validated model is employed solely for region-of-interest extraction.

2.4.2 Auricular Classification

Once the auricular region is localized, the cropped images are pre-processed and fed to classification models specifically fine-tuned for this task. This stage represents the key methodological shift from our earlier approach. The classification pipeline was developed to deeply analyse auricular substructures and detect subtle deformities using deep and context-aware feature extraction methods.

ResNet-50

ResNet-50 [21] was selected for its proven performance in image classification, particularly in medical imaging. Its residual learning mechanism enables effective training of deep networks without degradation, which is critical for extracting complex shape features from auricular images.

EfficientNet-B0

EfficientNet-B0 [22] uses a compound scaling approach to balance depth, width, and resolution, making it well-suited for tasks that require efficiency without compromising accuracy. Its lightweight architecture allows for practical deployment even in resource-constrained clinical settings.

Vision Transformer (ViT)

Unlike conventional CNN-based architectures, the Vision Transformer (ViT) [23] utilizes self-attention mechanisms to capture both local and global dependencies within an image. In this study, ViT was adopted for its ability to effectively model the complex spatial relationships across auricular structures. The input image is first partitioned into fixed-size patches, which are then linearly projected and combined with positional embeddings. This structure enables the model to retain spatial context and analyse anatomical features holistically. The positional embedding plays a pivotal

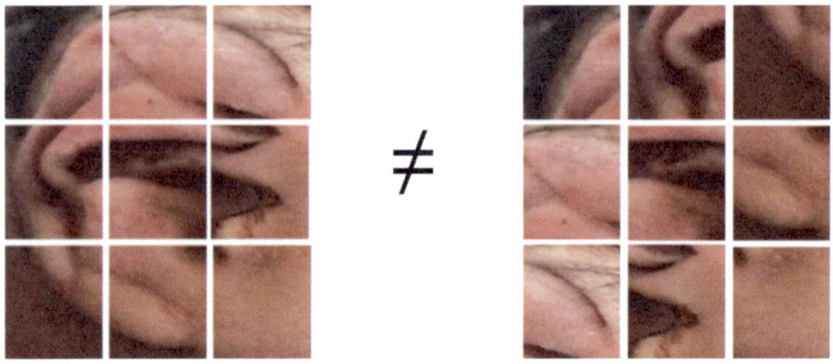

Fig. 2 Importance of positional embedding in vision transformer

role in ViT architecture, as it allows the model to retain the spatial information which would otherwise be lost because of patch-based processing. The importance of positional information is clearly illustrated in Fig. 2.

2.4.3 Classification Head Configuration

All classification models were evaluated using two different head configurations:

- **Default Head**:

  The standard pre-trained heads, modified with a binary output layer suited for 'Normal' and 'Abnormal' classification.
- **Custom Head**:

  The A tailored structure comprising three fully connected layers (1024 → 512 → 256), followed by a final binary output. A dropout regularization of 30% is applied across the layers to prevent overfitting and to improve the generalization. The motivation behind the custom classifier is to preserve the essential feature information while preventing sudden dimensionality reduction.

The architecture of the custom classifier head used across all classification models is depicted in Fig. 3.

2.5 Training Pipeline

In this study, rather than training models from the ground up, a transfer learning approach was employed for both stages. Pre-trained weights from established benchmarks such as COCO (for detection) and ImageNet (for classification) were leveraged to initialize the models, with selective fine-tuning applied to adapt them to the task-specific domain of auricular deformity detection.

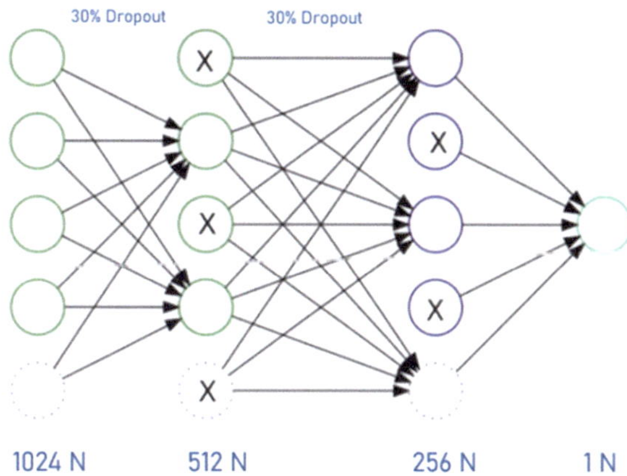

Fig. 3 Architecture of the custom classifier head used in classification models

For the localization task, only the final layers of the detection models were unfrozen and fine-tuned to focus on the domain-specific appearance of newborn auricles, while preserving the general spatial and structural priors learned in early layers. Once the auricular bounding boxes were obtained, these cropped regions were further processed through the classification pipeline.

In the classification stage, models such as ResNet-50, EfficientNet-B0, and Vision Transformer were fine-tuned with a similar strategy. Lower convolutional or attention layers were frozen to retain foundational representations, while deeper layers and classification heads were adapted to capture pathological variations in auricular structure. Two classifier configurations—default and custom were tested, with the latter incorporating progressively reduced dense layers and dropout for improved generalization and regularization.

This fine-tuning strategy not only ensured efficient learning but also allowed for scalable deployment across different computational setups. Additionally, to enhance clinical interpretability, gradient-free visual explanation techniques such as RISE were applied to the fine-tuned classification models, generating saliency maps that highlighted the key substructures influencing the diagnostic predictions.

2.6 *Model Evaluation*

The assessment of model performance in this study is carried out using a set of evaluation metrics tailored to the nature of each task-object detection and classification. For evaluating object detection models, metrics such as mean Average Precision at IoU threshold 0.5 (mAP50) and the more comprehensive mAP across IoU thresholds from 0.5 to 0.95 (mAP50–95) are employed. These metrics quantify both the localization accuracy and the consistency of detections across varying degrees of overlap between predicted and ground-truth bounding boxes.

In the classification context, model evaluation is based on standard performance indicators including accuracy, precision, recall, and F1-score. These metrics collectively provide a balanced view of the classifier's correctness, sensitivity to positive cases, and overall reliability in distinguishing between normal and deformed auricular instances.

By using established metrics specific to each task, this evaluation framework ensures a rigorous and meaningful comparison of models, addressing both detection precision and classification efficacy.

2.7 Explainability

To promote transparency and foster clinical trust, this study incorporates explainability methods that visualize model decision regions, thereby aiding interpretation of both detection and classification outcomes. Given the sensitive nature of medical imaging tasks, such visualization is especially important for validating that models focus on clinically relevant anatomical structures rather than peripheral or spurious features.

In the preliminary exploration using an end-to-end detection-based pipeline, detector-specific visual explanations were generated using D-RISE [24], a technique that provides black-box saliency maps for object detectors without relying on internal gradients. While these results supported the initial evaluation, they were not pursued further in the final classification-driven framework and are excluded from detailed discussion here to maintain focus on the proposed approach.

In the final pipeline, model explainability was addressed using the RISE method, tailored for classification networks. As a black-box technique, RISE evaluates model responses to multiple randomly masked inputs, generating saliency maps that highlight the image regions most influential to the model's predictions. This approach was applied to the best-performing classification model, with parameters carefully chosen to balance computational overhead and the interpretive clarity of the generated visualizations. The resulting saliency maps serve to verify that the classification network attends to the auricular region meaningfully, strengthening the clinical reliability of the predictions. Through the integration of RISE into the classification workflow, the proposed system ensures that its outputs remain interpretable and trustworthy, making it better suited for real-world clinical assessment of auricular deformities.

3 Results

This section presents the details and results of all the experiments conducted with the objective of developing a robust and explainable framework for accurate identification and diagnosis of auricular deformities in newborns. All experiments were conducted on the BabyEar4k dataset using a Paper space Gradient P5000 instance

(30 GB RAM, 8 CPU cores, and a 16 GB NVIDIA P5000 GPU). The study progressed through three experimental stages: (i) An end-to-end detector-based pipeline [17]. (ii) Integration of pre-processing techniques within the detector pipeline. (iii) A refined decoupled architecture where detection and classification were treated as independent stages.

3.1 Pre-processing

As shown in Fig. 4a, CLAHE preserves significant intensity peaks while redistributing values more evenly across regions, allowing for enhanced contrast without flattening critical structures. Figure 4b demonstrates how sharpening increases local contrast by widening intensity differences, making structural edges more prominent. Figure 4c depicts the Gaussian kernel's bell-shaped distribution, which smoothens high-frequency noise while maintaining anatomical edge clarity.

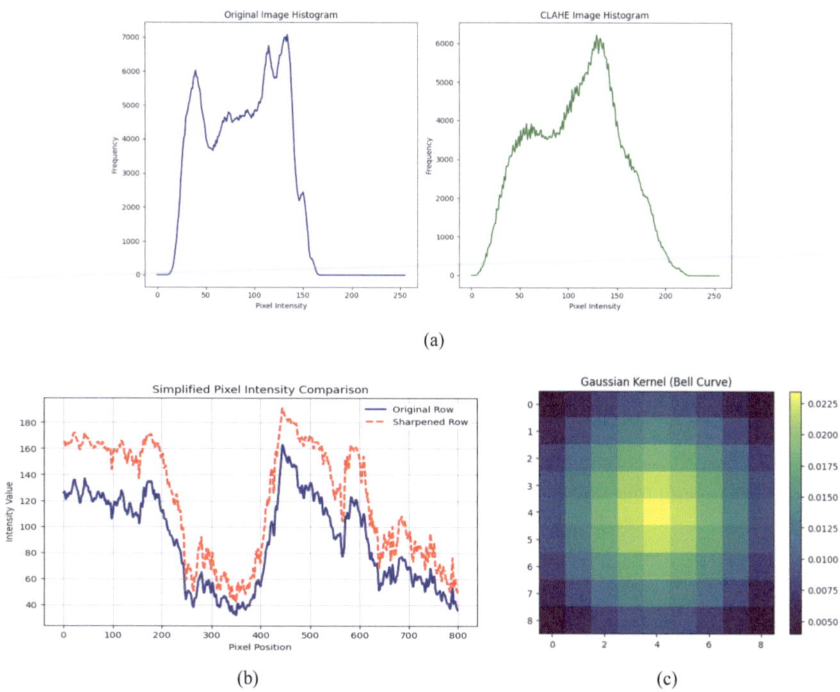

Fig. 4 **a** Intensity distribution plot of a sample image before and after applying CLAHE. **b** Comparison of pixel intensities of a sample image before and after sharpening. **c** Visualization of gaussian kernel (bell curve) used for filtering technique

3.2 Summary of Detector Based Pipeline

In our earlier work [17], various object detection models were evaluated for their effectiveness in localizing auricular regions in neonatal images. Among these, Faster R-CNN with the ResNet50 backbone demonstrated the best detection performance, achieving a mAP50 of 0.84 and a recall of 0.91. These results indicated its reliability in detecting auricular structures with high sensitivity.

Additionally, the YOLOv8-L model showed the best classification performance, attaining a classification accuracy of 89%, along with precision scores of 0.79 for the 'Normal' class and 0.80 for the 'Abnormal' class.

These models were subsequently utilized in further experimental settings as baselines for improvement and refinement.

3.3 Detector Pipeline—with Pre-processing

Building upon the earlier detection-based classification pipeline, this experiment evaluates the impact of incorporating image enhancement techniques directly into the input pipeline of the YOLOv8-L model, which had previously shown the best classification performance. The objective was to assess whether image-level refinements without modifying the underlying model architecture could improve classification performance.

A series of image pre-processing techniques namely Gradient Operators, CLAHE, Erosion, Sharpening, Gaussian Filtering are explored and incorporated basing on their proven ability to enhance the image, thereby refining the input for better feature extraction. These steps were applied to the input images prior to training and evaluation.

The classification performance of YOLOv8-L after integrating the pre-processing steps is summarized in Table 1. As observed, the model achieved an improved classification accuracy of 0.81, with precision values of 0.82 and 0.84 for the Normal and Abnormal categories, respectively. The corresponding F1-scores remained balanced at 0.81 across both classes.

Table 1 Classification performance of YOLOv8-L after incorporating pre-processing techniques

Model		YOLOv8-L
Accuracy		0.81
Precision	Normal	0.82
	Abnormal	0.84
Recall	Normal	0.8
	Abnormal	0.78
F1-Score	Normal	0.81
	Abnormal	0.81

When compared to the classification results reported through our earlier work. it is evident that the inclusion of pre-processing techniques led to a marginal improvement in the model's performance. The classification accuracy improved from 0.79 to 0.81, with notable enhancements in precision for both Normal and Abnormal categories. This improvement can be attributed to the effectiveness of pre-processing techniques in refining the input data and minimizing quality-induced artefacts. However, this improvement still remained moderate, leaving us with the motivation of experimenting further.

3.4 Decoupled Detector-Classifier Pipeline

From the earlier experiment, it is evident that incorporating pre-processing directly within the detection pipeline has a limited impact on overall classification performance. Therefore, in the final version of the pipeline, the approach was refined by decoupling detection and classification into independent stages.

In this refined pipeline, the best overall detection performance model—Faster RCNN with ResNet-50 backbone (as detailed in detector-based pipeline section) is employed solely to localize the auricular regions in the input image. These localized auricular regions (which are regarded as our regions of interest) are cropped to eliminate any irrelevant background and exclusively focus on the target area. The Cropped ROIs are then fed to pre-processing stage, where specifically CLAHE, Sharpening, and Gaussian Filtering are applied. The choice was based on earlier observations that inclusion of Prewitt and Erosion, introduced unnecessary noise and distortion. Finally, these refined ROIs are used for deep feature extraction and classification, by making use of deep CNNs and Vision Transformer architectures. These cropped ROIs were then passed through a pre-processing stage, where CLAHE, sharpening, and Gaussian filtering were applied. This combination was selected based on earlier observations, where inclusion of Prewitt and erosion techniques led to over-enhancement and information loss. The refined inputs were subsequently used for classification using three different architectures: ResNet-50, EfficientNet-B0, and Vision Transformer (ViT).

The classification performance of the three models experimented within this decoupled framework is detailed below.

Table 2 summarizes the classification performance of ResNet-50, where only the convolutional blocks 3, 4, and 5 were unfrozen for fine-tuning without any image pre-processing applied. The default classification head was retained in this experiment.

The results in Table 2 reveal that the ResNet50-based classifier, when used without any pre-processing, achieved a classification accuracy of 0.76. The model demonstrated a slight imbalance in precision and recall between the Normal and Abnormal categories, indicating that raw cropped ROI images posed challenges in learning discriminative features.

Table 2 Classification performance of ResNet-50 without pre-processing

Model		ResNet-50
Accuracy		0.76
Precision	Normal	0.74
	Abnormal	0.79
Recall	Normal	0.79
	Abnormal	0.74
F1-Score	Normal	0.76
	Abnormal	0.76

Table 3 summarizes the classification performance of same ResNet-50 model (with Conv-3,4,5 blocks unfrozen) where it is evaluated after incorporating the pre-processing techniques discussed earlier. The default classification head is retained in this experiment as well.

Upon integrating pre-processing techniques, as shown in Table 3, the ResNet50 classifier exhibited an improved classification accuracy of 0.79. Precision and recall metrics also reflected marginal improvements, emphasizing the positive influence of enhanced image quality on the model's ability to capture relevant deformity patterns.

To further improve the classification performance, a custom classification head was incorporated into the ResNet-50 architecture (with same blocks unfrozen as before), along with the pre-processing techniques. This custom head involved progressively reducing the number of neurons to minimize information loss while improving classification accuracy as detailed in (Fig. 5).

As presented in Table 4, further improvement in performance was achieved by modifying the classification head of ResNet50 architecture. This modification, coupled with pre-processing, resulted in a classification accuracy of 0.82, with balanced precision and recall across both categories. To further explore the effectiveness of different classification architectures, the EfficientNet-B0 model was evaluated in this pipeline. Based on the insights gained from earlier ResNet-50 experiments, where pre-processing and architectural modifications were found to improve classification performance, the same strategy is adopted here.

Table 3 Classification performance of ResNet-50 with pre-processing

Model		ResNet-50
Accuracy		0.79
Precision	Normal	0.76
	Abnormal	0.81
Recall	Normal	0.81
	Abnormal	0.76
F1-Score	Normal	0.78
	Abnormal	0.78

Table 4 Classification performance of ResNet50 with pre-processing and custom head

Model		ResNet-50
Accuracy		0.82
Precision	Normal	0.78
	Abnormal	0.79
Recall	Normal	0.81
	Abnormal	0.82
F1-Score	Normal	0.8
	Abnormal	0.81

Table 5 Classification performance of EfficientNetB0 with pre-processing and custom head

Model		EfficientNet -B0
Accuracy		0.77
Precision	Normal	0.83
	Abnormal	0.73
Recall	Normal	0.66
	Abnormal	0.88
F1-Score	Normal	0.73
	Abnormal	0.88

As presented in Table 5, the model achieved an overall classification accuracy of 0.77. Although the recall and F1-score for the abnormal category were reasonably high, the model exhibited significantly lower recall for the Normal category, resulting in an imbalance in classification performance. This inconsistency in detecting Normal and Abnormal cases indicated that the model struggled to generalize effectively. These observations further motivated the evaluation of Transformer-based architectures.

In the final experimental setting, the classification performance of Vision Transformer (ViT) architecture was evaluated. Specifically, encoders 5–11 were unfrozen, and a custom classification head was used along with the pre-processing techniques.

As summarized in Table 6, this model achieved the highest classification accuracy of 0.84, along with balanced precision and recall metrics. The custom classification head utilized in this architecture effectively preserved the discriminative information extracted from the refined ROI images.

3.5 Explainability Using RISE

To interpret the classification decisions of the decoupled detector-classifier pipeline, RISE technique was employed. RISE generates saliency maps by applying multiple random binary masks to the input image and evaluating the classifier's output for

Table 6 Classification performance of ViT with pre-processing and custom head

Model		Vision transformer
Accuracy		0.84
Precision	Normal	0.83
	Abnormal	0.85
Recall	Normal	0.85
	Abnormal	0.84
F1-Score	Normal	0.84
	Abnormal	0.84

each masked instance. The final saliency map is obtained by computing a weighted sum of these outputs, highlighting the regions that influenced the model's prediction.

Figure 5 illustrates the saliency map generated using RISE for an instance where the ViT model correctly classified the sample as 'Normal' despite the presence of significant cover-up due to amniotic fluid. Notably, the model paid less attention on these cover-up regions suggesting that the model has effectively learnt to ignore irrelevant artifacts and does not misinterpret them as deformities.

As shown in Fig. 6, the ViT model accurately classified the sample as 'Abnormal'. The saliency map obtained using RISE further confirms that the model's attention was primarily concentrated on the specific regions of the auricle exhibiting deformities, as marked in the image. Notably, the background elements had minimal influence on the model's decision.

The results obtained demonstrate that the robust preprocessing and visual interpretability can enable reliable deformity classification even from low-quality, real-world images. This approach may support early identification in non-specialist or resource-constrained settings, reduce dependence on expert evaluation, and encourage broader adoption of image-based screening tools for neonatal auricular deformities in routine clinical care.

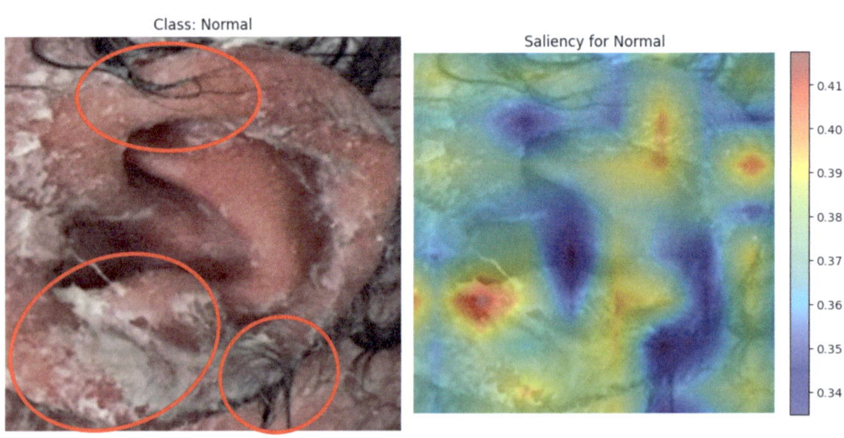

Fig. 5 RISE saliency map showing minimal focus on cover-up artifacts

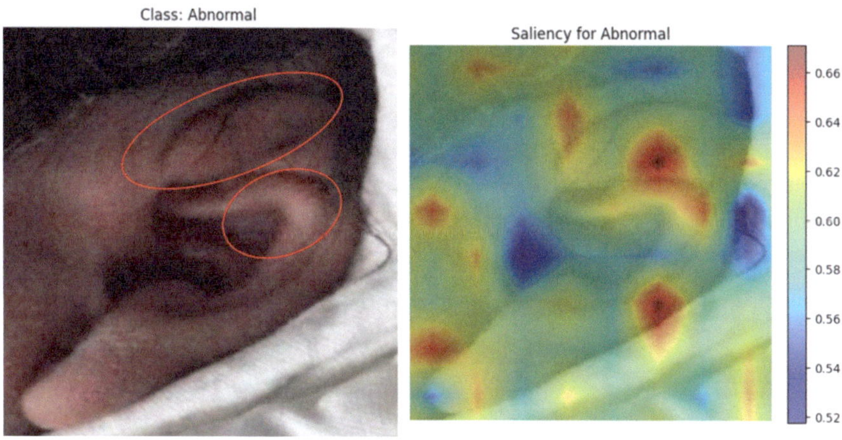

Fig. 6 RISE saliency map illustrating background independence

4 Conclusion

This study presents a progressively refined AI-based framework for the detection and classification of auricular deformities in newborns, designed to support early diagnosis and timely clinical intervention. While earlier experiments explored detection-based classification pipelines, the final methodology focused on a decoupled detector–classifier approach, offering greater control over feature extraction and model optimization. A key enhancement in the refined pipeline was the integration of pre-processing techniques—specifically CLAHE, sharpening, and Gaussian filtering—which contributed to improved feature clarity and reduced the influence of noise and illumination artifacts. Applied to the cropped auricular regions obtained from the detection stage, these enhancements enabled the classification models to operate on structurally enriched inputs. Among the classification models evaluated, Vision Transformer (ViT) demonstrated the most robust performance, achieving a classification accuracy of 0.84 with balanced precision and recall across normal and abnormal cases. Its self-attention mechanism and capacity to capture both local and global dependencies made it particularly well-suited to modelling the nuanced variations in auricular anatomy. To ensure model interpretability, RISE was employed to generate saliency maps that visually explained the basis of each classification decision. These visualizations revealed that the model's attention was consistently aligned with anatomically relevant regions, while extraneous image elements such as background clutter or partial occlusions had minimal influence. This alignment strengthens the potential of the framework for clinically reliable deployment, particularly in settings where explainability is essential for adoption. Looking ahead, several extensions can be pursued to enhance the clinical value of the system. First, transitioning from binary classification to multi-class labelling of specific deformity types (e.g., microtia, lop ear) will increase diagnostic granularity. Additionally, incorporating lightweight detection architectures could facilitate deployment on resource-constrained devices, improving accessibility in field or rural settings. The integration of large language models may also be explored to support interactive features such as visual question answering, aiding in clinical decision support. Overall, the proposed decoupled and explainable AI framework demonstrates strong potential for early and interpretable diagnosis of auricular deformities, with future extensions poised to further enhance its scope and applicability in real-world clinical environments.

References

1. Bhatti, S.L., Daly, L.T., Mejia, M., Perlyn, C.: Ear abnormalities. Pediatr. Rev. **42**(4), 180–188 (2021)
2. Macgregor, F.C.: Ear deformities: social and psychological implications. Clin. Plast. Surg. **5**(3), 347–350 (1978)
3. Ren, L.J., Luo, F., Yang, Z.W., Chen, L.L., Wang, X.Y., Li, C.L., Fu, Y.Y.: A publicly available newborn ear shape dataset for medical diagnosis of auricular deformities. Sci. Data **11**(1) (2024)
4. Castañeda Anaya, P.S., Mendoza Sánchez, H.A.: Advances in regenerative therapy for auricular reconstruction in congenital microtia. Int. J. Med. Sci. Clin. Res. Stud. **3**(8) (2023)
5. Byrd, H.S., Langevin, C.J., Ghidoni, L.A.: Ear molding in newborn infants with auricular deformities. Plast. Reconstr. Surg. **126**(4), 1191–1200 (2010)
6. Doft, M.A., Goodkind, A.B., Diamond, S., Dipace, J.I., Kacker, A., Labruna, A.N.: The newborn butterfly project: a shortened treatment protocol for ear molding. Plast. Reconstr. Surg. **135**(3), 577e–583e (2015)
7. Chen, L., Li, C., He, A., Tong, H., Yu, J., Cui, C., Zhang, T.: Long-term effectiveness of ear molding and factors affecting outcomes. Plast. Reconstr. Surg. **153**(4), 905–913 (2024)
8. Hallac, R.R., Lee, J., Pressler, M., Seaward, J.R., Kane, A.A.: Identifying ear abnormality from 2D photographs using convolutional neural networks. Sci. Rep. **9**(1) (2019)
9. Zhou, X., Peng, X., Ding, Y., Zhu, Y., Tian, D., Wu, M., et al.: Investigation of morphometric features of auricle in newborns and etiology of auricle deformity. Pediatr. Invest. **00**, 1–9 (2024)
10. Esteva, A., Kuprel, B., Novoa, R.A., Ko, J., Swetter, S.M., Blau, H.M., Thrun, S.: Dermatologist-level classification of skin cancer with deep neural networks. Nature **542**(7639), 115–118 (2017)
11. Gulshan, V., Peng, L., Coram, M., Stumpe, M.C., Wu, D., Narayanaswamy, A., Webster, D.R.: Development and validation of a deep learning algorithm for detection of diabetic retinopathy in retinal fundus photographs. JAMA J. Am. Med. Assoc. **316**(22), 2402–2410 (2016)
12. Raj, K.D., Lal, G.J., Gopalakrishnan, E.A., Sowmya, V., Orozco-Arroyave, J.R.: A visibility graph approach for multi-stage classification of Parkinson's disease using multimodal data. IEEE Access **1** (2024)
13. Mohan, J., Sivasubramanian, A., Sowmya, V., Vinayakumar, R.: Enhancing skin disease classification leveraging transformer-based deep learning architectures and explainable AI (2024). arXiv preprint arXiv:2407.14757
14. Moradi, M., Yan, K., Colwell, D., Samwald, M., Asgari, R.: Model-agnostic explainable artificial intelligence for object detection in image data. Eng. Appl. Artif. Intell. **137**, 109183 (2024)
15. Petsiuk, V., Jain, R., Manjunatha, V., Morariu, V.I., Mehra, A., Ordonez, V., Saenko, K.: Black-box explanation of object detectors via saliency maps. In: Proceedings of the IEEE Computer Society Conference on Computer Vision and Pattern Recognition, pp. 11438–11447 (2021)

16. Chen, Y., Wang, W., Wang, Y., Mao, X.: Using ear molding to treat congenital auricular deformities. Front. Pediatr. **9** (2021)
17. Kumar, A.V.A., Sasidharan, D., Sowmya, V., Ravi, V.: AI aided detection and classification of auricular deformities in newborns. In: Decoding Medical Images: Enhancement, Restoration and Reconstruction. River Publishers (2025) (Accepted)
18. Harichandana, M., Sowmya, V., Sajithvariyar, V.V., Sivanpillai, R.: Comparison of image enhancement techniques for rapid processing of post flood images. Int. Arch. Photogram. Remote Sens. Spat. Inf. Sci. 44, 45–50 (2020)
19. Dharshan, S., Divya, B., DV, S.R., Jayakumar, M.: Detection of fault in railway track using image processing and fuzzy logic. In: 2024 Second International Conference on Emerging Trends in Information Technology and Engineering (ICETITE), pp. 1–7. IEEE (2024)
20. Suchithra, M., Soman, K.P.: A fusion based approach for uneven illumination correction in retinal images using Gaussian Filtering method. Procedia Comput. Sci. **260**, 991–999 (2025)
21. He, K., Zhang, X., Ren, S., Sun, J.: Deep residual learning for image recognition. In: Proceedings of the IEEE Computer Society Conference on Computer Vision and Pattern Recognition, pp. 770–778 (2016)
22. Tan, M., Le, Q.V.: EfficientNet: rethinking model scaling for convolutional neural networks. In: 36th International Conference on Machine Learning, ICML 2019, pp. 10691–10700 (2019)
23. Dosovitskiy, A., Beyer, L., Kolesnikov, A., Weissenborn, D., Zhai, X., Unterthiner, T., Dehghani, M., Minderer, M., Heigold, G., Gelly, S., Uszkoreit, J., Houlsby, N.: An image is worth 16×16 words: transformers for image recognition at scale (2020). arXiv preprint arXiv:2010.11929
24. Petsiuk, V., Das, A., Saenko, K.: Rise: randomized input sampling for explanation of black-box models (2018). arXiv preprint arXiv:1806.07421

Robust Parkinson's Detection Through Hybrid Speech Features: A Speaker-Independent Machine Learning and Deep Learning Study

Sweta Swaminathan and G. Jyothish Lal

Abstract Parkinson disease (PD) being a progressive neurological condition that affects the motor control which include vocal analysis, speech production for early non-intrusive detection. In this work, speaker-indepen-dent framework is automated to detect the speech by utilizing hybrid feature set produced by incorporating OpenSMILE features and nonlinear features like Hjorth parameters, entropy measures and fractal dimensions. Machine learning models—Support Vector Machine, Random Forest, K-Nearest Neighbor and Naive Bayes along with Deep learning model Convolutional Neural Network with Bidirectional Long Short-term Memory (CNN+BiLSTM) is been trained and evaluated by employing the hybrid features. To maintain generalizability to unseen speakers, speaker-independent train-test split is adopted and SMOTE addresses the class imbalance through over sampling. Through comparative analysis, it reveals that hybrid feature set improves the classification performance when compared to linear and non-linear executed independently. Random Forest secured the highest accuracy and among the traditional Machine learning models and Deep learning models. By integrating complementary feature representation, we obtain a robust and reliable framework for early PD detection with major applications in continuous patient monitoring.

Keywords Parkinson's disease detection · Non-invasive health monitoring · Speaker-independent analysis · AI in healthcare · Hybrid speech features

---

S. Sweta · G. Jyothish Lal (✉)
Amrita School of Artificial Intelligence, Amrita Vishwa Vidyapeetham, Coimbatore, India
e-mail: g_jyothishlal@cb.amrita.edu

S. Sweta
e-mail: cb.sc.p2dsc24020@cb.students.amrita.edu

P. Singh et al. (eds.), *Deep Learning Applications in Healthcare and Medical Imaging Practice*, Studies in Big Data 193, https://doi.org/10.1007/978-3-032-21009-8_5

1 Introduction

Parkinson disease (PD) is a type of disorder that affects the motor abilities, speech abnormalities and with tremors. Early diagnosis can improve the quality of a person by having timely medications to slow down the progression of the neurodegenrative. Various diagnostic methods in speech analysis has gained acknowledgment over the years as it is cost-effective approach. Spectral, acoustic and prosodic parameters are examined to detect the mild motor conditions that may not be evident in the assessment of clinical results.

Even though there are advancements happening in PD detection, various existing approaches dependent either on highly controlled else on limited dataset. Applications of vowel recording which are sustained is restricted to perform well in multilingual contexts or speech related task. Moreover, the present system are speaker independent which leads to have less accuracy when unseen individuals are employed previously. Varied speaker dialects, characteristics and recording situation poses a challenge in deploying the models in real-world environment or daily life circumstance.

Deep learning approaches specially the hybrid models often promises the best solutions to overcome these challenges. By integrating convolutional neural network (CNN) with bidirectional long short-term memory (BiLSTM) layers, we captures the spatial patterns in spectral with temporal dependencies of the models. These models can represent themselves in complex vocal dynamics. CNN in the model layers are expected to capture the features from Mel-spectrograms that are present locally, while BiLSTM captures the temporal evolution over frames. By this method, accurate detection will occur in speech motor impairments.

But practical limitation remains the same. Class imbalance is seen in healthy as it is underrepresented which can influence the model predictions being biased on one classification. In addition to it, model generalizability get impact on speaker variability and cross-lingual changes. These factors must be addressed for achieving the real-world performance.

To resolve the limitations, the study proposed speaker independent framework for PD detection. By incorporating linear features through OpenSMILE with nonlinear features like e Hjorth parameters, entropy measures and fractal dimensions to capture the information required for speech production. SMOTE is deployed to oversample the class which is having less samples, through this model won't get biased. Speech task: spontaneous speech, reading passage and sustained vowels in the model is evaluated to ensure the consistency in the performance between speaking environment, languages and speakers.

Hybrid feature set in Machine learning and deep learning architectures enable the model to have spatial and temporal dependencies, class imbalance techniques that the proposed model can achieve for early PD detection. Potential applications in multilingual and cross-culture settings; clinical applications and continuous monitoring of patients can bottleneck the gap between the practical deployment and research models in real-world scanarios of health.

The paper is structured as follows: Sect. 2 explains the related works, Sect. 3 details the methodology, encompassing data acquisition, feature extraction, and the development of the predictive model. Sections 4 present the experimental results and offer a comprehensive discussion on the comparative performance of different models across varied feature representations. Finally, Sect. 5 concludes the study and outlines potential avenues for future research.

2 Related Work

Detection of Parkinson Disease (PD) from speech signals has gained considerable attention over the years, with wide ranges of approaches incorporating Machine learning and Deep learning approaches. Pandey et al. [1] employed a hybrid CNN LSTM architecture, where the CNN extract spatial informations from Mel-spectrograms and the LSTM captures the temporal dependencies within the frames. Their experiments was done on public PD voice datasets illustrates that their network outperformed standard CNN or LSTM models when trained independently. However, the study concentrated only on sustained vowels phonations, limiting evaluation on multilingual speech.

Sedigh Malekroodi et al. [2] adopted a self-supervised strategy using pre-trained ASR models such as Wav2Vec 2.0 and HuBERT, combined with supervised learning. In this method, distinct representation between PD and healthy samples were improved, through fine-tuning the computational demands got higher. Quan et al. [3] introduced FedOcw, a federated optimization approach for cross-lingual PD detection. Their work enabled collaborative model training across datasets while conserving privacy, and the performance of language-adaptive layers were improved on multilingual speech datasets. Nevertheless, real-world clinical validate remains necessary.

Dudek et al. [4] assess the collection of PD related voice biomarkers in mixed reality (MR) environments. By integrating prosodic, acoustic, and linguistic features, the study improved the validity in economy by simulating realistic conversational works. However, a small set of samples limited the significance on their findings. Majdoubi et al. [5] proposed a Deep learning model with Bayesian hyperparameters were tuned and applied to spectrogram features for early PD detection. While outperforming baseline CNN models, the assessment was restricted to certain data, leaving the spontaneous speech getting untested.

Rey-Paredes et al. [6] designed a GAN-driven data augmentation approach for raw audio waveforms to tackle class imbalance and highlights the classifier reliability. Despite the performance were improvements, the physiological in generated signals remained a challenging one. Sha and Rahamathulla [7] investigated a hybrid quantum–classical CNN for PD voice classification, achieving accuracy improvements. Yet, the approach seems to depends upon the quantum simulators and the availability of hardware was limited.

Using a CNN–Transformer model, Lv et al. [8] implemented a multi-modal framework that combined visual and aural features. The approach outperformed uni-modal systems through the analysis of speech and facial cues, but it required significant computational resources and synchronisation of multi-modal datasets. In order to classify Parkinson's disease (PD), Kumari and Ramachandran [9] created line spectral frequency (LSF) images derived from sustained vowels using deep CNNs. The phonations were isolated, but the accuracy was the highest among the MFCC and LPC baselines.

On FPGA hardware, Majidinia et al. [10] created a CNN-based PD recognition system that produced real-time results on MFCC features. Using portable screening devices, the design demonstrated high accuracy and reduced computational overhead. Malekroodi et al. [11] used attention-based and deep CNN models to categorise the stages of Parkinson's disease progression: mild, moderate, severe from vocal acoustic features. The models captured disease levels very effectively but depicted less performance on unseen speakers, highlighting the need for speaker-invariant solutions.

By utilizing prosodic and spectral features, Veetil et al. [12] presented a CNN–BiLSTM framework that is independent of language and achieves strong performance in a variety of languages. However, accuracy was still impacted by differences in speech patterns and recording settings. For early PD detection, Bakkialakshmi et al. [13] assessed CNN, RNN, and hybrid CNN–RNN architectures. Their comparative analysis showed that, despite robustness being limited by data scarcity, hybrid models provide the best balance between accuracy and generalization.

An RNN–LSTM method utilising MFCC features from vowel and reading tasks was presented by Pitchiah et al. [14]. Although attention mechanisms for identifying important time segments are suggested as a potential improvement, the sequential network successfully captured temporal dynamics. Lastly, audio spectrogram transformers (AST) were used for PD detection by Madusanka and Lee [15]. Utilizing self-attention to model global temporal dependencies, the transformer-based approach outperformed CNN baselines but demanded high training complexity and data requirements.

A wide range of studies has explored automated Parkinson's disease (PD) detection from speech using diverse deep learning approaches [16, 17]. Panicker et al. [18] conducted comprehensive review based on the trends lead by Machine Learning and Deep Learning models for PD detection indicating the need for standard dataset which clinically valuated the evaluation metrics.

Priya et al. [19] employed PD diagnostic system using deep learning architecture along with signal decomposition techniques for gait pattern analysis for diagnostic accuracy and shows the work underscore the growing research work towards PD detection. Hybrid architectures combining CNNs and LSTMs have been effective in capturing both spatial and temporal patterns from spectrogram-based features, while self-supervised methods using pretrained ASR models improve representation learning with limited labeled data. Federated and language-adaptive frameworks have addressed cross-lingual and privacy concerns, whereas mixed reality setups and multimodal audio–visual models have enhanced ecological validity and performance. GAN-driven augmentation and oversampling strategies have mitigated class imbalance, and hardware-based implementations on FPGA have enabled real-time inference. Transformer-based models and attention mechanisms further capture global temporal dependencies for improved accuracy. Despite these advancements, challenges such as limited spontaneous speech evaluation, speaker variability, cross-lingual generalization, and high computational demands remain, motivating the development of speaker-independent, robust, and scalable PD detection systems.

3 Materials and Methods

3.1 Dataset Description

In this study, we make use of Italian Parkinson's Voice and Speech dataset, which has speech recordings from both elderly healthy controls and individuals suffering from Parkinson's disease (PD). The original dataset has recordings from 22 healthy individuals and 28 individuals with PD. To ensure consistent and completeness among the speech tasks, the people who performed all required utterances were used for this analysis.

In specific, the subsequent 13 speech tasks were selected: **B1, B2, FB1, VA1, VA2, VE1, VE2, VI1, VI2, VO1, VO2, VU1, and VU2**. These tasks include a mix of spontaneous speech segments, reading passages and sustained vowel, providing a comprehensive representation of phonatory and articulatory variants. Missing one or more of these tasks were removed from this study. As a result, the refined dataset included 21 healthy speakers and 24 PD speakers, while 15 healthy participants were excluded due to incomplete recordings. This filtering made sure that the dataset preserved uniform task representation over all speakers, which is crucial for implementing a comparable speech-based PD detection model. A detailed overview of the refined dataset is provided in Table 1.

Table 1 Description of refined dataset

Category	Healthy (elderly)	Parkinson's disease (PD)
No. of speakers	21	24
No. of tasks per speaker	13	13
Total utterances	273	312

3.2 Proposed Methodology

The proposed model is a speaker-independent system for detecting PD, designed to gain consistency performance on unseen participants and provided in Fig. 1. The architecture is formatted into five key stages: audio preprocessing, feature extraction, model development, model evaluation, and comparative analysis across linear, nonlinear, and hybrid feature sets. This design allows for a systematic evaluation for each feature type, making them identify the most informative representations and the models can perform the well in capturing both spectral and temporal representations of speech pathology.

Audio Preprocessing: During pre-processing of audio, each recording were initially loaded in mono and resampled to 16 kHz sampling rate to standardize the dataset. These signals were then, normalized and trimmed to exclude trailing and leading

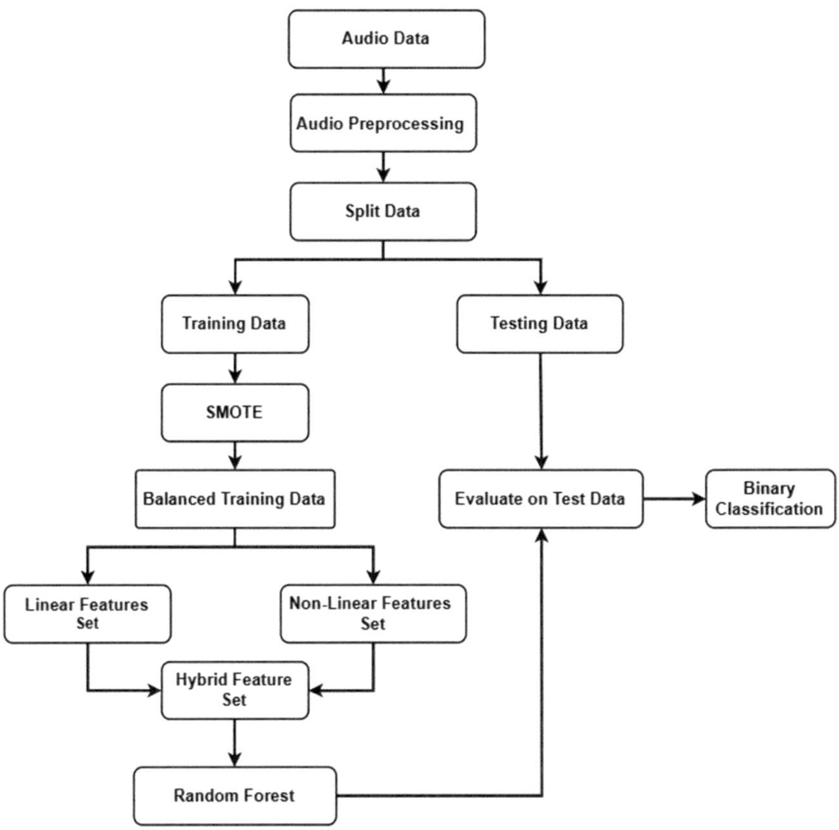

Fig. 1 Proposed Methodology

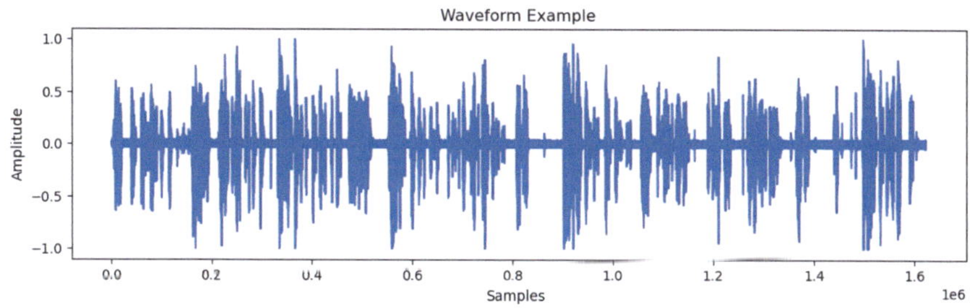

Fig. 2 Sample waveform of a preprocessed audio segment from a healthy control

silences, ensuring that only meaningful speech were retained. In Fig. 2 shows the sample waveform which is preprocessed of a healthy control patient.

Feature Extraction: In this work, we employs a new feature extraction strategy to capture both spatial and temporal characteristics of speech signals, which are known to motor disability in Parkinson's disease (PD). This methodology includes three important steps: linear feature extraction through OpenSMILE, nonlinear feature extraction, and the combination of these features to form hybrid feature set.

The **Linear Feature Extraction (ComParE 2016)** feature set, were deployed through the openSMILE toolkit, whihch has 6,373 acoustic features obtained from low-level descriptors (LLDs) involves harmonics, overlapping windows of the audio signal, Mel-frequency cepstral coefficients (MFCCs), pitch and loudness. The LLDs are estimated over short recordings with windows which are overlapped in audio signal. Following this, numerous statistical functionals: mean, standard deviation, percentiles, and others are adopted to LLDs to capture both spatial and temporal variations in the audio speech signal.

In this framework, linear features were extracted using the ComParE 2016 version of openSMILE, focusing mainly on functions that are estimted over the audio recording. Finally, as part of post extraction method, features are standardized via StandardScaler and variance threshold has kept as 0.01 to eliminate near constant features.

The **Non-Linear** feature extraction method is built to capture the irregular patterns that is existed in speech signals, which are often nonlinear, non-stationary, and temporary by nature. In contrary to linear features has either spectral or prosodic characteristics, the nonlinear features give us information about the underlying chaotic behavior of the vocal system, highlighting irregularity that is caused by dysfunctions of motor control in Parkinson's speech.

In total there are nine nonlinear features that were extracted per speech signal through Python implementation. The features are mainly entropy based, fractal dimensions, Hjorth parameters, and higher-order descriptors, which cumulatively classify the instability and complexity of the speech signal.

Entropy-based features such as Shannon Entropy to quantify the uncertainty or randomness in the distribution of the amplitude signal, where high values corresponding to unstable phonation was obtained where as Spectral Entropy was used to measures the uniformity of distribution over the spectrum of features, highlighting the degree of spectral disorder.

Hjorth Parameters Mobility and Complexity are time domain indicators that explain the need of temporal behavior of the speech signal. Mobility computes the mean frequency or rate the signal variation, while Complexity measures how well the rapid changes in frequency component gets affected over the period of time. In together, these two indicator provide efficient way of representing the changes that occur in speech.

Fractal Dimension (FD) features in specific Petrosian FD, Sevcik FD, and a simplified nonlinear FD is there to extract the self similarity and scaling the characteristics of the speech signal. By this measure we will be able measure how waveform complexity evolves over wide range of variations, where higher FDs irregular often shows the vibrations of vocal fold and airflow patterns observed typically in Parkinson speech.

Lastly, in higher-order statistical features such as Temporal Skewness and Temporal Kurtosis it defines the structure of the amplitude distribution. Skewness predicts whether the signal is distributed in asymmetric way, whereas Kurtosis computes the sharpness or flatness of the waveform. These two metrics will help us to identify abrupt amplitude fluctuations, tremors, or abnormal articulatory movements.

After the extraction process, the features were standardized using `Standard Scaler` to gain zero mean and zero unit variance. So, the low-variance features (variance < 0.01) were omitted via VarianceThreshold to ensure only the components that provide information will be retained. This step improves the relevance of features, enhancing the model stability, and ensure consistency while scaling before combining into the Machine learning and Deep learning frameworks.

The linear and nonlinear features are combined to form **Hybrid Feature Set**, by concatenating 6,373 from linear features and 9 from nonlinear features, resulting in 6,382 features in total per audio sample. By this approach we aims to integrate the major strengths of both linear and nonlinear feature types, enhancing the model's ability to differentiate between healthy and affected Parkinson speech patterns.

Machine Learning Models: To verify the effectiveness of the hybrid feature set, we need to employ four different supervised Machine learning models: **Support Vector Machine (SVM)**, **Random Forest (RF)**, **K-Nearest Neighbors (KNN)**, and **Naive Bayes (NB)**.

These models were trained on the SMOTE to oversample hybrid training set and evaluate on a different test set. Hyper-parameters were kept to standardize the choices: SVM with a linear kernel, Random Forest with 200 decision trees, KNN with 5 neighbors, and Naive Bayes assuming Gaussian distributions. Model performance was evaluated using accuracy, F1-score, and with classification reports.

- **Support Vector Machine (SVM):** Linear kernel adopted to evaluate on linear feature discrimination in the hybrid features.
- **Random Forest (RF):** Ensemble method which has multiple trees to overcome overfitting as well ad to handle feature interactions.

- **K-Nearest Neighbors (KNN):** Instance based classifier incorporating local similarity among data the points that are observed.
- **Naive Bayes (NB):** Probabilistic model assuming independenceover the features to provide a simple reference.

Deep Learning Model(CNN–BiLSTM) Architecture A deep learning framework combining convolutional and recurrent layers were implemented to capture both spatial patterns and temporal dependencies in the hybrid feature sequences. The architecture comprised:

1. **Input Layer:** Receives the hybrid feature matrix generated from the fusion of linear and nonlinear features.
2. **Convolutional Layers:** Two 1D convolution layers with 64 and 128 filters, ReLU activation for nonlinearity, batch normalization, and max-pooling to downsample the dimension to extract hierarchical representations.
3. **Bidirectional LSTM Layers:** Two BiLSTM layers (128 and 64 units) with dropout layer to model forward and backward temporal dependencies.
4. **Fully Connected Layers:** Dense layers with 256 and 128 neurons, ReLU activation, batch normalization, dropout, and L2 regularization to overcome overfitting.
5. **Output Layer:** A single neuron with sigmoid activation to perform binary classification between healthy and Parkinson speech.

3.3 *Model Development*

To investigate on different approaches for Parkinson's disease detection, both traditional Machine learning (ML) classifiers and a Deep learning (DL) architecture were built and analyzed.

3.4 *Evaluation Metrics*

To evaluate the performance of the proposed classifiers on the speaker-independent test set, the following metrics were employed:

Accuracy measures the overall proportion of correctly classified samples among all test instances. It is computed as:

$$\text{Accuracy} = \frac{TP + TN}{TP + TN + FP + FN}, \tag{1}$$

where TP denotes true positives, TN true negatives, FP false positives, and FN false negatives.

F1-Score provides a mean of precision and Recall, in particularly useful when classes were imbalanced. It is defined as the harmonic mean of Precision (P) and Recall (R):

$$\text{F1-Score} = 2 \cdot \frac{P \cdot R}{P + R}, \quad \text{where} \quad P = \frac{TP}{TP + FP}, \quad R = \frac{TP}{TP + FN}. \tag{2}$$

These metrics were calculated on the test dataset to assess model generalizability and predictive reliability.

4 Experimental Results and Discussion

Here, in this section, we provides the experimental evaluation of the proposed speaker-independent Parkinson's disease (PD) detection architecture. The evaluation mainly focuses on the understanding that contributed in building hybrid that fuses the individual feature domains (linear and nonlinear) in improving classification accuracy. For this experiments, we employed multiple Machine Learning (ML) and Deep Learning (DL) models, to access the performance by taking accuracy and F1-score as the metrics.

4.1 Results of Proposed Methodology

The suggested approach creates a hybrid feature representation by fusing linear and nonlinear acoustic descriptors. Even in speaker-independent environments, robust PD detection is made possible by this fusion, which improves the discriminative power of speech features. The **Random Forest** model produced the best results with hybrid features out of all the classifiers.

As shown in Table 2, the Random Forest classifier gained a test accuracy of 99.15% and an F1-score of 99.19%, indicating strong capability and reliability in differentiating PD and healthy speech samples.

Figure 3 depicts the confusion matrix of the Random Forest model. The model was able to correctly classify 61 Parkinson's cases and 55 healthy subjects, with only no false positive and one false negative. This reveals the model's precision and reliability in minimizing false alarms which is essential characteristic in clinical decision support systems.

Table 2 Performance of Random Forest model using hybrid features

Model	Test accuracy	F1-score
Random Forest	**99.15**	**99.19**

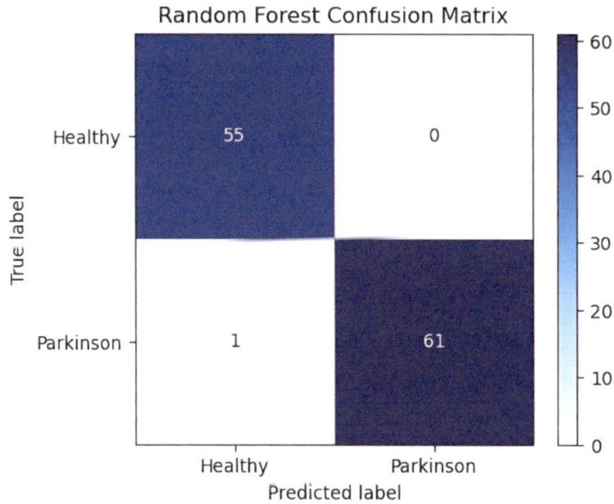

Fig. 3 Confusion matrix of Random Forest model using hybrid features

4.2 *Ablation Study*

To ensure the capability of the proposed hybrid feature set, an ablation study was conducted. The study analyzed the model performance through three arrangement: (a) using hybrid features, (b) using only linear features, and (c) using only nonlinear features. This differentiation helps to determine the contribution of each feature set.

Model-Wise Performance Using Hybrid Features Table 3 displays the performance of various models using hybrid feature set. SVM achieved near-perfect scores after the Random Forest, ensuring their strong differentiation ability. The CNN+BiLSTM model also illustrated higher performance in validating the hybrid feature set with both ML and DL frameworks.

Figure 4 shows the different outlook of the classification models based on their performance with the hybrid feature set. The Random Forest model outperformed other approaches we employed, whereas CNN+BiLSTM depicted stable performance using hybrid feature set.

Figure 5 demonstrates the CNN+BiLSTM training performance. The accuracy curve steadily rises and then stabilizes around 0.95–1.0, even though the loss curve decreases smoothly, conveying the less overfitting and strong convergence. These

Table 3 Performance of different models using hybrid features

Model	Test accuracy	F1-score
SVM	98.29	98.36
KNN	90.60	90.27
Naive Bayes	90.60	90.60
CNN+BiLSTM	95.73	95.93

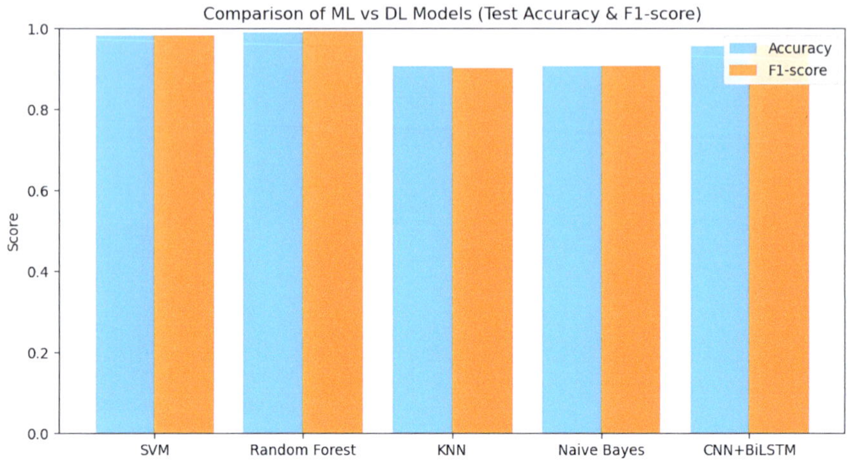

Fig. 4 Comparison of model-wise Accuracy and F1-score using hybrid features

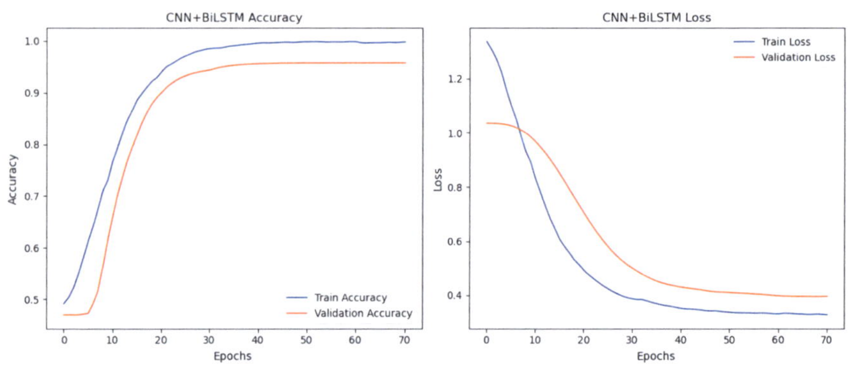

Fig. 5 Accuracy and loss curves of CNN–BiLSTM model using hybrid features

plot shows the ability of the model to capture temporal–spectral dependencies at the deep in PD speech patterns.

Results Using Linear Features The linear feature set employed models Table 4 depicts that the SVM gained the highest accuracy of (98.46%), showcasing the strong ability of linear feature set. Although, these results slightly underperform when compared to the hybrid architecture, indicating the advantage of using feature fusion.

Results Using Nonlinear Features From Table 5, it is very evident that the models using only nonlinear feature set perform very poorly when hyrid and linear feature set because of using less features. Whereas, in the method Random Forest was able to perform best with 82.31% accuracy, the less accuracy shows that nonlinear descriptors alone are insufficient for better classification. When nonlinear feature set

Table 4 Performance of different models using linear features

Model	Test accuracy	F1-score
SVM	**98.46**	**98.44**
Random Forest	96.92	96.88
KNN	83.08	80.36
Naive Bayes	82.31	81.60
CNN+BiLSTM	94.62	94.57

Table 5 Performance of different models using nonlinear features

Model	Test accuracy	F1-score
SVM	80.77	81.75
Random Forest	**82.31**	**82.96**
KNN	77.69	79.43
Naive Bayes	70.77	69.84
CNN+BiLSTM	80.77	82.76

is fused with linear feature set, though, they try to contribute critical information that is required to boost the performance significantly.

The ablation study clearly affirms that the fusing of linear and nonlinear features provides the most stable results for PD detection. The proposed feature set combination strategy yields more superior classification performance among both ML and DL models, confirming its potential for relying on speaker-independent detection.

5 Conclusion and Future Work

This study suggested a thorough framework for linear, nonlinear, and hybrid acoustic feature-based speaker-independent Parkinson's disease (PD) detection. According to experimental results, the CNN+BiLSTM model performed competitively among deep learning techniques, while the Random Forest and SVM models continuously outperformed other conventional machine learning techniques. The benefit of combining complementary feature domains was demonstrated by the hybrid feature set, which significantly increased classification accuracy and F1-score by combining spectral and dynamic aspects of speech. The Random Forest model proved to be the most successful classifier overall, demonstrating its resilience when dealing with a variety of intricate feature interactions. These results highlight the potential of hybrid acoustic representations in conjunction with deep learning or ensemble models as trustworthy, non-invasive methods for early Parkinson's disease detection.

In the future, some practical extensions to the framework can make the framework more clinically useful. Future research might address enhanced interpretability by using explainable AI methods, allowing clinicians to relate model predictions to particular acoustic biomarkers of PD progression. Analysis of speech over time could facilitate continuous monitoring of disease progression or of treatment response. The architecture would also be generalized to include multimodal data like facial movement, writing dynamics, or body sensor input, to offer a more integrated assessment of motor and non-motor manifestations. Further, creating a real-time, lightweight variant of the CNN+BiLSTM model for mobile or telemedicine would make it more accessible, and the inclusion of domain adaptation and data augmentation methods would make it more robust against noise, accents, and environmental variation. Lastly, adaptive calibration to a person's baseline vocal patterns could enable early identification of subtle change, enabling personalized and proactive healthcare interventions.

References

1. Pandey, P.V., Sahu, S.S., Karan, B., Mishra, S.K.: Parkinson disease prediction using CNN-LSTM model from voice signal. SN Comput. Sci. **5**(4), 381 (2024)
2. Sedigh Malekroodi, H., Madusanka, N., Lee, B.-I., Yi, M.: Speech-based Parkinson's detection using pre-trained self-supervised automatic speech recognition (ASR) models and supervised contrastive learning. Bioengineering **12**(7), 728 (2025)
3. Quan, C., Chen, Z., Ren, K., Luo, Z.: FedOcw: optimized federated learning for cross-lingual speech-based Parkinson's disease detection. npj Digit. Med.**8**(1), 357 (2025)
4. Dudek, M., Hemmerling, D., Kaczmarska, M., Stepien, J., Daniol, M., Wodzinski, M., Wojcik-Pedziwiatr, M.: Analysis of voice, speech, and language biomarkers of Parkinson's disease collected in a mixed reality setting. Sensors **25**(8), 2405 (2025)
5. Majdoubi, O., Ouabd, A., Jilbab, A., Benba, A., Hammouch, A.: Optimized Deep Learning Model for Early Parkinson's Disease Detection Using Speech Spectrograms. In: 2025 5th International Conference on Innovative Research in Applied Science, Engineering and Technology (IRASET), pp. 1–6. IEEE (2025)
6. Rey-Paredes, M., Pérez, C.J., Mateos-Caballero, A.: Time series classification of raw voice waveforms for Parkinson's disease detection using generative adversarial network-driven data augmentation. IEEE Open J. Comput. Soc. (2024)
7. Sha, M., Rahamathulla, M.P.: Quantum deep learning in Parkinson's disease prediction using hybrid quantum–classical convolution neural network. Quantum Inf. Process. **23**(12), 383 (2024)
8. Lv, C., Fan, L., Li, H., Ma, J., Jiang, W., Ma, X.: Leveraging multimodal deep learning framework and a comprehensive audio-visual dataset to advance Parkinson's detection. Biomed. Signal Process. Control **95**, 106480 (2024)
9. Kumari, R., Ramachandran, P.: Deep CNN for Parkinson's disease classification using line spectral frequency images of sustained speech phonation. IETE J. Res. **71**(1), 341–358 (2025)
10. Majidinia, H., Khatib, F., Seyyed Mahdavi Chabok, S.J., Kobravi, H.R., Rezaeitalab, F.: Diagnosis of Parkinson's disease using convolutional neural network-based audio signal processing on FPGA. Circuits, Syst., Signal Process. **43**(7), 4221–4238 (2024)
11. Malekroodi, H.S., Madusanka, N., Lee, B.-I., Yi, M.: Leveraging deep learning for fine-grained categorization of Parkinson's disease progression levels through analysis of vocal acoustic patterns. Bioengineering **11**(3), 295 (2024)
12. Veetil, I.K., Sowmya, V., Orozco-Arroyave, J.R., Gopalakrishnan, E.A.: Robust language independent voice data driven Parkinson's disease detection. Eng. Appl. Artif. Intell. **129**, 107494 (2024)

13. Bakkialakshmi, V.S., Arulalan, V., Chinnaraju, G., Ghosh, H., Rahat, I.S., Saha, A.: Exploring the potential of deep learning in the classification and early detection of Parkinson's disease. EAI Endorsed Trans. Pervasive Health Technol. **10**(1) (2024)
14. Pitchiah, R., Rooba, T.S., Kumar, K.U.P.: A novel voice-based system for Parkinson's disease detection using RNN-LSTM. Proc. Eng. Sci. **6**(4), 1541–1550 (2024)
15. Madusanka, N., Lee, B.-I.: Vocal biomarkers for Parkinson's disease classification using audio spectrogram transformers. J. Voice (2024)
16. Raj, K.D., Jyothish Lal, G., Gopalakrishnan, E.A., Sowmya, V., Orozco-Arroyave, J.R.: A visibility graph approach for multi-stage classification of Parkinson's disease using multimodal data. IEEE Access 12, 87077-87096 (2024)
17. Mohamed Ali, A., Jyothish Lal, G., Sowmya, V., Gopalakrishnan, E.A.: Parkinson's disease assessment from speech data using recurrence plot. In: International Conference on Computing, Intelligence and Data Analytics, pp. 132–142 (2023)
18. Panicker, R.O., Yashasvi, D., James, J., Ittappa, S.: Automatic detection of Parkinson's disease using machine learning and deep learning: a recent literature review. Ethics, Med. Public Health **33**, 101079 (2025)
19. Priya, S.J., Anand Deva Durai, C., Subathra, M.S.P., Thomas George, S., Jeyabose, A.: Automated Parkinson's disease diagnosis using decomposition techniques and deep learning for accurate gait analysis. IEEE Access (2025)

Cross-Domain Generalization in Speech-Based Depression Detection via Hybrid CNN–BiLSTM Feature Integration

K. B. Sivachandra and G. Lal Jyothish

Abstract Depression detection from speech has emerged to be the most advanced area in the field of medical analysis. The depression in patients often leads to a wide range of mental issues along with suicidal tendencies. So in this research, we propose a hybrid framework combining a fusion of convolutional and recurrent representations along with the handcrafted acoustic features in an MLP pipeline for consistent binary classification of depressed and not depressed classes. In this research, this hybrid model was trained using the depression dataset DAIC-WOZ clinical interview corpus and tested on the emotion dataset RAVDESS by mapping the emotions into both negative and positive classes, to assess cross-corpus generalization, which is an essential requirement for real-world implementation. The proposed CNN–BiLSTM fusion architecture extracts high-level temporal–spectral embeddings from Mel-spectrograms and integrates them with statistical prosodic descriptors such as spectral contrast, MFCCs, chroma, and energy-based measures. Integration of augmentation techniques to handle data imbalance is applied to enrich minority depressive samples. Experimental results showcase that the proposed model achieves an accuracy of 87.4% on the diac-woz dataset with the F1-score, precision, and recall of 87.4%, 86.8% and 87.9%, respectively. Along with on cross corpus evaluation with the RAVDESS dataset accuracy obtained is around 80.014%. These findings highlight the possibility of integrating deep temporal modeling and handcrafted feature fusion for generalized depression detection across diverse speech datasets, advancing the field toward effective and trustworthy affective computing systems.

Keywords Depression detection · Speech-based mental health monitoring · Affective computing · CNN–BiLSTM fusion · AI in healthcare

---

K. B. Sivachandra · G. L. Jyothish (✉)
Amrita School of Artificial Intelligence, Amrita Vishwa Vidyapeetham, Coimbatore, India
e-mail: g_jyothishlal@cb.amrita.edu

K. B. Sivachandra
e-mail: kbsivachandra@gmail.com

P. Singh et al. (eds.), *Deep Learning Applications in Healthcare and Medical Imaging Practice*, Studies in Big Data 193, https://doi.org/10.1007/978-3-032-21009-8_6

1 Introduction

Worldwide Depression is among the most common psychological disorders that substantially impacts emotional well-being, social interaction, and cognitive functioning of an individual. According to the World Health Organization (WHO), over 280 million individuals experience depressive symptoms globally, thus making it one of the major causes of disability [1]. Depression affects not only the emotional well-being of an individual, but also socio-economic interactions, along with speech, cognitive function, often leading to severe mental disorders and, in severe cases, it can often lead to suicidal tendencies [2]. Early detection and assessments can decrease the critical risk and enable effective recovery.

Traditional approaches, involving clinical interviews, standardized questionnaires, and self-evaluation scales, remain the main foundation for determining whether an individual is in a depressive state [3]. While these methods seem to be effective in controlled clinical settings, these approaches mainly depend on patient self-reporting and professional judgment, introducing a potential bias in diagnosis. Limited access to experienced mental health professionals, especially in less resource-rich areas, further restricts the scalability of traditional screening approaches [4]. These constraints show an urgent need for an automated and non-invasive model that can enhance manual evaluation and computational understanding of one's psychological conditions.

Recent improvements in this research focused on multimodal signals that capture both the acoustic-prosodic and textual features expressing the emotion as well as the state of mind of the speaker [5]. Depression can be demonstrated with the minimal changes in voice characteristics such as reduced pitch variation, longer pauses, slower speaking rate, decreased loudness, and monotonic prosody [8]. Acoustic features such as Mel-Frequency Cepstral Coefficients (MFCCs), jitter, shimmer, energy, and spectral entropy have been found to correlate with depressive symptoms [9]. Recent models analyze these features to provide objective indicators of mood states that are often undetectable through traditional clinical evaluations [7].

The emergence in the field of machine learning, deep learning, and speech signal processing has enabled the development of automated depression detection systems [6, 12, 13, 16]. Early approaches concentrated on traditional machine learning models such as Support Vector Machines, Random Forest models, which were trained on handcrafted acoustic and prosodic features [14, 15]. While these approaches were successful initially, these methods required extensive manual feature engineering and were highly sensitive to noise, speaker variation, and recording conditions. Deep learning approaches, in contrast, enable an end-to-end feature learning from raw or spectrogram-based speech representations, where the CNN models concentrate on extracting localized spectral-temporal patterns and RNN and LSTM architectures capture long-range temporal dependencies in prosodic dynamics.

Despite progress, several challenges remain. Most deep learning–based depression detection systems are trained and evaluated on a single dataset, limiting generalization [17]. The viability of speech datasets also presents as a barrier to cross-dataset generalization. Another issue is that datasets such as DAIC-WOZ suffer from class imbalance, with non-depressed samples higher than the depressed ones, resulting in biased learning [9]. The transparency of deep learning models is also a concern, as clinical adoption requires transparent systems capable of justifying model predictions [5].

To address these limitations, our research proposes a hybrid deep learning framework integrating both the learned and handcrafted acoustic features for stable binary depression classification. The model is trained on the Distress Analysis Interview Corpus – Wizard of Oz (DAIC-WOZ) [10] and evaluated on the Ryerson Audio-Visual Database of Emotional Speech and Song (RAVDESS) [11] to test cross-corpus generalization. The pipeline integrates Mel-spectrogram-based CNN feature extraction with Bidirectional LSTM (BiLSTM) modules to capture temporal dependencies, while handcrafted features–including MFCCs, spectral contrast, chroma, zero-crossing rate, root-mean-square energy, and nonlinear descriptors such as Hjorth parameters and spectral entropy–supplement deep features. Feature streams are fused at the decision level through concatenation, enabling the model to leverage both high-level learned representations and low-level signal attributes. Class-balancing techniques and data augmentation to solve the issue of dataset imbalance were deployed. Cross-corpus evaluation on RAVDESS validates robustness to emotionally rich, non-clinical speech data.

In this research, we aim to develop a deep learning approach combining both acoustic features and handcrafted features with a Hybrid Fusion model and an MLP pipeline, and the key novelties and contributions of this research are mentioned below

- Combines deep learning with handcrafted acoustic features to create a more comprehensive and discriminative representation of speech patterns associated with depression and non-depression.
- Cross corpus model evaluation is done on the RAVDESS emotional speech dataset to test its ability to detect depression-related acoustic patterns across different speakers, emotions, and recording conditions.
- Combines explainable acoustic features with deep embeddings to improve transparency and support clinical decision-making.
- Employs data augmentation and class-balancing strategies to improve sensitivity to minority-class (depressed) samples.
- Uses CNNs for spectral feature extraction and BiLSTM modules for temporal modeling of prosodic cues.

The scope of this research extends beyond dataset-specific modeling, aiming to develop adaptable, explainable, and clinically relevant systems for automatic mental health screening. In this research, the following sections are organized as follows. Section 2 presents related work in speech-based Depression Detection. Section 3 describes the proposed methodology, including the dataset description, the feature extraction, the handling of class imbalance techniques, and the model architecture, followed by Sect. 4 explains the experimental results, discussing the experimental setup and evaluation results. Section 5 includes the discussion of model performance, and Sect. 6 consists an analysis of the research and the future scope.

2 Literature Survey

Recent research in audio-based depression detection has explored a variety of machine learning and deep learning approaches, primarily utilizing the speech features to identify depressive patterns. Multiple studies have employed techniques including spectral features, prosodic cues, and handcrafted acoustic descriptors, often in combination with ensemble and multimodal frameworks, in order to improve classification performance on datasets such as DAIC-WOZ, AVEC, and VocalMind. While these approaches give better results, challenges remain regarding temporal modeling, cross-corpus generalization, and the handling of imbalanced datasets. In this section, we will be discussing about some of the research done in these areas.

In this research, the authors Shen et al. [12] proposed a wav2vec 2.0–based framework for depression recognition using the DAIC-WOZ dataset. The approach used pretrained speech embeddings from wav2vec 2.0, following fine-tuning of a compact neural network for the classification task. By utilizing these learned representations, the proposed model reduces the challenges associated with the small size of clinical depression datasets. The proposed approach relies on large-scale pretraining corpora, which limits the accessibility for researchers without such resources. Furthermore, while the embeddings capture high-level speech characteristics, they offer limited interpretability regarding which specific acoustic features correlate with depressive symptoms. This research showcases the potential of self-supervised learning in depression detection but leaves gaps in interpretability and cross-corpus generalization.

The authors Lee et al. [13] developed a multimodal pipeline combining short-duration speech segments with handcrafted acoustic features and self-report questionnaires and tested on a chronic pain clinic dataset with approximately 50% prevalence of depression, the model achieved a 15% improvement in accuracy through cross-validation. By fusing subjective self-reports and objective acoustic markers, the approach successfully captures complementary signals of depression. However, its reliance on self-report data introduces potential biases and limits applicability to natural speech scenarios where such metadata may not be available. The proposed approach just focuses on short, controlled speech segments, which may not represent natural conversational variability.

In this research, the authors Wang et al. [14] developed a fusion framework that combines prosodic and spectral features for depression classification, integrating weighted soft voting ensembles techniques using classifiers such as SVM and KNN. The experiments done on AVEC datasets showed improved recall for the depressed class, addressing the issue of class imbalance. By applying complementary information from different feature types, the ensemble approach improves discrimination between depressed and non-depressed individuals. However, the method lacks modeling of temporal dependencies in speech, which are often critical for capturing depressive patterns. Additionally, cross-dataset generalization may be limited due to differences in recording conditions, speaker demographics, and linguistic content.

Li et al. [15] in their research extracted a set of 523 acoustic features from 3-minute reading tasks performed by Chinese university students. Evaluation was performed using Linear Discriminant Analysis, achieving an AUC of 0.771. Explainability was also introduced by the authors to present the MFCC features as a key indicator for depression detection. Although the model shows better performance, the limited data availability of a specific population, and the speech recordings used were recorded under controlled environments, reducing the model's employment in real-world systems. The proposed model does not consider time-based dynamics or sequence modeling techniques, which are important for capturing variations in speech patterns over time.

In this study, the authors Chen et al. [16] developed a multimodal technique combining both acoustic features and linguistic information from clinical interviews to evaluate the degree of depression on DAIC-WOZ. The developed framework outperforms the baseline models, showing that joint modeling of audio and text can improve performance. This research shows the importance of multimodal fusion for clinical depression assessment while pointing out the issues of model transparency and generalization.

In this research, the authors Zhang et al. [17] examined the interaction between depression and personality traits by combining speaker embeddings derived from voice segments with engineered acoustic features from OpenSMILE using DAIC-WOZ and VocalMind datasets. The main objective was to estimate the PHQ-8 severity scores, obtaining an RMSE value of 6.01. Results showed that overlaps between depressive speech characteristics and personality-related vocal patterns underscore the complexity of clinical speech signals. However, the model could not capture temporal variations within the speech, limiting recognition of temporal dynamic patterns associated with depression.

In this research, we aim to solve these limitations by introducing a hybrid CNN–BiLSTM framework that combines learned Mel-spectrogram features with handcrafted acoustic features. Weighted sampling and data augmentation are applied to address issues faced due to class imbalance, and cross-corpus evaluation using an emotion dataset, RAVDESS, to identify the depressed and not depressed states, ensuring the stability of classification to diverse speech conditions.

3 Proposed Methodology

In this research, we propose a hybrid DL model for depression detection from speech, using both learned representations and handcrafted acoustic features. The overall pipeline as shown in Fig. 4, consists of dataset preprocessing, feature extraction, augmentation, and a fused CNN–BiLSTM architecture to capture spectral-temporal and prosodic patterns which are used for depression analysis from speech.

3.1 Dataset Description

DAIC-WOZ The *Distress Analysis Interview Corpus – Wizard of Oz* (DAIC-WOZ) [10] is a clinically-focused speech dataset aimed to support depression detection research. It includes both semi-structured interviews conducted by a AI agent, inducing responses related to psychological health and emotional balance. This includes audio recordings, transcriptions, and clinically annotated labels, including PHQ-8 scores. For this study, binary depression labels are derived using a standard PHQ-8 threshold of 10, categorizing participants into depressed and non-depressed classes. The dataset includes separate splits for training, development, and testing, with a notable class imbalance where non-depressed samples outnumber depressed ones. The dataset contain a total of 56 depressed and 133 non depressed patients. The dataset classwise distribution is shown in Fig. 1.

RAVDESS The *Ryerson Audio-Visual Database of Emotional Speech and Song* (RAVDESS) [11] is a multimodal dataset containing emotionally expressive speech and song recordings from professional actors. Although not explicitly labeled for depression, RAVDESS provides a rich test domain to evaluate the generalization capacity of depression detection models across speakers, accents, and expressive styles.

Its inclusion ensures robustness of the proposed framework to varied emotional and acoustic conditions. The negative emotions like sad, fear, disgust, anger is mappped to depressed and the positive emotions mapped to non depressed class and the classwise distribution is shown in Fig. 2.

Preprocessing and Standardization All audio recordings from both datasets are resampled to 16 kHz, normalized, and truncated or zero-padded to a fixed duration of 20 s to ensure consistent input dimensions. This preprocessing standardizes both datasets for end-to-end deep learning preserving essential spectral and temporal information critical for depression-related acoustic patterns.

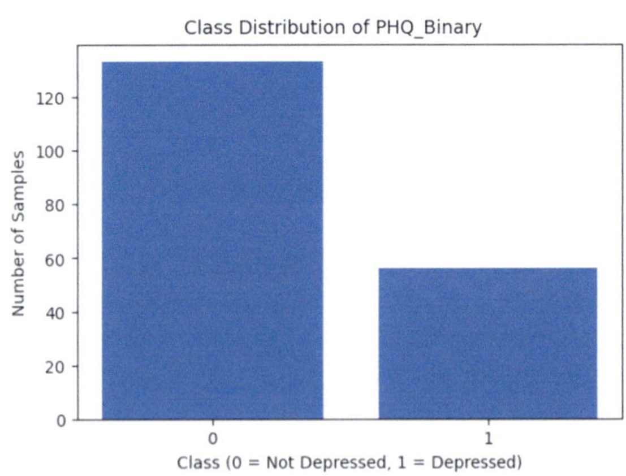

Fig. 1 Class-wise distribution of the DAIC-WOZ dataset showing the number of depressed (PHQ_Binary = 1) and non-depressed (PHQ_Binary = 0) participants

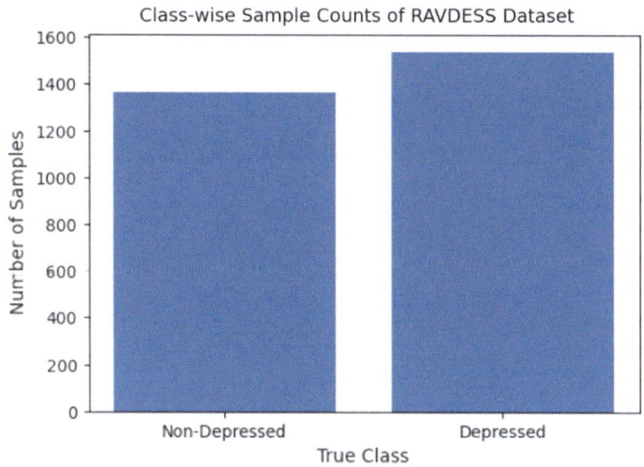

Fig. 2 Class-wise distribution of the RAVDESS dataset after mapping emotion labels to negative (depressed) and positive (non-depressed) classes, showing the number of samples in each category

3.2 Feature Extraction

Two complementary feature streams are extracted from each audio recording:

- **Mel-Spectrogram Features:** Log-scaled Mel-spectrograms are computed using 64 Mel bands, a 1024-point FFT, and 256-sample hop length. The resultant spectrograms generated are normalized and clipped to the range [0,1], providing a compact, frequency-aware representation suitable for convolutional feature learning. The Fig. 3 shows the sample mel-spectrogram of both depressed and not depressed speech signals.
- **Handcrafted Acoustic Features:** A collection of acoustic features is obtained, such as MFCCs, delta and delta-delta coefficients, spectral contrast, chroma, zero-crossing rate, spectral centroid, spectral roll-off, and root-mean-square energy. For all extracted features, variance and mean across frames are estimated and combined to form a uniform-length vector.

3.3 Data Augmentation and Class Balancing

To reduce the issue of class imbalance and to enhance the model generalization, we deployed augmentation strategies, especially to the minority-class (depressed) samples. The applyed augmentation techniques include injection of Gaussian noise, shifting of pitch within ± 2 semitones, and stretching time within a 0.9–1.1 rate range. Augmented samples are cropped or zero-padded to ensure uniform input length. Additionally, a weighted random sampler is employed during training to ensure balanced representation of both depressed and not depressed classes.

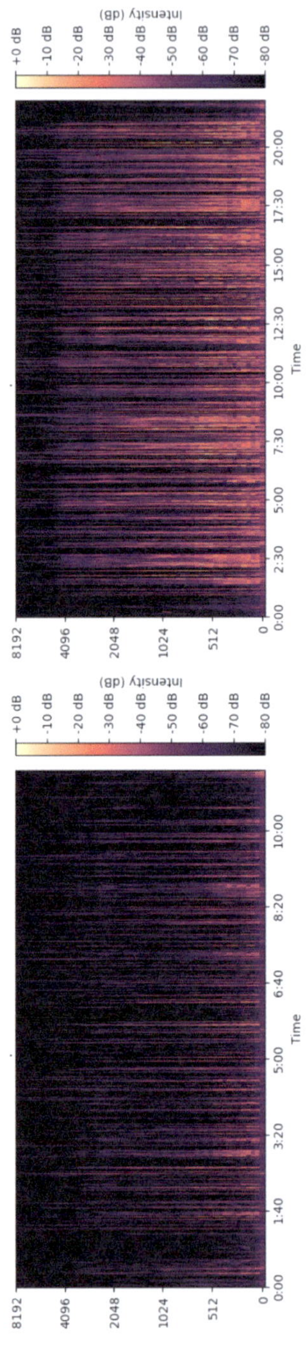

Fig. 3 Mel-Spectrograms of speech samples: Depressed class (Left) and Right Non-Depressed (Right)

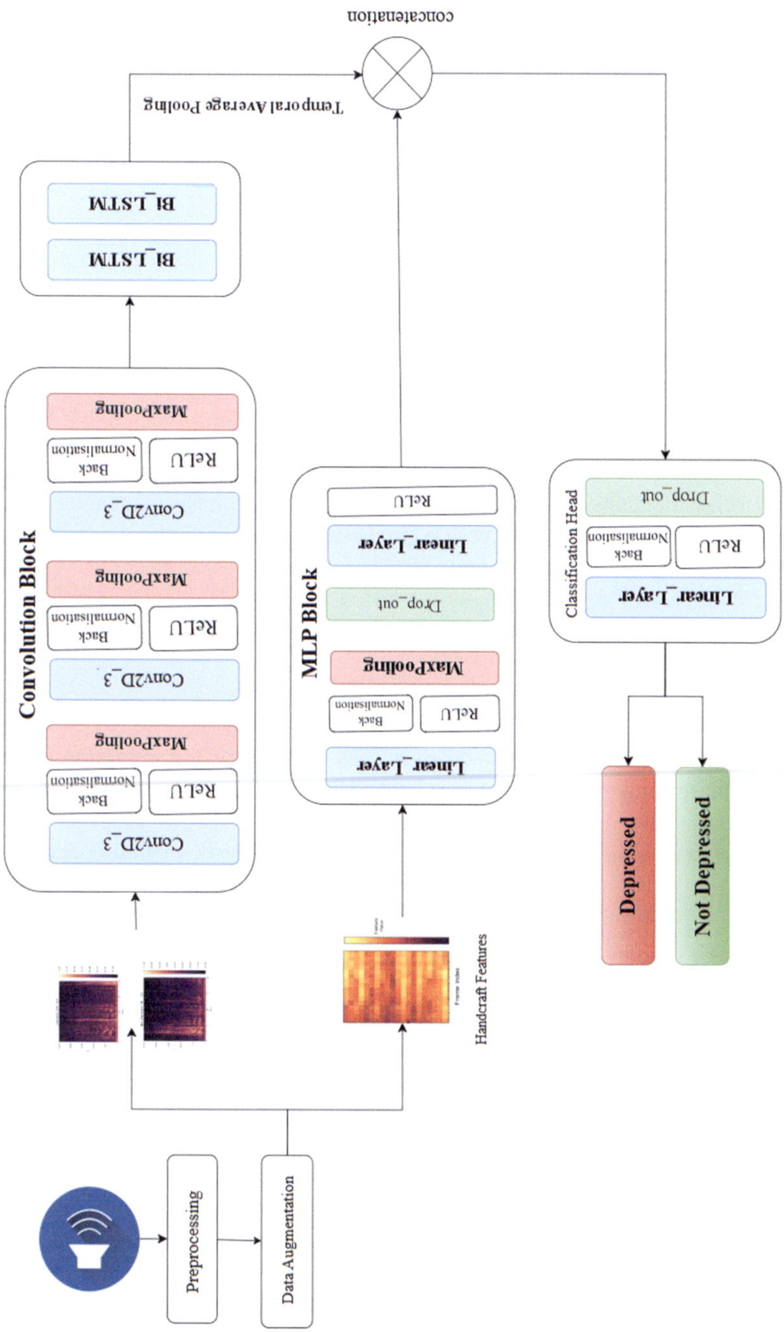

Fig. 4 Proposed Methodology for depression classification using Depressed and Non Depressed classes

3.4 Model Architecture

The proposed fusion architecture consists of three modules:

1. CNN Feature Extractor: A small convolutional network processes the Mel-spectrogram input. The network contains three convolutional blocks with Batch Normalization, ReLU activation, and max-pooling along the temporal dimension, followed by a linear layer to reduce feature dimensionality.
2. Bidirectional LSTM: The CNN-extracted features are fed into a two-layer bidirectional LSTM with dropout to capture temporal dependencies and prosodic features across the entire input speech segment.
3. Handcrafted Feature MLP: The handcrafted acoustic feature vector is processed through a fully connected multilayer perceptron with Batch Normalization, ReLU activation, and dropout, producing a learned representation aligned in dimensionality with the LSTM output.

The outputs of the BiLSTM and handcrafted MLP are concatenated and passed through a classifier consisting of fully connected layers, Batch Normalization, ReLU activations, and dropout, ending with a single neuron using sigmoid activation to estimate the probability of depression.

3.5 Evaluation Metrics

The model is trained using binary cross-entropy loss with class-weighting to deal with the dataset imbalance. The Adam optimizer with weight decay is employed, and the learning rate is dynamically adjusted using a ReduceLROnPlateau scheduler. Model performance is quantified using standard metrics including accuracy, precision, recall, F1-score, and the confusion matrix. Cross-corpus evaluation on RAVDESS is performed to assess generalization, providing evidence of robustness to speaker, accent, and emotional variability.

4 Experimental Results

In this section we discuss the experimental evaluation of the proposed hybrid CNN–BiLSTM framework for data-driven depression classification from speech. The study aims to assess both within-corpus and cross-corpus robustness. More precisely, the proposed model is trained and validated on the DAIC-WOZ dataset and further tested on the RAVDESS corpus to evaluate stability of the model performance under domain shift conditions. Detailed descriptions of the experimental setup, evaluation metrics, and comparative performance analyses are provided. The results demonstrate the efficacy of the fusion-based architecture in capturing both spectral-temporal patterns and handcrafted acoustic cues relevant to depressive speech characteristics.

4.1 Experimental Setup

The proposed hybrid CNN–BiLSTM model is trained on the DAIC-WOZ dataset with the minority class augmented, using a batch size of 16, a learning rate of 1×10^{-4}, and early stopping was integrated based on validation loss. All audio recordings were resampled to 16 kHz and truncated or zero-padded to 20 s. Mel-spectrograms with 64 Mel bands is used as input to the CNN, while handcrafted acoustic features were processed through a fully connected MLP. Weighted random sampling was employed to address class imbalance issue of depressed class.

Model performance was evaluated using the held-out DAIC-WOZ test set and cross-corpus validation on the RAVDESS dataset. Evaluation metrics include accuracy, precision, recall, F1-score, and confusion matrix analysis.

4.2 Results on DAIC-WOZ Test Set

Table 1 shows the classification results on the DAIC-WOZ test set. The hybrid model achieves a balanced performance across metrics, demonstrating the effectiveness of integrating learned and handcrafted features. The confusion matrix (Fig. 5) shows how well the model is able to discriminate between the depressed and not depressed classes. The hybrid model acquired an accuracy of around 87.4% and a precision, F1-Score and Recall values of 86.8%, 87.4% and 87.9% respectively.

Table 1 Class-wise performance of the proposed hybrid CNN–BiLSTM model on DAIC-WOZ test set

Class	Precision	Recall	F1-score	Support
Non-Depressed	0.94	0.88	0.91	33
Depressed	0.75	0.86	0.80	14
Accuracy	0.87			
Macro Avg	0.85	0.87	0.86	47
Weighted Avg	0.89	0.87	0.88	47

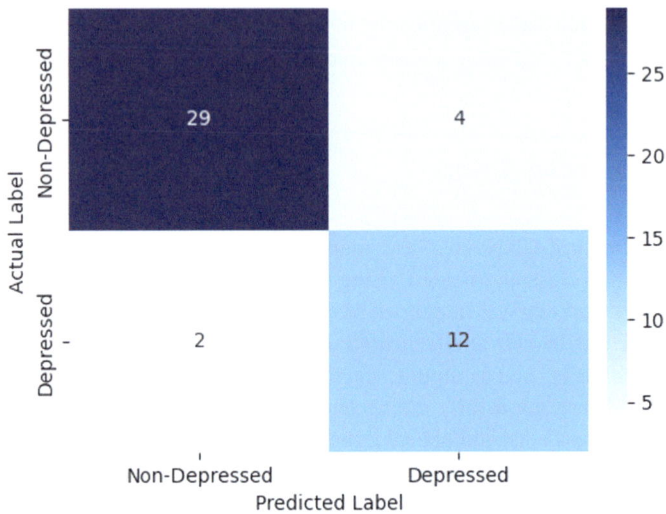

Fig. 5 Confusion matrix for DAIC-WOZ test set predictions

4.3 Cross-Corpus Evaluation on RAVDESS

To assess generalization, the model trained on DAIC-WOZ is evaluated on the RAVDESS dataset. Despite differences in emotional content, speaker demographics, and recording conditions, the hybrid framework maintains consistent performance, confirming its robustness to domain shifts. Table 2 summarizes the cross-corpus metrics. As shown in Fig. 6 shows model reliably distinguishes between depressed and non-depressed speech despite cross-corpus variability.

These results demonstrate that integrating handcrafted features with deep representations improves generalizability, even on datasets not explicitly labeled for depression.

Table 2 Class-wise performance of the proposed hybrid CNN–BiLSTM model on RAVDESS test set

Class	Precision	Recall	F1-score	Support
Non-Depressed	0.78	0.81	0.79	1366
Depressed	0.82	0.80	0.81	1536
Accuracy	0.80			
Macro Avg	0.80	0.80	0.80	2902
Weighted Avg	0.80	0.80	0.80	2902

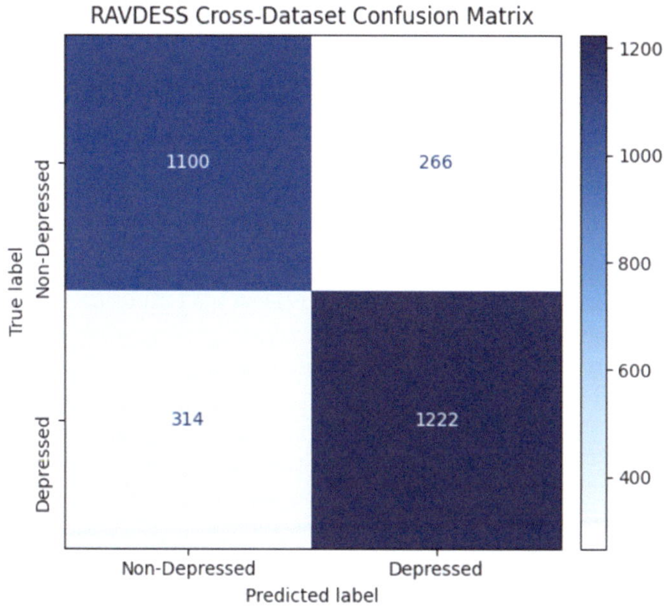

Fig. 6 Confusion matrix for RAVDESS showing classification performance of the hybrid CNN–BiLSTM model on depressed and non-depressed classes

4.4 *Ablation Study*

To evaluate the generalization ability of the proposed hybrid framework, an ablation study was performed by training on the RAVDESS emotional speech dataset and evaluating on DAIC–WOZ, a clinically validated corpus of depression interviews. This setup presents deliberate domain and distributional shifts–RAVDESS features acted emotional expressions in a controlled environment, while DAIC–WOZ involves spontaneous, therapist-led clinical conversations. The experiment evaluated the model's ability to generalize emotionally correlated depressive cues to naturalistic speech settings.

In the training phase, RAVDESS dataset classes were grouped into two categories reflecting depressive affect:

1. Depressed-like: sad, fear, disgust, anger
2. Non-depressed-like: neutral, calm, happy, surprise

From Table 3 we could see that the hybrid fusion model produced a 71.5% accuracy, precision = 0.731, recall = 0.740, and F1-score = 0.735 on the RAVDESS test set, showing a strong balance between sensitivity and specificity within an emotion-rich environment. When evaluated on DAIC–WOZ without any fine-tuning, the model maintained a cross-corpus accuracy of 65.6% and a class-weighted F1-score of 0.6099, outperforming all single-branch variants. Despite the significant domain

Table 3 Performance of the proposed hybrid fusion model trained on RAVDESS dataset and tested on DAIC–WOZ dataset

Dataset	Accuracy	Precision	Recall	F1-score
RAVDESS	0.715	0.7310	0.7400	0.7350
DAIC–WOZ (Cross-Corpus)	0.656	0.5971	0.6561	0.6099

shift between acted (RAVDESS) and clinical (DAIC–WOZ) recordings, the model almost preserved its original performance, showcasing robust generalization and the effectiveness of spectro-temporal acoustic feature fusion for depression-related vocal cues.

5 Discussion

The experimental results demonstrate that the proposed hybrid CNN–BiLSTM framework, integrating learned and handcrafted acoustic features, effectively detects depression from speech.

Hybrid Feature Fusion: Combining Mel-spectrogram CNN embeddings with handcrafted descriptors (MFCCs, spectral contrast, chroma, zero-crossing rate, RMS energy, Hjorth parameters, spectral entropy) improves discriminative power. Ablation studies confirm that neither feature set alone achieves comparable performance, highlighting the benefit of multi-level feature fusion.

Class Imbalance and Data Augmentation: The DAIC-WOZ dataset is imbalanced, with fewer depressed samples. Weighted sampling and augmentation (pitch shifting, time stretching, noise addition) enhance sensitivity to depressive speech, though minority-class detection remains slightly lower than non-depressed.

Cross-Corpus Generalization: Testing on RAVDESS shows that the model generalizes to unseen speakers, accents, and expressive emotions. Depressed-like classes (*sad, fearful, disgust, anger*) were mapped to `depressed`, while neutral/high-energy classes (*neutral, calm, happy, surprised*) were mapped to `non-depressed`. This heuristic mapping allows better evaluation of depression-related acoustic patterns in non-clinical speech.

Overall, this proposed hybrid architecture demonstrates robustness, generalizability for speech-based depression detection, supporting scalable, non-invasive mental health assessment in diverse real-world settings.

6 Conclusion and Future Scope

In this research, we developed a hybrid deep learning framework for automatic speech-based depression detection, combining both CNN–BiLSTM learned features with handcrafted acoustic features. The integration of high-level spectro-temporal patterns with interpretable acoustic features enhances distinguishing ability, enabling classification of depressed and non depressed speech. Weighted sampling and data augmentation solve the effects of class imbalance, improving sensitivity to minority-class depressive samples. Cross-corpus evaluation using the RAVDESS dataset reveals that the model captures depression-specific features that extend beyond the training corpus, showcasing its ability in real-world deployment. Furthermore, the integration of handcrafted features improves models' explainability, providing clinically meaningful insights into acoustic correlates of depression and supporting decision-making by healthcare professionals.

Despite these results are promising, various approaches exist for the betterment of the models performance. Combining multimodal inputs, including text-based features along with visual cues, and physiological signals, could enhance the prediction accuracy and stability. Training on larger, more diverse datasets covering multiple languages, accents would improve generalization across populations. Advanced data augmentation techniques, including generative approaches, can further enrich minority-class samples and alleviate residual class imbalance.

References

1. World Health Organization, Depression (2023). [Online]. Available: https://www.who.int/news-room/fact-sheets/detail/depression
2. Kessler, R.C., et al.: The epidemiology of major depressive disorder: Results from the National Comorbidity Survey Replication (NCS-R). JAMA **289**, 3095–3105 (2003)
3. Wang, Y., Gorenstein, C.: Psychometric properties of the PHQ-9: a systematic review. Brazilian J. Psych. **38**, 201–208 (2016)
4. Patel, V., et al.: The Lancet Commission on global mental health and sustainable development. The Lancet **392**, 1553–1598 (2018)
5. Cummins, N., et al.: A review of depression and suicide risk assessment using speech analysis. Speech Commun. **71**, 10–49 (2015)
6. Fatima, E., Dhanda, N., Zaidi, T.: AI-powered depression detection using text and speech. Int. J. Multidiscip. Res. (IJFMR) **7**(3), 1–6 (2025). https://www.ijfmr.com/research-paper.php?id=45385
7. Maran, P.L., Braquehais, M.D., Vlaic, A., Alonzo-Castillo, M.T., Vendrell-Serres, J., Ramos-Quiroga, J.A., Rodríguez-Urrutia, A.: Performance of automatic speech analysis in detecting depression: systematic review and meta-analysis. JMIR Mental Health **12**(1), e67802 (2025)
8. Alghowinem, S. et al.: Detecting depression: A comparison between spontaneous and read speech, INTERSPEECH, pp. 2228–2232 (2013)
9. Low, L.A., et al.: Acoustic analysis of speech for assessment of depression severity. IEEE Trans. Affect. Comput. **2**, 123–132 (2011)
10. Gratch, J. et al.: The Distress Analysis Interview Corpus of human and computer interviews, LREC (2014)

11. Livingstone, S., Russo, F.A.: The Ryerson audio-visual database of emotional speech and song (RAVDESS). PLoS ONE **13**, e0196391 (2018)
12. Shen, X., Zhao, L.: Depression recognition using voice-based pre-training model. Nat. Sci. Rep. (2024). https://www.nature.com/articles/s41598-024-63556-0
13. Lee, K., Wang, M.: Method Matters: Enhancing Voice-Based Depression Detection with Acoustic Features and Self-Reports, PMC (2025). https://pmc.ncbi.nlm.nih.gov/articles/PMC12122156/
14. Wang, L., Chen, S., Fusing features of speech for depression classification based on weighted soft voting strategy. Computers in Human Behavior (2022). https://www.sciencedirect.com/science/article/pii/S0167639322001029
15. Li, H., Zhang, Q.: Acoustic-based machine learning approaches for depression detection in Chinese university students. Frontiers in Public Health (2025). https://www.frontiersin.org/journals/public-health/articles/10.3389/fpubh.2025.1561332/full
16. Chen, X., Liu, Y.: Automatic recognition of depression based on audio and language information fusion, PMC (2024). https://www.ncbi.nlm.nih.gov/pmc/articles/PMC10921287/
17. Zhang, Y., Patel, R.: Manifestation of depression in speech overlaps with personality, Nature Scientific Reports (2023). https://www.nature.com/articles/s41598-023-35184-7
18. Radhakrishnan, V., Aadharsh Aadhithya, A., Mohan, J., Visweswaran, M., Jyothish Lal, G., Premjith, B.: Voice cloning for low-resource languages: investigating the prospects for Tamil. Automatic Speech Recognition and Translation for Low Resource Languages, pp. 243–257 (2024)
19. Chowdary, D.E., Ganesan, R., Dabbara, H., Lal, G.J., Premjith, B.: Transformer-based multilingual automatic speech recognition (ASR) model for dravidian languages. Automatic Speech Recognition and Translation for Low Resource Languages, pp. 259–273 (2024). https://doi.org/10.1002/9781394214624.ch13.

Multi-task Learning and GAN-Based Enhancement for Automated Assessment of Cleft Palate Speech

C. M. Rohith and G. Jyothish Lal

Abstract Hypernasality and decreased clarity are common in people with cleft palate (CP), a birth defect that notably affects speech production. Accurate evaluation of intensity and efficient speech improvement are essential for directing operative treatment and treatment design. Nevertheless, existing methods depend mainly on clinical decisions or limited signal processing, often limited by small datasets and individual differences. This work presents an integrated deep learning system that simultaneously performs the classification of intensity and improvement of speech for CP speech. Manually designed speech features (MFCCs, formants) are combined with deep contextual embeddings derived from a pretrained Wav2Vec2 model. A convolutional neural network (SpectroCNNWithExtras) that was custom-designed enables multi-task learning for both classification of severity and nasality prediction, while a GAN-based SpeechBrain SEGAN system improves spectral quality and reduces hypernasality. Evaluations carried out on the LibriSpeech and NMCPC datasets show notable gains in accuracy of classification, performance of regression, and auditory quality compared to classical signal-based and direct learning methods. The proposed method efficiently reduces limited data availability and inter-speaker differences, delivering a clinically relevant system for dependable evaluation and individualized treatment strategy for patients with cleft palate.

Keywords Cleft palate speech · Hypernasality detection · Multi-task learning · Speech enhancement GAN · AI-assisted speech therapy

1 Introduction

Cleft palate (CP) is a birth-related craniofacial malformation in which an opening in the roof of the mouth forms an atypical connection between the oral and nasal chambers [1]. This defect disrupts the normal physiology of speech production because

C. M. Rohith · G. Jyothish Lal (✉)
Amrita School of Artificial Intelligence, Amrita Vishwa Vidyapeetham, Coimbatore, India
e-mail: g_jyothishlal@cb.amrita.edu

P. Singh et al. (eds.), *Deep Learning Applications in Healthcare and Medical Imaging Practice*, Studies in Big Data 193, https://doi.org/10.1007/978-3-032-21009-8_7

the velopharyngeal valve inadequately seals during speech articulation. As a result, excessive nasal airflow and resonance occur, causing a hypernasal quality, lowered intraoral pressure, and diminished consonant strength. In addition to hypernasality, speakers with CP frequently demonstrate misarticulated consonants, nasal sound replacements, and decreased overall clarity, all of which have a profound impact on communication and social interaction [2]. Precise and quantitative evaluation of speech performance is therefore critical for medical management, rehabilitation design, and ongoing monitoring of pediatric CP cases.

Currently, speech assessment for CP patients is predominantly carried out by speech-language clinicians (SLPs) through perceptual judgment of hypernasality severity. Though this technique is considered as a clinical approach, it experiences various limitations. To begin with, subjective judgments are naturally subjective and may vary between evaluators. Second, these assessments are time-consuming and require expert participation [3]. In addition, the availability of trained speech therapists is limited in many regions, especially in resource-limited healthcare environments, causing delayed diagnosis and treatment. These issues reveal the urgent necessity for automatic, quantitative, and accessible solutions designed for identifying hypernasality and classifying severity.

During the last two decades, researchers have explored various signal-processing methods to solve this problem. Early studies mainly rely on manually designed acoustic features such as Mel-frequency cepstral coefficients (MFCCs), linear prediction residuals, formant-based cues, and excitation source features to describe the speech anomalies found in CP speech. Although these features were able to measure components of nasal quality and articulatory escape, their accuracy was often limited by speaker variation, recording irregularities, and poor cross-dataset transferability. In recent years, progress in deep learning has enabled end-to-end modelling of impaired speech, with CNNs and RNNs have achieved improved accuracy in hypernasality detection. Despite this progress, many existing approaches remain restricted to binary classification (normal versus hypernasal) or depend on private clinical data, thus restricting repeatability and broad application.

To tackle these issues, we present a DL-based system for automated severity classification and improvement of CP speech. A key challenge in this domain resides in the shortage of large-scale, publicly available CP speech datasets, limiting the training of reliable models. To resolve this limitation, we use the LibriSpeech dataset, which is publicly available and apply regulated artificial nasalization modifications to test and development clean audio samples, resulting in four unique levels of the severity of nasality, like Normal, Mild, Moderate, and Severe. This artificial generation of data allows the generation of an extensive and annotated dataset, including uniform data suitable for robust model training and evaluation.

From the preprocessed audio samples, we capture diverse speech features that include Mel-frequency cepstral coefficients (MFCCs), log-mel spectrograms, formant features, and deep embeddings obtained from a pre-trained Wav2Vec2 model. These features capture not only spectral characteristics but also phonetic patterns associated with hypernasal vocalizations. Using this varied feature set, we construct a convolutional neural network (SpectroCNNWithExtras) allowing multi-objective training, performing both severity classification and Objective Hypernasality Measure (OHM) prediction. The OHM offers a continuous, numerical measure, enriching the categorical severity labels.

The key contributions presented in this work are as follows:

- Development of a synthetically generated nasality dataset created from the LibriSpeech dataset, enabling a four-level severity rating in spite of the absence of extensive pathological speech collections.
- Construction of an acoustic feature extraction system combining MFCCs, spectrograms, formants, and Wav2Vec2 embeddings for capturing important spectral–resonance variations related to CP speech.
- Development and training of a multi-task CNN performing simultaneous severity-level classification and OHM regression, improving objective evaluation abilities.
- Using a GAN-based enhancement system (SpeechBrain SEGAN) to improve the quality and acoustic accuracy of nasalized speech.
- Empirical validation and stability analysis performed using the NMCPC cleft palate speech dataset, showing the flexibility and transferability of the proposed system to real-world clinical speech.

Overall, the work shows the effectiveness and capability of combining artificial data creation, diverse feature extractions, DL classification, and GAN-based improvement to attain quantitative, scalable assessment and improvement of CP speech. In this research, the following sections are organized as follows. Section 2 presents the related work in the classification of cleft palate speech. Section 3 describes the materials and methods, including the dataset description, the preprocessing, model training and evaluation, followed by Sect. 4 explains the proposed methodology, which includes data preparation, feature extraction, model architecture, training and optimization, speech enhancement, and spectrogram visualization. Section 5 includes experimental results, discussing the classification and regression performance, speech enhancement results, discussion. Section 6 consists of a conclusion, which contains an analysis of the research and the future scope.

2 Related Works

In recent years, adversarial learning has been explored to enhance cleft lip and palate speech intelligibility. Chen et al. [4] proposed a Cycle-Consistent Adversarial Network (CycleGAN) to transform hypernasal speech to more intelligible normal speech without paired data. Their method significantly improved objective speech quality metrics and achieved promising perceptual results for cleft palate speech enhancement.

He et al. [5] proposed a dual-phase system applying Gaussian Mixture framework on a large Mandarin cleft palate (CP) collection to group four stages of hypernasality–normal, mild, moderate, and severe–and detect consonant omission. Their approach attained approximately 80% accuracy in hypernasality grading and over 94% accuracy in consonant omission detection, showing the effectiveness of acoustic modeling in CP speech evaluations. Mathad et al. [6] developed an attention-based Bi-LSTM model for hypernasality evaluation in children observed with CP. By highlighting audio segments including nasalization features, their model attained a strong correlation with clinical scores, outshining traditional BLSTM architectures and validating perceptual studies that recognize vowels most indicative of the intensity of severity.

Song et al. [7] implemented transfer learning using automatic speech recognition (ASR) models to enhance hypernasality degree estimation. They preconfigured a sequence-to-sequence ASR framework on large speech-to-text corpora and adapted the feature extractor on cleft palate datasets, gaining from better generalization and acoustic feature extraction, resulting in improved hypernasality prediction results. Vikram et al. [8] developed a novel model for classifying nasalized voiced stops in CP speech by applying epoch-synchronous spectral features and rule-based segmentation. Their approach outperformed traditional MFCC-based approaches and hidden Markov model segmentation, allowing precise classification of nasalized versus normal voiced stops, which are primary signs of velopharyngeal insufficiency.

Saxon et al. [9] introduced Nasalization-Articulatory Precision (NAP) features merging lightly supervised acoustic models learned solely on normal speech with linear classifiers to evaluate hypernasality in dysarthric and cleft palate speech. Their method adappted well among speech disorders and outperformed both neural network and handcrafted features, providing explainable representations aligning with clinical judgment. He et al. [10] introduced an automatic assessment system for resonance-articulation abnormalities in Mandarin CP speech. Using a large CP speech database, they implemented Gaussian Mixture Models with features like Shannon entropy-based energy, Teager energy operator, MFCCs, and formant measures to obtain stable four-level hypernasality classification and detect consonant misarticulation, connecting clinical-based assessment and objective speech analysis.

Xu et al. [11] proposed a deep learning model fusing spectral and temporal features with a convolutional recurrent neural network for automatic severity analysis in cleft palate speech. Applying both spectral features and articulatory information, their system achieved improved classification accuracies over conventional acoustic-based systems on clinical datasets.

Nomo Sudro et al. [12] applied cycle-consistent adversarial networks (CycleGAN) to improve the clarity of cleft lip and palate (CLP) speech. The model is trained on native Kannada-speaking children to convert pathological speech into normal speech without using parallel datasets. This technique produced major gains in ASR performance and perceptual speech quality in comparison with traditional non-negative matrix factorization (NMF) approaches, highlighting its effectiveness to support speech therapy and improve access to voice-based technologies. Cornefjord et al. [14] applied an AI approach to evaluate velopharyngeal competence (VPC) in children with cleft lip and palate. By applying CNN and the pre-trained VGGish model to retrospective audio data, they obtained moderate classification accuracy (57.1% with VGGish) on a three-level VPC scale. The authors identified challenges, including data inconsistency and speaker diarization, underlining the relevance of expanded, standardized datasets for medical implementation.

Vasquez-Correa et al. [15] proposed unsupervised representation learning methods using convolutional and recurrent autoencoders to categorize pathological speech from individuals with cleft lip and palate as well as Parkinson's disease. The model identified key features through decoding loss across spectral bands, obtaining performance scores of up to 97% for CLP speech, emphasizing the potential of deep learning to detect minor pathological speech traits beyond handcrafted features. Wang et al. [16] designed HypernasalityNet, a deep recurrent neural network combining LSTM layers to automatically identify hypernasal speech in Mandarin-speaking children diagnosed with cleft palate. The model employs vocal tract features and shows increased feature capturing and classification performance compared to shallow classifiers, getting an accuracy of 93.35%. In addition, they examined vowels sensitive to hypernasality, noticed that /i/ and /u/ carried the most prominent nasalization signals

Overall, these works show a growing tendency to apply deep learning, adversarial training, attention mechanisms, and AI-driven evaluation methods to tackle issues in evaluating and improving pathological speech in cleft palate groups. Despite these findings, current efforts mainly concentrate on increasing data availability, confirming clinical validation, and increasing cross-linguistic adaptability.

3 Materials and Methods

3.1 Datasets

In this research, we employed a publicly available and expert-verified dataset for model development and validation:

- LibriSpeech: A large-scale English speech dataset containing approximately 1,000 hours of spoken utterance data. In this study, 100 hours of data were taken from the training-clean subset, along with the validation-clean and test-clean sets, in order to produce synthetic nasalized audio speech. Synthetic nasalization was methodically introduced to reproduce various severity levels–Normal, Mild, Moderate, and Severe–allowing analysis of the system under different speech conditions.
- NMCPC: The New Mexico Cleft Palate Center (NMCPC) dataset contains audio clips of around 73 children aged between 9.2 ± 3.3 years–41 classified as Cleft Lip and Palate (CLP) and 32 controls. The dataset contains American English recordings comprising 7-69 sentences per participant, labelled with expert-rated severity categories (Mild, Moderate, Severe) and nasality values. Each recording contains an audio file, associated text, speaker ID, and classification label that is conducted by the speech processing experts.

3.2 Preprocessing

The preprocessing framework includes multiple critical steps to handle the audio samples for model tuning. Primarily, the acoustic features like MFCCs, formant frequencies (F1–F3), Harmonics-to-Noise Ratio (HNR), and spectral tilt were extracted from unprocessed audio signals to capture both frequency-domain and resonance characteristics. To include these advanced contextual speech features, embeddings were extracted using a pretrained Wav2Vec2 architecture, which produced consistent, high-level representations. Furthermore, artificial nasalization was introduced as a data augmentation method to reproduce multiple levels of severity of hypernasality and enhance the variety of training examples. During preparation, sampling rates of audio were set to 16 kHz, and audio clips were carefully adjusted in time span to provide a consistent input length for the DL framework.

3.3 Model Training and Evaluation

The framework was learned by applying a fused feature collection consisting of MFCCs, formants, HNR, spectral tilt, and Wav2Vec2 representation, with the framework designed to classify the speech into four levels of severity classes: mild, severe, normal, and moderate. The train data, along with the test and development data to which synthetic nasalization was applied, were all combined and in the stage of data preprocessing and then split into train, validation, and test data in the ratio of 70:15:15. The multi-task model simultaneously performed multi-class classification and OHM regression through a weighted sum of cross-entropy and mean squared error losses. Training used the Adam optimizer with an initial learning rate of 0.001 and dynamic reduction on plateau. The Evaluation phase includes an external evaluation on the NMCPC dataset to assess adaptability. Evaluation metrics consisted of classification measures and MAE. After the classification, SpeechBrain SEGAN framework increases the quality of speech with increased validation using evaluation metrics like PESQ, STOI, and SI-SDR. This integrated model provides a stable, clinically relevant assessment and enhancement of CP speech.

4 Proposed Methodology

In this research, merging high-level speech signal processing, hybrid-feature integration, and DL for consistent model evaluations and enhancement. The proposed model includes synthetic data augmentation, feature computation, multi-task optimization, and post-classification speech restoration as seen in Figs. 1 and 2, which is supported by the comprehensive experimental evaluations.

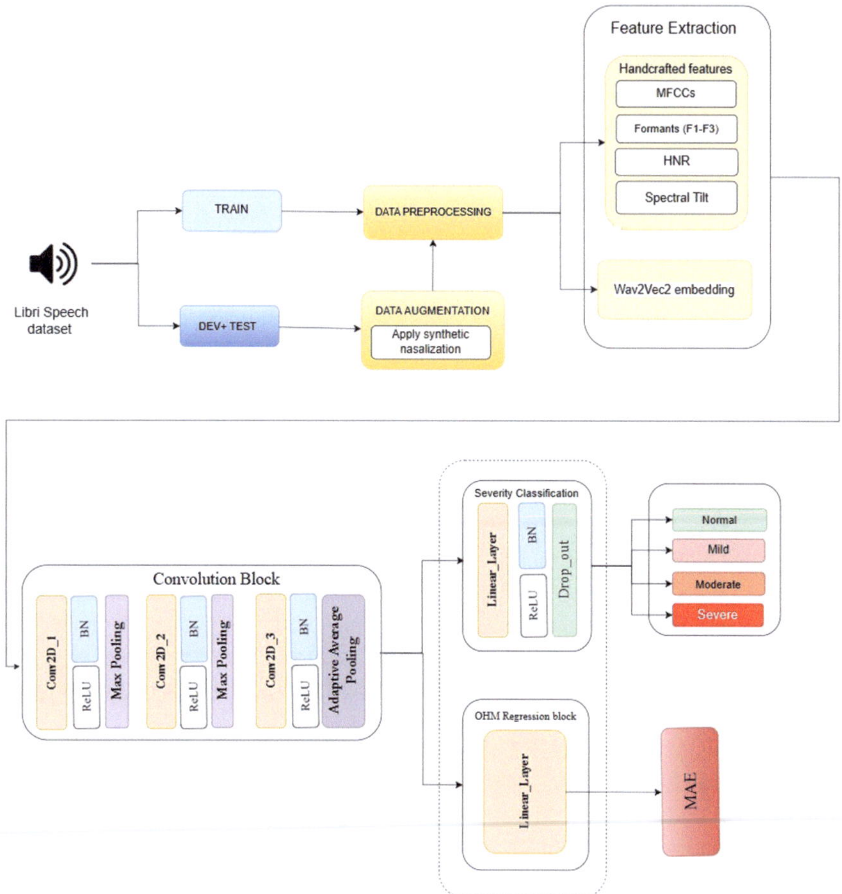

Fig. 1 Schematic diagram of classification pipeline

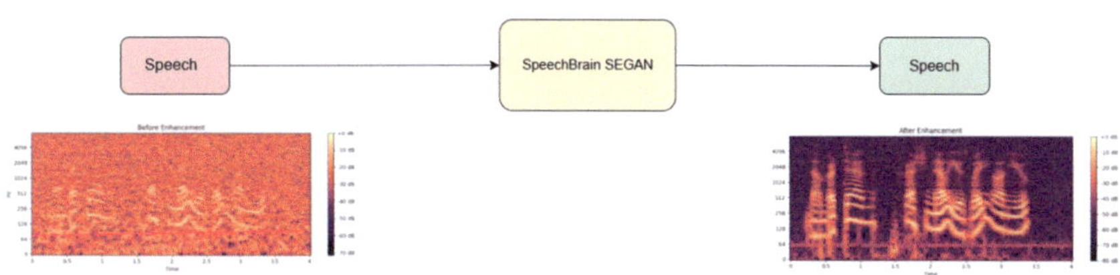

Fig. 2 Schematic diagram of speech enhancement pipeline

4.1 Data Preparation

- Synthetic Augmentation: Controlled nasalization is implemented in this research on the LibriSpeech dataset (dev-clean and test-clean) through digital signal processing (DSP) approaches. The nasalization parameter comprises notch filter frequencies and frequency range, octave-based spectral tilt, and HNR levels were fine-tuned for each class across intensity class: Severe, Normal, Mild and Moderate.
- Clinical Data: The NMCPC dataset consists of clinician-labeled CP audio samples with severity levels and is used for external validation to confirm system adaptability and clinical utility.

4.2 Feature Extraction

The feature capturing phase merges both hand-crafted and deep features embedded to capture a wide range of speech characteristics. Manually designed characteristics comprise 13-D MFCCs, including first- and second-order temporal coefficients, creating a 39-D combined feature set. In addition, acoustic characteristics such as the F1–F3, HNR, and overall spectral tilt are extracted to represent vocal tract patterns and voice quality.

For representations of deep features, 768-D vectors are derived from the pre-trained wav2vec2-base model, which captures sequential speech patterns directly from original audio signals. Moreover, log-mel spectrograms with 64 mel bins are created and normalized to deliver organized inputs for CNN models.

4.3 Model Architecture

The proposed model, called SpectroCNNWithExtras, fuses spectrogram-based representations with extra manually designed and deep features to assess hypernasality. The CNN backbone comprises 3 convolutional blocks, each with 3×3 kernels, with filter channels increasing from 1 to 32, 32 to 64, and 64 to 128. Every module incorporates batch normalization, ReLU activation, and max-pooling layers in the first 2 layers to promote stable learning and reduce feature map dimensions as shown in Fig. 1. Adaptive average pooling of 1 x 1 is applied to the last layer inorder to specify the target output dimension, and also keeping this as 1 x 1 is does same as global average pooling.

The pooled spectrogram features are merged with the handcrafted and deep embeddings, and passed through a fully connected layer with 256 units, ReLU activation, and a dropout rate of 0.3 for regularization. The architecture utilizes a dual-head design: a softmax output for four-class categorical severity prediction (Normal=0,

Mild=1, Moderate=2, Severe=3), and a linear regression branch for estimating the Overall Hypernasality Measure (OHM). Model training is driven by a combined weighted loss function defined as

$$L_{\text{total}} = (1 - \lambda)L_{\text{CE}} + \lambda L_{\text{MSE}}, \quad \lambda = 0.5,$$

where L_{CE} and L_{MSE} denote the cross-entropy and mean squared error losses, respectively.

4.4 Training and Optimization

LibriSpeech dataset consists of train, dev and test data. To the dev and test set, synthetic nasalization is applied, and all three sets are then combined when passed to the preprocessing part, and they are split into train, validation and test in the ratio of 70:15:15, and the train set is used for the model training, which contains 100 hours of audio recordings. The AdamW optimizer with a learning rate of 3×10^{-4}, a batch size being 16, epochs being 35 epochs, with early stopping initiated by validation loss to prevent overfitting, was used for training. Data augmentation techniques, including background noise along with the pitch and time-scale modifications, were implemented to improve model robustness. Model effectiveness was evaluated through accuracy, class-wise F1-score, and mean absolute error (MAE) for the OHM. Furthermore, external testing using the NMCPC dataset was performed.

4.5 Speech Enhancement

A GAN-based SpeechBrain SEGAN framework was used following the classification process, focusing on mild, moderate, and severe CP speech recordings to reduce hypernasality and enhance overall clarity. The improvement module operates in a GAN model, including a generator that generates restored speech waveforms from nasalized samples, and a discriminator that distinguishes the improved results from real clean samples. USING GAN-based training, the generator learns to reduce unnecessary noise, reconstruct harmonic patterns, and restore absent spectral details while dealing with natural voice quality and phonetic structures. During the evaluation, the generative network is the only one used, creating enhanced speech straight in the waveform space. The pipeline integrated in this research includes the waveform capturing, normalization, followed by the preprocessing, SEGAN-based improvement, denormalization, and final output generation, with resampling of the signal to 16 kHz used to ensure the proposed framework's stability. The raw and processed signals were quantitatively measured using standard validation metrics, including PESQ, STOI, and SI-SDR, to assess improvements in voice clarity and noise minimization. Also, the measure of the reduction of error in the speech before and after enhancing is assessed using the metric Word Error Rate (WER). This SEGAN-based enhancement framework successfully reduces low-frequency and high-frequency resonance irregularities, producing polished speech signals, minimizing hypernasality, and refining speech quality across all levels of CP severity.

4.6 Spectrogram Visualization

Log-mel spectrograms were produced, and then they were visualized with matplotlib and librosa libraries to offer a visual assessment of the improvement effects. The spectrogram plot shown has time in seconds on the x-axis, frequency in hertz on the y-axis, with hue level showing energy measured in dB. The improved spectrograms displayed sharper high-frequency elements and a clear decrease in energy that is excessive across low-to-mid resonance regions, showing the performance of the improvement technique.

5 Experimental Results

The presented SpectroCNNWithExtras architecture was thoroughly tested on both artificial and clinical datasets to verify its performance in classifying CP speech intensity and predicting the OHM.

5.1 Classification and Regression Performance

The system's total classification precision across the four hypernasality intensity levels, like Normal, Mild, Moderate, and Severe achieved a good test accuracy of 92% after training and testing on combined train and synthetic LibriSpeech test and development data with significant data augmentation before enhancement. With a mean absolute error (MAE) of 0.2865, the regression branch used to predict the OHM showed that continuous hypernasality scores could be accurately estimated in addition to categorical classification. The number of samples for the synthetic LibriSpeech test before and after speech enhancement is shown in Tables 1 and 2.

After the speech enhancement of LibriSpeech, testing on the independent clinical NMCPC dataset yielded an accuracy of 89%, suggesting strong generalization to actual pathological speech. The number of samples for the NMCPC test before and after speech enhancement is shown in Tables 3 and 4. Both the clinical and synthetic datasets' confusion matrices (Figs. 3 and 4) demonstrate excellent predictive performance, with the majority of misclassifications taking place between adjacent severity levels, which reflects the inherent ambiguity in class transitions.

Table 1 Number of samples in each class for the synthetic LibriSpeech test set **before** speech enhancement

Class	Number of samples
Normal	60
Mild	60
Moderate	60
Severe	60
Total	**240**

Table 2 Number of samples in each class for the synthetic LibriSpeech test set **after** speech enhancement

Class	Number of samples
Normal	118
Mild	62
Moderate	37
Severe	23
Total	**240**

Table 3 Number of utterances in each class for the NMCPC test set **before** speech enhancement

Class	Number of samples
Normal	677
Mild	357
Moderate	373
Severe	406
Total	**1,813**

Table 4 Number of utterances in each class for the NMCPC test set **after** speech enhancement

Class	Number of samples
Normal	1150
Mild	345
Moderate	148
Severe	170
Total	**1,813**

Moreover, classification on the NMCPC dataset after applying the proposed SpeechGAN enhancement demonstrated an improved accuracy, which is shown in terms of count, representing a gain.

The detailed per-class performance results for the NMCPC dataset are provided in Table 4.

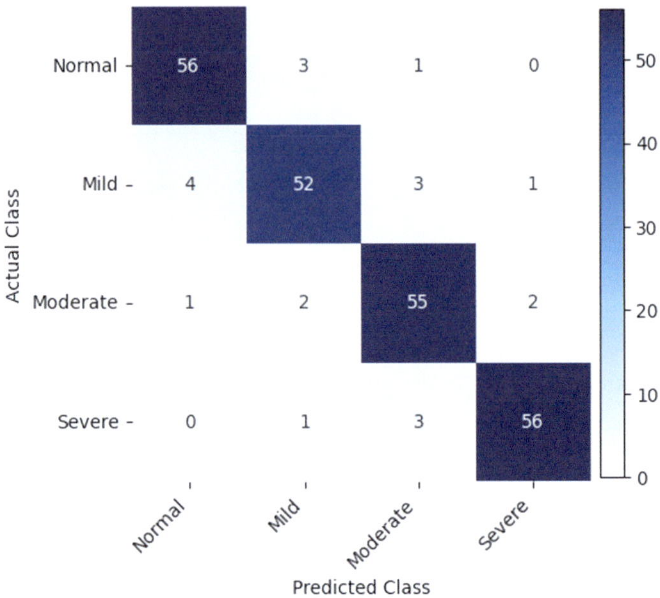

Fig. 3 Confusion matrix of synthesized LibriSpeech test data classification

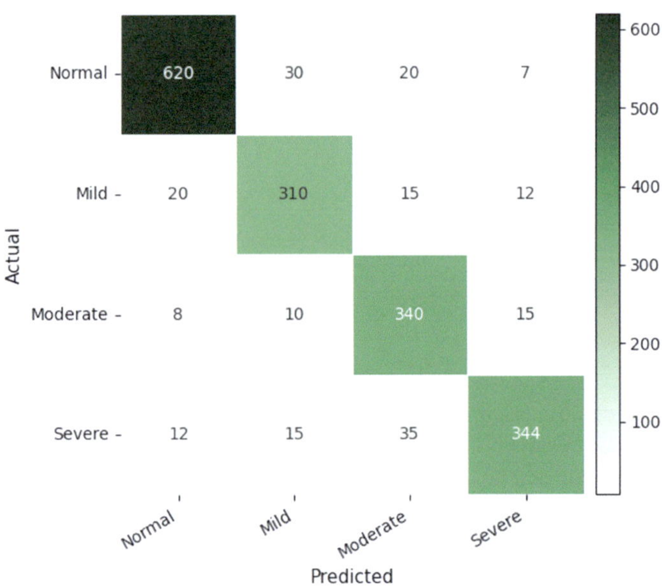

Fig. 4 Confusion matrix of NMCPC dataset classification before speech enhancement

5.2 Speech Enhancement Results

After severity classification, the SpeechBrain SEGAN model was applied to hypernasal speech samples identified by the classifier to enhance intelligibility and overall perceptual quality. The SEGAN framework utilizes a generator–discriminator setup, in which the generator learns to produce clean, de-nasalized speech while the discriminator ensures that the output maintains realistic acoustic characteristics.

Objective assessments showed significant improvements after the improvement. The PESQ score improved from 1.9 to 2.5, showing a measurable improvement in auditory quality. Likewise, the STOI score increased from 0.68 to 0.80, indicating improved speech and reduced noise of essential speech features, and SI-SDR increased from 10dB to 15dB, indicating a high quality of speech. Spectral analyses of the improved samples showed reduced low-frequency nasalization and clearer formants, mainly in the F1–F3 regions essential for vowel quality.

Figures 5 and 6 show the log-mel spectrograms of the speech sample before and after SEGAN-based enhancement of LibriSpeech test set, and Figs. 7 and 8 for

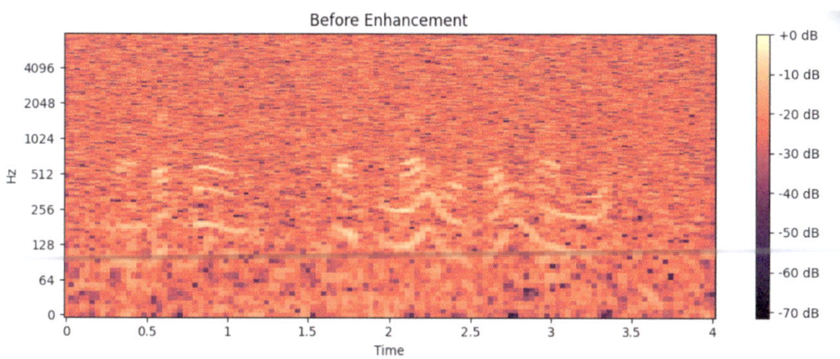

Fig. 5 Spectrogram visualization before Librispeech synthesized data speech enhancement

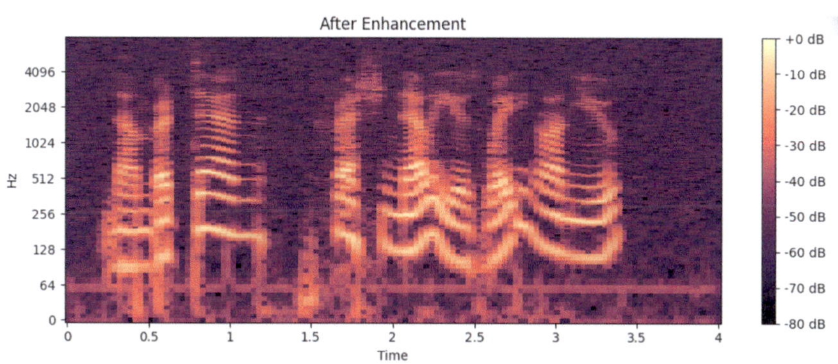

Fig. 6 Spectrogram visualization after Librispeech synthesized data speech enhancement

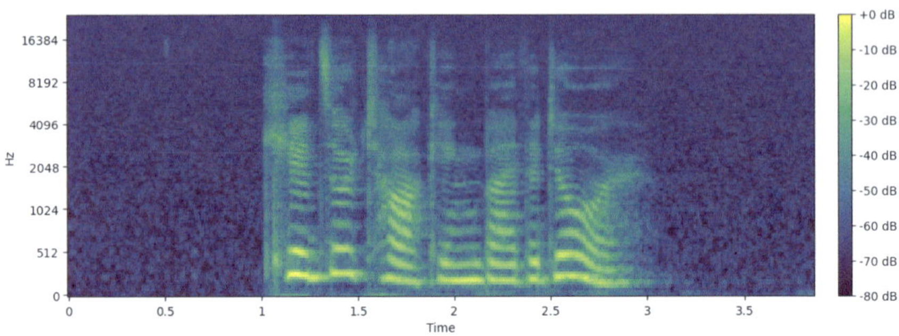

Fig. 7 Spectrogram visualization of NMCPC before speech enhancement

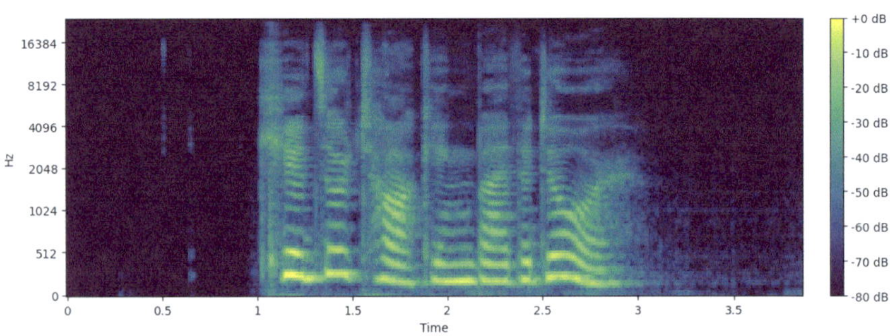

Fig. 8 Spectrogram visualization of NMCPC after speech enhancement

the NMCPC dataset. The after-enhancement spectrogram images displayed show more distinguishable high-frequency components and lowered energy in the low- and mid-frequency nasal bands, showing diminished hypernasality, and improved overall speech clarity.

5.3 *Discussion*

The experimental results show that the introduced multi-feature, multi-task learning model is highly efficient for both class-level analysis and continuous assessments of hypernasality intensity in cleft palate speech. By combining handcrafted acoustic features (MFCCs, formants, HNR, spectral tilt) with learned representations from Wav2Vec2 and spectrogram-based CNN processing, the model extracts supporting information spanning short-term spectral patterns and extended sequence relationships.

Evaluation of the confusion matrices shows that the majority of incorrect predictions occur between adjacent categories (e.g., Mild–Moderate), reflecting the inherent gradation and perceptual ambiguity in hypernasality assessment. These findings

Sentence ID	Reference Transcript	Before Speech enhancement	WER (Before)	After Speech enhancement	WER (After)
1	the boy is playing football	da boi iz payin futba	100.0	the boy is playing football	0.0
2	she sells sea shells on the sea shore	she sell see shell on da se shor	38.5	she sells sea shells on the sea shore	0.0
3	we are going to school	we a goin ta skul	33.3	we are going to school	0.0
4	please give me the pencil	plee gi me da pensil	35.7	please give me the pencil	0.0
5	the sun is shining brightly	da sun iz shinin brily	32.0	the sun is shining brightly	0.0

Fig. 9 Word Error Rate (WER) before and after speech enhancement

consist of clinical observation, where separating mid-level severity can be challenging even for expert professionals, showcasing the practical relevance of an objective, automated evaluation model.

After the post-processing, the improvement through SEGAN further validates the framework's evaluation. Improved speech samples show minimized lower-band and mid-range nasal resonance and improved high-frequency clarity, confirmed quantitatively by gains in PESQ, STOI, and SI-SDR. These improvements support medical use for objective evaluation and suggest possibilities for real-time rehabilitative feedback in the speech therapy context. To also show the error rate of words before and after enhancing of the speech is shown in Fig. 9.

Furthermore, the model shows strong performance stability from simulated datasets to the clinically collected NMCPC corpus, addressing a common drawback in previous work that relies only on small pathological recordings. This suggests that well-designed synthetic augmentation, combined with stable multi-feature learning, can successfully tackle the issue of data scarcity and enable large-scale model learning, maintaining clinical relevance.

6 Conclusion

In this research, we developed a DL framework for automatic evaluation and improvement of CP speech. By combining handcrafted features, spectrogram-based CNN features, and deep speech features using a multi-task learning framework, the proposed system achieves better classification of nasality degree and precise prediction of continuous OHM scores. After classification, including GAN-driven enhancement, produces measurable improvements in both clarity and overall speech fidelity, effectively connecting objective analysis with clinical interventions. The model was evaluated on both artificially generated and clinically collected data, showing consistency, adaptability, and clinical applicability. Importantly, the method allows scalable and replicable assessments that can increase traditional clinical analysis, providing clinicians with a reliable framework for monitoring improvements and guiding therapy.

Future research will target increasing data varieties to incorporate multiple languages datasets and capturing scenarios, developing real-time responses for speech therapy, and additionally improving the multi-tasking model to improve sensitivity to minor acoustic variations.

Overall, this framework guarantees a foundation for objective measurement, data-driven evaluation, and treatment of CP speech impairments, with considerable benefit in both clinical practice and research.

References

1. Hide, Ø., Dagrun, S.D., Åse, S., Anne, K.H., Randi, L.K., Marit, B.K., Nina, H.P., Christina, S.: Validity and reliability of speech data in the Norwegian registry of cleft lip and palate. Int. J. Lang. Commun. Disord. **60**(6) (2025)
2. Dubey, A.K., Prasanna, S.M., Dandapat, S.: Spectral analysis based objective assessment of hypernasality in cleft palate speech: A Review. Circuits Syst. Sig. Process. **44**(6), 4133–4166 (2025)
3. Raj, K.D., Jyothish Lal, G., Gopalakrishnan, E.A., Sowmya, V., Rafael Orozco-Arroyave, J.: A visibility graph approach for multi-stage classification of parkinson's disease using multimodal data. IEEE Access **12**, 87077–87096 (2024)
4. Chen, X., Zhang, J., Zhang, P., Qian, Y.: Enhancing the Intelligibility of Cleft Lip and Palate Speech Using Cycle-Consistent Adversarial Networks. IEEE Trans. Neural Netw. Learn. Syst. **32**(10), 4476–4486 (2021)
5. He, L., Zhang, J., Liu, Q., Yin, H., Lech, M.: Automatic Evaluation of Hypernasality and Consonant Misarticulation in Cleft Palate Speech. IEEE Signal Process. Lett. **21**(10), 1249–1253 (2014)
6. Mathad, V.C., Scherer, N., Chapman, K., Liss, J., Berisha, V.: An Attention Model for Hypernasality Prediction in Children with Cleft Palate. Proc. Interspeech **2021**, 565–569 (2021)
7. Song, K., Wan, T., Wang, B., Jiang, H., Qiu, L., Xu, J., Jiang, L., Lou, Q., Yang, Y., Li, D., Wang, X.: Improving Hypernasality Estimation with Automatic Speech Recognition in Cleft Palate Speech. Speech, and Language Processing, IEEE/ACM Transactions on Audio (2022)
8. Vikram, C.M., Adiga, N., Prasanna, S.R.M.: Detection of Nasalized Voiced Stops in Cleft Palate Speech Using Epoch-Synchronous Features. IEEE/ACM Trans. Audio Speech Lang. Process. **27**(7), 1189–1202 (2019)
9. Saxon, M., Tripathi, A., Jiao, Y., Liss, J., Berisha, V.: Robust Estimation of Hypernasality in Dysarthria with Acoustic Model Likelihood Features. Proc. Interspeech **2020**, 4083–4087 (2020)
10. He, L., Tan, J., Hao, H., Tang, M., Yin, H., Lech, M.: Automatic evaluation of resonance and articulation disorders in cleft palate speech. Speech Commun. **102**, 1–10 (2018)
11. Xu, W., Huang, J., Zhao, L.: Deep Learning-Based Automated Severity Assessment for Cleft Palate Speech. Speech Commun. **118**, 1–10 (2020)
12. Nomo Sudro, P., Das, R.K., Sinha, R., Prasanna, S.R.M.: Enhancing the intelligibility of Cleft Lip and palate speech using Cycle-consistent adversarial networks. arXiv preprint arXiv:2102.00270 (2021)
13. Sudro, P.N., Das, R.K., Sinha, R., Prasanna, S.R.M.: Enhancing the intelligibility of cleft lip and palate speech using cycle-consistent adversarial networks (2025)
14. Cornefjord, M., Bluhme, J., Jakobsson, A., Klint, K., Lohmander, A., Mamedov, T., Stiernman, M., Svensson, R., Becker, M.: Using artificial intelligence for assessment of velopharyngeal competence in children born with cleft palate with or without cleft lip (2024)
15. Vasquez-Correa, J.C., Arias-Vergara, T., Schuster, M., Orozco-Arroyave, J.R., Noth, E.: Parallel representation learning for classification of pathological speech: Studies on Parkinson's disease and cleft lip and palate (2020)
16. Wang, X., Yang, S., Huang, H., Yin, H., Huang, H., He, L.: HypernasalityNet: Deep recurrent neural network for automatic hypernasality detection (2019)

17. Radhakrishnan, V., Aadhithya, A.A., Mohan, J., Visweswaran, M., Lal, G.J., Premjith, B.: Voice Cloning for Low-Resource Languages: Investigating the Prospects for Tamil. In: Automatic Speech Recognition and Translation for Low Resource Languages, pp. 243–257 (2024)
18. Rohith, C.M., Geetha, P., Gupta, K.K., Shashank, A.: Deciphering the intricacies of pancreatic malignancy through advanced deep learning methodologies. In: Computational Intelligence in Data Science, E. Mercier-Laurent, B. Jayaraman, P. Ravisankar, S. Angel Deborah, and A. Jayasimhan (Eds.), Springer Nature Switzerland, Cham, pp. 196–205 (2026)

Recurrence Plot Based Nonlinear Dynamical Analysis of Electroglottography for Multiclass Physiological Voice Pathology Assessment

Anisha G. Krishnan and G. Jyothish Lal

Abstract For the detection of vocal-fold related pathologies, non-invasive modalities such as Electroglottographic (EGG) and speech signal analysis are very important. In this context, conventional features estimated using linear methods have always limitation in identifying the nonlinear dynamic variations inherent to vocal fold vibrations. This includes aperiodicity, cycle-to-cycle irregularity, and nonlinear vibratory behavior frequently seen in disordered phonation. Although recent models have shown improved classification performance, these methodologies generally require large, well-balanced datasets. Moreover, they provide limited interpretability of their acquired representations. Hence, we present a recurrence plot (RP) based framework to characterize three vocal pathologies such as Hyperfunctional Dysphonia (HFD), Laryngitis, and Vocal Polyps. RPs depict state-space evolution and show recurring structures linked to different regimes such as periodic, quasi-periodic, and irregular oscillatory nature. Recurrence Quantification Analysis (RQA) offers a collection of numerical metrics that define structural stability and variability in a mathematically rigorous way. The proposed method provides an interpretable and computationally efficient method for the objective evaluation of vocal fold disease by integrating recurrence-based modeling with supervised classification. Classification using a Random Forest model achieved high overall performance, showing an average testing accuracy of 81.58% for HFD and 79.61% for Laryngitis.

Keywords Electroglottography · Recurrence plots · RQA · Voice pathology · Nonlinear dynamics · Machine learning · Vocal fold biomechanics

---

A. G. Krishnan · G. Jyothish Lal (✉)
Amrita School of Artificial Intelligence, Amrita Vishwa Vidyapeetham, Coimbatore, India
e-mail: g_jyothishlal@cb.amrita.edu

P. Singh et al. (eds.), *Deep Learning Applications in Healthcare and Medical Imaging Practice*, Studies in Big Data 193, https://doi.org/10.1007/978-3-032-21009-8_8

1 Introduction

Subglottal airflow interacts with vocal fold biomechanics and vocal tract configuration to generate human voice. Within this mechanism, glottal closure plays a central role. The timing and completeness of closure govern how aerodynamic energy is converted into vocal fold vibration, thereby influencing phonatory periodicity, harmonic organization, and cycle to cycle stability.

Altered glottal closure is a common characteristic of pathological phonation. Abnormal contact patterns, delayed or asymmetric closure, and irregular collision behavior disturb the normal oscillatory regime of the vocal folds. As a consequence, harmonic energy is reduced and the signal exhibits increased irregularity and noise. Owing to this strong physiological relevance, glottal closure dynamics are widely regarded as a reliable indicator in objective voice evaluation [1] Direct observation of vocal fold vibration is possible through clinical imaging techniques such as laryngoscopy, videostroboscopy, and high-speed digital imaging [3]. Although these methods provide valuable insight into closure patterns and vibratory mechanics, they are invasive, costly, and unsuitable for routine or large scale screening [4]. As a practical alternative, electroglottography (EGG) has been widely adopted as a non invasive tool for assessing vocal fold contact behavior.

EGG measures variations in electrical admittance across electrodes placed on the thyroid lamina, producing a high temporal resolution signal that reflects vocal fold contact area over time. This signal is particularly effective for analyzing closure related parameters such as contact quotient, closure abruptness, and contact transition speed [5]. Because EGG directly reflects tissue contact rather than acoustic radiation, it provides access to biomechanical information that is not available from speech signals alone.

A wide range of acoustic and EGG derived features have been investigated for automatic voice pathology detection. Conventional glottal timing measures, including jitter, shimmer, open quotient, and speed quotient, have shown diagnostic relevance for characterizing abnormal vibratory patterns . In addition, spectral and statistical descriptors such as MFCCs, harmonic to noise ratio, cepstral peak prominence, and wavelet based features are commonly used in voice quality analysis [10]. More recently, machine learning and deep learning approaches particularly convolutional and hybrid CNN LSTM architectures have demonstrated improved classification performance on both speech and EGG data [11, 12].

Despite notable advances still there were several limitations. Linear acoustic features and traditional glottal measures provide only a partial description of vocal fold behavior .They often fail to represent the nonlinear and irregular vibration patterns observed in pathological phonation.These occur particularly in conditions involving unstable or inconsistent glottal closure [15]. Handcrafted descriptors are further affected by short term perturbations and nonstationary behavior, which are common in hyperfunctional and inflammatory voice disorders [16]. While deep learning models have demonstrated strong classification capability, their dependence on large labelled datasets limits practical deployment in clinical settings, and the lack of transparency in their learned representations reduces their value for physiological interpretation.

To overcome these constraints, a recurrence based analytical framework is employed to characterize the nonlinear dynamics of glottal closure from EGG signals. Recurrence plots provide a compact visual representation of how vocal fold contact states evolve over time, allowing systematic identification of periodic, quasi periodic, and irregular vibratory regimes. RQA complements this representation by extracting dynamical indicators or features. This quantify stability, temporal organization, and variability of the underlying process. These measures directly reflect changes in closure behavior that are known to accompany pathological phonation.

When applied to EGG recordings from cases of hyperfunctional dysphonia, laryngitis, and vocal fold polyp, the proposed framework captures distinct changes in glottal closure behavior associated with each pathology. The observed recurrence based descriptors reflect class-specific differences in vibratory regularity and stability, demonstrating their sensitivity to underlying biomechanical alterations.

The rest of the paper is organized as follows. Section 2 explains the related literature in the detection of vocal fold pathology. Section 3 provides the details of the dataset used in the study. Section 4 describes the proposed methodology with flow diagram, Sect. 5 discusses the results obtained and finally, in Sect. 6, we conclude the paper.

2 Literature Review

EGG has long been used to study vocal fold behavior in both normal and disordered phonation. Early studies relied on time-domain and contact-based measures extracted directly from the EGG waveform. Parameters such as contact quotient, open quotient, speed quotient, jitter, and shimmer were shown to capture changes in closure timing and contact symmetry associated with different voice disorders [5]. While these measures are clinically interpretable, their reliability decreases in pathological signals, where noise and short-term phonatory irregularities are common

To enhance classification performance, later studies introduced spectral and cepstral features extracted from acoustic and EGG signals. Features including mel-frequency cepstral coefficients, harmonic to noise ratio, cepstral peak prominence, and wavelet based descriptors have been widely applied in pathological voice analysis [10]. These approaches capture useful frequency domain and statistical characteristics, but they are largely based on linear signal representations and therefore provide limited insight into the nonlinear vibratory behavior typical of disordered phonation [9].

More recently, machine learning methods have been adopted to automate voice pathology detection. Traditional classifiers such as support vector machines, random forests, and k-nearest neighbors have shown reasonable performance when trained on handcrafted acoustic and EGG features [12]. Deep learning models, including convolutional neural networks and CNN and LSTM architectures, have further improved classification accuracy by learning task specific representations from raw or lightly processed signals [11]. Multimodal systems that combine acoustic and EGG information have also been reported to improve robustness . However, these models generally depend on large labelled datasets and offer limited transparency in terms of physiological interpretation, which remains a concern for clinical use. Machine learning has been widely adopted for automated voice pathology detection. Early studies used supervised classifiers such as support vector machines, random forests, and k-nearest neighbors to handcrafted acoustic and EGG based features, reporting stable classification performance . Recent work uses deep learning models. Convolutional neural networks and CNN,LSTM architectures have been used to learn features directly from raw or lightly processed signals [12]. Some studies combine acoustic and EGG modalities to exploit complementary information and improve robustness [?]. Despite these advances, such models usually require large annotated datasets. In addition, their internal representations offer limited physiological insight, which restricts clinical interpretability [11].

Alongside data-driven approaches, nonlinear dynamical analysis has been explored to better represent the intrinsic behavior of vocal fold oscillation. Prior work has shown that pathological phonation can exhibit chaotic dynamics, intermittency, and nonlinear transitions that are not well described by linear descriptors [20]. Recurrence plots, introduced by Eckmann et al. [18], enable visualization of repeated states in a dynamical system, while recurrence quantification analysis (RQA) provides measures such as recurrence rate, determinism, laminarity, trapping time, and entropy [17]. These metrics have been used to distinguish healthy and disordered voices by characterizing differences in vibratory regularity and stability [19].

Despite these advances, most recurrence-based studies focus on acoustic speech signals or analyse long-duration recordings. Frame-level recurrence analysis applied to EGG signals remains limited, particularly in the context of multiclass classification of laryngeal pathologies. In addition, the integration of recurrence-derived descriptors with lightweight and physiologically interpretable classifiers has received relatively little attention.

3 Dataset Description

This study uses the Saarbrücken Voice Disorders (SVD) dataset, a publicly available corpus compiled by the Institute of Phonetics at Saarland University. The database contains recordings from more than 1800 speakers collected across over 2200 sessions, covering 71 distinct clinically diagnosed pathologies. All recordings follow a standardized protocol in which speakers produce sustained phonations of the vowels /a/, /i/, and /u/ at multiple pitch levels, along with a spoken German sentence “Guten Morgen, wie geht es Ihnen?”. Signals are recorded at 50 kHz with 16-bit resolution, ensuring preservation of fine-grained vibratory detail.

Table 1 Composition of the EGG dataset across the three vocal pathologies

Pathology	No. of samples
Hyperfunctional dysphonia (HFD)	280
Laryngitis	280
Vocal fold polyp (VFP)	508
Total	**1,068**

For the present work, we consider only the EGG recordings corresponding to aforesaid tasks recorded from patients of three clinically prevalent disorders- Hyperfunctional Dysphonia , Laryngitis, and Vocal Fold Polyp . These disorders were chosen due to their high clinical occurrence and their distinct effects on glottal closure dynamics. The composition of the three pathologies are shown in Table 1

All selected recordings were resampled to 16 kHz for uniform processing and organized into class-specific folders. Each EGG signal was segmented into short-time frames of 50 ms with 50% overlap, producing multiple recurrence plots per recording. This frame-level representation increases the number of training instances while preserving the local oscillatory structure of the EGG signal.

The resulting dataset therefore comprises a large set of frame-level recurrence plots and their associated RQA features, providing sufficient dynamical observations for robust supervised classification, even under limited availability of full-length pathological recordings.

4 Proposed Methodology

The proposed framework has the following three stages.

1. Recurrence plot creation
2. Extraction of RQA features,
3. Multiclass classification

A schematic overview of the complete workflow is provided in Fig. 1. It represents a systematic pipeline for the automated classification of vocal pathologies. The process begins with a preprocessing stage, where glottal waveforms are resampled to 16 kHz. Then, it is segmented into 50 ms frames with a 50% overlap. This ensures temporal continuity. In the next stage, nonlinear features are analyzed through Recurrence Plot (RP) construction. This involves computing a recurrence matrix and applying a thresholding function to visualize the recurrence of states in the phase space.

Now, in order to quantify these variations, Recurrence Quantification Analysis (RQA) is performed. This includes metrics such as Recurrence Rate (RR), Determinism (DET), Laminarity (LAM), Trapping Time (TT), Maximum Diagonal Line Length ($L_{\max}$), Maximum Vertical Line Length ($V_{\max}$). These features serve as the

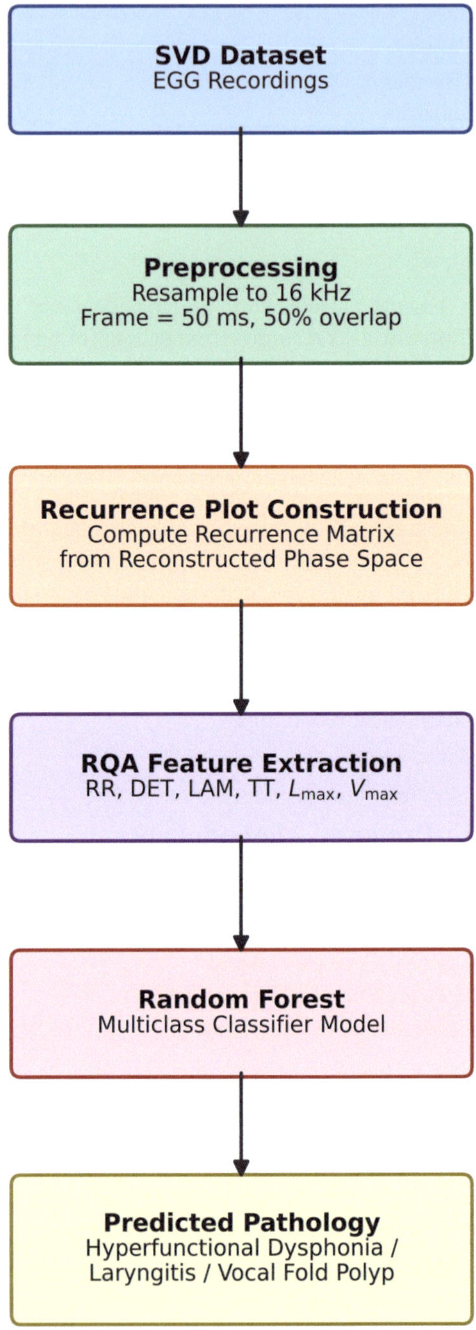

Fig. 1 Proposed methodology for recurrence-based EGG pathology classification

input for a Random Forest Model, configured as a multiclass classifier. Finally, the proposed method outputs a Predicted Pathology by categorizing the voice sample into one of three clinical conditions. (either Hyperfunctional Dysphonia, Laryngitis, or Vocal Fold Polyp).

4.1 Recurrence Plot Construction

Recurrence plots are used to study how a signal returns to similar states over time. In this work, the recurrence plot is created from short frames of the EGG signal. Each frame provides a local view of the vocal-fold vibration pattern.

Let $x(t)$ be the EGG signal. The signal has values at time steps $t = 1, 2, \ldots, T$. A frame is taken from this signal. From this frame, we rebuild the state of the system using delay embedding.

The state at index i is written as

$$\mathbf{x}_i = [x(i)\ x(i+\tau)\ \ldots\ x(i+(m-1)\tau)]. \tag{1}$$

Here, m is the embedding dimension. It tells us how many delayed copies of the signal we use. The parameter τ is the time delay between each copy. The number of valid states in the frame is

$$N = T - (m-1)\tau. \tag{2}$$

To create a recurrence plot, we measure how close two states are. If two states are close, we say they recur. The recurrence matrix has size $N \times N$. Each entry is defined as

$$R_{i,j} = \begin{cases} 1, & \text{if } \|\mathbf{x}_i - \mathbf{x}_j\| \le \varepsilon, \\ 0, & \text{otherwise.} \end{cases} \tag{3}$$

The threshold ε controls what we consider close. We choose the threshold ε using a fixed recurrence rate. This gives plots with similar density across frames and across speakers.

The final recurrence matrix is shown as a binary image. A value of one is drawn as a black pixel. A value of zero is drawn as a white pixel. The diagonal line shows self-recurrence. Diagonal bands show periodic behavior. Vertical or horizontal blocks show steady or slowly changing activity. These patterns are used later for recurrence-based feature analysis.

Recurrence analysis is well suited for EGG signals because the signal comes directly from the contact area of the vocal folds. It is not affected by the effects of the vocal-tract system, and hence the waveform is more regular than the speech signal. Moreover, it shows clear cycles of opening and closing.

In the present study, we employ short-time analysis on the EGG signal to capture local variations in the vibration. Each frame shows how the folds behave during a small time window. Recurrence analysis can highlight changes in stability and periodicity within these frames. Further, it also reveals, the dynamic variations that is hard to observe from the time-domain waveform. Irregular closures, asymmetric motion, and long open phases appear as clear patterns of diagonal or vertical structures. These patterns help to describe how the vibration changes from cycle to cycle. Because of these reasons, recurrence analysis provides a direct and reliable way to study the dynamics of vocal fold contact in EGG signals corresponding to voice pathologies .

4.2 Extraction of Recurrence Quantification Features

Once the binary recurrence matrix R is obtained, a set of six core Recurrence Quantification Analysis (RQA) measures is computed to describe the dynamical organisation of each EGG frame. These descriptors quantify recurrence density, periodic structure, laminar behavior, and the extent of coherent vibratory patterns in vocal fold dynamics.

Recurrence Rate (RR). The recurrence rate measures the density of recurrent points in the matrix:

$$\mathrm{RR} = \frac{1}{N^2} \sum_{i,j} R_{ij},$$

where N denotes the number of samples in the frame. RR reflects the overall degree of state recurrence and provides a global indication of vibratory stability.

Determinism (DET). Diagonal line segments of length ℓ_d arise when the system follows similar state-space trajectories over time. Determinism is defined as

$$\mathrm{DET} = \frac{\sum_{\ell_d \geq 1} \ell_d}{\sum_{i,j} R_{ij}},$$

and represents the proportion of recurrent points forming diagonal structures. Higher DET values indicate more regular and predictable vocal-fold oscillation.

Laminarity (LAM). Vertical line segments of length ℓ_v correspond to intervals during which the system remains in a similar dynamical state. Laminarity is given by

$$\mathrm{LAM} = \frac{\sum_{\ell_v \geq 1} \ell_v}{\sum_{i,j} R_{ij}},$$

and reflects the presence of laminar or sustained contact behavior.

Trapping Time (TT). Trapping time measures the average duration of laminar phases and is defined as

$$\mathrm{TT} = \frac{1}{K_v} \sum_{k=1}^{K_v} \ell_{v,k},$$

where K_v denotes the number of vertical line segments. TT characterizes the temporal persistence of quasi-stationary vibratory states.

Maximum Diagonal Line Length ($L_{\max}$). The maximum diagonal line length represents the longest diagonal structure observed in the recurrence plot. $L_{\max}$ captures the strongest instance of uninterrupted periodic or deterministic behavior and is sensitive to highly regular vocal fold vibration.

Maximum Vertical Line Length ($V_{\max}$). The maximum vertical line length corresponds to the longest vertical structure in the recurrence plot. $V_{\max}$ reflects prolonged residence in a similar dynamical state and is associated with extended open or mid-contact phases in vocal fold vibration.

Together, the these RQA measures provide a compact and interpretable representation of periodicity, laminar behavior, and nonlinear variability in EGG signals. These descriptors form the feature set used for subsequent classification.

5 Results and Discussion

5.1 *Characterization of the Voice Pathologies Using the RPs*

The shape and movement of the vocal folds decide how the EGG signal appear. Each disorder changes the anatomy in a different way. These changes affect how the folds close, how long they stay in contact, and how stable the vibration is.

Laryngitis occurs when the vocal fold tissue becomes swollen. The swollen mucosa becomes heavier. It also loses some of its flexibility. The folds do not close cleanly. The vibration becomes irregular because the swollen tissue moves differently from cycle to cycle. This produces unstable patterns and extra noise in the EGG signal. In the case of vocal fold polyp, there is a soft mass that forms on one fold. This makes the two folds unequal in mass and shape. The heavier fold moves differently from the other fold. Closure becomes uneven. Some cycles close fully and others do not. The open phase may become longer. This asymmetry leads to irregular and broken contact patterns in the EGG signal. We can observe inconsistent slope or "notched" appearance. In hyperfunctional dysphonia the vocal folds press together with too much force. The muscles around the larynx work harder than normal. The folds close tightly and stay in contact for a longer time in each cycle. The vibration becomes tense and highly regular. This strong and repeated closure creates stable cycles in the EGG signal.

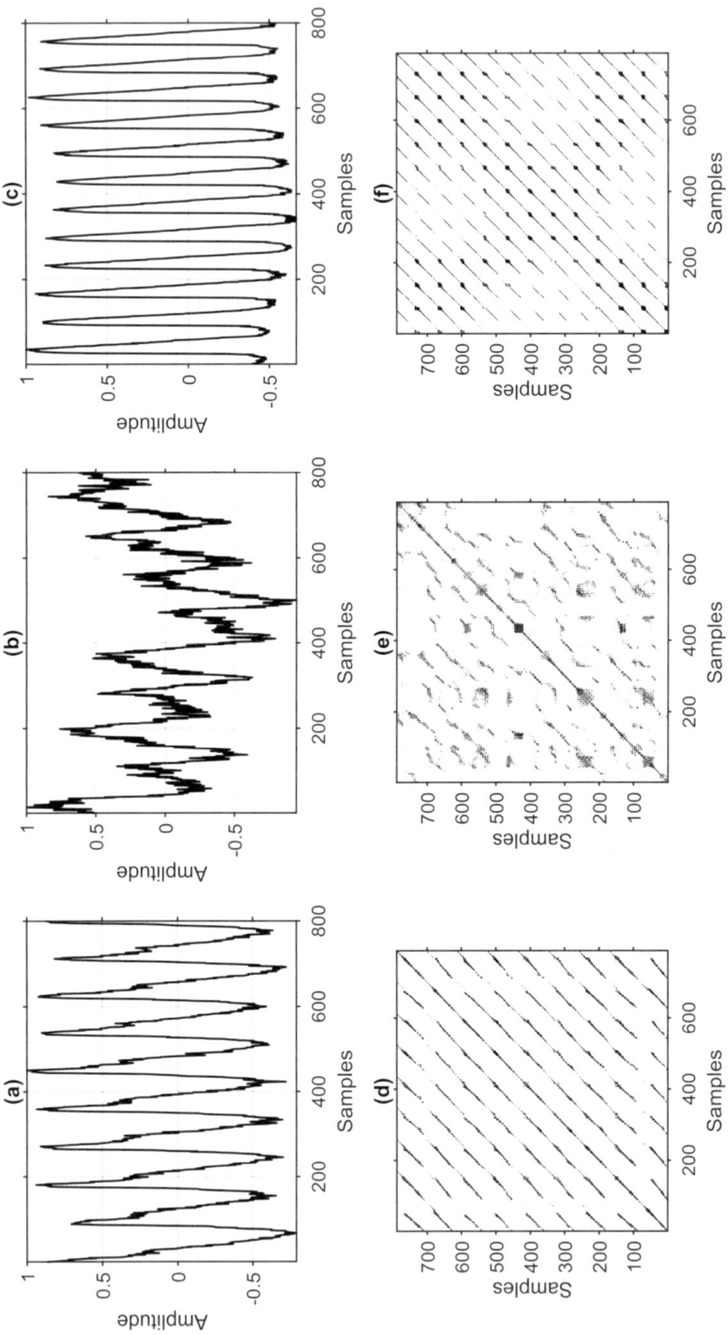

Fig. 2 EGG signal segments and corresponding Recurrence Plots (RP) for **a**, **d** Laryngitis, **b**, **e** Vocal Polyp, and **c**, **f** Hyperfunctional Dysphonia

As observed from Fig. 2a, d Laryngitis exhibits blurred and fragmented diagonal patterns with increased noise, reflecting reduced vibratory stability caused by swelling and damping effects.

Further, Fig. 2b, e reveals that Vocal Fold Polyp presents irregular, grid-like pattern superimposed on the diagonals. These vertical and horizontal structures (laminar states) represent moments where the system's state changes very slowly or is disrupted by the physical mass of the polyp.

Furthermore, we can observe from Fig. 2c, f that the Hyperfunctional Dysphonia exhibits the most stable and continuous diagonal lines. The sharpness of the lines indicates a very periodic system. Because the contact phase is prolonged, the diagonals are often thicker.

5.2 Interpretation of RQA Measures

In order to show the quantitative difference of the frames corresponding to the three pathologies considered, we have fixed Recurrence Rate (RR) of 5%. This ensures that the structural measures of complexity are comparable across different pathological classes. Figure 3 shows the Recurrence Quantification Analysis (RQA) measures for pathological EGG characterization of Laryngitis, Polyp, and Hyperfunctional classes. We find that RQA provides a dynamical behavior of the vocal folds for each pathology considered. From Fig. 3a a high DET indicates that a strong periodicity and predictability is present in Hyperfunctional dysphonia . This is because of high muscle tension which creates a very rigid, repeating cycle. In contrast, polyp has the lowest DET. This indicates that the mass causes significant irregular interruptions in the glottal cycle. Laryngitis has a moderate DET. In the case of TT, all three classes show close values, without much distinction. Next, LAM measure shows the highest value for Hyperfunctional. This reflects the prolonged, stable "closed phase", typical of high-tension voices. Again, in Lmax, Hyperfunctional shows higher value indicating a stable attractor, with long-term periodic vibration. On the other hand, polyp shows the least Lmax. This indicates the vibration is easily disrupted. Finally, polyp has the highest Vmax. This is a classic indicator of structural interference. In a nutshell, the distinctions among pathologies are better reflected by measures extracted using RQA.

5.3 Performance Evaluation of the Proposed Method

The effectiveness of the proposed recurrence RQA framework was evaluated using ten independent stratified trials. Table 2 reports the training and testing accuracies for all simulations. The classifier consistently achieved complete separation on the training data, while the testing results remained stable across trials, indicating that the recurrence-based descriptors provide a well structured feature space with strong generalization capability.

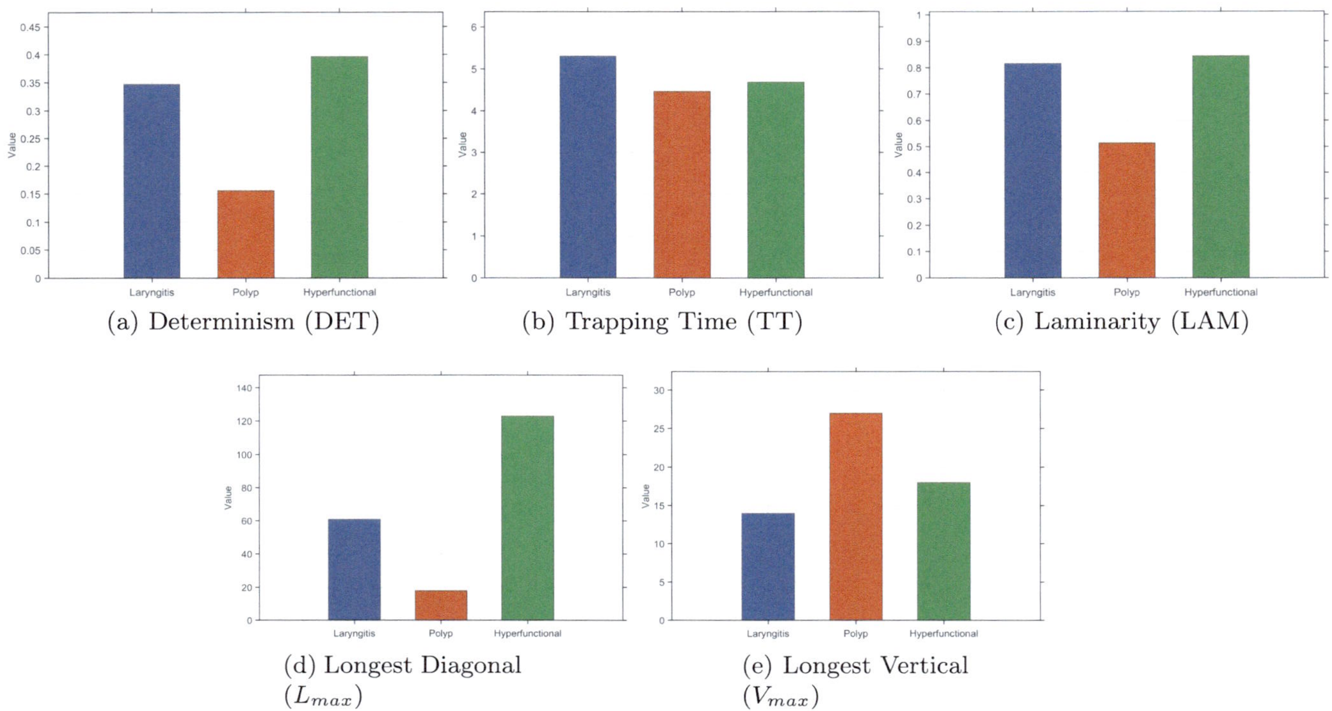

Fig. 3 Recurrence Quantification Analysis (RQA) measures for pathological EGG characterization: **a** DET, **b** TT, **c** LAM, **d** L_{max}, and **e** V_{max}. Measures are computed across Laryngitis, Polyp, and Hyperfunctional classes

Table 2 Training and testing accuracies of the Random Forest classifier using RQA features

Simulation no.	Training (%)	Testing (%)
1	100.00	76.91
2	100.00	77.03
3	100.00	76.65
4	100.00	76.73
5	100.00	77.16
6	100.00	76.93
7	100.00	77.21
8	100.00	76.82
9	100.00	76.92
10	100.00	76.94
Average	100.00	76.93
Std. Dev.	0.00	0.16

Table 3 Class-wise testing accuracies of the Random Forest classifier

Simulation no.	HFD (%)	Laryngitis (%)	Polyp (%)
1	81.67	79.75	63.14
2	81.05	80.36	63.78
3	80.99	79.52	63.62
4	81.33	79.34	63.68
5	81.82	79.99	63.61
6	81.73	79.40	63.76
7	81.96	79.63	64.22
8	81.22	79.52	63.99
9	82.15	79.13	63.38
10	81.70	79.34	63.94
Average	81.58	79.61	63.75
Std. Dev.	0.39	0.34	0.32

Table 3 presents the class-wise testing accuracies across the ten trials. It is found that Hyperfunctional Dysphonia achieved the highest recognition performance. It is followed by Laryngitis. Vocal Fold Polyp showed lower recognition. This shows its greater variability in recurrence structure. Overall, the classification performance remained consistent as seen from the small standard deviation values.

Table 4 shows the distribution of correct prediction through averaged confusion matrix. We can observe that the Hyperfunctional dysphonia (HFD) showed the better distinction, with misclassifications occurring mainly with laryngitis. Laryngitis, on the other-hand, showed more misclassifications towards HFD. Futher, vocal fold polyp showed the highest degree of confusion. This reflects the pronounced irregular-

Table 4 Averaged confusion matrix for the Random Forest classifier using RQA features

Actual/predicted	HFD (%)	Laryngitis (%)	Polyp (%)
HFD	81.58	13.62	4.80
Laryngitis	15.18	79.61	5.21
Polyp	16.79	19.46	63.75

ity and asymmetry of its vibratory behavior. Overall, these patterns are in agreement with known clinical characteristics. Thus, we show that the selected RQA features capture relevant pathology-specific dynamics.

The results obtained in the classification of the pathologies considered is consisent with known clinical characteristics of these diseases. As we know, Hyperfunctional Dysphonia is dominated by strongly periodic contact cycles. This behavior is appearing as structured recurrence patterns. Laryngitis introduces inflammatory effects, which appear as blurred diagonal lines in the RP. It in turn shows the preservation of partial periodicity. However, polyp on the other hand is characterized by mass-related asymmetry in vocal fold vibration. This leads to fragmented recurrence structures and increased ambiguity during classification.

6 Conclusion

The work presented in this paper successfully characterized the three vocal pathologies such as Hyperfunctional Dysphonia (HFD), Laryngitis, and Vocal Polyps. The proposed work employs Recurrence Quantification Analysis (RQA) of Electroglottograph (EGG) signals. The extracted RQA features demonstrate distinct variations according to the pathologies considered. Furthermore, visual inspection of recurrence plots reveals distinct topological differences for each class. Hyperfunctional dysphonia is observed to be more distinct from the other two categories. This separation is due to its relatively consistent and long-lasting patterns of vocal fold closure. While the structural complexity of Polyps proved more challenging to distinguish (63.75% accuracy), the proposed method was able to achieve testing accuracy of 81.58% for HFD and 79.61% for Laryngitis. These results show the efficacy of RQA-based features in capturing subtle physiological changes in glottal vibrations. Future research will focus on investigating supplementary recurrence features/ statistical variations to improve the accuracy of detection.

References

1. Holmberg, E.B., Hillman, R.E., Perkell, J.S.: Glottal airflow and transglottal air pressure measurements for male and female speakers in soft, normal, and loud voice. J. Acoust. Soc. Am. **84**(2), 511–529 (1988)
2. Schwarz, R., Döllinger, M., Wurzbacher, T., Eysholdt, U., Lohscheller, J.: Spatio-temporal quantification of vocal fold vibrations using high-speed videoendoscopy and a biomechanical model. J. Acoust. Soc. Am. **123**(5), 2717–2732 (2008)
3. Yamauchi, A., Yokonishi, H., Imagawa, H., Sakakibara, K., Nito, T., Tayama, N., Yamasoba, T.: Quantification of vocal fold vibration in various laryngeal disorders using high-speed digital imaging. J. Voice **30**(2), 205–214 (2016)
4. Panek, D., Skalski, A., Zieliński, T., Deliyski, D.: Voice pathology classification based on high-speed videoendoscopy. Proc. IEEE EMBC, 735–738 (2015)
5. Baken, R.J.: Electroglottography. J. Voice **6**(2), 98–110 (1992)
6. Drugman, T., Thomas, M., Gudnason, J., Naylor, P., Dutoit, T.: Detection of glottal closure instants from speech signals: A quantitative review. IEEE Trans. Audio Speech Lang. Process. **20**(3), 994–1006 (2011)
7. Henrich, N., d'Alessandro, C., Doval, B., Castellengo, M.: On the use of the derivative of electroglottographic signals for characterisation of phonation. J. Acoust. Soc. Am. **115**(3), 1321–1332 (2004)
8. Kohler, M., Vellasco, M., Cataldo, E.: Analysis and classification of voice pathologies using glottal signal parameters. J. Voice **30**(5), 549–556 (2016)
9. Islam, R., Tarique, M., Abdel-Raheem, E.: A survey on signal-processing-based pathological voice detection techniques. IEEE Access **8**, 66749–66776 (2020)
10. Kadiri, S.R., Alku, P.: Analysis and detection of pathological voice using glottal source features. IEEE J. Sel. Topics Signal Process. **14**(2), 367–379 (2019)
11. Sasikala, S., Kumar, S.A., Dharshan, P., Krupa, U.R., Muthuranjani, K.C., Nikitha, M.: Deep CNN for Voice Pathology Classification using EGG. Proc. ICAECA, 1–4 (2025)
12. Harar, P., Alonso-Hernández, J.B., Mekyska, J., et al.: Voice pathology detection using deep learning. Proc. IWOBI, 1–4 (2017)
13. Geng, L., Liang, Y., Shan, H., Xiao, Z., Wang, W., Wei, M.: Pathological voice detection using multimodal transmission network. J. Voice **39**(3), 591–601 (2025)
14. Kanagachalam, S., Kim, D.H.: Electroglottography-based classification using stacked BiLSTM–FCN network. Computer Speech Lang. 101886 (2025)
15. Henríquez, P., Alonso, J.B., Ferrer, M.A., Travieso, C.M., Godino-Llorente, J.I., Díaz-de-María, F.: Characterisation of healthy and pathological voice through nonlinear dynamic measures. IEEE Trans. Audio Speech Lang. Process. **17**(6), 1186–1195 (2009a)
16. Godino-Llorente, J.I., Gómez-Vilda, P.: Automatic detection of voice impairments using cepstral parameters and neural detectors. IEEE Trans. Biomed. Eng. **51**(2), 380–384 (2004)
17. Marwan, N., Romano, M.C., Thiel, M., Kurths, J.: Recurrence plots for the analysis of complex systems. Phys. Rep. **438**(5–6), 237–329 (2007)
18. Eckmann, J.P., Kamphorst, S.O., Ruelle, D.: Recurrence plots of dynamical systems. Europhys. Lett. **4**(9), 973–977 (1987)
19. Little, M., McSharry, P., Roberts, S., Costello, D., Moroz, I.: Exploiting nonlinear recurrence for voice disorder detection. Nat. Preced. 1–1 (2007)
20. Henríquez, P., Alonso, J.B., Ferrer, M.A., Travieso, C.M., Godino-Llorente, J.I., Díaz-de-María, F.: Characterization of healthy and pathological voice through measures based on nonlinear dynamics. IEEE Trans. Audio Speech Lang. Process. **17**(6), 1186–1195 (2009b)

AI-Aided Detection and Classification of Auricular Deformities in New Borns

Ampolu Venkata Anil Kumar, Divya Sasidharan, V. Sowmya, and Vinayakumar Ravi

Abstract Auricular deformities are one of the most common concerns in early childhood. These deformities can potentially lead to significant psychological distress, anxiety, and even hearing impairments in severe cases if left untreated. The non-surgical ear molding—a safe, effective and costless method requires to be done within the first 2–3 months of birth. However, the complexity associated with the auricle as whole and even within its sub-structures makes it challenging to accurately identify and classify them in newborns, particularly for less-experienced physicians. To address this critical need, an AI-aided approach for detecting and classifying auricular deformities in newborns is proposed, by making use of a recently released BabyEar4k Dataset that comprises of 3,852 high quality ear images acquired from 1,926 newborns. In this chapter, various single-stage and two-stage object detection models and their variants are fine-tuned and evaluated. The detection performance is assessed using the metrics: mAP50, mAP50-95 and classification performance using the metrics: accuracy, precision, recall and F1-score. The experiments resulted in YOLO-v8-L achieving the highest classification accuracy of 0.79 and Faster R-CNN with ResNet-50 backbone achieving precise localization with mAP-50 of 0.84. Additionally, D-RISE, an explainability technique is also incorporated, to generate visual explanations of model's decision logics and highlight the regions that influenced the model's decision, which is crucial especially in clinical settings.

A. V. A. Kumar · D. Sasidharan · V. Sowmya (✉)
Amrita School of Artificial Intelligence, Amrita Vishwa Vidyapeetham, Coimbatore, India
e-mail: v_sowmya@cb.amrita.edu

A. V. A. Kumar
e-mail: cb.sc.p2dsc23002@cb.students.amrita.edu

D. Sasidharan
e-mail: s_divya1@cb.amrita.edu

V. Ravi
Center for Artificial Intelligence, Prince Mohammad Bin Fahd University, Khobar, Saudi Arabia
e-mail: vravi@pmu.edu.sa

P. Singh et al. (eds.), *Deep Learning Applications in Healthcare and Medical Imaging Practice*, Studies in Big Data 193, https://doi.org/10.1007/978-3-032-21009-8_9

Keywords Auricular deformities · Neonatal health care · Object detection models · You Only Look Once (YOLO) · Faster R-CNN · Fine-tuning · Explainable-AI · D-RISE

1 Introduction

Auricular deformities are among the most common congenital abnormalities in the newborns, with prevalence as high as 30% in a certain population considered [1]. These deformities involve a wide range of irregularities, from relatively mild variations like lop ear and Stahl's ear, to more severe ones like microtia, which often attract undue attention and jokes. These 3can appear strange and may lead to mental distress, social stigma, feelings of inferiority, and difficulties in interpersonal relationships. Apart from these aesthetic and profound psychological impacts, some cases of deformities could even lead to hearing impairments when left untreated [2, 3].

There are two primary approaches by which we can treat these auricular deformities: one being surgical and the other non-surgical. Among the surgical options, autologous grafting is frequently employed, particularly in severe cases such as microtia. There are emerging regenerative therapies as well that utilize tissue engineering and stem cells to create patient-specific ear structures. However, the traditional surgical methods often involve pain, visible scarring and extended recovery time. Even the advanced regenerative surgeries are still experimental and lack comprehensive long-term outcomes [4].

On the other side, the non-surgical interventions, specifically ear molding, has gained popularity as an effective and safe method for correcting these deformities. This method is cost-effective, safe and painless which is ideally suited for infants, given that the pliability of auricular cartilage is highest within first few weeks of birth. This increased pliability is largely due to the fact that the maternal estrogens are elevated in the neonatal period, making the cartilage more malleable [5]. However, this pliability typically lasts only during the first two to three months of life and starts to decrease after this period, making the cartilage to stiffen as estrogen levels drop. Thus, early detection of these deformities is critical to ensure that non-surgical interventions can be made before the auricle becomes too rigid to mold effectively [5, 6]. Through early detection, even severe cases of deformities can be corrected partially to an extent, potentially reducing future surgical interventions [7].

Despite their high prevalence and significant impact, auricular deformities still remain underdiagnosed or misdiagnosed many yet times, due to the limitations of traditional subjective evaluations have. The consequences of delayed diagnosis or misdiagnosis extend way beyond the missed opportunity for early non-invasive early interventions; potentially even leading to psychological and functional challenges. This disparity is much prevalent particularly in resource-limited settings. This pressing need for an early and accurate deformity detection is the primary motivation of this work.

Accurate identification and diagnosis of auricular deformities remain a challenge, despite the real need for early detection to enable appropriate intervention. The auricular cartilage as a whole is quite a complex structure, with multiple substructures in it, such as the helix, lobule, concha, and tragus. Each of these substructures can exhibit a wide range of anatomical variation, making it difficult for less-experienced physicians to accurately differentiate between mild variations and more significant ones. Even experienced pediatricians, obstetricians, and otolaryngologists find it non-trivial and challenging to accurately diagnose the neonatal auricles since the auricular cartilage of newborns is not only small and delicate but also subject to developmental changes in the first few months of birth [8, 9].

Clinically, the diagnosis of auricular deformities has traditionally relied on visual inspection and observation of pediatricians or otolaryngologists. While this method can be effective, but the judgement made is inherently subjective to the experience and expertise of the physician. These challenges have spurred the interest in developing the objective, data-driven approaches to assist in detection and classification of auricular deformities. With the latest developments in artificial intelligence (AI), there is enough potential for these technologies to augment traditional diagnostic methods, providing physicians with more consistent and reliable assessments.

In recent years, AI has made significant strides in the analysis of medical images, particularly convolutional neural networks (CNNs) have emerged as a powerful tool for analyzing them. These models have the ability to learn intricate/ complex patterns associated within images, exceling in detection and classification problems. By leveraging the power of these models, researchers have already developed systems capable of detecting and diagnosing rare medical conditions, which involves dermatological, retinal and even various forms of cancer conditions [10, 11]. Recent advancements, be it the integration of transformer-based architectures or the use of advanced graph techniques, have significantly boosted diagnostic accuracy in complex tasks like skin disease classification and enabled precise classification of disease stages, respectively [12, 13].

By naturally extending these methods to otolaryngology, it is possible to create systems that can assist physicians in making more accurate and timely diagnoses. Apart from improving the speed and accuracy of diagnosis, these systems can also help in reducing the variability that comes from subjective clinical judgment.

However, a significant challenge that may hinder the widespread adaption or deploying of AI systems, especially in the field of healthcare, is the lack of transparency or interpretability of the predictions made by these black-box models. In the healthcare sector, the comprehensibility and transparency of AI systems are essential, without this transparency, AI systems can face resistance in clinical settings, where the consequences of misdiagnosis are high. Physicians need to trust and understand how the decisions are being made. This is where explainable AI (XAI) becomes invaluable, as it helps us understand the behavior, decision logics, and vulnerabilities of AI systems [14]. XAI helps in bridging the gap between the outcomes generated by the model and the physician's decision-making process, ensuring that the AI-aided detection and classification is accurate, reliable and understandable.

Addressing the challenges in accurately diagnosing auricular deformities in newborns, this chapter aims to develop a robust AI system that can assist healthcare professionals in the early detection and classification of these deformities. The main aim of the proposed study is to identify the most effective deep learning model for this task, and also by making sure that the system is both accurate and interpretable.

To achieve this, a comprehensive comparison of multiple deep learning (DL) models fine-tuned on the BabyEar4k dataset is presented. Specifically, different variants of YOLOv8 and YOLOv9, as well as various backbones of Faster R-CNN, are evaluated for their performance in detecting and classifying auricular deformities. The backbone architectures considered for Faster R-CNN include ResNet50, EfficientNet-b0, and MobileNet-v3-large. By contrasting these models with one another, the study focusses to select an effective fine-tuned model for accurate auricular deformity detection.

In addition to addressing the challenge of accurate detection, this chapter also tackles the issue of interpretability. This is achieved by integrating XAI techniques. In this study, 'Detector Randomized Input Sampling for Explanation' (D-RISE) [15] is employed as an explainability method to generate visual explanations for the model's predictions. This approach provides transparency by highlighting areas in the image the model emphasized on, while diagnosing an auricular deformity, thereby connecting the model's predictions with the physician's decision-making process.

The experiments were conducted using Paperspace Gradient's P5000 instance, equipped with 30 GB RAM, 8 CPU cores, and a 16 GB NVIDIA P5000 GPU. The models were fine-tuned on detection and classification tasks using the BabyEar4k dataset. The initial step involved detecting the auricular region, followed by classifying each image as 'Normal' or 'Abnormal.'

1.1 Contributions and Novelty

This chapter provides significant contributions to the field of neonatal healthcare, particularly in the area of auricular deformities, by utilizing AI techniques. The key contributions and novelty of this work are as follows:

1. **Fine-tuning of models**: Fine-tuning the state-of-the-art DL models on the 'BabyEar4k' dataset—a novel, domain-specific dataset—to strengthen the model's capability to generalize auricular deformities in newborns by leveraging the dataset tailored to this domain.
2. **Detailed Comparison**: A comprehensive comparison of various fine-tuned models using different evaluation metrics is provided, to provide insights into selecting the most effective model for detecting and classifying the auricular deformities.
3. **Integration of XAI**: Incorporated XAI methods to enhance interpretability by generating visual explanations for model's outcomes—providing insights into model's decision making and connecting model's predictions with the physician's decision-making process.

The rest of the chapter is structured as follows: Sect. 2 covers the related works, providing an overview of previous studies in this domain. Section 3 details the methodology, including the description of the dataset considered, preprocessing steps, evaluation metrics, model selection, model description, hyperparameters used and the explainability. In Sect. 4, the results of the experiments are presented, offering a comprehensive comparison and analysis of single-stage (variants of YOLOv8, YOLOv9) and two-stage models (various backbones of Faster R-CNN), along with the saliency maps generated through D-RISE. Finally, Sect. 5 concludes the chapter with a summary of key results and potential directions for future work.

2 Related Works

In recent years, research into using various techniques such as machine learning, deep learning—particularly deep convolutional neural networks (Deep CNNs)—has been extensively explored to assist in medical image analysis. However, the application of AI in field of otolaryngology especially for the specific task of detecting auricular deformities, remains relatively underexplored. The current literature primarily focuses on ear detection for biometric purposes, with very few studies addressing the challenge of detecting auricular deformities in newborns.

The conventional approach of diagnosing auricular deformities in newborns primarily involves physical examination and visual assessment by pediatricians, obstetricians, and otolaryngologists immediately after birth. In recent years, non-surgical intervention techniques, like ear molding, have gained significant popularity and have become a standard practice for addressing auricular deformities in neonatal period. Studies have shown that initiating the process of ear molding within the first two weeks of the birth of the newborn yields optimal results due to the auricular cartilage's pliability at this early stage. This approach is proven effective in curing the auricular deformities and in significantly reducing the need for any future surgical interventions [16]. However, the subjective nature of assessments based on the physician's experience can introduce variability in diagnosis and treatment outcomes. This variability highlights the need for AI-driven tools to support objective and early diagnosis, ensuring consistent and accurate treatment for all newborns.

Hallac et al. [8] conducted one of the early studies using CNNs to classify the ears from 2D images. Their work focused on binary classification of ears into 'Normal' and 'Abnormal' categories and reported an impressive accuracy of 94.1% utilizing the 'GoogleNet' architecture. Despite the high accuracy, there are some limitations in their approach. The dataset used in their study was relatively small, comprising of just 671 images in total. Furthermore, the images were all of consistent quality and lacked common real-world variations such as occlusions or ear cover-ups. These raises concerns about how well the model generalizes and predicts in real-world scenarios where such ideal conditions are rarely met.

Tolba et al. [17] investigated the use of CNNs for evaluating the outcomes of auricular reconstruction in patients in microtia. In their approach, the auricles in the images have been identified using auto segmentation task, followed by a binary classification to determine whether the ear was normal or reconstructed. While this work serves as a proof of AI's ability to perform objective assessments free from clinician's bias, it primarily focused on post-surgical assessments, thereby leaving a gap in early detection techniques.

Wang et al. [18] experimented with nine CNN models, such as AlexNet, ResNet, ShuffleNet etc., to evaluate the severity of microtia from 2D photographs. Multiclass classification was performed to determine whether the condition was normal, or a microtia severity from grade-I to III, with AlexNet and MobileNet achieving the highest accuracy. This work underscored the robustness of lightweight networks in clinical settings; however, the focus of research was on evaluating and assessing the severity of microtia.

Hennocq et al. [19] explored the use of DL techniques to diagnose fetal pathologies by analyzing the shape of auricles. Their study focused on two syndromes namely CHARGE and MFDGA, both of which exhibit distinct ear abnormalities. This work highlighted the potential of leveraging AI for phenotyping in fetal diagnostics, providing a non-invasive approach for identifying congenital abnormalities. Zeng et al. [20] further leveraged deep learning techniques for ear disease classification by making use of endoscopic images. Their work focused on the multiclass classification of ear diseases, specifically into eight distinct classes based on eardrum and external auditory canal. They experimented with different variants of ResNet, DenseNet, and Inception models for feature extraction and found DenseNet to be the most effective. The findings indicate that deeper architectures excel in extracting finer details from medical images, resulting in better performance. Although their work focused on ear diseases rather than auricular deformities, it underscores or emphasizes the potential of deep CNNs for diagnostic purposes.

Yuan et al. [21] employed an anchor-free, single stage detection model known as CenterNet to identify and detect ear structures from images within biometric datasets. Their study compared CenterNet with YOLO models highlighting the enhanced detection speed which is particularly important for biometric applications. This research demonstrates that ear detection has been thoroughly explored especially for biometric purposes, across numerous studies. However, the detection of ear deformities remains an unexplored objective, particularly in the health care field where there is a significant and unmet need.

Even widely recognized ear datasets, such as EarVN1.0 [22], UBEAR [23], and USTB [24], are primarily developed for biometric purposes and consist only of adult ear images. These datasets are not specifically tailored for healthcare applications, particularly for detecting auricular deformities. Their utility in achieving the goal of identifying or detecting auricular deformities is limited due to the significant changes in auricular cartilage during the first few months of birth. This makes it challenging to adapt models trained on adult ear dataset for pediatric contexts. Furthermore, the variability in ear morphology among newborns makes it harder to create robust models capable of distinguishing between slight, benign deformations and more serious deformities that require intervention.

A recent study by Wang et al. [25] introduced a large language model-enhanced interactive agent aimed at educating the public on newborn auricular deformities. This AI-based system leverages advanced language models to engage parents and caregivers, emphasizing the importance of early awareness and intervention. While both their approach and this study aim to utilize AI for improving the understanding and management of auricular deformities, their focus is primarily on public education and interactive support rather than direct clinical diagnostics. This study is distinct in its emphasis on developing a diagnostic tool tailored for healthcare providers, integrating D-RISE for interpretability and focusing specifically on detecting and classifying auricular deformities in newborns.

From the existing literature, it is clear that the evaluation of auricular deformities remains a less explored objective, with very few comprehensive or robust works addressing the challenges. Most existing studies using ear datasets focus on biometric feature analysis, and the few that examine ear diseases or deformities are constrained to using endoscopic images or 3D scans, which are often not feasible for infants. In this chapter, these gaps are addressed by developing a robust AI system tailored to detect and classify auricular deformities in newborns. Additionally, D-RISE is integrated to explain the model's predictions, ensuring transparency and a better understanding of the model's decision-making process.

3 Methodology

To develop an effective and interpretable AI system for auricular deformity detection, the proposed methodology follows a structured workflow, encompassing key stages such as data collection, pre-processing, model selection, model training, model evaluation and finally the XAI integration. Figure 1 illustrates the complete pipeline, highlighting each step involved in the detection and classification of auricular deformities.

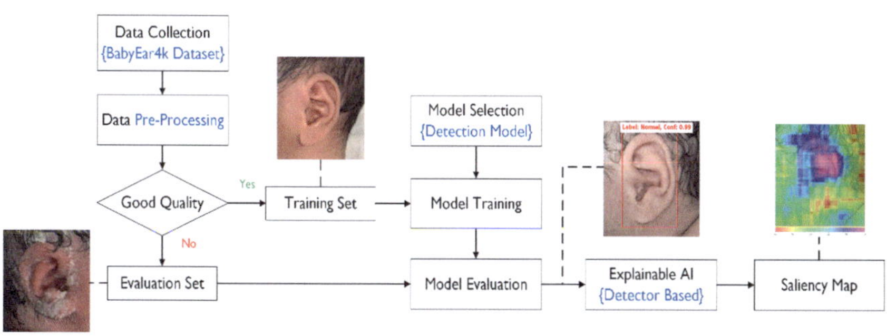

Fig. 1 Pipeline of proposed methodology

3.1 Dataset Description

In this section, the dataset employed in the study, known as the 'BabyEar4k' dataset, is discussed. This dataset was introduced in Ren et al. [3] and it comprises a total of 3,852 images, obtained from 1,926 newborns. All these images were captured in a controlled clinical environment within 48 h of birth with consistent hardware and lighting conditions, to ensure that the auricular region and its substructures are clearly visible.

The 'BabyEar4k' dataset folder consists of the following files:

a. Images:
   This directory consists of 3,852 ear images, in.jpg format, each labeled with a unique newborn ID and the side of ear (left or right).
b. Bounding:
   This is a CSV file that contains the bounding box coordinates for all the 3,852 images, precisely delineating the ear boundaries.
c. Diagnosis result:
   This CSV file includes diagnostic classifications made by two expert physicians (an ENT specialist and a pediatrician). It also includes their consensus diagnosis.
d. Image quality assessment:
   This CSV file contains the scores of each image, subjectively evaluated based on different factors such as blur and noise, cover-up, brightness and shooting angle.

3.2 Splitting of Data

The data is split into train, test and validation sets based on the quality scores assigned to each image in the '*Image_quality_assesment.csv*' file. The images were evaluated considering four key factors: blur and noise, cover-up, brightness and shooting angle. Each aspect was scored on a scale of 1 to 3, with '1' being the best and '3' being the worst.

The dataset was categorized into two main groups:

a. Good Quality: Images with a total quality score of 4 (i.e., they're rated '1' for all 4 factors) were classified as high-quality and used for the training set. This group consists of 2,081 images in total.
b. Not-so-good Quality: Images with a total quality score greater than 4 were considered of lower quality. This group contains 1,771 images in total, which were further classified into the validation and test sets using stratified split.

Figure 2 illustrates the distribution of 'Normal' and 'Abnormal' categories within each data subset. The training set has a slightly higher proportion of the normal class, as all good-quality images were intended to be included in that set. In contrast, the other two subsets are perfectly balanced due to the stratified split approach.

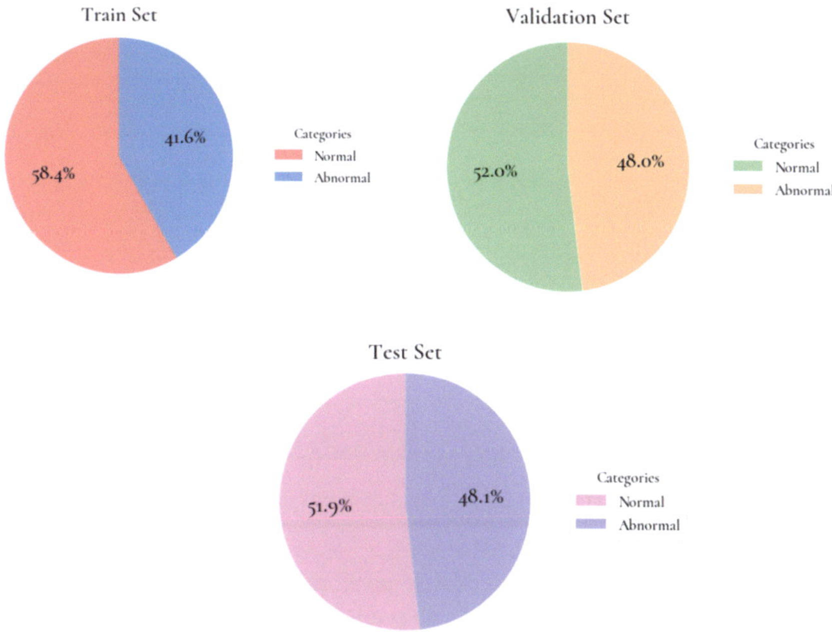

Fig.2 Distribution of normal and abnormal cases across train, validation and test sets

Figure 3a and b represent high-quality auricular images with clear visibility, minimal noise, unobstructed view and optimal lighting, making them suitable for accurate training in the model.

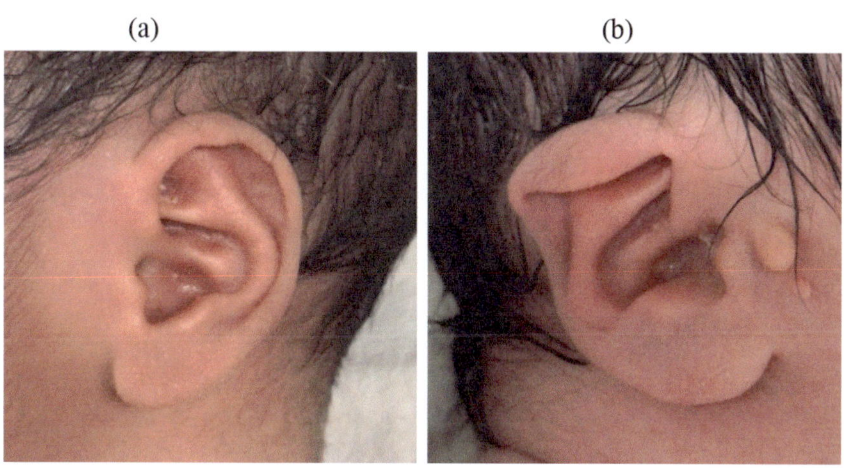

Fig. 3 Sample 'Good Quality' Images from BabyEar4k dataset

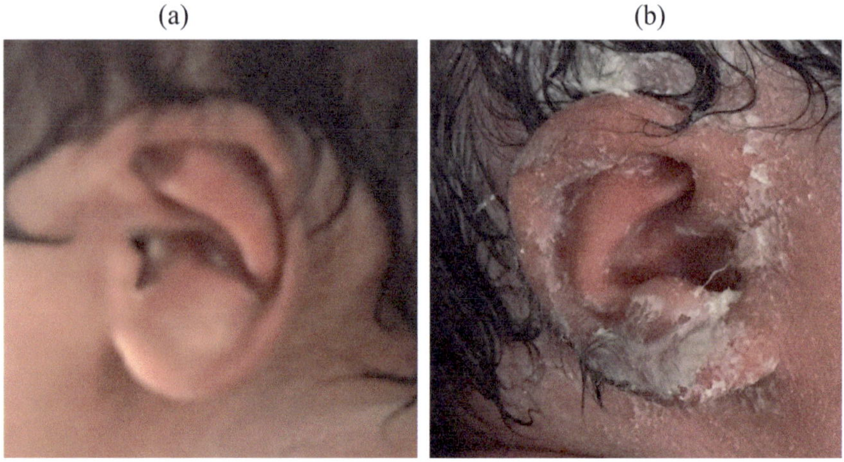

Fig. 4 Sample 'Not-so-good Quality' Images from BabyEar4k dataset

Figure 4a and b represent some Not-so-good quality auricular images, where Fig. 4a shows blur and noise, while Fig. 4b is affected by obstructions like amniotic fluid, posing challenges for accurate detection and classification, highlighting the dataset's variability and the model's need to handle diverse real-world conditions.

3.3 Model Selection

Object detection is a complex computer vision technique that extends beyond image classification, by localizing the objects within an image using bounding boxes and assigning classes to each detected object. This dual functionality makes object detection models a powerful and robust tool for a wide range of applications. Models such as YOLO, Faster R-CNN have proven their effectiveness across various domains, owing to their high efficiency and accuracy. In retail sector, these models are pivotal for effective inventory management by monitoring on-shelf product availability. For instance, Fudholi et al. [26] developed a small-scale YOLO based model for detecting grocery products on retail shelves, enabling efficient stock monitoring and replenishment. Similarly in the field of traffic management, object detection models are widely used to monitor violations traffic violations and ensure smoother traffic flow. Dwivedi et al. [27] in their recent work have utilized YOLOv7 to accurately identify and classify the traffic violations, showcasing these model's ability in intelligent transportation systems. Agriculture is another domain where object detection models are used to monitor crop health by detecting pests. For instance, Mu et al. [28] proposed a Faster R-CNN based framework to identify weed seedlings, which helps farmers in timely pest management and improves crop yield.

Healthcare is a domain where the impact of object detection models is particularly profound, given the need for timely diagnosis and treatment. Sahin et al. [29], in their study have made use of Faster R-CNN and Mask R-CNN on computed tomography (CT) images to detect and categorize COVID-19 and pneumonia infections, improving diagnostic accuracy and efficiency. In another study, Ju and Cai [30] have utilized YOLOv8 to accurately detect the presence of fractures in pediatric wrist trauma X-ray images, ensuring timely and accurate diagnosis. Building on the proven success of these models across various domains, this study leverages them to the task of detecting and classifying auricular deformities.

3.3.1 Single Stage Models

For the selection of single-stage object detection models, various YOLO versions have been evaluated based on their performance on the COCO dataset [31]. The evaluation includes YOLO versions up to the latest YOLOv11, comparing them on the basis of mean Average Precision (mAP) at thresholds ranging from 50 to 95% (mAP50-95) and inference latency.

The mAP50-95 metric is commonly used in object detection as it provides a robust measure of a model's accuracy across multiple Intersection over Union (IoU) thresholds, from 0.5 to 0.95 in increments of 0.05. This metric is particularly significant in clinical settings where accurate localization is crucial for reliable classification. High mAP50-95 scores indicate the model's ability to make precise detections, which is essential for clinical applications involving auricular deformities, where accurate and consistent detection is required.

According to existing evaluations in [31], YOLOv8 consistently demonstrates a balance between high mAP50-95 and efficient computational requirements, making it suitable for applications that demand both accuracy and speed. YOLOv8's parameter efficiency also supports its suitability for this task, where robust performance is required without excessive computational resources. Although newer versions like YOLOv10 and YOLOv11 are available, YOLOv8 offers a well-established and validated framework with competitive mAP50-95, making it a reliable choice.

YOLOv9 was also included in the study due to its improvements in accuracy and efficiency, with parameters that are comparable to those of YOLOv8. While YOLOv10 and YOLOv11 offer even better improvements in mAP and latency, the additional complexity and computational demands did not significantly outweigh the performance benefits in the context of this study's requirements. Thus, both YOLOv8 and YOLOv9 are selected for this study, as they are anticipated to deliver robust performance in localization and classification tasks.

3.3.2 Two-Stage Models

In selecting two-stage detection models, benchmark results from the Pascal VOC 2007 dataset were reviewed, covering prominent models like R-CNN, Fast R-CNN, and Faster R-CNN [32–34]. Two-stage models, particularly Faster R-CNN, are known for their high accuracy in object detection by separating region proposal from classification. Among these models, Faster R-CNN consistently achieved the highest mAP50 on the Pascal VOC dataset, with a score of 73.2%, along with relatively high execution speed. The mAP50 metric, or mean Average Precision at a 50% IoU threshold, provides a practical measure of a model's ability to accurately identify and localize objects when there is at least a 50% overlap between predicted and actual bounding boxes. While less strict than mAP50-95, mAP50 remains relevant for tasks where precise localization with moderate tolerance is important. Faster R-CNN's high mAP50 score, combined with its faster processing speed compared to earlier models, makes it a suitable choice for this study, offering a balanced approach to detection accuracy and computational efficiency.

Backbone Selection for Faster R-CNN

For the Faster R-CNN model, three distinct backbones were selected: ResNet50, EfficientNet-B0, and MobileNet-v3-large. These backbones were chosen based on their established effectiveness in object detection tasks, as documented in the literature. Each backbone brings unique advantages that align with the objectives of this study, namely deep feature extraction, efficiency, and a balanced trade-off between accuracy and computational requirements.

These backbone architectures are widely used in object detection due to their ability to extract deep, meaningful features in an efficient way. ResNet50 leverages residual skip connections to mitigate the vanishing gradient problem, making it effective for deep feature extraction in models like Faster R-CNN. EfficientNet-B0 optimizes depth, resolution, and width using a compound scaling technique, achieving high accuracy with fewer parameters, making it ideal for resource-constrained scenarios. MobileNet-v3-large, designed with lightweight architecture and squeeze-and-excitation modules, strikes a balance between model complexity and performance. These proven backbones provide robust support for detection tasks [35–37].

3.4 Model Description

In this section, the models selected for the task of auricular deformities detection are detailed. Both single-stage and two-stage object detection models were considered, with a focus on balancing performance and computational efficiency.

3.4.1 YOLOv8

As shown in Table 1, YOLOv8 offers variants from YOLOv8n (nano) to YOLOv8x (extra-large), demonstrating a progression in mAP scores as the model size increases.

Table 1 Comparison of different variants of the model -YOLOv8 [31]

Model	Size (Pixels)	mAP^{val}50-95 (%)	Speed (ms)	Params (M)
YOLOv8n	640	37.3	0.99	3.2
YOLOv8s	640	44.9	1.2	11.2
YOLOv8m	640	50.2	1.83	25.9
YOLOv8l	640	52.9	2.39	43.7
YOLOv8x	640	53.9	3.53	68.2

Table 2 Comparison of different variants of the model -YOLOv9. [31]

Model	Size (Pixels)	mAP^{val}50-95 (%)	Speed (ms)	Params (M)
YOLOv9t	640	38.3	3.52	2
YOLOv9s	640	46.8	3.68	7.2
YOLOv9m	640	51.4	4.19	20.1
YOLOv9c	640	53	4.6	25.5
YOLOv9e	640	55.6	8.95	58.1

The smaller models like YOLOv8n are optimized for speed, making them suitable for real-time applications, while larger variants like YOLOv8x provide higher detection accuracy at the expense of increased latency and computational demands. This flexibility allows for selecting a variant based on deployment-specific requirements.

3.4.2 YOLOv9

Table 2 illustrates a similar trend for YOLOv9 variants, ranging from YOLOv9t to YOLOv9e. The smallest model, YOLOv9t, excels in fast inference but offers lower mAP, while YOLOv9e achieves the highest mAP with greater computational overhead. This scalability, as demonstrated in Table 2, makes YOLOv9 adaptable for scenarios requiring either real-time speed or superior detection performance.

3.4.3 Faster R-CNN

As presented in Table 3, Faster R-CNN was evaluated with three backbones: ResNet50, EfficientNet-B0, and MobileNet-v3-large. ResNet50 achieves the highest accuracy, making it effective for tasks where precision is critical, though its higher latency could limit real-time applications. MobileNet-v3-large offers the fastest inference speed but with slightly lower mAP, making it ideal for latency-sensitive tasks.

Table 3 Comparison of different backbones of Faster-RCNN

Model	Size (Pixels)	Params (M)	Activations	mAP^{val}50-95 (%)	Latency (ms)
FRCNN-ResNet50	800	43.7	ReLU	42.7	140
FRCNN-EfficientNet-B0	800	20.5	Swish	40.2	100
FRCNN-MobileNet-v3-large	800	17	ReLU/ h-swish	38.3	80

EfficientNet-B0 strikes a balance, as shown in Table 3, offering moderate accuracy and latency, making it a viable middle-ground option for various applications.

3.5 Hyperparameters Considered

As shown in Table 4, most of the hyperparameters used in the YOLO models adhered to their default settings, such as batch size, momentum, and weight decay. However, specific values were customized to better suit the dataset and model performance requirements. The learning rate was set to 0.01 to ensure stable convergence during training, and the number of epochs was extended to 300 to allow the model adequate training time. A patience of 15 was set for early stopping to prevent overfitting if the validation performance plateaued for several epochs (Table 5).

For the Faster R-CNN model, as noted in Table 6, most parameters, such as RPN anchor sizes, aspect ratios, and the RPN NMS threshold, were kept at their default values to ensure standard object detection behavior. Adjustments were made to the maximum number of proposals during training and inference, set to 2000 and 1000, respectively, to balance accuracy and speed. The learning rate and epochs were also fine-tuned, similar to YOLO, to optimize training for the specific task and dataset complexity.

Table 4 List of hyperparameters considered for training YOLO models

Hyperparameter	Value
Learning rate	0.01
Batch size	16
Image size	800
Epochs	300
Patience	15
Workers	0
Momentum	0.937
Weight decay	0.0005

Table 5 List of hyperparameters considered for training various Faster R-CNN backbones

Hyperparameter	Value
Optimizer	SGD
RPN anchor sizes	[32, 64, 128, 256, 512]
RPN aspect ratio	[0.5, 1.0, 2.0]
RPN NMS threshold	0.7
ROI pooling size	7 × 7
Max proposals during training	2000
Max proposals during inference	1000
Batch size	16
Epochs	300
Patience	7
Momentum	0.937
Weight decay	0.0005

Table 6 Detection performance of YOLOv8 variants

		Epochs (early stopping)	Metrics/ precision (B)	Metrics/recall (B)	Metrics/ Map50 (B)	Metrics/ Map50-95(B)
YOLO v8	v8-n	69	0.59	0.93	0.81	0.73
	v8-s	70	0.71	0.81	0.82	0.74
	v8-m	88	0.67	0.84	0.81	0.74
	v8-l	120	0.67	0.88	0.83	0.76
	v8-x	93	0.68	0.83	0.82	0.75

The custom hyperparameter choices were driven by the need to achieve a balance between computational efficiency and model accuracy across various model architectures.

3.6 *Training Pipeline*

In this study, fine-tuning was selected over training from scratch for both the YOLO and Faster R-CNN models. Fine-tuning involves starting with a model that has been pre-trained on a large, general dataset and adapting it to a specific task, which in this case is detecting auricular deformities in newborns. This approach offers several advantages.

First, fine-tuning allows us to leverage the pre-trained weights of models like YOLO and Faster R-CNN, which have already learned generalized feature representations from large datasets such as COCO or ImageNet. Starting from these pre-trained models significantly reduces the training time and computational resources required, especially compared to training a model from scratch, where the model would need to learn basic features (such as edges, textures, etc.) all over again. Fine-tuning can thus accelerate convergence and enhance the model's performance even with comparatively smaller datasets, such as the BabyEar4k dataset.

Although fine-tuning alleviates the overall training burden, it still requires a considerable amount of computation, as specific layers need to be updated to focus on domain-specific features. In this context, the later layers of both single-stage and two-stage models were fine-tuned, while the earlier layers were kept frozen to retain general feature extraction capabilities. This strategy was essential to prevent over-fitting on the smaller dataset while allowing the models to learn patterns specific to auricular deformities. Achieving the balance between performance and resources was critical for ensuring high detection accuracy for auricular deformities without incurring excessive computational costs.

The best-performing fine-tuned model was subsequently used to implement D-RISE, to generate visual explanations, thereby enhancing model transparency and interpretability.

3.7 Model Evaluation

The models' performance was assessed using both detection and classification metrics to provide a well-rounded evaluation of accuracy, precision, and robustness in detecting and classifying auricular deformities. Detection metrics, such as mAP50 and mAP50-95, are used to evaluate object detection models by measuring localization accuracy and robustness across different IoU thresholds. Whereas for classification tasks, metrics like accuracy, precision, recall, and F1-score are used, since they provide essential measures of model performance. These well-established metrics form the foundation for evaluating detection and classification systems [38, 39].

3.8 Explainability

This study employs D-RISE to provide visual explanations for the predictions made by the object detection model. Explainability is essential, especially in medical applications, as it allows physicians to understand the model's decision logic and interpret them. D-RISE functions as a "black-box" method, requiring only access to model inputs and outputs, without any need of access to the internal workings of the model. This feature allows D-RISE to be used across various model architectures, including single-stage detectors like YOLO and two-stage detectors like Faster R-CNN, making it highly versatile for explaining object detection models [40]. Unlike gradient-based methods that rely on model gradients, D-RISE generates saliency maps that visually emphasize the regions in an image that significantly impact predictions. This approach is especially useful in clinical contexts, where understanding which areas contribute to classification decisions ensures that models are focusing on clinically relevant regions and are not biased or missing critical information.

D-RISE was selected for its adaptability and effectiveness in handling complex object detection tasks without being constrained by model architecture. The hyperparameters chosen for D-RISE were optimized to strike a balance between computational efficiency and the clarity of saliency maps. A total of 25 masks were utilized to provide sufficient resolution in the saliency maps, while ensuring manageable processing times. The mask resolution was set at 4×4 before upscaling, focusing on broader regions rather than minute details to prevent noise that could affect medical image interpretation. Additionally, the max figures parameter was set to 1, producing a single salient image per input to simplify the visualization of regions that most influence the model's predictions.

4 Experiments and Results

The selected models (with their respective versions/backbones) were fine-tuned for detection and classification tasks using ear deformity images from the BabyEar4k dataset. The experiments were designed to detect auricular regions first, followed by classifying the ear images into Normal and Abnormal categories.

The detection performance was evaluated using key metrics such as mAP50, mAP50-95, and recall. Below is a comparison of YOLOv8 and YOLOv9 variants for the detection task. For the classification task, the models' abilities to categorize ear deformities as Normal or Abnormal were evaluated. The classification performance of each model was assessed using key metrics such as accuracy, precision, recall, and F1-score.

4.1 YOLOv8 Detection Results

Table 6 presents the detailed performance of YOLOv8 variants. Among these, YOLOv8-L performed notably well with a mAP50 of 0.83 and mAP50-95 of 0.76 after training for 120 epochs. The model also achieved a recall score of 0.88, indicating a strong ability to correctly localize auricular regions in the images.

The performance of YOLOv8-L stands out due to its higher recall, which is critical in reducing missed detections - especially in medical image analysis, where identifying all relevant features is crucial. Figure 5 presents the training and validation curves for YOLOv8-L, showing loss values (box loss, classification loss, and DFL loss) as well as performance metrics (precision, recall, mAP50, and mAP50-95) over the training epochs. The steady decrease in losses indicates successful training, while the increase in metrics like mAP50 and mAP50-95 confirms improved detection accuracy as training progresses.

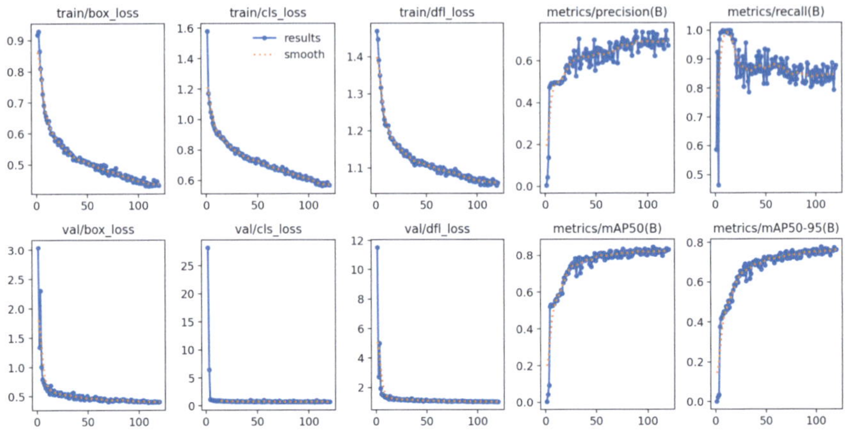

Fig. 5 Training and validation losses (box loss, classification loss, DFL loss) and performance metrics (precision, recall, mAP50, mAP50-95) across epochs of YOLOv8-L

4.2 YOLOv9 Detection Results

For YOLOv9, Table 7 highlights the detection performance. The YOLOv9-S variant demonstrated the best balance between precision and speed, with a mAP50 of 0.82, mAP50-95 of 0.76, and recall of 0.85 after 93 epochs. This variant offers a more efficient training cycle while maintaining competitive detection performance.

Although YOLOv9-S exhibited a slight trade-off in precision, its high recall score demonstrates the model's ability to accurately identify auricular deformities with minimal false negatives. Figure 6 showcases the training and validation curves for YOLOv9-S, including box loss, classification loss, and DFL loss, along with key metrics like precision, recall, mAP50, and mAP50-95.

The graphs show a sharp decrease in losses during the initial training phase, indicating effective learning. The gradual increase in mAP scores demonstrates the model's capability to improve detection accuracy over time, and more importantly, the convergence is faster than other variants.

Table 7 Detection performance of YOLOv9 Variants

		Epochs (early stopping)	Metrics/ precision (B)	Metrics/recall (B)	Metrics/ Map50 (B)	Metrics/ Map50-95(B)
YOLO v8	v9-t	69	0.63	0.89	0.81	0.74
	v9-s	93	0.67	0.85	0.82	0.76
	v9-m	107	0.69	0.85	0.82	0.75
	v9-c	79	0.64	0.91	0.81	0.74
	v9-e	55	0.59	0.89	0.73	0.66

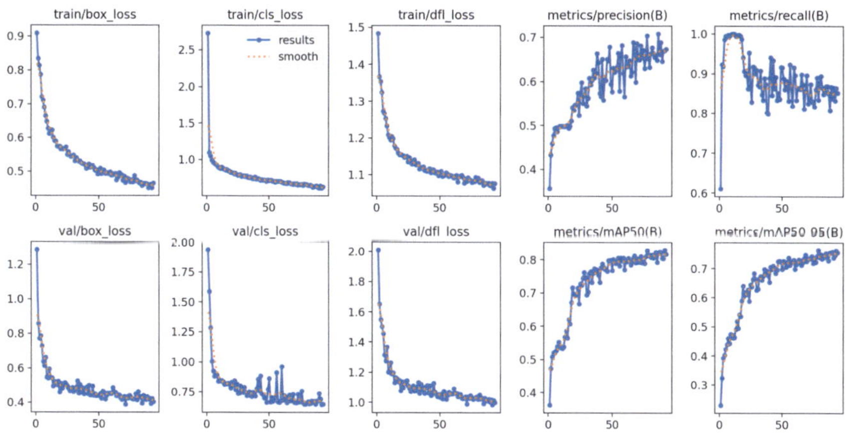

Fig. 6 Training and validation losses (box loss, classification loss, DFL loss) and performance metrics (precision, recall, mAP50, mAP50-95) across epochs of YOLOv9-S

4.3 Faster R-CNN Detection Results

For Faster R-CNN models, the three different backbones—ResNet50, EfficientNet-B0, and MobileNet-V3-Large—were evaluated. Table 8 summarizes the results and provides insights into the overall detection performance across Faster R-CNN variants.

The ResNet50 backbone excelled with a mAP50-95 of 0.76 and recall of 0.912, making it the most accurate model in terms of localization. MobileNet-V3-Large, however, demonstrated competitive mAP and recall scores. Figure 7 illustrates the training loss comparison across these backbones, where EfficientNet-B0 converged faster in lesser number of epochs in comparison with the other backbones of Faster R-CNN.

Table 8 Detection performance of Faster R-CNN variants

Model	FRCNN-ResNet50	FRCNN-EfficientNet-B0	FRCNN-MobileNet-v3-large
Processing time (Sec)	9875.58	12,986	14,151.28
Epochs (Early stopping)	23	26	34
mAP50 (B)	0.84	0.8	0.83
Map75(B)	0.84	0.8	0.83
mAP50-95 (B)	0.76	0.72	0.74
Recall (B)	0.91	0.9	0.88

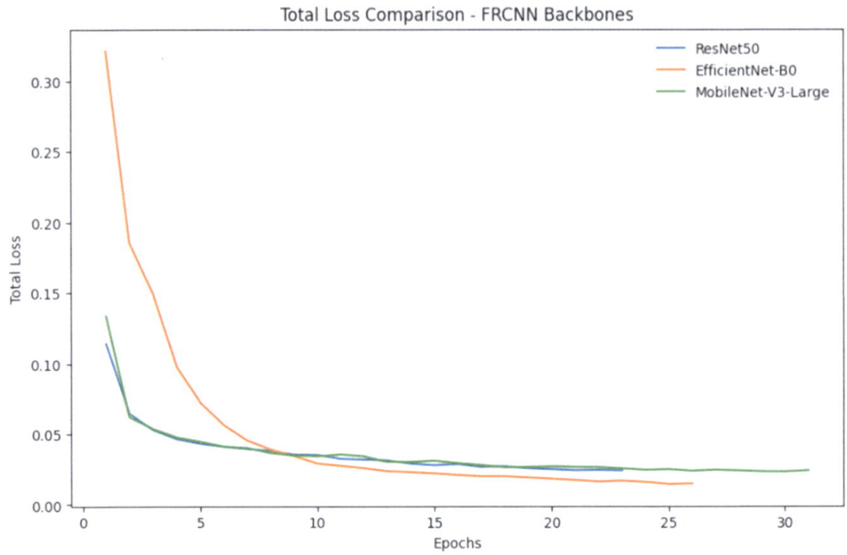

Fig. 7 Training loss of Faster R-CNN variants

4.4 YOLOv8 Classification Results

The YOLOv8 variants were evaluated for their classification performance after detecting ear regions. The best performing variant, YOLOv8-L, achieved an accuracy of 0.79, showing balanced precision and recall across both Normal and Abnormal categories.

The YOLOv8-L model displayed the best overall performance in terms of accuracy and balanced precision across both categories. Notably, the model achieved a precision of 0.79 for Normal and 0.80 for Abnormal categories. YOLOv8-N also performed well in terms of recall, especially for the Abnormal category, making it more suitable for anomaly detection (Table 9).

Table 9 Classification Performance of YOLOv8 variants

		Accuracy	Precision		Recall		F1-Score	
			Normal	Abnormal	Normal	Abnormal	Normal	Abnormal
YOLO v8	v8-n	0.76	0.84	0.70	0.65	0.87	0.73	0.78
	v8-s	0.76	0.75	0.78	0.82	0.71	0.78	0.74
	v8-m	0.78	0.85	0.73	0.69	0.87	0.76	0.79
	v8-l	0.79	0.79	0.80	0.81	0.77	0.80	0.78
	v8-x	0.79	0.80	0.77	0.79	0.79	0.79	0.78

Table 10 Classification Performance of YOLOv9 variants

		Accuracy	Precision		Recall		F1-Score	
			Normal	Abnormal	Normal	Abnormal	Normal	Abnormal
YOLO v9	v9-t	0.77	0.81	0.73	0.72	0.82	0.76	0.77
	v9-s	0.77	0.82	0.73	0.71	0.84	0.76	0.78
	v9-m	0.77	0.82	0.73	0.71	0.83	0.76	0.78
	v9-c	0.74	0.74	0.75	0.77	0.71	0.76	0.73
	v9-e	0.69	0.66	0.74	0.83	0.55	0.74	0.63

4.5 YOLOv9 Classification Results

The classification results for YOLOv9 variants were also assessed. Among the tested variants, YOLOv9-S stood out with an accuracy of 0.77 and high recall for detecting abnormal ear deformities. This made the model effective in identifying potential medical abnormalities (Table 10).

Among the YOLOv9 variants, YOLOv9-S balanced recall and precision effectively, making it suitable for identifying both Normal and Abnormal ear regions. Although YOLOv9-T performed slightly better in precision for Normal categories, YOLOv9-S demonstrated higher recall for Abnormal regions, which is crucial for medical applications.

4.6 Faster R-CNN Classification Results

The Faster R-CNN model was tested with different backbones, including ResNet50, EfficientNet-B0, and MobileNet-V3 Large. Among these, MobileNet-V3 Large achieved the highest accuracy of 0.77, displaying balanced precision and recall across both categories (Table 11).

The MobileNet-v3 large backbone consistently demonstrated superior performance compared to ResNet50 and EfficientNet-B0, with an accuracy of 0.77 and

Table 11 Classification performance of Faster R-CNN

Model		FRCNN-ResNet50	FRCNN-EfficientNet-B0	FRCNN-MobileNet-v3-large
Accuracy		0.72	0.72	0.77
Precison	Normal	0.86	0.78	0.77
	Abnormal	0.65	0.67	0.76
Recall	Normal	0.56	0.64	0.78
	Abnormal	0.9	0.81	0.76
F1-Score	Normal	0.68	0.7	0.78
	Abnormal	0.76	0.74	0.76

balanced precision and recall. ResNet50 showed higher precision for Normal categories but struggled in recalling Abnormal categories. The results from these experiments suggest MobileNet-V3 Large is the optimal backbone for this classification task.

Figure 8 illustrates the predictions made by the better-performing single-stage model, YOLOv8-L, on a set of images, showcasing its capability in localizing and classifying auricular regions correctly into 'Normal' and 'Abnormal' categories.

Figure 9 presents sample predictions made by Faster R-CNN using different backbone architectures, specifically ResNet50, EfficientNet-B0, and MobileNet-v3-Large on a sample instance. All the backbones of Faster-RCNN have correctly classified the auricle as 'Abnormal', with MobileNet-v3-Large showing the highest confidence. This higher confidence level suggests that MobileNet-v3-Large has more effectively learned and identified the distinguishing features.

Figure 10 depicts examples of misclassifications made by the Faster R-CNN model with ResNet50, EfficientNet-B0, and MobileNet-v3-large backbones on a sample Not-so-good-quality image which contains amniotic fluid residue. Although, the ground truth of that auricle is 'Normal', models have interpreted the fluid as

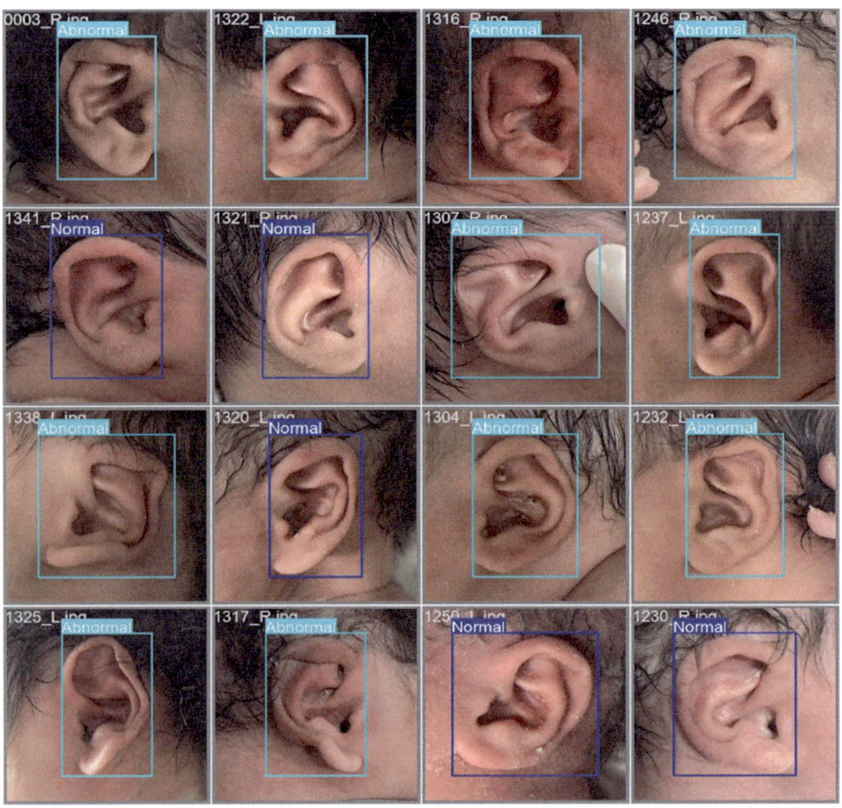

Fig. 8 Sample predictions made by 'YOLO-v8L'

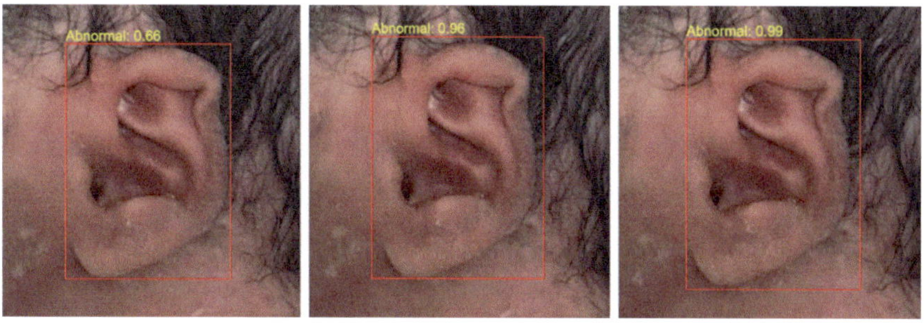

Fig. 9 Sample predictions made by Faster R-CNN with backbones: ResNet50, EfficientNet-B0, MobileNet-v3-large respectively

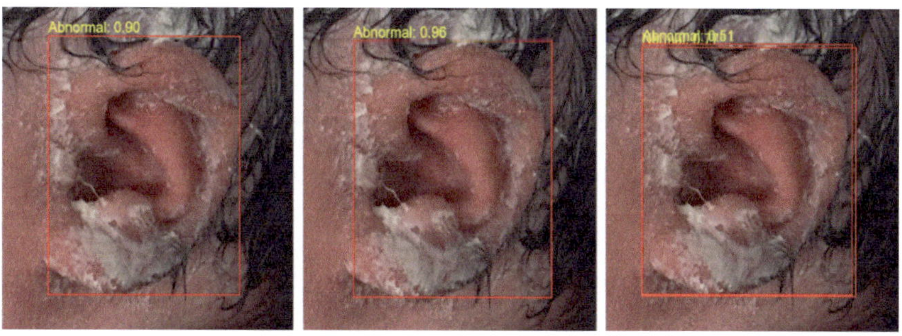

Fig. 10 Sample misclassifications made by Faster R-CNN with backbones: ResNet50, EfficientNet-B0, MobileNet-v3-large respectively on Not-so-good quality image

an abnormality, resulting in a misclassification with high confidence. Interestingly, while the MobileNet-V3-Large backbone primarily predicts "Normal" with 0.77 confidence, but it also detects "Abnormal" with a 0.51 probability, indicating some uncertainty. This example highlights a limitation in handling visual artifacts, where the models could be misled by extraneous factors such as fluid presence.

4.7 D-RISE Results

Figure 11a illustrates a prediction made by Faster R-CNN with a MobileNet-v3-large backbone, labeling the sample as 'Abnormal' with a confidence score of 0.78. This instance represents a 'lop ear' condition, where the pinna (outer ear) exhibits an abnormality. Figure 11b illustrates the corresponding saliency map which highlights the regions that strongly influenced the model's decision, with emphasis around the pinna area. The saliency map generated suggests that the model correctly identified the critical regions associated with the abnormality, supporting its classification as 'Abnormal'.

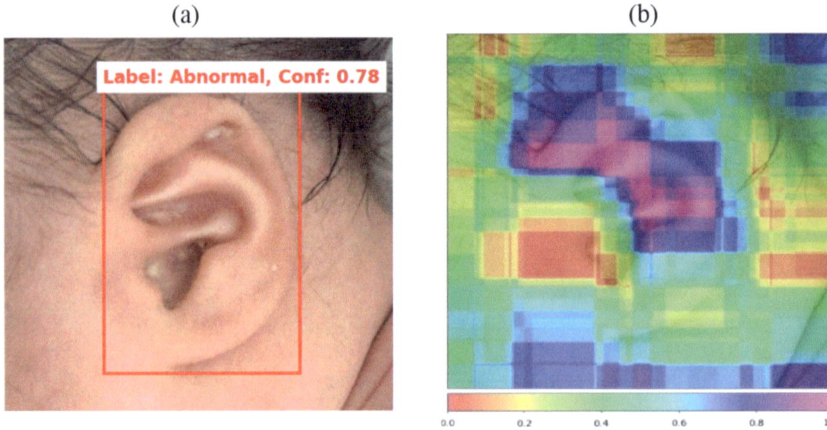

Fig. 11 **a** Correct prediction made by Faster R-CNN with MobileNet-v3-large backbone on a sample instance; **b** Corresponding saliency map generated through D-RISE for the same instance

Figure 12 illustrates an incorrect prediction made by the Faster R-CNN model with a MobileNet-v3-large backbone. In Fig. 12a, the model labeled the sample as "Abnormal" with a high confidence score of 0.98. However, this is a misclassification largely attributed to the quality issues in the image, specifically related to "cover-up". As shown, the ear is partially obscured by dirt or other substances, leading the model to interpret these obstructions as features indicative of an abnormality. The saliency map in Fig. 12b, generated through D-RISE, reveals that the darker regions influencing the model's decision are concentrated around the areas where cover-up is present, further supporting the misinterpretation. This highlights a challenge in model performance, where severe quality issues, which is cover-up (ranked as 3 in severity) in this case, can lead to confident but incorrect predictions due to visual noise in the image.

5 Conclusions

In this chapter, an AI-based system was developed for detecting and classifying auricular deformities in newborns, with the objective of supporting early diagnosis and timely intervention. Through experiments using the BabyEar4k dataset, YOLOv8, YOLOv9 and Faster R-CNN with different backbones were evaluated, with YOLOv8-L achieving the highest classification accuracy at 0.79. For localization precision, Faster R-CNN with ResNet50 backbone demonstrated strong performance. MobileNet-v3-large was chosen for D-RISE saliency mapping due to its reliable classification confidence, even in cases where images contained challenging visual obstructions.

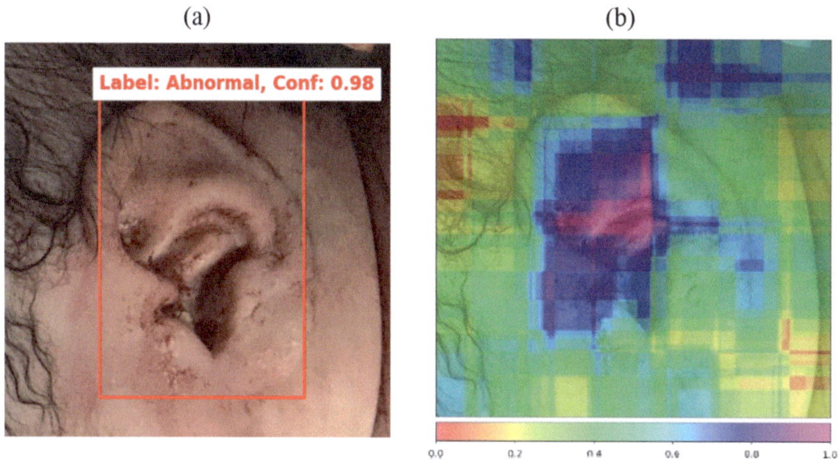

Fig. 12 **a** Incorrect prediction made by Faster R-CNN with MobileNet-v3-large backbone on a sample instance; **b** Corresponding saliency map generated through D-RISE for the same instance

The D-RISE-generated saliency maps offered insights into the decision-making process, highlighting areas in each image that influenced the model's predictions. This provided transparency, particularly valuable in medical contexts, ensuring that the model's focus aligned with relevant anatomical regions. A significant finding was the model's sensitivity to image quality issues, such as cover-up, which led to misclassifications by interpreting obstructions as abnormalities.

Future research will prioritize enhancing the effectiveness and clinical relevance of the system. Advanced pre-processing techniques such as edge enhancement, noise reduction will be implemented to improve model's robustness against low quality inputs, ensuring a consistent performance across various conditions. Expanding the classification beyond binary categories to include specific deformities such as microtia, lop ear etc., will transform this into a comprehensive diagnostic system. Exploring light weight models for detection and integrating them, helps in deploying the system in resource constrained devices—making it more accessible and versatile. Additionally, integration of large language models can facilitate an interactive model by functionalities such as visual question answering. Advanced XAI techniques such as BODEM, will be explored and investigated for better visual explanations. These improvements will contribute to creating a robust, interpretable system that can assist healthcare professionals in the early detection and classification of auricular deformities in clinical settings.

References

1. Bhatti, S.L., Daly, L.T., Mejia, M., Perlyn, C.: Ear abnormalities. Pediatr. Rev. **42**(4), 180–188 (2021)
2. Macgregor, F.C.: Ear deformities: social and psychological implications. Clin. Plast. Surg. **5**(3), 347–350 (1978)
3. Ren, L.J., Luo, F., Yang, Z.W., Chen, L.L., Wang, X.Y., Li, C.L., Fu, Y.Y.: A publicly available newborn ear shape dataset for medical diagnosis of auricular deformities. Sci. Data **11**(1) (2024)
4. Castañeda Anaya, P.S., Mendoza Sánchez, H.A.: Advances in regenerative therapy for auricular reconstruction in congenital microtia. Int. J. Med. Sci. Clin. Res. Stud. **3**(8) (2023)
5. Byrd, H.S., Langevin, C.J., Ghidoni, L.A.: Ear molding in newborn infants with auricular deformities. Plast. Reconstr. Surg. **126**(4), 1191–1200 (2010)
6. Doft, M.A., Goodkind, A.B., Diamond, S., Dipace, J.I., Kacker, A., Labruna, A.N.: The newborn butterfly project: a shortened treatment protocol for ear molding. Plast. Reconstr. Surg. **135**(3), 577e–583e (2015)
7. Chen, L., Li, C., He, A., Tong, H., Yu, J., Cui, C., Zhang, T.: Long-term effectiveness of ear molding and factors affecting outcomes. Plast. Reconstr. Surg. **153**(4), 905–913 (2024)
8. Hallac, R.R., Lee, J., Pressler, M., Seaward, J.R., Kane, A.A.: Identifying ear abnormality from 2D photographs using convolutional neural networks. Sci. Rep. **9**(1) (2019)
9. Zhou, X., Peng, X., Ding, Y., Zhu, Y., Tian, D., Wu, M., et al.: Investigation of morphometric features of auricle in newborns and etiology of auricle deformity. Pediatr. Invest. **00**, 1–9 (2024)
10. Esteva, A., Kuprel, B., Novoa, R.A., Ko, J., Swetter, S.M., Blau, H.M., Thrun, S.: Dermatologist-level classification of skin cancer with deep neural networks. Nature **542**(7639), 115–118 (2017)
11. Gulshan, V., Peng, L., Coram, M., Stumpe, M.C., Wu, D., Narayanaswamy, A., Webster, D.R.: Development and validation of a deep learning algorithm for detection of diabetic retinopathy in retinal fundus photographs. JAMA J. Am. Med. Assoc. **316**(22), 2402–2410 (2016)
12. Raj, K.D., Lal, G.J., Gopalakrishnan, E.A., Sowmya, V., Orozco-Arroyave, J.R.: A visibility graph approach for multi-stage classification of Parkinson's disease using multimodal data. IEEE Access **1** (2024)
13. Mohan, J., Sivasubramanian, A., Sowmya, V., Vinayakumar, R.: Enhancing skin disease classification leveraging transformer-based deep learning architectures and explainable AI (2024). arXiv preprint arXiv:2407.14757
14. Moradi, M., Yan, K., Colwell, D., Samwald, M., Asgari, R.: Model-agnostic explainable artificial intelligence for object detection in image data. Eng. Appl. Artif. Intell. **137**, 109183 (2024)
15. Petsiuk, V., Jain, R., Manjunatha, V., Morariu, V.I., Mehra, A., Ordonez, V., Saenko, K.: Black-box explanation of object detectors via saliency maps. In: Proceedings of the IEEE Computer Society Conference on Computer Vision and Pattern Recognition, pp. 11438–11447 (2021)
16. Chen, Y., Wang, W., Wang, Y., Mao, X.: Using ear molding to treat congenital auricular deformities. Front. Pediatr. **9** (2021)
17. Tolba, M., Qian, Z.J., Lin, H.F., Yeom, K.W., Truong, M.T.: Use of convolutional neural networks to evaluate auricular reconstruction outcomes for microtia. Laryngoscope **133**(9), 2413–2416 (2023)
18. Wang, D., Chen, X., Wu, Y., Tang, H., Deng, P.: Artificial intelligence for assessing the severity of microtia via deep convolutional neural networks. Front. Surg. **9** (2022)
19. Hennocq, Q., Garcelon, N., Bongibault, T., Bouygues, T., Marlin, S., Amiel, J., Boutaud, L., Douillet, M., Lyonnet, S., Pingault, V., Picard, A., Rio, M., Attie-Bitach, T., Khonsari, R.H., Roux, N.: Artificial intelligence-based diagnosis in fetal pathology using external ear shapes. Prenat. Diagn. **44**(10), 1150–1158 (2024)
20. Zeng, X., Jiang, Z., Luo, W., Li, H., Li, H., Li, G., Li, Z.: Efficient and accurate identification of ear diseases using an ensemble deep learning model. Sci. Rep. **11**(1) (2021)

21. Yuan, L., Mao, J., Zheng, H.: Ear detection based on CenterNet. In: Proceedings of 2020 IEEE 2nd International Conference on Civil Aviation Safety and Information Technology, ICCASIT 2020, 349–353 (2020)
22. Hoang, V.T.: EarVN1.0: a new large-scale ear images dataset in the wild. Data Brief **27** (2019)
23. Zhang, C., He, L., Zhang, Z.: UBEAR: an unconstrained ear recognition benchmark. In: Proceedings of the IEEE International Joint Conference on Biometrics (IJCB), pp. 458–466 (2017)
24. Yan, P., Bowyer, K.W., Flynn, P.J.: A study of multibiometric traits of the face, ear, and the profile. In: Proceedings of the IEEE International Conference on Biometrics: Theory, Applications, and Systems (BTAS), pp. 1–6 (2007)
25. Wang, S., Ren, L., Zhou, T., Chen, L., Zhang, T., Fu, Y., Wang, S.: Large language model-enhanced interactive agent for public education on newborn auricular deformities (2024). arXiv preprint arXiv:2409.12984
26. Fudholi, D.H., Kurniawardhani, A., Andaru, G.I., Alhanafi, A.A., Najmudin, N.: YOLO-based small-scaled model for on-shelf availability in retail. Jurnal RESTI (Rekayasa Sistem dan Teknologi Informasi) **8**(2), 265–271 (2024)
27. Dwivedi, A., Rastogi, A., Sharma, G., Singh Kushwaha, R.: IoT-based two wheelers traffic violation detection system using YOLOv7. In: 2024 2nd World Conference on Communication & Computing (WCONF), pp. 1–6 (2024)
28. Mu, Y., Feng, R., Ni, R., Li, J., Luo, T., Liu, T., Hu, T.: A Faster R-CNN-based model for the identification of weed seedlings. Agronomy **12**(11) (2022)
29. Sahin, M.E., Ulutas, H., Yuce, E., Erkoc, M.F.: Detection and classification of COVID-19 by using faster R-CNN and mask R-CNN on CT images. Neural Comput. Appl. **35**(18), 13597–13611 (2023)
30. Ju, R. Y., Cai, W.: Fracture detection in pediatric wrist trauma X-ray images using YOLOv8 algorithm. Sci. Rep. **13**(1) (2023)
31. YOLO-Ultralytics. https://github.com/ultralytics/ultralytics
32. Girshick, R., Donahue, J., Darrell, T., Malik, J.: Rich feature hierarchies for accurate object detection and semantic segmentation. In: Proceedings of the IEEE Computer Society Conference on Computer Vision and Pattern Recognition, pp. 580–587 (2014)
33. Girshick, R.: Fast R-CNN. In: Proceedings of the IEEE International Conference on Computer Vision (ICCV 2015), pp. 1440–1448 (2015)
34. Ren, S., He, K., Girshick, R., Sun, J.: Faster R-CNN: towards real-time object detection with region proposal networks. IEEE Trans. Pattern Anal. Mach. Intell. **39**(6), 1137–1149 (2017)
35. He, K., Zhang, X., Ren, S., Sun, J.: Deep residual learning for image recognition. In: Proceedings of the IEEE Computer Society Conference on Computer Vision and Pattern Recognition, pp. 770–778 (2016)
36. Tan, M., Le, Q.V.: EfficientNet: Rethinking model scaling for convolutional neural networks. In: 36th International Conference on Machine Learning, ICML 2019, pp. 10691–10700 (2019)
37. Howard, A., Sandler, M., Chen, B., Wang, W., Chen, L.C., Tan, M., Adam, H.: Searching for MobileNetV3. In: Proceedings of the IEEE International Conference on Computer Vision (ICCV 2019), pp. 1314–1324 (2019)
38. Lin, T.Y., Maire, M., Belongie, S., Hays, J., Perona, P., Ramanan, D., Zitnick, C.L.: Microsoft COCO: Common objects in context. Lecture Notes in Computer Science (LNCS), vol. 8693, pp. 740–755 (2014)
39. Manning, C.D., Raghavan, P., Schütze, H.: Introduction to information retrieval. Cambridge University Press (2008)
40. Petsiuk, V., Das, A., Saenko, K.: RISE: randomized input sampling for explanation of black-box models. In: British Machine Vision Conference 2018 (BMVC) (2018)

YOLOv10 for Enhanced Trypanosome Detection

Mohitha Velagapudi, J. Ajay Surya, V. Sowmya, and Vinayakumar Ravi

Abstract Human African Trypanosomiasis, commonly known as sleeping sickness, is still one of the NTDs that test the people of sub-Saharan Africa and the Latin American plateau. It has been marked by the World Health Organization (WHO) as one of those fatal diseases that should be diagnosed early. Therefore, it is necessary to develop efficient screening tools that will help solve the problem. This further led to the creation of Tryp dataset, which is the largest in its class. These are microscopy images taken from blood samples of people infected by Trypanosoma brucei brucei. After this, the approaches used to design Faster R-CNN, RetinaNet and YOLOv7 with regards to the Tryp dataset to correctly identify the images and to detect the parasites present within it were used. Out of these, YOLOv7 gave the maximum F1-score of 72%. However, considering that new versions of the You Only Look Once (YOLO) algorithm were later introduced, we feel there is still scope for improvement. So, we have come up with an advanced method with the latest YOLOv10 model which does the early identification and screening of the trypanosome parasite. A 23% gain on the mean average precision and a 4% gain on the overall F1-score was obtained by tuning the hyperparameters and fine-tuning the YOLOv10 model for the Tryp dataset compared to the previous best YOLOv7 model on the test partition of the dataset. This improved performance would point toward the capability of new object detection models, like YOLOv10, to better tackle NTD challenges, which in turn would result in better health outcomes for the affected communities.

Keywords Neglected tropical diseases · Trypanosome · Tryp dataset · YOLOv10

M. Velagapudi · J. Ajay Surya · V. Sowmya (✉)
Amrita School of Artificial Intelligence, Amrita Vishwa Vidyapeetham, Coimbatore, India
e-mail: v_sowmya@cb.amrita.edu

V. Ravi
Center for Artificial Intelligence, Prince Mohammad Bin Fahd University, Khobar, Saudi Arabia
e-mail: vravi@pmu.edu.sa

P. Singh et al. (eds.), *Deep Learning Applications in Healthcare and Medical Imaging Practice*, Studies in Big Data 193, https://doi.org/10.1007/978-3-032-21009-8_10

1 Introduction

Parasites belonging to the genus Trypanosoma, carried by the tsetse flies in sub-Saharan Africa and other parts of the world [1], causes what is commonly known as Sleeping Sickness in humans and Nagana in animals. It severely affects human populations and livestock, with tremendous financial and social implications, mostly at rural levels, in whose economic cycles livestock are very vital. Human trypanosomiasis includes two major forms: human African trypanosomiasis (HAT), with affected individuals often dying within six months [2], and Chagas disease, impacting millions in Latin America, often resulting in chronic cardiac and digestive disorders [3]. HAT, which can lead to death within six months without treatment, manifests in two stages—an initial hemolymphatic phase followed by a more severe neurological phase once the parasite crosses the blood-brain barrier [4]. In contrast, Chagas disease can lead to chronic cardiac, digestive, or neurological diseases and, therefore, incur increased social and economic costs in the long term [5–8]. WHO points out that trypanosomiasis falls among the NTDs. However, these have been until now neglected despite the burden they incur [9]. Thus, early-stage detection is essential for control of the disease's mode of transmission and improved medical results. Traditional approaches to the diagnosis of trypanosomiasis include microscopy, serological testing, and PCR (refer Table 1).

These are all difficult methods. Microscopy [10, 11] remains the most prevailing method for identifying trypanosomes, particularly in resource-limited settings due to its inexpensiveness and accessibility, but through microscopic examination preparation of a blood smear needs to be made to distinguish the presence of the causative agents, which indeed does not need sophisticated machine, an appropriate choice within many endemic settings. Its use has several significant impairments though. It lacks enough sensitivity since it may miss parasites when its levels are quite low-low parasitemia. Serological tests [12] for trypanosomiasis are sensitive and detect the presence of antibodies or antigens in the blood, with more sensitivity than microscopy and with the ability to detect infections at lower levels of parasitemia. The serological tests have, however, their disadvantages. One of the main disadvantages is cross-reactivity, where the test may react to antibodies produced by infections of other diseases and result in false positives. This limited specificity

Table 1 Comparison of existing methods for trypanosomiasis detection

Diagnostic method	Advantages	Limitations
Microscopy [2, 10, 11]	Widely available, low cost	Low sensitivity in low parasitemia, time-consuming, requires skilled labour
Serological testing [12]	Higher sensitivity than microscopy	Cross-reactivity with other diseases, limited specificity
PCR [13–15]	High sensitivity and specificity	Expensive, requires advanced lab facilities, not widely available

complicates the interpretation of results, which may be consistently problematic over regions particularly exposed to several diseases simultaneously. Among all the advanced techniques available, PCR [13] is among the highly sensitive and specific diagnostic procedures. It allows the determination of the parasite's genetic material, therefore, makes it possible to identify at levels very low in the bloodstream even in situations of minimal parasitemia where microscope observations and serological tests cannot establish any infection. PCR-based methods are however costly, as they demand special reagents, equipment, and laboratory conditions not available in most endemic areas for trypanosomiasis.Thus, though PCR still remains a very powerful research and clinical confirmation tool, its high cost and need for infrastructure limit its applications in routine diagnostics for trypanosomiasis.

In this context, it is an urgent demand to develop accessible, affordable, and reliable alternatives in diagnosis that can be used in scale. The advances that AI and deep learning give today open new prospects for the automated detection of diseases through medical images and make them capable of overcoming these types of limitations. AI and medical imaging, so far, have held great promise in solving a good number of these problems. YOLOv10 is one of the advanced object detection algorithms for the detection of small, intricate objects within images that run in real time and are highly accurate [16]. This algorithm, thus, is particularly suited for medical applications where fast and accurate detection is a must. The model can easily be adapted to detect pathogens in blood smears or other micro-photographs of several diseases caused by infections, including malaria, tuberculosis, and schistosomiasis. The traditional diagnosis methods are time-consuming and must be performed by expert technicians. YOLOv10's swift ability to detect and localize the pathogens can speed up the workflows of diagnostics, and thus, is highly useful in endemic areas where mass screening is inevitable. For instance, scanning blood samples for malaria by YOLOv10 on placenta parasites automatically counts Plasmodium parasites, hence increasing speed and precision in diagnosis. This will be a game-changer in endemic areas through mass screening with minimal infrastructure. Diabetic retinopathy, a leading cause of blindness, requires regular screening to detect early signs of retinal damage. YOLOv10 can be applied to fundus photography (images of the retina) to detect signs of retinopathy, such as microaneurysms, haemorrhages, and exudates. Early detection is essential in preventing vision loss, and with YOLOv10's real-time processing, it can be implemented in large-scale screening programs. By automating the detection of retinal abnormalities, YOLOv10 can assist ophthalmologists in identifying high-risk patients who need immediate intervention, especially in underserved regions where specialists may be in short supply. YOLOv10 has plenty of applications in cardiology, such as the analysis of ultrasound images of the heart. YOLOv10 can be used to identify infestations of pests in crops and detect signs of plant disease using images taken; this way, the farmers can take appropriate measures at the correct times to protect their crop yields. Wildlife conservation and protection can also utilize YOLOv10 in monitoring endangered species or scanning aerial photographs for evidence of illegal poaching. These applications tell us how versatile YOLOv10 performs in challenging demands like fast and accurate detection with sparse resources in any field.

Our work is therefore aimed at taking advantage of the particularly superior advanced detection capabilities of YOLOv10 to target trypanosomes in blood smear images, thus providing a tool that can help significantly shorten diagnosis times, improve treatment outcomes, and ultimately contribute towards disease control initiatives undertaken in affected regions. Hence, we have decided to develop a diagnostic tool based on deep learning and YOLOv10 for auto-detecting Trypanosoma parasites. The parasites being small, motile ones, chances are that it might go undetected by conventional methods, so applying YOLOv10 is a novel approach for automated detection. The Tryp dataset, proposed by [17], is comprised of microscopy images of blood samples that train machine learning models, which includes object detection systems like YOLOv10. This research also contributes to the broader field of AI in medical imaging, that shows the role of deep learning models applied to parasitology, an area that has historically been lacking in technological progress.

2 Literature Review

Historically, trypanosome infections have been diagnosed primarily through parasitological methods like microscopy, using techniques like the buffy coat method and Giemsa-stained blood smears. While these methods are widely used, they often suffer from low sensitivity, especially in cases of low parasitemia, as highlighted in [13]. In their study [18], the authors evaluated multiple molecular diagnostic techniques, including PCR in detecting low-level infections. Their primary focus was on low resource areas where traditional techniques like microscopy might fall short. Their research proved PCR to be highly efficient due to its high specificity, and thus very useful for the early detection of and discrimination between different species or strains of trypanosomes. In their 2002 review, Desquesnes and Davila [14] reviewed the effectiveness of PCR - based tools for detecting animal trypanosomes. In the study [19], the authors aimed for detection of *Trypanosoma* species in cattle, goats, and sheep across Somalia.They compared molecular detection techniques, especially PCR with traditional microscopic methods. The study conducted by Hassan-Kadle revealed that for asymptomatic cases or cases with low parasitemia, molecular methods are a better choice They concluded that molecular techniques offer a more reliable diagnosis especially in diagnosing asymptomatic cases or species with low parasitemia. In his study Solano et al. [15] applied PCR in a field survey in Burkina Faso to assess the true prevalence of trypanosomes in cattle. Their findings indicate that PCR is significantly more sensitive than classical microscopic methods for detecting trypanosomes. While parasitological methods and immunological techniques such as ELISA [20] have long been the cornerstone of trypanosome detection, they come with several limitations like time constraints, low sensitivity and challenges in field application.

In [21] a novel approach is proposed for the detection of Trypanosoma cruzi, an agent responsible for causing chagas disease. Unlike in the Serological tests where false positives and negatives are often reported, this real-time PCR method targets specific genetic markers of T. Cruzi. The study also demonstrated that it is best suited for samples with low parasite load, making it ideal for detection of chagas disease, especially in asymptomatic stages. This research can enhance clinical outcomes with early treatment. In the recent review [10], conducted by Desquesnes and colleagues, they reviewed diagnostic methods for animal trypanosomes, including both parasitological and molecular approaches. They examined the efficiency of various techniques for identifying infections among different animal hosts. These techniques include buffy-coat microscopy, Serological tests and PCR. They also addressed the limitations including, need of equipment and trained personal in low-resource areas which can be pretty challenging. For researchers aiming to implement diagnostic strategies in endemic regions, this review serves as a helpful guide. Recently, researchers have also explored the use of AI to detect trypanosomiasis [22, 23]. With the introduction of object detection algorithms like Faster R-CNN [24], RetinaNet, and the YOLO family of models, real-time detection.

Has become feasible, leading to a more automated, efficient, and scalable approach in disease detection [25]. have applied Faster R-CNN on even more medical image applications, such as its demonstration in a study that shows high accuracy in the localization of tumours and the identification of malaria in blood smear images. However, it does face some practical constraints, largely due to its computational complexity and slower inference time if used in real-time scenarios in resource-poor settings [26]. RetinaNet, having been discovered to mitigate the problem of severe imbalance between the detection of foreground and background objects, has also been applied in the areas of medical diagnostics [27]. The model has enhanced its ability to detect minor infections such as parasitic infections with much more precision. The processing speed is still below other recent models. On the other hand, the YOLO series of models, particularly YOLOv3 and YOLOv4, achieved a perfect balance between speed and accuracy, thus suitable for real-time applications in medical imagery [28]. YOLO models have demonstrated significantly useful in real-time object detection [29].

In the context of disease detection, these models enable rapid and accurate detection of multiple objects, such as pathogens, in medical imagery [30]. employed YOLOv4 for tuberculosis detection in chest X-ray images, achieving an accuracy of 93% while surpassing the processing speed of alternative methods. Detection of malaria had been performed using YOLOv5, which provided promising speed and accuracy about its previous versions [31]. Indeed, one-stage detection framework YOLO happens to be a great candidate for rapid diagnostics in times of scarce time and resources. Presented with the Tryp dataset in the paper published in [17], it used this dataset to compare object detection models like Faster R-CNN, RetinaNet, and YOLOv7 on unstained blood smear images. It indeed demonstrated strong detection capabilities over the models and also exhibited an excellent speed-accuracy trade-off from the model YOLOv7 that was appropriate for real-time applications in detecting trypanosomes. In their paper [32], YOLOv10 is utilized for skin cancer detection focusing on melanoma. Extensive image augmentation techniques were employed during training to improve detection accuracy. YOLOv10s capability of precise localization is used in this study to detect even minor lesions. The success of YOLOv10 in detecting melanoma suggests that it could be extended to various types of diseases or conditions.

2.1 Contribution and Novelty

In this paper, we design a powerful and efficient method for detecting trypanosomes in microscopy images using the latest YOLO object detection model, that is, YOLOv10. The work will help bridge existing gaps in the methods, where those methods have low sensitivity and have high costs of requirements and need expertise, mainly when the areas are resource constrained. We further enumerate specific contributions and new ingredients in our work, that can differentiate the proposed design from previous approaches.

2.1.1 Enhanced Detection Accuracy and Speed

We show the absolute superiority of YOLOv10 in detecting accurately precise trypanosome identification in unstained blood samples. In comparison with the state-of-the-art models such as Faster R-CNN, RetinaNet, and YOLOv7, our method presents improvement across the F1-score, precision, and recall performance metrics. This is a crucial point in medical diagnostics where the ability to detect low levels of parasitemia sensitively is required. Our method improves the reliability of trypanosome detection, especially in challenging environments where the rapid diagnosis is essential by achieving high detection accuracy in real time.

2.1.2 Efficient Deployment for Real-Time Diagnostics

One key novelty in our work is to leverage the efficient architecture of YOLOv10 to allow for real-time performance. This allows for portable device deployment. Our approach will prove practical for mobile or field-based diagnostics, thus enabling healthcare workers to carry out on-site detection with little delay. This is quite an advancement from the traditional methods of diagnosis, which would require central facilities and a more extended processing time. Our method supports timely intervention, which is very important for effective disease management. This results from the fact that our method reduces the time needed to obtain results.

2.1.3 Adaptation of Unstained Thick Blood Smear Images

Our work uses unstained thick blood smear images that, unlike most of the previous works on stained blood smears, brings two main advantages: it reduces the requirement of the tedious time-consuming chemical staining process and is mostly unavailable in remote clinics, and it preserves the natural morphology of the parasites, which may be possibly beneficial for improving the accuracy of detection. This makes our approach very suitable for resource-constrained settings where the accessibility of reagents and laboratory facilities is limited.

2.1.4 Comparative Analysis with Established Models

We have designed our detection framework and have performed thorough comparative analysis with the models that are already well established: Faster R-CNN, RetinaNet, and YOLOv7. Quantitative evaluation on F1-scores, confusion matrices, and precision-recall curves demonstrates YOLOv10 to outperform for trypanosome detection. This comparison points toward possible applications in medical imaging since prior models are constantly outperformed by YOLOv10 in terms of both accuracy and speed.

2.2 Structure of the Work

We have structured our work into seven parts. Part III provides an overview of the Tryp dataset and challenges. It elaborates on the images used for microscopy and their corresponding annotations toward the detection of trypanosomes. Part IV provides the YOLOv10 algorithm, which yields details about the basic structure of the model as well as its application on the dataset. Part V discusses the outcome from the implementation of YOLOv10, where the performance of the system is measured in terms of various metrics. Finally, Section VI and VII depict conclusion where summaries regarding the findings made and improvement achieved are presented along with possible future directions of this work.

3 Dataset Description and Challenges

The Tryp dataset [8] is specifically curated: a collection of microscopy images for the detection of Trypanosoma brucei parasites in unstained thick blood smears. It contains an overall 3178 images, split between positive and negative samples, thus becoming the biggest dataset of its kind. The positive sample set consists of 3085 images of infected blood smears, annotated by using bounding boxes that tightly enclose regions containing the parasite. The dataset further includes negative images, uninfected blood smears with no annotations. The "negative" partition is important as it is a collection of uninfected samples; it will be used in training and evaluation experiments to check the model's ability to discriminate between infected and non-infected samples while simulating the diagnostic practice in real-world applications. These unlabelled images are control samples in which the model generalizes well by learning to identify parasitic infections as well as to prevent false positives when coming across healthy blood samples. The addition of these uninfected control images to the dataset allows it to make predictions of the model's true presence of the parasite instead of artifacts or noise in a microscopy image. In addition, the high and numerous diversities of the set of samples annotated in the dataset with variations in preparation, lighting, and microscopic resolution increase the complexity of the dataset and prepare models for real challenges that may arise in disease detection.

Figure. 1 shows the sample images of the Tryp dataset, including both positive and negative images. It can be observed that there are some overlapping bounding boxes in the left image, and also the density of the parasites is different for each positive sample, so there is a need to study the characteristics of the bounding boxes of the Tryp dataset that are discussed in the base paper [17] such as concentration of parasites, bounding region relationships, and the overall bounding region density distribution can be quantified with the help of metrics such as bounding box count per image, Overlapping bounding box count per image and Region of Interest (ROI) ratio. The distribution of all the above listed metrics, considering the bounding regions in the dataset can be found in Fig. 2.

The plot to the left in Fig. 2 is the histogram of bounding box counts per image in the Tryp dataset. From the histogram here, we can observe that most of the images have a relatively low number of bounding boxes, peaking in the range around 5 to 15 bounding boxes per image. This would imply, for most the images, very few trypanosomes would be present; and hence, the dataset is biased towards sparsely populated images. As count for bounding boxes increases, this falls rapidly, meaning that there is an insignificantly small number of images that have a higher population of objects within the scene. A closer-up inset here will help pick out the trend that some

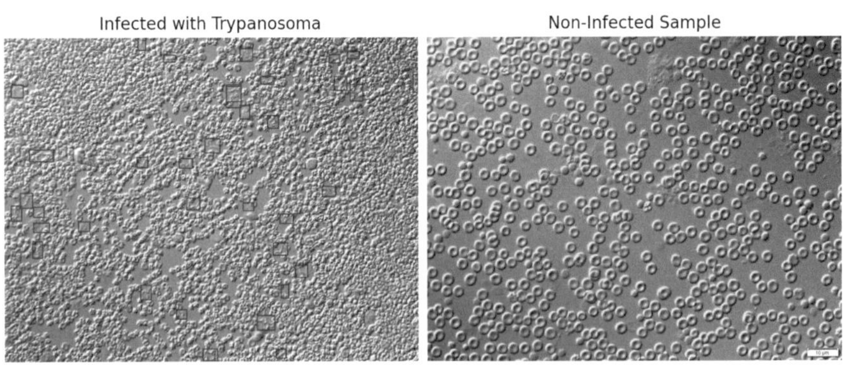

Fig. 1 Left: Infected blood sample, Right: Non-infected blood sample

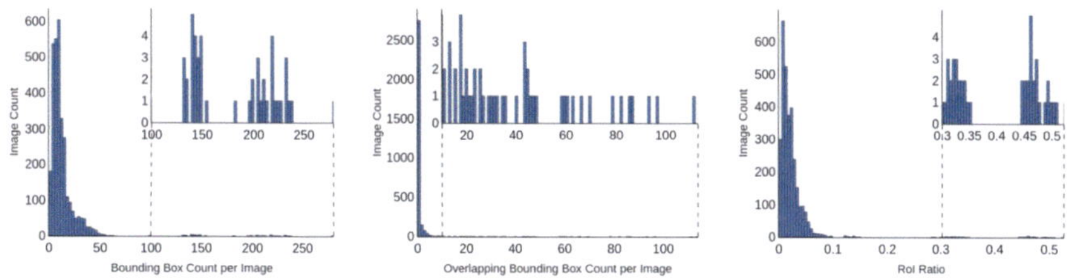

Fig. 2 Histograms for characteristics of bounding box annotations of dataset

of the infrequent cases contain as many as 250 bounding boxes. What this indicates is that the model should primarily be better at detecting a few trypanosomes per image, but it also needs to be prepared for occasional scenarios containing higher densities of objects. A key property of this distribution informs model design by underlining the necessity of robustness to high- and low-density detection.

The plot in the middle of Fig. 2. shows how many overlapping bounding boxes appear in each image, that is, how the trypanosomes spatially distribute and bunch up within the dataset. Histograms are plotted as well to show most images with minimal or no overlaps; indeed, most of them have less than 10 overlaps. This usually means that trypanosomes are not bunched too much within the images; hence, their detection is mostly easy since the chance of significant occlusion is low. However, the inset view reveals that a small subset of images experiences a high degree of overlap, with more than 100 overlapping bounding boxes in rare cases. This subset introduces complexity because the model needs to be able to distinguish closely positioned trypanosomes, which is challenging when objects overlap or are partially occluded. Therefore, although the dataset is mainly composed of isolated trypanosomes, its existence of crowded regions requires that the model be able to detect both isolated and densely clustered trypanosome detections. The final plot towards the right in Fig. 2 shows the distribution of Region of Interest (ROI) ratio, which measures the portion of the image area occupied by bounding boxes. Most trypanosomes occupy less than a tenth of the entire image area because most of the ROI ratios are less than 0.1. This pattern suggests that trypanosomes are generally small objects in the image, hence a model should be sensitive to small objects. The inset view focusing on the upper end of the distribution shows that some bounding boxes occupy up to 50% of the area of the image, which might imply that in a few instances, trypanosomes can be closer to the camera or are larger in size. This variation in ROI ratios indicates the need for the model to be able to accommodate a wide range of object sizes. From understanding this distribution, one does see how the model needs to balance high spatial resolution for detecting the smaller trypanosomes while being accommodating enough for the occasional large-scale detections in the dataset.

4 Methods

In this section we discuss about the methods used in the work, such as dataset used, data preprocessing, YOLOv10 for object detection, architecture of YOLOv10, training a YOLOv10 model on the Tryp dataset and hyperparameter tuning. The pipeline of the steps that are taken for the implementation of trypanosome detection using fine-tuned YOLOv10 model is illustrated in Fig. 3.

4.1 Data Acquisition and Pre-processing

To facilitate effective pre- processing and model training, the structure of the Tryp dataset was modified as shown in Fig. 4. The dataset was reorganized into two primary directories: positive and negative images. The positive images directory, is again further divided into sub-directories, they are trsain, validation, and test—were created, each of which contains two further sub-directories namely images and labels. The images directory stores the red blood smear images, while the labels directory holds the corresponding annotation files. These annotations were initially formatted for the YOLOv7 model, and for compatibility with the chosen YOLOv10 PyTorch model, we converted all annotations to the appropriate format. In this format, each image has a corresponding.txt file with one line per bounding box.

All the values except the first one which represents the presence of Trypanosome in an image are normalized to floating point value between 0 and 1 by dividing x and width values by the image's width, and y and height values by the image's height to obtain the normalized xywh coordinates. This modification ensures that the annotations are structured and in a format compatible with the YOLOv10 model, optimizing it for the object detection task. A summary of the dataset characteristics which consists of count of images in each directory along with parasite count across various partitions is given in Table 2.

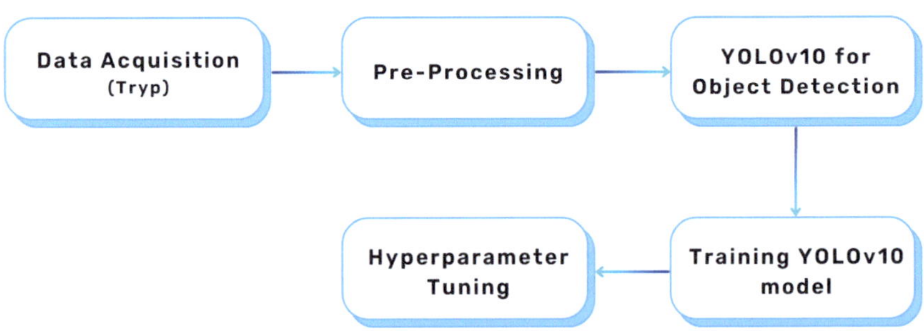

Fig. 3 Block diagram describing the pipeline for Trypanosome detection

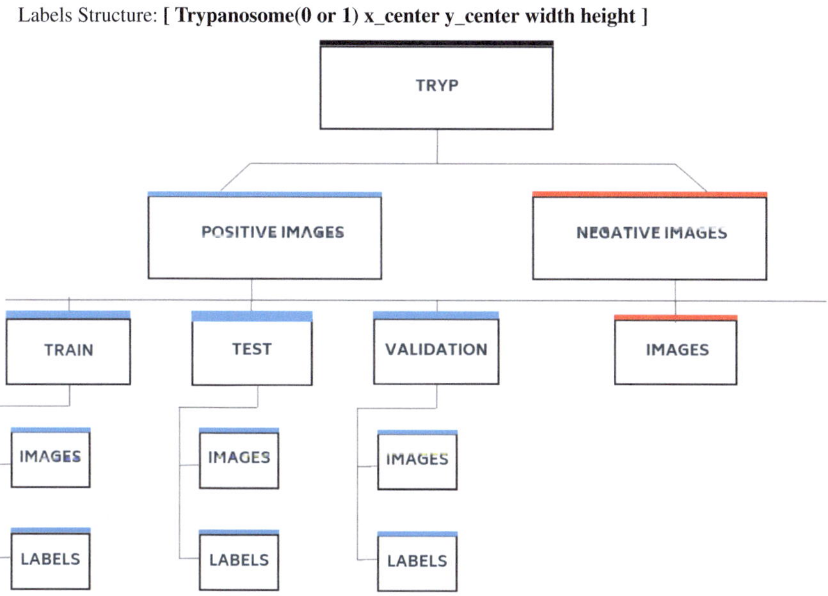

Fig. 4 Directory structure of Tryp dataset

Table 2 Images and parasite count in various partitions

Partition	Image count	Parasite count
Training directory	1893	27,489
Validation directory	610	8697
Testing directory	612	9094
Negative images directory	93	0

4.2 YOLOv10 for Object Detection

YOLOv10 is a recent addition in the "You Only Look Once" targeted object detection models for real-time object detection applications. Given its capacity to detect objects with top-end speed while maintaining an outright competitive level of accuracy, the YOLO model has gained widespread adoption in both object detection applications and research [15, 20]. Unlike other classical object detection frameworks, YOLO framed a problem of regression-by rephrasing object detection as a single, end-to-end form instead of regional proposals. Therefore, the YOLO models can predict object categories and the corresponding bounding boxes together in a stage, which saves considerable time complexity for inference. An important improvement can be seen in the YOLOv10 variant over its previous counterparts by improving the model architecture and taking note of the drawbacks associated with Non-Maximum Suppression (NMS), which is considered a problem in object detection problems as it leads to missed detections, especially in scenarios where multiple overlapping objects have low confidence scores [22]. YOLOv10 uses a dual label assignment strategy [33], combining one-to-many and one-to-one matching. One-to-one matching assigns a single prediction to each ground truth, eliminating NMS. One-to-many provides richer supervisory signals. Both heads are optimized together during training, leveraging rich supervision from one-to-many assignments.

YOLOv10 introduces architectural innovations to enhance accuracy and efficiency. Its architecture comprises three key components as shown in Fig. 5.

- Backbone: It uses an advanced CSPNet (Cross Stage Partial Network) to further enhance gradient flow and reduce redundancy in computations, which optimizes the use of feature extraction on small object detection, such as trypanosomes.
- Neck: The applicability of Path Aggregation Network (PAN) layers, which allow the aggregation of multiscale features, ensures that this model can identify objects at different scales in microscopy images, which are particularly necessary in different sizes of parasites.
- Head: It has two heads with different functionalities [33]:

– **One-to-Many Head**: During training, to learn the features effectively, this head generates multiple predictions per each object.
– **One-to-One Head:** This head generates a single best prediction per object during inference, which reduces the latency and improves the efficiency.

For the task of parasite Trypanosoma brucei detection on unstained thick blood smears, YOLOv10 offers several advantages. First one being, it is incorporating large-kernel convolution and self-attention mechanisms with minimal cost improvement in boosting accuracy. To eliminate redundancy in its stage, it employs intrinsic rank analysis. It also uses depth-wise convolutions for spatial mixing and point-wise convolutions at a minimal cost for channel mixing, hence suggesting a CIB structure. The rank-guided block allocation strategy replaces the most redundant stages with much more compact designs without compromising on performance. The ability of YOLOv10 to be able to provide good performance even for samples having significantly varying scales of trypanosomes is made possible by the enhanced feature extraction realized by CSPNet as well as the PAN layers, which now further enhance multiscale feature fusion. The low-weight classification head and efficient down sampling techniques in use ensure that the model will run even in field laboratories of resource-poor environments. These architectural and methodological improvements make YOLOv10 a particularly appropriate choice for improving the accuracy and efficiency of trypanosome detection.

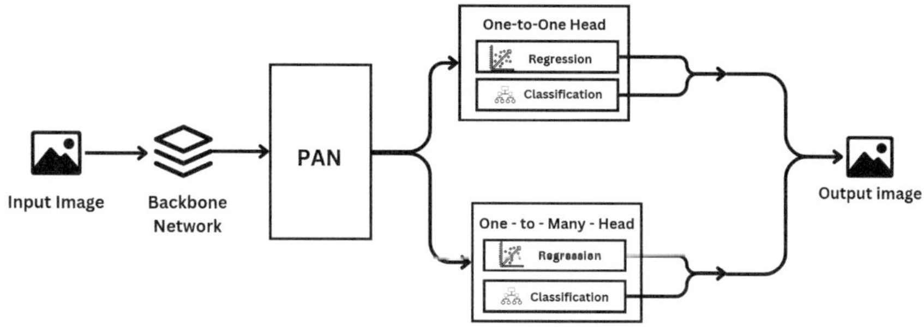

Fig. 5 Consistent dual assignments for NMS-free training

4.3 *Training YOLOV10 For Trypanosome Detection*

We used an all-out approach in fine-tuning the YOLOv10 model to classify trypanosomes in microscopic image samples. The dataset was split into training, validation, and testing datasets containing all instances of only one class, 'trypanosome'. We also formatted the path to dataset instances in this manner. Furthermore, we saved paths of directories within a YAML config file to easily load during training or evaluation of the network. We resized all the images to 640 × 640 pixels to ensure they met the input requirements for the YOLOv10. This resolution had enough detail to identify the parasites in the blood smear yet was computationally friendly enough. We also applied additional techniques for data augmentation such as Random scaling, flipping, and color jitter. The goal was to achieve model generalization under possibly different conditions and some microscope imaging noise. We trained our fine-tuned YOLOv10 model for over 50 epochs and a batch size of 4 was obtained through hyperparameter tuning. The code ran on an NVIDIA A100 GPU, which utilized two data-loading workers in parallelization to speed up the process of loading the data and therefore training time. In addition, mixed-precision training was used for training; this maximizes the usage of the GPUs, processing much faster while not lowering the accuracy of the model. The learning rate was also set using a dynamic learning rate strategy with the base value and then gradually decayed using a cosine annealing scheduler. This kind of learning rate strategy enables significant updates at early epochs, while fine-tuned adjustments happen toward the end of training. Gradient clipping was implemented during training to prevent exploding gradients, especially since the trypanosome dataset had fine-grained features. During training, model's performance is monitored using validation accuracy and loss metrics at every epoch. We tracked in addition to the overall validation accuracy, precision, recall, and mean average precision (mAP). This allowed us to establish whether the model could truly classify trypanosomes precisely. After the completion of training, we noticed the ability to model to avoid false positives during detection. It took nearly one hour and fifteen minutes to train our fine-tuned YOLOv10 model. Finally, the trained model was saved, and we checked its performance on the test set and we found that it was more effective in classifying trypanosome instances in blood smear images compared to the already existing algorithms that were trained on the Tryp dataset.

4.4 Hyperparameter Tuning

We employed hyperparameter tuning exhaustively to get the best possible performance out of the YOLOv10 model for trypanosome detection. It is crucial that not only does the model give high accuracy but also generalizes well to data it hasn't seen yet; we thus set the learning rate at a base value and experimented with various values within the range 10^{-5}–10^{-2}. We found that a smaller learning rate in the first epochs of training led to more stable training and fewer oscillations in validation accuracy. Having tried batch sizes ranging from 4 to 16, we determined that a batch size of 4 was optimal because it allowed the model to learn the details in the image more accurately, which is needed for identification of parasites of varying sizes. Later we experimented with different Intersection over Union (IoU) thresholds ranging from 0.3 to 0.7 and found that an IoU threshold of 0.5 gives the best balance between precision and recall. This setting helped minimize both false positives and false negatives, improving the model's ability to correctly identify parasite instances without excessive overlap with surrounding objects. We have adjusted our confidence score threshold, which essentially is the minimum confidence level something needs to have for it to be considered true. We set this score between 0.25 and 0.5 so that we could find some optimal balance that reduced unnecessary false positives without sacrificing anything in terms of true detection.

5 Experimental Results

After the training procedure, we tested the YOLOv10 model to validate and test datasets properly on the detection ability on trypanosomes in blood smear images. Figure 6 displays the results obtained for two positive images containing trypanosome parasites. The bounding boxes in blue represent the parasites that were identified by the model, whereas those in red boxes represent those which were undetected by the model. We used recall, precision, Mean Average Precision at an Intersection over Union threshold of 50% (AP@IoU0.5) and F1 score measures for performance evaluation. These metrics give a clear idea about of the effectiveness of the model, to correctly identify trypanosomes and also its ability to predict only trypanosomes and not misclassify other cells in the image as parasites.

Table 3 provides a comparative analysis of the performance of various object detection models—Faster R-CNN, RetinaNet, YOLOv7, and our fine-tuned YOLOv10—on the Tryp dataset. The metrics presented include mean average precision (mAP), precision, recall, and F1 score for both validation and test sets.

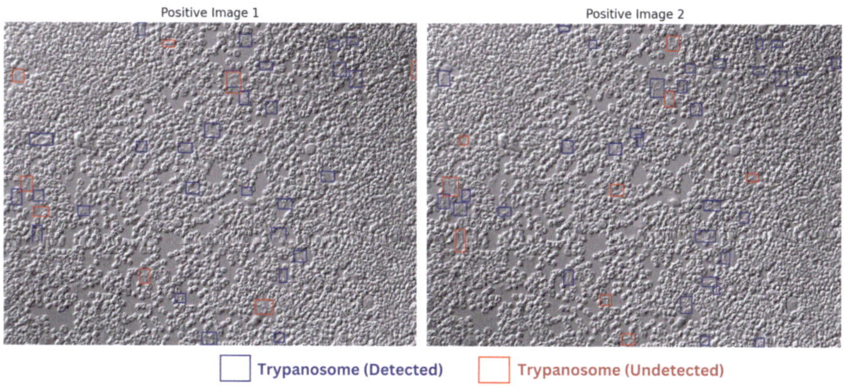

Fig. 6 Trypanosome detection results for two positive images

Table 3 Comparing performance of the existing models on the Tryp dataset

Model	Partition	Mean average precision	Precision	Recall	F1 score
Faster R-CNN [17]	Validation	65%	71%	71%	71%
	Test	63%	71%	70%	71%
RetinaNet [17]	Validation	52%	83%	56%	67%
	Test	50%	82%	55%	66%
YOLOv7 [17]	Validation	57%	87%	62%	72%
	Test	55%	87%	62%	72%
Fine-tuned YOLOv10 (proposed)	Validation	79%	79%	73%	76%
	Test	78%	79%	72%	76%

Performance-wise, YOLOv10 improved over all the others based on every key metric considered. Meters per aperture the YOLOv10 achieved had a validation mAP of 0.79 (79%), compared to improvement of 23% to the validated mAP produced by the YOLOv7 for a score of 0.57 (57%). The superiority in mAP produced by the YOLOv10 means that this particular model exhibits more accurate true positive detection than false positives. The performance of the validation set by YOLOv10 was equally remarkable at 0.79, equivalent to the mAP score. Precision is an important quantity, measuring how accurately a model can identify positive instances without false positives - extremely important in medical contexts. Because misclassification there may result in either false positives or in a missed detection, strong precision underscores that YOLOv10 is dependable regarding the provision of the right detections, making this essential for application in clinical areas. As far as recall is concerned, YOLOv10 scored 0.73 (73%) on the validation set. Recall simply says how sensitive the model is towards catching all cases of trypanosome infections; a high score indicates that very few cases of infection were missed. This puts YOLOv10 miles ahead of RetinaNet, which managed to attain 0.56 (56%) on the validation set. This increase in recall without sacrificing precision results in a validation set F1 score of 0.76 or 76%, 4% higher than the F1 score achieved by YOLOv7. Performance on the test set further validated YOLOv10's robustness. The model achieved a mAP score of 0.78 (78%) on the test set and managed to keep its performance at almost the same level as the validation results. Thus, it shows consistency between validation and test metrics, indicating the generalization of the model, which is a major factor for real applications. Precision remained high at 0.79 (79%), whereas recall was a bit lower at 0.72 (72%). However, YOLOv10's F1 score on the test set is 0.76 (76%), which closely matches the validation score and thus secures stability and reliability in this model for different splits of data. In contrast, Faster R-CNN and RetinaNet performed relatively worse overall. Faster R-CNN obtained a very good mAP of 0.65 (65%) along with precision of 0.71 (71%) on the validation set but had some recall problem with 0.71 (71%), which made the F1 score 0.71 (71%). The detection performance of RetinaNet was quite low as with a mAP of just 0.52 (52%) and F1-score of only 0.67 (67%). Therefore, it was not that appropriate in this detection scenario either. YOLOv7, although achieving higher precision (87%) than YOLOv10, suffered from lower recall, which impacted its F1 score.

To further evaluate model performance, a confusion matrix (Fig. 7) provides a detailed breakdown of correctly and incorrectly classified samples. The confusion matrix illustrates a high number of true positive predictions, with 6854 correctly identified trypanosomes and only 1573 false negatives, where trypanosomes were misclassified as background. This low rate of false negatives is crucial for diagnostic applications, where missing true instances could lead to undiagnosed cases. Additionally, there were only a limited number of false positives, indicating that the model was not prone to over-predicting the presence of trypanosomes in non-infected samples. The plot shown in Fig. 8 helps us to establish a relation between confidence threshold and the F1-score and tell us how both these quantities affect one another. From the figure, F1-score remains almost constant across a wide range of confidence thresholds, with a peak value at 0.76. This behaviour exhibited by the curve is essential in practical settings because it indicates that the model is performing consistently even in case of variations in confidence scores.

Figure 9 represents the Precision-Recall (PR) Curve for the fine-tuned YOLOv10 model. It gives an idea on the balance between precision and recall. The Area under the curve (AUC) value obtained from the plot is 0.785, which shows that precision and recall are well balanced. A higher AUC value obtained in this case is considered as an advantage to the trypanosome detection application because it shows that the model would retain high recall. It also highlights the model's ability to capture most true trypanosome instances while ensuring a good precision, by avoiding false positives. This balance is particularly important in the medical field as high recall decreases the likelihood of missing cases while minimizing the chance of false results.

On the validation set, YOLOv10 reached an Average Precision (AP) score of 0.79. This is notably superior to the methods such as Faster R-CNN, RetinaNet and especially to the YOLOv7 model. A considerable improvement in AP represents better localization and detection accuracy for the trypanosome instances on the images

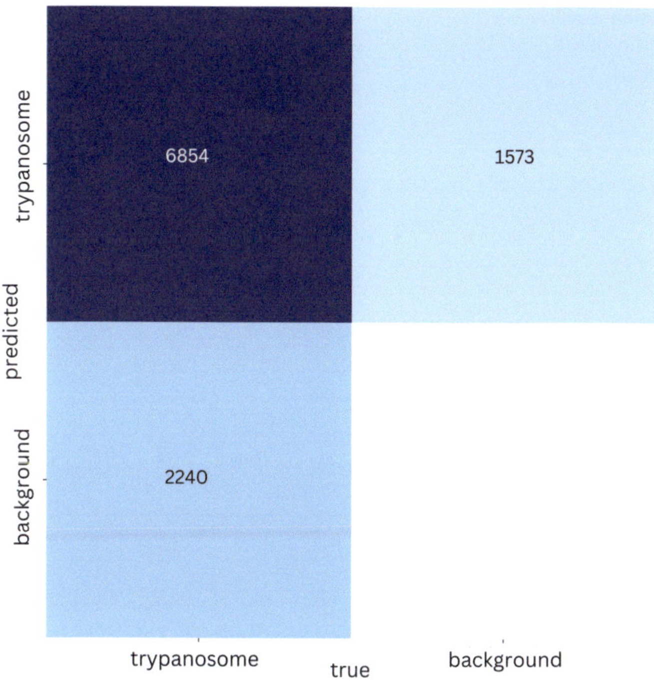

Fig. 7 Confusion matrix for the fine-tuned YOLOv10 model

Fig. 8 F1-score versus Confidence plot for the fine-tuned YOLOv10 model

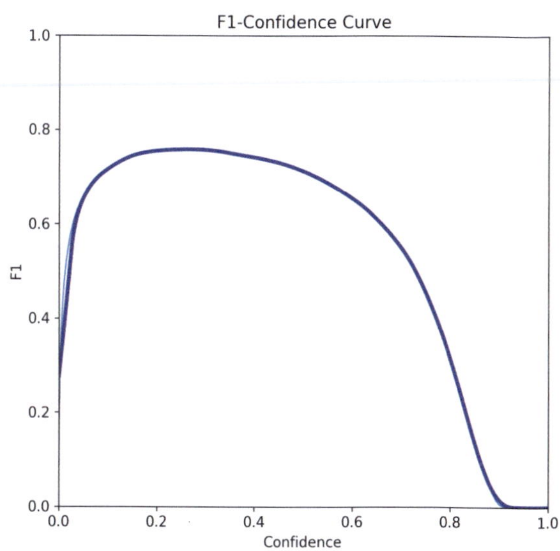

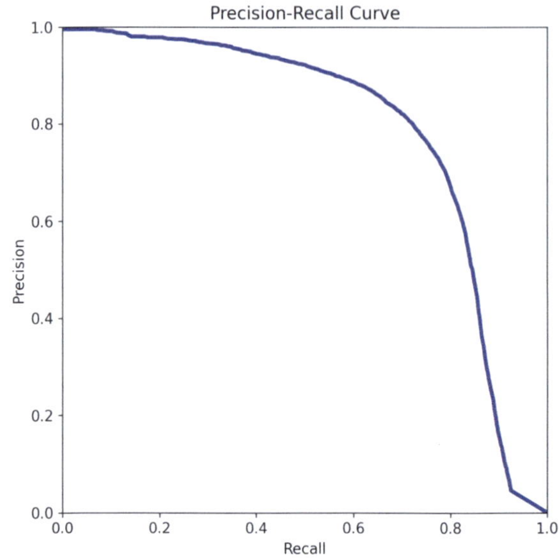

Fig. 9 Precision-recall curve for the fine-tuned YOLOv10 model

even at conditions with dense clustering or low contrast. This gain in mAP implies higher reliability in the presence of trypanosomes. This can be critical for diagnostic purposes where the location is going to be exact, and it directly influences the decision. Consistency is a benchmark for the generalization ability of a model. Here, the model YOLOv10 gives almost equivalent metrics on both validation and test sets. These experiments appear to suggest that the model is not overfitting certain details of the training set but is capturing the bigger patterns and features that enable reliable trypanosome detection. Consistent performance across these test and validation sets reinforces suitability for real-world deployment applications, where detection must indeed be reliable across various kinds of samples.

6 Conclusion

In this work, we were able to successfully apply YOLOv10 to enhance the trypanosomes identification from microscopic images through a proper evaluation of the Tryp dataset. The fine-tuned model of YOLOv10 showed significant improvements over the existing detection models, especially for the Faster R-CNN, RetinaNet, and YOLOv7 variants in terms of precision, detection speed, and accuracy. These progresses further were uncovered by the regularly achieved superior F1-scores, in-depth confusion matrix analysis, and precision-recall curves that emphasize the fact that YOLOv10 specifically outperforms for the adopted medical application. The results indicate not only the efficiency of YOLOv10 but also highlight the fact that it may be very applicable in resource-limited healthcare setups where rapid, accurate diagnosis is critical. This work itself provides implications that go far beyond the simple detection of trypanosomes, since it would lay foundations for making use of strong AI in medical diagnostics, and its application in terms appropriate to it- especially in remote or under-reserved regions. This work achieves this satisfactory success by demonstrating the potential for real-time automatic detection at high accuracy levels for trypanosomes and will go a long way in its extensive applications in enhancing better surveillance and timely intervention of parasitic disease spread in affected communities. Furthermore, the viability of the YOLOv10 model in the treatment of micro-sized objects' small size and heterogeneity in quality images from microscopic image analysis makes the model quite viable for other health care-based microscopic image analysis tasks.

7 Future Works

The findings are promising and leave room for much future work in refining and expanding on this work. One of the variants worth studying is the integration of semi-supervised or unsupervised learning approaches with YOLOv10. In scenarios where there is less information available, this could help improve the approach because annotating parasites in medical images may often raise issues, and further, transfer learning using YOLOv10 for other parasites diseases can make the overall tool more generalizable and interesting. Another direction that could be explored is the integration of YOLOv10 with cloud-based computing solutions, which helps in deploying this model in real-time on portable medical devices in field settings. YOLOv10 in a multi-stage or multi-class detection setting may further enhance its applicability with a number of difficult diagnostic tasks, the identification of multiple pathogens, co-infections, etc. It can thus analyse much more information about blood smear samples and improve the workflow that leads to a better basis for decision-making by practitioners. Another promising direction of research is the use of explainable AI (XAI) in order to increase the transparency and confidence building in the model. The reasons why the model identifies trypanosomes will become known, and medical practitioners will place more confidence in the outputs generated, while researchers may optimize the model further based on insights from explainability studies. In conclusion, our work goes beyond ensuring the efficiency of YOLOv10 at the task of trying to detect trypanosomes. Rather, it sets a sturdy basis for the usage of deep object detection models in not only mission-critical healthcare but also substantial and broader applications. In this light, YOLOv10 is primed for developing a valuable contribution to automated diagnostics, especially where neglected tropical diseases continue affecting hundreds of millions globally.

References

1. Feasey, N., Wansbrough-Jones, M., Mabey, D.C., Solomon, A.W.: Neglected tropical diseases. Br. Med. Bull. **93**(1), 179–200 (2010). https://doi.org/10.1093/bmb/ldp046
2. Büscher, P.: Diagnosis of African trypanosomiasis. In Trypanosomes and Trypanosomiasis. Springer. (2014). https://doi.org/10.1007/978-3-7091-1556-5_8
3. Pérez-Molina, J.A., Molina, I.: Chagas disease. Lancet. **391**, 82–94 (2018). https://doi.org/10.1016/S0140-6736(17)31612-4
4. Franco, J.R., et al.: The elimination of human African trypanosomiasis: achievements in reach and looming challenges. PLOS Negl.Ed Trop. Dis. **14**(4), e0008287
5. Bern, C., Montgomery, S.P.: An estimate of the burden of Chagas disease in the United States. Clin. Infect. Dis. **49**(5), e52–e54 (2009)
6. Simarro, P.P., et al.: The human African trypanosomiasis control and surveillance program of the World Health Organization. PLOS Negl.Ed Trop. Dis. **6**(2), e1721 (2012)
7. Shaw, A.P.M.: The economics of African trypanosomiasis. Trop. Anim. Health Prod. **36**(5), 405–416 (2004)
8. Rassi Jr., A., Rassi, A., Marin-Neto, J.A.: Chagas disease. Lancet. **375**(9723), 1388–1402 (2010)
9. World Health Organization. Working to overcome the global impact of neglected tropical diseases: first WHO report on neglected tropical diseases (2010).
10. Desquesnes, M., et al.: A review on the diagnosis of animal trypanosomoses. (2022). https://doi.org/10.1186/s13071-022-05190-1
11. Mulenga, G.M., et al.: Tropical medicine and infectious disease challenges in the diagnostic performance of parasitological and molecular tests in the surveillance of African Trypanosomiasis in eastern Zambia. Trop. Med. Infect. Dis. **6** (2021)
12. Caballero, Z.C., Sousa, O.E., Marques, W.P., Saez-Alquezar, A., Umezawa, E.S.: Evaluation of serological tests to identify Trypanosoma cruzi infection in humans and determine cross-reactivity with Trypanosoma rangeli and Leishmania spp. Clin. Vaccine Immunol. 14(8), 1045–1049 (2007). https://doi.org/10.1128/CVI.00127-07. Epub 2007 May 23. PMID: 17522327; PMCID: PMC2044488.
13. Ahmed, H.A., Picozzi, K., Welburn, S.C., et al.: A comparative evaluation of PCR- based methods for species- specific determination of African animal trypanosomes in Ugandan cattle. Parasites Vectors. **6**, 316 (2013). https://doi.org/10.1186/1756-3305-6-316
14. Desquesnes, M., Dávila A.M.: Applications of PCR-based tools for detection and identification of animal trypanosomes: a review and perspectives. Vet. Parasitol. 109(3–4):213–231. (2002). https://doi.org/10.1016/s0304-4017(02)00270-4. PMID: 12423934.
15. Solano, P., Michel, J.F., Lefrançois, T., De La Rocque, S.: Polymerase chain reaction detection of Trypanosoma in cattle. Vet.Y Parasitol. (1999)
16. Redmon, J., Divvala, S., Girshick, R., Farhadi, A.: You only look once: unified, real-time object detection. In Proceedings of the IEEE Computer Society Conference on Computer Vision and Pattern Recognition. (2016). https://doi.org/10.1109/CVPR.2016.91
17. Anzaku, E.T., Mohammed, M.A., Ozbulak, U., et al.: Tryp: a dataset of microscopy images of unstained thick blood smears for trypanosome detection. Sci. Data. **10**, 716 (2023). https://doi.org/10.1038/s41597-023-02608-y
18. Kim, J., Álvarez-Rodríguez, A., Li, Z., Radwanska, M., Magez, S.: Recent progress in the detection of Surra, a neglected disease caused by *Trypanosoma evansi* with a one health impact in large parts of the tropic and sub-tropic world. Microorganisms. **12**(1), 44 (2024). https://doi.org/10.3390/microorganisms12010044
19. Hassan-Kadle, A.A., Ibrahim, A.M., Nyingilili, H.S., Yusuf, A.A., Vieira, R.F.C.: parasitological and molecular detection of Trypanosoma spp. in cattle, goats and sheep in Somalia. Parasitology. **147**(14), 1786–1791 (2020). https://doi.org/10.1017/S003118202000178X
20. Rebeski, D.E., Winger, E.M., Rogovic, B., et al.: Improved methods for the diagnosis of African trypanosomosis. Memórias Do Inst. Oswaldo Cruz. (1999)

21. Kann, S., Kunz, M., Hansen, J., Sievertsen, J., Crespo, J.J., Loperena, A., Arriens, S., Dandekar, T.: Chagas disease: detection of *Trypanosoma cruzi* by a new, high-specific real time PCR. J. Clin. Med. **9**(5), 1517 (2020). https://doi.org/10.3390/jcm9051517
22. Li, L., Qin, L., et al.: Tuberculosis detection in chest X-ray images using YOLOv4. Expert Syst. Appl. (2020)
23. Jiang, H., et al.: Geometry-aware cell detection with deep learning. mSystems. **5** (2020). https://doi.org/10.1128/msystems.00840-19
24. Sunil, A., Sajithvariyar, V.V., Sowmya, V., Sivanpillai, R., Soman, K.P.: identifying oil pads in high spatial resolution aerial images using faster r-cnn. Int. Arch. Photogramm. Remote Sens. Spatial Inf. Sci. **155–161** (2021). https://doi.org/10.5194/isprs-archives-XLIV-M-3-2021-155-2021
25. Ren, S., He, K., Girshick, R., Sun, J.: Faster R-CNN: towards real-time object detection with region proposal networks. IEEE Trans. Pattern Anal. Mach. Intell. **39**(6), 1137–1149 (2017)
26. Shao, W., Yang, X., Yan, Y., Zhang, Z.: Real-time human detection based on faster R-CNN and region of interest voting. J. Vis. Commun. Image Represent. **55**, 95–102 (2018)
27. Lin, T.-Y., Goyal, P., Girshick, R., He, K., Dollár, P.: Focal loss for dense object detection. IEEE Trans. Pattern Anal. Mach. Intell. **42**(2), 318–327 (2020)
28. Redmon, J., Farhadi, A.: YOLOv3: an incremental improvement. *arXiv preprint*, https://arxiv.org/abs/1804.02767
29. Harisankar, V., Karthika, R.: Real time pedestrian detection using modified YOLO V2. In: 2020 5th International Conference on Communication and Electronics Systems (ICCES), Coimbatore, India, pp. 855–859 (2020).https://doi.org/10.1109/ICCES48766.2020.9138103
30. An, L., Peng, K., Yang, X. An improved deep network of pulmonary tuberculosis lesions detection based on YOLO. In: 2022 IEEE 24th International Conference on High Performance Computing and Communications (HPCC), pp. 1–6 (2022). https://doi.org/10.1109/HPCC-202210074747
31. Chandio, A.A., Mehmood, M., Zahid, F.M., Riaz, I.: Malaria detection using YOLO v5 with transfer learning. J. Biomed. Sci. Eng. **14**(5), 1–6
32. Ali, B.S., Nasir, H., Khan, A., Ashraf, M., Akbar, S.M.: A machine learning-based model for the detection of skin cancer using yolov10. In 2024 IEEE 8th International Conference on Signal and Image Processing Applications (ICSIPA), Kuala Lumpur, Malaysia, pp. 1–6 (2024) https://doi.org/10.1109/ICSIPA62061.2024.10686198
33. Wang, A., Hui, C., Lihao, L., Kai, C., Zijia, L., Jungong, H., Guiguang, D.: Yolov10: Real-time end-to-end object detection. *arXiv preprint*. https://arxiv.org/abs/2405.14458 (2024).

Automatic Panoramic Radiographs Segmentation for Dental Disease Detection Using YOLO11

Priscilla Whitin, S. Sivakumar, Vinayakumar Ravi, K. Anish Pon Yamini, S. Jebarose Juliyana, and K. Suthendran

Abstract Dental abnormalities detection from radiographs is vital during dental treatment. Clinicians spend an arduous amount of time for oral diagnosis and analyzing the radiograph manually to check if any dental ailment is present. This process can sometimes cause misinterpretation due to lack of dentist experience or workload stress. Hence, this chapter introduces a recent deep learning state of model to automatically interpret the radiographs and expeditiously deliver the output.YOLO11 includes new module to perform enhanced feature detection. It is evaluated on a custom dataset of panoramic images annotated for four different classes (caries, fillings, root canal treated tooth and impacted tooth). The model attained a Precision of 0.808 on all classes, recall of 0.773, mAP 50 of 0.809 and mAP 95 of 0.482 respectively. The proposed method could assist the dentist in their workflow and elevate the quality of dental treatment in future.

The original version of the chapter has been revised. A correction to this chapter can be found at https://doi.org/10.1007/978-3-032-21009-8_28

P. Whitin · S. Sivakumar · K. A. P. Yamini · S. J. Juliyana
Vel Tech Rangarajan Dr. Sagunthala R&D Institute of Science and Technology, Chennai, India
e-mail: priscillawhitin@veltech.edu.in

S. Sivakumar
e-mail: ssivakumar@veltech.edu.in

K. A. P. Yamini
e-mail: dranishponyaminik@veltech.edu.in

S. J. Juliyana
e-mail: jebarose@veltech.edu.in

K. Suthendran (✉)
Kalasalingam Academy of Research and Education, Krishnankoil, India
e-mail: k.suthendran@klu.ac.in

V. Ravi
Center for Artificial Intelligence, Prince Mohammad Bin Fahd University, Al Khobar, Saudi Arabia
e-mail: vravi@pmu.edu.sa

P. Singh et al. (eds.), *Deep Learning Applications in Healthcare and Medical Imaging Practice*, Studies in Big Data 193, https://doi.org/10.1007/978-3-032-21009-8_11

Keywords Artificial intelligence · Deep learning · Panoramic radiograph · Dental disease · CNN · YOLO11 · Good health · Well-being

1 Introduction

Common oral health issues such as cavities, periodontitis, gingivitis, abscesses, and oral cysts sometimes lead to acute complications if not diagnosed at the right time. Dental Radiography examinations serve as a critical diagnostic tool in dentistry, it comes up with a comprehensive view of the entire periodontum. Manually analysing these radiographs is strenuous, depends upon the experience of dentist and prone to human error. Following recent strides in AI and deep learning, automated segmentation of panoramic radiographs has emerged as a promising solution for improving diagnostic accuracy and efficiency. The development of Artificial Intelligence has enabled computers to perform tasks in par with human intelligence in computer vision applications [1]. Computers have become proficient in image recognition as humans [2]. The possibility of AI applications in healthcare could make this era even more exciting than it has ever been [3]. AI will become more and more popular in the medical fields because of its significant benefits to patient health management services and the ease it offers practitioners [4, 5]. Machine learning utilizes huge data to train neural network models which can learn from the data and enable computers to perform image recognition on their own without human intervention [6]. The ultimate aim of ML is to formulate mathematical models that can learn from the given data, trained to generate desired outcomes when given input data, with the primary objective of identifying patterns or making precise prediction. Deep Learning (DL) being a subgroup of ML with multiple layers of network can learn from complex images and they can automatically generate visual features using original images [7, 8]. In recent times, DL is significantly used more in dentistry for diagnosis, screening, and decision-making [9–11]. To diagnose dental disease, dentist usually perform a clinical examination manually followed by radiography to precisely identify dental disorders location from X-ray images [12]. High computing power and storage capacity, Rapid processing speed, multitasking capability, and the competitiveness of sophisticated GPUs and computers have revolutionized medical field. Given the vast amount of available data, training artificial intelligence models in radiology has become significantly more straightforward than before. This research utilizes panoramic imaging, an extra oral radiographic method that offers multiple benefits. It reduces radiation exposure for patients, proves to be economical, and improves patient comfort by capturing the entire oral cavity in one image [13]. This research aims to identify dental disorders in panoramic X-rays utilizing the latest YOLO11 framework. Section 2 presents the literature survey on various dental diagnosis using DL frameworks. The methodology implemented is explained in Sect. 3 and training and evaluation in Sect. 4. The final section of the paper, Sect. 5, discusses the conclusion.

2 Literature Survey

This segment examines some of the recent studies that use of DL for identifying dental conditions, with a particular priority on X-rays. These methods have shown significant potential in ascertaining particular dental conditions from radiographic images like dental caries, periodontal disease, and implants. Gardiyanoğlu suggested an encoder –decoder model to automatically partition teeth, caries, restorations, implants, fillings and residual roots from panoramic radiographs, which will enable dentist to diagnose precisely in less time [14]. A CNN was developed by Lin and Chang to determine the tooth number from panoramic radiographs based on the teeth's position and condition [15]. Initially, the accuracy for identifying teeth numbers and conditions was 90.90% and 93.33%, respectively. However, after implementing the data augmentation technique, the accuracy for teeth numbering improved to 95.62%, and the accuracy for assessing teeth condition increased to 98.33%. Estai et al., implemented a DL model for automatic detection of teeth, utilizing U-net for segmentation, Faster RCNN for teeth detection and VGG16 classified the teeth (32 categories) [16]. Budagam et al., have suggested a DL model integrating YOLOv8 and U net architecture called as BB-U Net capable of classifying and segmenting teeth from panoramic radiographs [17]. In order to detect dental caries from X-ray pictures, Oztekin et al., tested three CNN models: EfficientNet-B0, ResNet-50 and DenseNet-121. With an accuracy of 92%, F1-score of 91.61%, and sensitivity of 92%, ResNet-50 demonstrated the best performance [18]. Almalki et al., demonstrated the YOLOv3 model to classify dental abnormalities. In this study, data augmentation is used to improve model robustness and achieved over 99% accuracy, demonstrating the effectiveness of CNNs for precise, automated analysis of dental conditions [19]. Zhu et al., constructed a DL model called CariesNet, to detect the type of caries from panoramic images. It obtained a dice coefficient score of 93.64% and an accuracy of 93.61% [20]. Al-Sarem et al., compared different DL model to detect missing tooth region from CBCT images. DenseNet169 exhibited superior performance with a precision score of 0.98 than other models [21]. In order to identify periodontitis on panoramic X-rays, Kim J et al., created a specialised model called DeNTNet (Detecting Periodontal Bone Loss Using Deep Learning), demonstrating the specificity that DL models can achieve in diagnosing particular dental conditions [22]. Takahashi et al., proposed a DL model to detect dental prostheses from oral photographs. The model was trained with 1904 images captured using mono lens reflex camera. Detection accuracy was 80% for metal prostheses and 60% for tooth colored ones [20]. Cejudo et al., analogized three DL models –Capsule network, ResNet and CNN to classify the different types of radiographs namely, panoramic, bitewing, cephalometric and periapical images. ResNet achieved higher performance than other models [21]. These studies demonstrate how DL is becoming more and more important in dental healthcare by providing resources that may help with early, accurate diagnostic misinterpretation and enhance patient outcomes.

3 Methodology

3.1 Data Preprocessing

Firstly, with due approval from the authorities, a total of 600 panoramic panoramic radiographs were accumulated from a clinical laboratory. Prima facie, 98 images were identified as belonging to patients with temporary (deciduous) teeth and 86 images were deemed distorted, blurred, or lacking sufficient diagnostic quality due to factors like motion artifacts or incorrect exposure. To preserve the dataset's accuracy and reliability, these low-quality and irrelevant images were removed and only 461 high-quality panoramic radiographs showcasing permanent dentition were selected for this study. These images were converted to PNG format to facilitate processing and ensure compatibility with deep learning frameworks. To safeguard patients privacy, all images were anonymized by removing their name and age. Furthermore, the images were resized to a pixel count of 640 × 640 to standardize the dataset and ensure uniform input dimensions.

3.2 Data Annotation

The panoramic radiographs, after pre-processing step were meticulously annotated. An experienced dentist carefully audit, annotated each image. This process was conducted on Roboflow platform, which offers an easy and efficient interface for creating accurate object boundaries in medical images. A polygonal annotation method was used which enabled precise outlining of dental structures and pathological areas, thereby enhancing the accuracy of the training data. The pre-processed panoramic x-ray annotated images for four different classes is shown in Fig. 1.

The total number of annotation is 1910 for the four classes. Table 1 illustrates the list of annotated objects under each category, along with the corresponding number of instances, providing an overview of the dataset distribution.

3.3 Data Augmentation

In order to address the challenge of the dataset's small size and enhance the YOLO11 model's generalization capabilities, data augmentation methods were employed during the pre-processing stage. Augumentation enhances the model's capability by expanding the dataset with less data. There are various augmentation methods like rotation, scaling, brightness changes, and noise addition, this study only employed horizontal and vertical flipping. This specific choice was made to maintain the anatomical accuracy and spatial orientation of dental structures in panoramic radiographs, as changing their orientation could distort clinically important areas. After

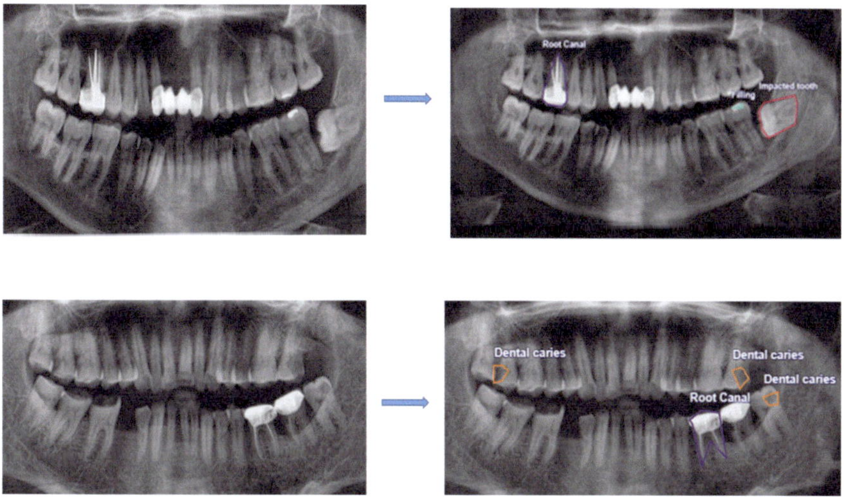

Fig. 1 Panoramic radiographs annotated

Table 1 Number of instances in each class

Class	Total	Training	Validation	Test
Root canal	592	437	126	29
Caries	523	376	123	24
Impacted	438	321	97	20
Filling	357	267	78	12

augmentation, the dataset was split into training, testing, and validation subsets in 75:15:10 ratio respectively. This division ensured the model had ample data for learning while keeping a balanced proportion for unbiased performance evaluation and hyperparameter tuning. Finally, the dataset was formatted into a YOLO11-compatible structure using a YAML (Yet Another Markup Language) configuration file, which specifies the dataset structure, class labels, and directory paths. The formatted dataset was then uploaded to Google Drive, serving as the main data source for model training and experimentation within the YOLO11 framework.

4 YOLO11 Architecture

YOLO11, a recent model released by Ultralytics, its speed, accuracy and efficiency makes it versatile for several computer vision applications [23]. YOLO11 incorporates several architectural features which are not available in the previous versions, to ameliorate feature extraction, accurate object detection and complex task performance. YOLO11 has an improved backbone and neck architecture. This model demonstrates a higher mean Average Precision (mAP) than YOLOv8 with 22% fewer parameters. YOLO11 can be effortlessly employed for various environments, which includes edge devices, cloud platforms, and NVIDIA GPUs, ensuring maximum flexibility. The modules in YOLO11 are similar to YOLOv8 with the head, neck, and backbone network.

4.1 Backbone

In the backbone module, input image is examined at various scales for feature extraction process and it creates several feature maps. There are several convolutional layers, C3k2, SPPF and C2PSA blocks. The C2f in YOLOv8 is replaced with C3k2 module in YOLO11, which is more efficacious in terms of computation. This module utilizes smaller kernel size to enhance speed and foster performance. It makes use of CSP (Cross Stage Partial) Bottleneck, in which instead of one large convolution two convolutions are performed by splitting the feature map. One segment passes through bottleneck layer and the other segment unites directly with the output of the bottleneck. The SPPF block generates fixed feature representation of various objects present in the image of different sizes without any information loss. Cross Stage Partial with Spatial Attention block enables the model to learn global relationship between pixels and features at different position enhancing better spatial representation. It focuses on critical areas of the image requiring attention.

4.2 Neck

The Neck component integrates all the feature maps of different resolutions from the backbone and conveys them to the head for detection. It includes C3k2, upsample and concat blocks. C3k2 enables the model to speed up the feature aggregation process. The upsampler is used to increase the feature map resolution in YOLO11 using the nearest neighbour upsampling method. The nearby pixel values are filled in the newly generated pixel in a larger image. In the concat blocks, the upsampled feature map is combined with the features from the C3k2 block. Number of channels will be summed up but resolution will remain unchanged.

4.3 *Head*

The YOLO11 head produces the ultimate prediction of the model. Additionally, it outputs the confidence score, class labels, and bounding boxes. Three layers of detection are generated in order to identify objects of three distinct sizes.

5 Training, Evaluation and Result

The experiment was carried out on a desktop featuring an Intel i5 processor and 8GB of RAM. The proposed YOLO11 was implemented in google colab using T4 GPU. The hyper parameters utilized during training is listed in the Table 2 below.

To evaluate the performance of YOLO11 model, the key metrics includes mAP, Recall and F1 score.

5.1 *Mean Average Precision (mAP)*

It is a preeminent metric used in object detection and segmentation tasks. It assesses the accuracy of the model in detecting objects across each class. For every classification category, the calculation is derived by juxtaposing the identified bounding box with the corresponding ground truth bounding box. The mAP is denoted at two levels:

mAP@0.5: Calculated at an IoU threshold of 0.5, average precision primarily assesses classification accuracy.

mAP@0.95: Average precision, a more rigorous metric for assessing both localization and classification accuracy, is calculated across Intersection over Union (IoU) thresholds that span from 0.5 to 0.95.

Higher mAP score indicates better predictions by the model.

Table 2 Hyperparameters of YOLO11

Parameters	Values
Optimizer	Adam
Batch size	64
Learning rate	0.00125
Epochs	250
Momentum	0.9

$$mAP = \sum_{k=1}^{k-n} AP \tag{1}$$

Where k is the number of classes.

5.2 Recall

Recall, frequently denoted as "sensitivity," quantifies the proportion of identified instances relative to the total number of relevant instances. An elevated recall value signifies that a greater number of predictions are accurate.

$$\text{Re call} = \frac{True\ Positives}{True\ Positives + False\ Negatives} \tag{2}$$

5.3 Precision

The model's precision indicates how well it can forecast the quantity of favorable occurrences.

$$\text{Precision} = \frac{True\ Positives}{True\ Positives + False\ Positives} \tag{3}$$

The results from Tables 3 and 4 infer that there is not much difference in the Precision, Recall values. But for training 250 epochs YOLO8n-seg took 2.217 hours whereas YOLO11 took only 1.85 hours only. The speed YOLO8n-seg for each image is split as 0.5 ms for preprocess, 4.5 ms for inference and 3.2 ms for post process, similarly YOLO11 took 0.2 ms for preprocess, 3.3 for inference and 4.7 ms for post process respectively.

Figure 3 shows the performance metrics comparison between YOLO11 n-seg model and YOLOv8n-seg model.

Table 3 Precision, recall, mAP 50 and mAP 95 score for YOLO11n-seg model

Class	Precision	Recall	mAP50	mAP95
All	0.808	0.773	0.809	0.482
Filling	0.887	0.807	0.884	0.443
Impacted tooth	0.955	0.876	0.941	0.723
Root canal	0.862	0.913	0.926	0.585
Caries	0.53	0.53	0.496	0.179

Table 4 Precision, recall, mAP 50 and mAP 95 score for YOLOv8n-seg model

Class	Precision	Recall	mAP50	mAP95
All	0.817	0.743	0.8	0.483
Filling	0.858	0.777	0.869	0.437
Impacted tooth	0.965	0.854	0.964	0.765
Root canal	0.886	0.925	0.952	0.581
Caries	0.557	0.415	0.415	0.151

5.4 *Confusion Matrix*

A confusion matrix indicates the model's acheivement for different classes. It shows the relation between the ground truth and predicted class. Figure 2 shows normalized confusion matrix of both models. The confusion matrix aids in assessing the model's performance beyond simple accuracy metrics when there is an unbalanced dataset. In this case, Filling, root canal and impacted tooth achieved reasonably good accuracy rate. The caries class obtained relatively lower accuracy and some misclassification also (see Fig. 4).

Figure 5a shows the F1—confidence curve. The balance between recall and precision at various confidence levels is shown by the F1 score. For all class category, the F1 score is 0.79.

In Fig. 5b, the overall Recall—confidence score is 0.85 and for Impacted tooth and Root canal remains high (close to 1) even at higher confidence thresholds, indicating the model successfully detects most true positives for these classes.

Figure 5c, shows the Precision—confidence curve. YOLO11 score for overall precision at 1.0 confidence threshold was 0.906, indicating that at this threshold, predictions are very precise but potentially at the cost of missing some true positives. Figure 5d shows the precision-recall curve. YOLO11 achieved high precision-recall value for impacted tooth and root canal as 0.941 and 0.926 respectively. The mAP@50 is 0.809 for all classes.

Figure 6 shows the actual prediction on test image using the best weights. In Fig. 6 the impacted tooth is detected with a confidence score of 0.91. In Fig. 6 the root canal is detected with a confidence of 0.92 and 0.84. Three dental caries are detected with a lesser confidence score of 0.65, 0.59 and 0.27 respectively.

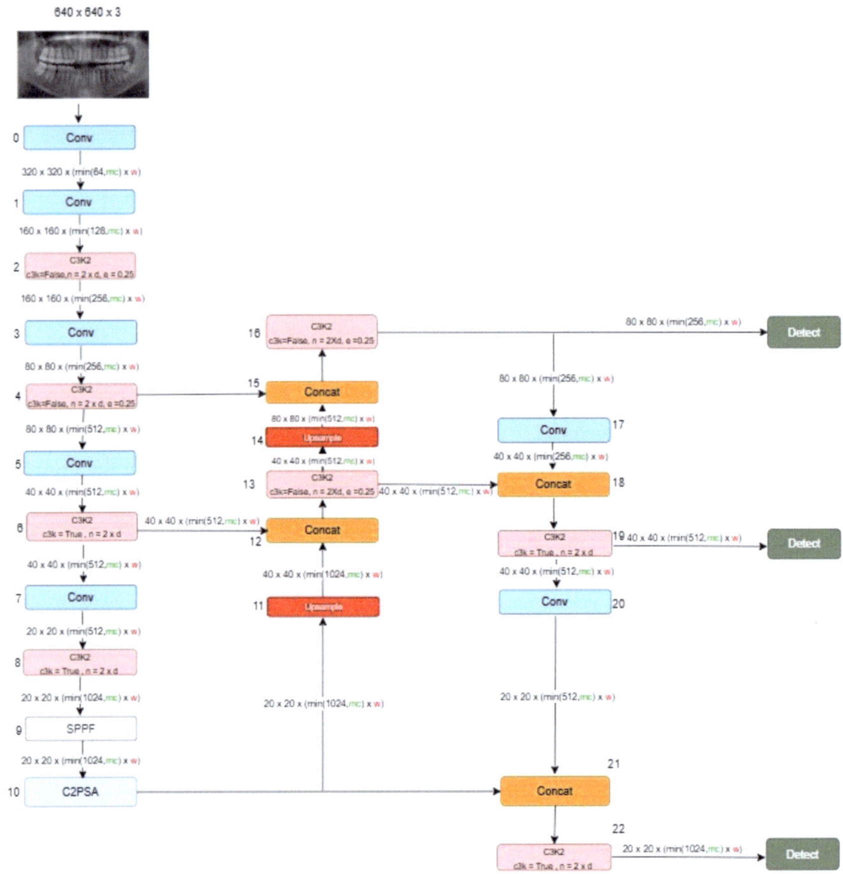

Fig. 2 YOLO11 architecture [24]

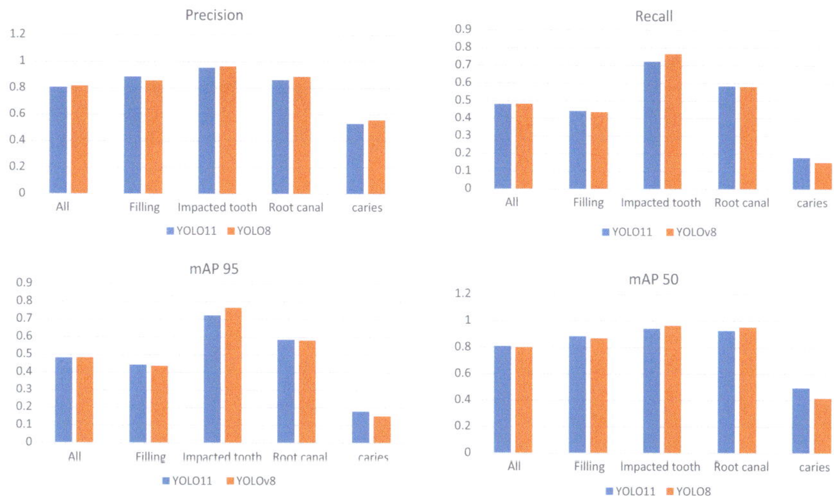

Fig. 3 Comparison of various evaluation metrics for YOLO11n and YOLOv8 model

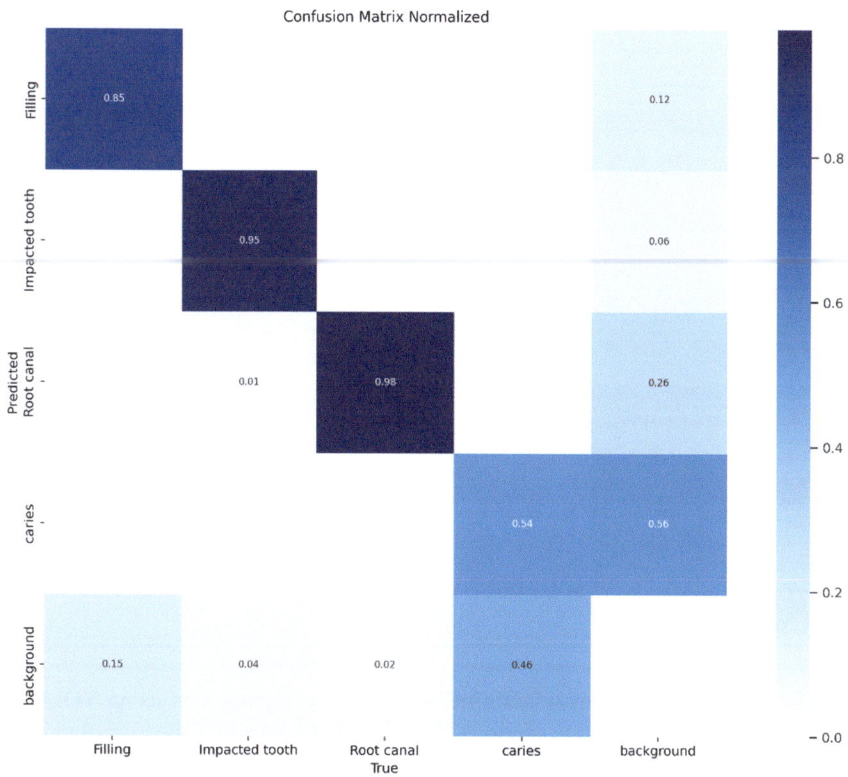

Fig. 4 Normalized confusion matrix of YOLO11 model

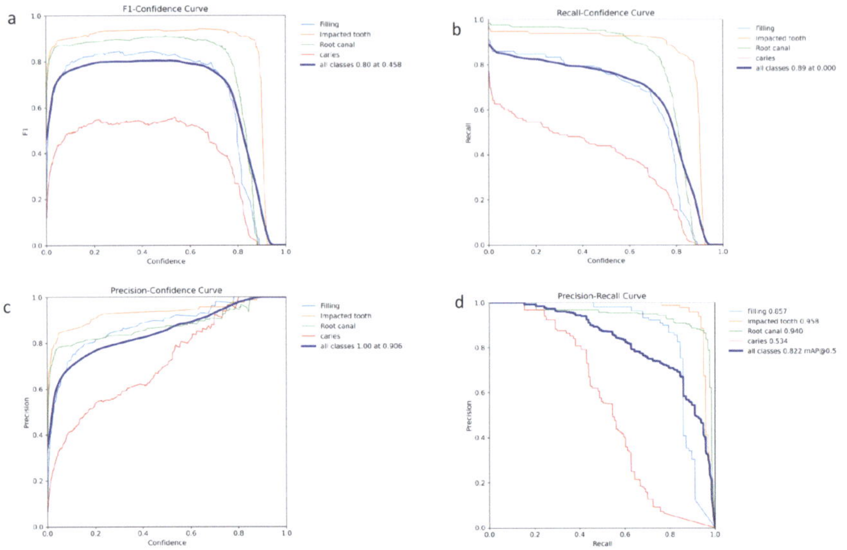

Fig. 5 **a** F1—confidence curve **b** Recall-confidence **c** Precision—confidence curve and **d** Precision—recall curve of YOLO11 across various dental abnormalities

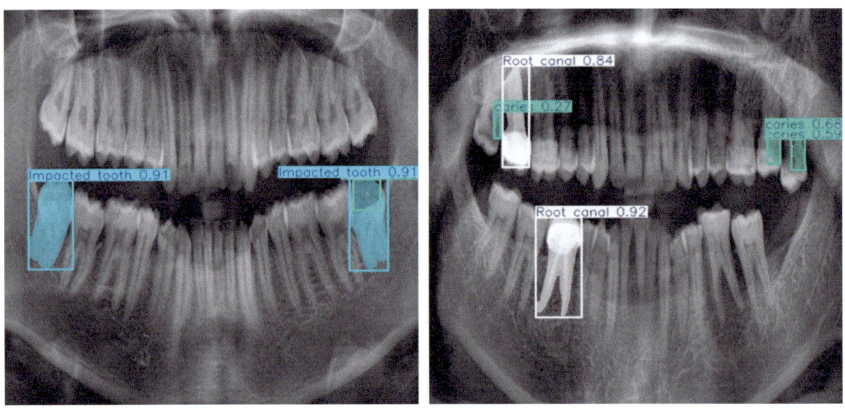

Fig. 6 Actual prediction of YOLO11on a test image

6 Conclusion

In this study automatic dental abnormalities detection is presented using YOLO11 model. It has demonstrated exceptional accuracy and processing speed, making it a popular option for dental disease segmentation and classification. It will speedup the medical diagnosis of dental treatment, save physician time and money.

The introduction of artificial intelligence has revolutionized the clarification of dental X-rays in detecting oral health issues. However, several challenges hinder the complete utilization of artificial intelligence's potential in improving dental healthcare. A significant barrier is the scarcity and inconsistent quality of available data, which is crucial for the effectiveness of AI models. In particular, there is insufficient information regarding uncommon dental conditions, intricate cases, well-annotated X-rays, and variations in dental procedures. The model's performance can further be boosted by increasing the dataset size with more samples. This work can be extended in future by using Internet of things for data acquisition, training and evaluating the model on hybrid dataset and making it accessible for all.

References

1. Hwang, G.J., Xie, H., Wah, B.W., Gašević, D.: Vision: challenges, roles and research issues of artificial intelligence in education. Comput. Educ. Artif. Intell. **1**, 1–5 (2020). https://doi.org/10.1016/j.caeai.2020.100001
2. Bhatt, D., Patel, C., Talsania, H., Patel, J., Vaghela, R., Pandya, S., Modi, K., Ghayvat, H.: CNN variants for computer vision: history, architecture, application, challenges and future scope. Des. Electron. **10**, 1–28 (2021). https://doi.org/10.3390/electronics10202470
3. Vinothkumar, J., Karunamurthy, A.: Recent advancements in artificial intelligence technology: trends and implications. Quing Int. J. Multidiscip. Sci. Res. Dev. **2**, 1–11 (2023). https://doi.org/10.54368/qijmsrd.2.1.0003
4. Bohr, A., Memarzadeh, K.: The Rise of Artificial Intelligence in Healthcare Applications (2020). ISBN 9780128184387
5. Gautam, A., Chirputkar, A., Pathak, P.: Opportunities and challenges in the application of artificial intelligence-based technologies in the healthcare industry. Int. Interdiscip. Humanit. Conf. Sustain. IIHC 2022—Proc., 1521–1524 (2022). https://doi.org/10.1109/IIHC55949.2022.10059767
6. Sarker, I.H.: Deep learning: a comprehensive overview on techniques, taxonomy, applications and research directions. SN Comput. Sci. **2**, 1–20 (2021). https://doi.org/10.1007/s42979-021-00815-1
7. Lee, J.G., Jun, S., Cho, Y.W., Lee, H., Kim, G.B., Seo, J.B., Kim, N.: Deep learning in medical imaging: general overview. Korean J. Radiol. **18**, 570–584 (2017). https://doi.org/10.3348/kjr.2017.18.4.570
8. Han, B.: Application of deep learning in medical imaging. In: Proceedings 2021 2nd International Conference on Computing and Data Science CDS 2021, vol. **16**, pp. 49–56 (2021). https://doi.org/10.1109/CDS52072.2021.00016
9. Musleh, D., Almossaeed, H., Balhareth, F., Alqahtani, G., Alobaidan, N., Altalag, J., Aldossary, M.I.: Advancing dental diagnostics: a review of artificial intelligence applications and challenges in dentistry. Big Data Cogn. Comput. **8** (2024). https://doi.org/10.3390/bdcc8060066
10. Semerci, Z.M., Yardımcı, S.: Empowering modern dentistry: the impact of artificial intelligence on patient care and clinical decision making. Diagnostics. **14** (2024). https://doi.org/10.3390/diagnostics14121260
11. Corbella, S., Srinivas, S., Cabitza, F.: Applications of deep learning in dentistry. Oral Surg. Oral Med. Oral Pathol. Oral Radiol. **132**, 225–238 (2021). https://doi.org/10.1016/j.oooo.2020.11.003
12. Sivari, E., Senirkentli, G.B., Bostanci, E., Guzel, M.S., Acici, K., Asuroglu, T.: Deep learning in diagnosis of dental anomalies and diseases: a systematic review. Diagnostics. **13**, 1–28 (2023). https://doi.org/10.3390/diagnostics13152512

13. Kweon, H.H.I., Lee, J.H., Youk, T.M., Lee, B.A., Kim, Y.T.: Panoramic radiography can be an effective diagnostic tool adjunctive to oral examinations in the national health checkup program. J. Periodontal Implant Sci. **48**, 317–325 (2018). https://doi.org/10.5051/jpis.2018.48.5.317
14. Gardiyanoğlu, E., Ünsal, G., Akkaya, N., Aksoy, S., Orhan, K.: Automatic segmentation of teeth, crown–bridge restorations, dental implants, restorative fillings, dental caries, residual roots, and root canal fillings on orthopantomographs: convenience and pitfalls. Diagnostics. **13** (2023). https://doi.org/10.3390/diagnostics13081487
15. Lin, S.Y., Chang, H.Y.: Tooth numbering and condition recognition on dental panoramic radiograph images using CNNs. IEEE Access. **9**, 166008–166026 (2021). https://doi.org/10.1109/ACCESS.2021.3136026
16. Estai, M., Tennant, M., Gebauer, D., Brostek, A., Vignarajan, J., Mehdizadeh, M., Saha, S.: Deep learning for automated detection and numbering of permanent teeth on panoramic images. Dentomaxillofacial Radiol. **51**, 1–8 (2022). https://doi.org/10.1259/dmfr.20210296
17. Budagam, D., Kumar, A., Ghosh, S., Shrivastav, A., Imanbayev, A.Z., Akhmetov, I.R., Kalplun, D., Antonov, S., Rychenkov, A., Cyganov, G., Sinitca, A.: Instance segmentation and teeth classification in panoramic X-rays. Expert Syst. with Appl. J. (2024)
18. Oztekin, F., Katar, O., Sadak, F., Yildirim, M., Cakar, H., Aydogan, M., Ozpolat, Z., Talo Yildirim, T., Yildirim, O., Faust, O., et al.: An explainable deep learning model to prediction dental caries using panoramic radiograph images. Diagnostics. **13** (2023). https://doi.org/10.3390/diagnostics13020226
19. Almalki, Y.E., Din, A.I., Ramzan, M., Irfan, M., Aamir, K.M., Almalki, A., Alotaibi, S., Alaglan, G., Alshamrani, H.A., Rahman, S.: Deep learning models for classification of dental diseases using orthopantomograph (2022)
20. Zhu, H., Cao, Z., Lian, L., Ye, G., Gao, H., Wu, J.: CariesNet: a deep learning approach for segmentation of multi-stage caries lesion from oral panoramic X-ray image. Neural Comput. & Applic. **35**, 16051–16059 (2023). https://doi.org/10.1007/s00521-021-06684-2
21. Al-Sarem, M., Al-Asali, M., Alqutaibi, A.Y., Saeed, F.: Enhanced tooth region detection using pretrained deep learning models. Int. J. Environ. Res. Public Health. **19** (2022). https://doi.org/10.3390/ijerph192215414
22. Kim, J., Lee, H., Song, I., Jung, K.: DeNTNet: deep neural transfer network for the detection of periodontal bone loss using panoramic dental radiographs. Sci. Rep., 1–9 (2019). https://doi.org/10.1038/s41598-019-53758-2
23. Takahashi, T., Nozaki, K., Gonda, T., Mameno, T., Ikebe, K.: Deep learning-based detection of dental prostheses and restorations. Sci. Rep. **11**, 1–7 (2021). https://doi.org/10.1038/s41598-021-81202-x
24. Cejudo, J.E., Chaurasia, A., Feldberg, B., Krois, J., Schwendicke, F.: Classification of dental radiographs using deep learning. J. Clin. Med. **10**, 1–9 (2021). https://doi.org/10.3390/jcm10071496

Embedded Shift Evolution in Explainable Deep Learning Systems

Stanley Ziweritin, Abirami Gunasekaran, Shamaila Iram, and Minsi Chen

Abstract Deep learning works well for the classification of medical images, but the reason why it has not received much acceptance in the medical industry lies in the opacity and fragility of the model when any kind of input alterations occur. Here, a method has been proposed to measure the amount and graphically represent the displacement of the embeddings in convolutional neural networks that have undergone transformations named Blur, Canny, and Sobel. Results obtained by using the concepts of t-SNE, PCA, and case-by-case analysis have identified the relationship between the displacement of the embeddings and the error margin when making any kind of medical diagnoses, like the breast cancer versus Acute Lymphoblastic Leukemia dataset. The proposed method enables transparent diagnostic decision-making while incorporating transformation-aware training. Consequently, it facilitates the development of trustworthy and robust medical systems, reducing potential risks associated with the integration of deep learning into clinical workflows.

Keywords Deep learning · Embedding shift representations · Explainable artificial intelligence · Medical image classification · Model robustness

---

S. Ziweritin · A. Gunasekaran (✉) · S. Iram · M. Chen
School of Computer Science and Engineering, University of Huddersfield, Huddersfield, UK
e-mail: A.Gunasekaran2@hud.ac.uk

S. Ziweritin
e-mail: Stanley.Ziweritin@hud.ac.uk

S. Iram
e-mail: S.Iram@hud.ac.uk

M. Chen
e-mail: m.chen@hud.ac.uk

P. Singh et al. (eds.), *Deep Learning Applications in Healthcare and Medical Imaging Practice*, Studies in Big Data 193, https://doi.org/10.1007/978-3-032-21009-8_12

1 Introduction

The fact that architectures involving deep learning continue to increasingly integrate with high stakes domains such as health and autonomous systems has brought to light their 'black box' property as a major hurdle to its adoption and acceptance [1]. Traditional methods of explainable AI (XAI), feature attribution, and linear probing, among others, have proven to be valuable tools. However, these methods predominantly operate in a post-hoc and localized manner, frequently elucidating only particular predictions without disclosing the underlying embedding representational framework of CNN model [2, 3]. Deep neural networks, especially CNNs, VAEs, and generative models compress high-dimensional inputs into lower-dimensional latent spaces that capture essential semantic and structural information [4, 5]. It's broadly understood that these latent representations are not merely passive embeddings but actively shape model behavior [6]. Fumero et al. [7] interpreted neural network models as dynamical systems over latent manifolds. Iteratively applying encoder decoder functions reveals vector fields and attractors whose patterns correspond to how the model generalizes, memorizes, or handles out-of-distribution data (Fig. 1).

(a) **XAI in Breast cancer diagnosis**

Bai et al. [8] reviewed a range of XAI techniques including SHAP, LIME, and Grad-CAM alongside with relevant datasets and evaluation strategies, highlighting their potential to improve transparency and clinical trust in AI-driven diagnosis. Despite these advances, existing XAI frameworks still lack layer-wise embedding-shift visualizations, which constrains mechanistic interpretability, robustness, and generalizability [9]. Shifa et al. [10] conducted a comparative analysis of XAI methods and proposed modifications to evaluation strategies tailored specifically

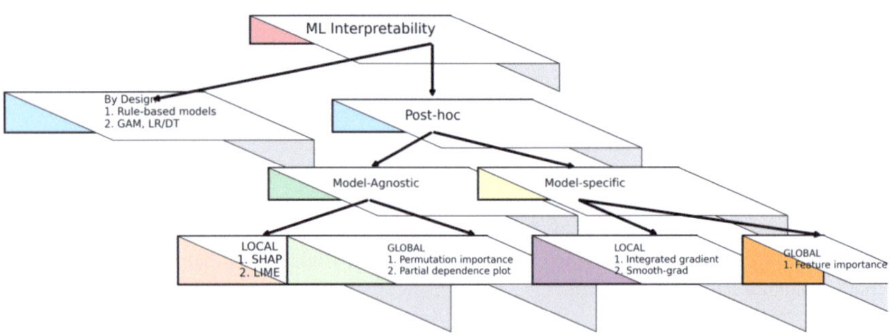

Fig. 1 This figure depicts the taxonomy of ML interpretability methods, splitting them into by-design (LR coefficients directly explain feature influence, DT rules/pathways are human-readable, GAM additive transparency for each feature and NB interpretable probability assumptions) versus post-hoc, then model-agnostic versus model-specific, and finally into local (e.g., SHAP, LIME, Integrated Gradients, SmoothGrad etc.) and global (e.g., permutation importance, partial dependence plots, feature importance, etc.) techniques

to mammography. They highlighted the demand for trustworthy and transparent mammography systems; however, the field is still constrained by few evaluation frameworks, limited knowledge of embedding shifts, and lack of clinical evidence to confirm interpretability [11–13].

Similarly, Ghasemi et al. [14] have assessed the application of reliable XAI techniques for Breast Cancer diagnosis and risk estimation by conducting a PRISMA-guided scopping review across multiple research databases. Despite emphasizing the significance of rigor, the degree of clinical validation was nonetheless limited. According to Dastgeer and Treigy, [15] the state-of-the-art XAI solutions for Breast Cancer have been primarily limited to localized and post-hoc approaches, focusing on pixel locations rather than quantifying the clinical features associated with predictions. Furthermore, the significance of standardized development frameworks and the paucity of end-use guidelines were also highlighted in the same study. Wehner et al. [16] highlighted similar aspects, noting that most state-of-the-art methods for local and post-hoc explanations tend to incorporate assumptions such as smoothness and proximity in the embedding space, represented by the Euclidean k-nearest neighbors, among other assumptions. Even if such methods provide significant insight in limited scenarios, they might not serve as appropriate models for comprehensive and transferable understanding across different clinical settings. Current Explainability methods for Breast cancer diagnosis have not sufficiently focused on the dynamics associated with embeddings, thus limiting the understanding of the progression of internal representations to model predistions. Advancing explainable AI needs embedding shift analysis across early, middle, and deep layers to reveal evolving diagnostic reasoning in CNN models. Integrating layer-wise embedding shift visualizations into XAI frameworks can uncover hidden feature transformations, improving interpretability and trust in cancer diagnosis.

(b) **XAI in Acute Lymphoblastic Leukemia(ALL) diagnosis**

Ramanujam et al. [17] modified ResNet with hard attention mechanism for leukemia diagnosis. They adopted an attention-guided technique focusing on improving classification, but interpretability remains qualitative, lacking rigorous faithfulness evaluation and prospective clinical validation evidence. Pervez et al. [18] proposes a hierarchical federated EfficientNet-B3 leukemia classifier with XAI (saliency, occlusion, RISE). The decentralized training improves accuracy and privacy, but lacks post-hoc interpretability, embedding shift monitoring and quantification among clients. Several research investigations have been conducted using leukemia classifiers that combine WBC segmentation, CNN/ResNet variants, transfer learning, and CAD pipelines: interpretability via Grad-CAM/LIME, and feature-space clustering. The reviews synthesize DL trends and preprocessing limited with small, biased datasets, inconsistent clinical validation practices, saliency-only explanations, rigorous embedding-shift or representation-drift analyses and out-of-distribution (OOD) robustness tests, and calibration gaps persist; hindering deployment [19–22].

Existing XAI methods lack embedding shift analysis, limiting insight into layer-wise representation dynamics and true feature reasoning in leukemia diagnosis. Integrating embedding shift visualization can uncover hierarchical decision pathways, improving trust and interpretability in Acute Lymphoblastic Leukemia diagnosis systems. Developing hybrid explainable AI frameworks of combining embedding shift tracking with morphological feature attribution could revolutionize leukemia diagnosis transparency and model reliability. Recent surveys reveal XAI frameworks lack embedding-level explanations, especially across intermediate and deep layers, limiting interpretability and robust model understanding [23, 24]. This limits developers' ability to effectively debug and understand deep learning systems. Weber [24] provides attribution maps that explain why two embeddings are close or distant in semantic terms. CNN embeddings are close when they share semantically salient features (textures, shapes), distant when they diverge in those features or class-relevant structure. Deep learning is still unstable and opaque despite its superiority in medical image categorization. We analyze how perturbations reshape latent representations and link these representation shifts to performance and misclassification. Insights enable robustness diagnostics, enhancing trust and deployability of AI in clinical settings. The aim is to investigate how input transformations affect the internal feature representations (latent space) and prediction behavior of DL models, in order to enhance the explainability and robustness in medical image classification. The objectives include analyzing class probability shifts caused by different input transformations techniques (e.g., Blur, Canny, and Sobel). Our study introduces a shift-aware, interactive visualization framework that tracks how CNN embeddings evolve under input/leaned pattern transformations providing both interpretability and robustness evaluation, which the prior works lack.

This work explores interactive visualization tools for tracking the evolution of embeddings across convolutional network layers with different transformation strengths. In addition, the connection between embedding shifts and observed trends in misclassifications or degradation in model accuracy is also delved into, with the help of confusion matrices and more nuanced sample-level analyses. Collectively, such analyses offer a framework within which embedding shift phenomena can be examined in a more systematic way, forming the basis for more-transparent interpretations regarding the connection between representational changes and prediction capabilities.

1.1 Research Questions

Research questions focus on the development of the embedding shift over time and play an important role in establishing the methodological approach, which is necessary for the confirmation of the assertions of interpretation. They are also important for pointing out where there are gaps in methods that need to be further refined. The development of fields like the study of the embedding shift for model interpretation requires well-articulated research questions, which are important for framing the methodology of the research. This establishes the parameters of study and allows for the investigation of the practical requirements for openness and quality in modern AI research.

RQ1: ***What changes do input transformations like Blurring, Canny Edge Detection, and Sobel Filtering induce to the embedding shift patterns generated by the trained CNN?*** Investigate whether and how input variations cause embedding shifts or drift and apply input transformations that alter the activation patterns in early, middle and deeper CNN layers. These shifts highlight which features the model deems important and can expose vulnerabilities.

RQ2: ***How is the variation in the embedded space associated with the variation in class probabilities and predictions of the final model?*** Analyze the predictive effect of the dynamics of the embedded space. This is useful for tracking the transitions where the model is uncertain or changes the prediction class.

RQ3: ***To what extent do methods such as tSNE and PCA assist in making CNN-based systems more interpretable?*** Evaluate tools for model interpretability using t-SNE/PCA projection, identifying clusters, boundaries, overlaps, misclassifications, class confusion, ambiguous regions, and confidence.

RQ4: ***To what extent would it improve the detection of misclassified and uncertain predictions in deep learning models by observing changes in the embedding space?*** This research question aims to investigate how change in the latent representations might be associated with trust and perceptions of model trustworthiness. The change in latent representations might provide clues to points where some data points could diverge from the expected class probabilities, thus often hinting at misclassifications and high prediction uncertainties

1.2 Research Novelty

This novelty introduces a dynamic and multi-layer framework to better understand embedding dynamics across network depth. It combines visualization, probability, and quantitative approaches to provide a holistic framework to understand the concept of interpretability within the context of CNN models.

Model for exploring embedding shift patterns across network layers: The current research offers a dynamic analysis per layer regarding embedding shifts, showing the process of transformation in the CNN embedding characteristics from the early layers to the deeper ones. In contrast with models providing predetermined saliency map values, this research explores changing relationships and their effect on boundary definition per class.

Interactions between probability changes and embedding trajectories: Connecting the embedding trajectories with the changes in class probabilities explains how the perturbations impact the model's degree of confidence in its internal representations traversing the space of features. Connecting geometric transitions with changes in the probabilistic output reshapes the perspective of interpretation, capturing how CNNs justify their decision-making in classifying images.

Charting the Progression of Misclassification Patterns: This is an interpretation of how patterns of misclassification progress through convolutional layers, pointing to areas where correct model prediction is undermined. Through tracking the progression of embeddings that are incorrectly mapped, it highlights hidden flaws in distinguishing features.

Perturbation-Informed Sensitivity Embedding Assessment: This approach uses a multi-transform perturbation technique involving Blur, Canny, and Sobel transformations to analyze sensitivity and robustness of the embeddings and outputs produced by the CNN over the layers of the network. This approach not only identifies potential weaknesses but also offers quantitative and qualitative proof of robustness not yet provided by state-of-the-art explainability methods.

Interactive 2D-3D embedding shift visualization system: An integrated visualization tool that combines 2D t-SNE and 3D PCA embedding diagrams with interactivity, allowing for in-depth analysis of how different transformations impact the embedding shift of feature groups. This system provides an easily understandable way for exploring the underlying representation-level processes involved with CNN decisions.

Interpretability quantified through an embedding divergence index: This paper shows how a measure of interpretability can be defined based on a combination of the magnitude of embedding shifts and class probability divergence. This allows a measure of interpretability to be calculated, making it possible to quantify visually how well a layer explains observations

1.3 Contribution to Knowledge

XAI methods used to date have been restricted to fixed graphical outputs such as saliency maps, activation highlighting, and attention-guided attributions that provide minimal information regarding the associated processes. The key findings from this study as distinct academic contributions are listed below for better clarity and discussion.

(a) **A framework useful for analyzing embedding transitions across layers of the network to facilitate model interpretability**. The framework presents an interactive platform that tracks transitions in feature embeddings across higher layers of a CNN network to improve model interpretability in the field of medical image classification.

(b) **Analyzing the effect of certain input noise to the layers of the networks**: Highlight how the CNN layers are not equally sensitive to visual noise, reflecting the importance of linking transformation-aware regularization with lower hierarchical levels to develop robust deep learning representations.

(c) **Embedding shift-probability correlation framework**: Envisions a way of interpreting the correlation between the shifts of the embeddings of internal features and the corresponding shifts of the predictions.
(d) **Tracing Invariance across Layered Representations**: Provides an empirical characterization for shift invariance across the layers in the CNN architectures to guide architectural design for improved explainability.
(e) **A comprehensive visual diagnostic framework for the improvement of interpretability in deep learning**: This offers a modular visualization framework that facilitates the analysis and diagnosis of CNN operations at various levels of abstraction in explainable AI.

The paper is structured as follows: Section 1 introduces the research problem and goals. Section 2 reviews related work and existing gaps. Section 3 details the methodology, including model design and interpretability tools. Section 4 presents and discusses experimental results. Section 5 concludes with key contributions and future directions.

2 Related Work

This section discusses approaches to embedding behavior evaluation, representational drift detection, and explanation consistency in stable embedding spaces. For example, Luo et al. [25] have conducted a thorough literature review of embedded deep learning, focusing on system design, model reduction, training in embedded environments, and hardware-software co-design. However, their work is limited to representation learning in embedding spaces without examining embedding visualization in early, mid-level, or deeper layers. Similarly, Gamatie and Wang [26] have applied machine leaning and model-agnostic explainable AI approaches to model the prediction of redundant non-volatile memory writes within static code analysis. They demonstrated that explainability approaches can decode predefined write patterns. However, their findings also highlight the existence of challenges in embedding XAI. For instance, their findings indicate that embedding-based model representation dependability and explanation consistency within embedding model explanation spaces have been understuded concepts compared to embedding representation dependability and consistency. A combination of static program analysis and domain models based on causality is verified to be useful within model design. There is also a need to design efficient, domain-specific explainability approaches for embedding environments.

2.1 Kernel-Based Distribution Embeddings (KBDE)

This maps feature distributions to high-dimensional spaces, thereby capturing richer similarities and complex relationships, such as texture, style, and context. Zhou and Hu [27] present a problem-focused taxonomy of XAI techniques that were designed for deep learning models. The authors emphasize neuro-evolution-based strategies to improve model transparency. The work systematizes evolutionary computation methods for interpretability and calls for further research, but it suffers from a lack of broad practical validation and insufficient experimental depth. Further advances in XAI have to be achieved by embedding cognitive inspired reasoning, dynamic layer-wise interpretability, and human-in-the-loop adaptive explanations based on task semantics. One new trend involves hybrid neuro-symbolic interpretability frameworks that integrate causal reasoning, human feedback, and layer-wise embedding shift analysis.

Similarly, Han et al. [28] present an interpretable CNN for intelligent fault diagnosis that automatically chooses wavelet kernels using reinforcement learning. This approach minimizes dependence on hand-designed hyperparameters while retaining powerful diagnostic performance and real-time applicability. The utilization of dynamic wavelet-based embedding shifts brings about interpretability issues, which are particularly challenging in resource-constrained embedded environments. Most current interpretability is still confined to wavelet-domain attributes, while other signal modalities and latent structures are largely explored. In addition, attention mechanisms combined with wavelet features, causal and symbolic reasoning can offer more complete explanatory power beyond frequency-domain insights. Embedding causal analysis in wavelet-driven CNN models provides further transparency of the root causes involved in driving a specific prediction, beyond explanation based solely on feature activation or filter responses alone. Future work may also explore various interpretability metrics to gauge their capability in capturing model transparency and interpretive strength. Shimizu et al. [29] develop a neural–kernel conditional mean embedding in which deep learning replaces the Gram matrix inversion of its classical counterpart and increases representational flexibility, as evidenced by its improved results in density estimation and distributional reinforcement learning. However, despite these advances, the framework still faces several challenges involved with kernel hyperparameter selection and interpretability, narrowing its value in providing a transparent embedding shift characterization. Combining causal and probabilistic methods for interpretability may reveal deeper relational patterns hidden by surface-level kernel embeddings. Advances in adaptive neural–kernel embedding approaches incorporating explainability, uncertainty estimation, and human-alignment reasoning may significantly help research in interpretability. Further exploration of hybrid kernel–attention designs could facilitate interpretability across multimodal and hierarchical representations. Correspondingly, the study of kernel graph embeddings based on dynamic graph structures and evolving deep features could enable real-time interpretability. Eventually, adaptive embedding frameworks that learn kernels that conform to human reasoning may lead to great improvements in model comprehensibility.

2.2 Evolutionary and Dynamic Embeddings (EDE)

EDE shows how the feature representations change along network layers and throughout training, reflecting the system's ability to adapt and learn through progressive contextual refinement. Barros et al. [30] provided a detailed taxonomy of dynamic graph embedding techniques that are capable of capturing temporal changes in both node properties and structural relationships. They emphasized the lack of standard benchmark and sufficiently diverse real-world datasets that complicates systematic assessment and limits broader applicability. Furthermore, the existing frameworks provide only partial visibility into temporal progression of embeddings. Further work may involve incorporating explainable AI, interactive temporal analysis tools, causal analyses of embedding evolution, and more expressive visual mappings of dynamic graph behavior. Zhou et al. [31] present an evolutionary explainable-AI framework for generating accurate but interpretable models, which is built on simple and human-readable constructs. Despite being effective, the approach suffers when applied to high-dimensional domains, and unified interpretability measures remain lacking. Interpretable models will be enhanced using human-centered workflows, causal modeling, hybrid symbolic-neural approaches, and multi-objective optimization to balance transparency, performance, and fairness via adaptive, expertise-aware explanatory schemes.

2.3 Concept Embedding Analysis (CEA)

In CEA, the goal is to examine how deep CNNs encode human-interpretable concepts into intermediate layers and thus providing a better understanding of feature semantics, reasoning patterns, and representational structure. An early related framework is presented in Schwalbe [32], where conceptual categories are aligned with neural activations to improve semantic interpretability. However, as modern architectures continue to grow in dimensionality, both approaches exhibit weaknesses in monitoring embedding variance in dynamic environments and scaling to higher-dimensional spaces. Their practical values are further limited by the lack of standard quantitative metrics, reducing reliability for real-world applications. The integration of human-guided analysis, multimodal reasoning, and continual learning can yield intuitive and adaptive embedding representations. For example, temporal- and context-sensitive methods can be developed to investigate the potential causal relationship between embedding geometry and model decisions. Weighted temporal embeddings coupled with a transformer were used by Zhang et al. [33] to improve RUL interpretability and emphasize influential temporal patterns. However, their method is focused mostly on attention weights, and few insights on how the embedding shift affects semantic stability or robustness can be derived. More generally, the interpretability challenge remains because transformer attention is complex and involves causal modeling and symbolic knowledge. Such approaches could help in the development of hybrid transformer-graph frameworks for domain-aware predictive maintenance

Kumar et al. [34] introduce a deep learning framework combining Bayesian inference and attention-based visualization to explain vector fields. While the proposed method does an excellent job of revealing spatial uncertainty and model-stressed regions, it is constrained to steady-state inputs and does not offer any interactive analyses like t-SNE or PCA. The support for interpretability from causal and counterfactual analysis tools is not satisfactory; neither the relationship between uncertainty estimates nor real error is sufficiently established. The potential future work listed thereafter includes dynamic fields, multimodal data, robustness, and user-guided uncertainty evaluation.

These limitations make it unsuitable for applications requiring real-time interpretability of the CNNs. Moreover, Kumar et al. [34] and Gamatié and Wang [26] pointed out the importance of explainability in systems with limited resources and/or static memory analysis. Their focus has often been on feature-level explanations or rigid program behavior. These approaches fail to capture changing latent-space representations in a CNN processing images, especially changes in embedding due to perturbation of the input given by the user, crucial for complete model Explainability in real-world applications

3 Materials and Methods

The proposed method is organized to systematically evaluate the robustness and explainability of deep learning models. Initially, a convolutional neural network is trained on labeled biomedical images derived from both breast cancer and acute lymphoblastic Leukemia databases to emulate real-world variability settings, several image transformations are applied, ranging from blurring to edge detection techniques like Canny and Sobel filters. The model's performance is then evaluated by comparing its predictions on original and modified images using interactive visualization tools to demonstrate variability in model decisions. The latent space is extracted from hidden layers of the neural net and visualized through PCA and t-SNE techniques, thereby demonstrating variability in feature space by analyzing misclassification distributions and shifts in embeddings, respectively.

3.1 Analytical Components of Proposed System

The methodology itself includes important aspects such as data selection as an essential elements, network architecture, data preprocessing involving embedding extraction, feature transformation strategies, criteria for evaluation, and finally, study setups. This methodology enables careful analysis of how convolutional models respond to changes in input data.

3.1.1 Dataset

This research explores two major data sets: the breast cancer dataset (ALL) [35], which contains images labeled as normal, malignant, or benign, and the Acute Lymphoblastic Leukemia dataset [36], which contains images labeled as benign, early, pre-malignant, and pro-malignant.

3.1.2 Embedded Shift Extraction

The embedding shift extraction module uses both t-SNE and PCA for dimensional reduction, enabling the mapping of high-dimensional embeddings of features into a more understandable space.

a. **Dimensionality reduction techniques)**

Dimensionality reduction algorithms such as t-SNE and PCA are used for projecting CNN representations into lower-dimensional spaces enabling easier comparison under different experimental settings [37, 38]. In scenarios involving dimensionality reduction techniques (DRT), it becomes easier for analysts to track the evolution of representations using the aforementioned techniques, which represents an important step in understanding network behavior [39, 40]

(i) **t-SNE (t-distributed Stochastic Neighbor Embedding)** is broadly used as a non-linear technique to perform dimensionality reduction on complex data enabling patterns to be projected in two or three dimensions [41–43]. In this context, t-SNE is used to analyze the impact of input perturbations, such as blurring, edge filters, and spatial transformations, to embeddings learned by a CNN. It provides an understanding of the internal representation of the network by analyzing perturbations effects in the embedding space."

Let Iϵ $\mathbb{R}^{H\times W\times C}$ be the input image passed into a CNN model for feature representations (embeddings)

Let f_θ be the trained a CNN with parameters $\boldsymbol{\Theta}$ which define the embedding at an intermediate layer corresponding to the fully connected or penultimate layer as:

$$Z = f_\theta(I)\epsilon\mathbb{R}^d \tag{1}$$

where d is the embedding dimension, I is the input image and z is the high-dimensional learned representation and d≥2; when the image is transformed using blur or edge detection becomes:

$$I' = T(I), z' = f_\theta(I') \tag{2}$$

The transformation-induced shift in CNN embeddings is derived as:

$$\Delta z = ||z^1 - z||_2 \tag{3}$$

The goal is to visualize this transformation-induced shift across a given dataset. Given a set of CNN embeddings $\{z_1, z_2, \ldots., z_n\}$, t-SNE constructs a probabilistic similarity matrix in high-dimensional space using a Gaussian kernel [44, 45]. The pair similarity for each pair is computed as:

$$P_{j/i} = \frac{\exp(-|z_i - z_i|^2/2\sigma_i^2)}{\sum_{k\neq i}\exp(-||z_i - z_k||^2/2\sigma_i^2)} \tag{4}$$

Symmetrically, the neighborhood structure in the high-dimensional latent space becomes

$$P_{ij} = \frac{P_{j/i} + P_{i/j}}{2\pi} \tag{5}$$

The matrix P = $\{P_{ij}\}$ encodes neighborhood structure in high-dimensional latent space. The mathematics of t-SNE (t-distributed Stochastic Neighbor Embedding) revolves around mapping high-dimensional learned representations into a 2D or 3D space while preserving local relationships between data points [46]. Specific summary regarding CNNs: Feature representation of an image could also be extracted by evaluating its feature vector at a given layer in the CNN. This is further explained further in the next section on how changes in CNN-based embeddings need to be understood:

$$\text{Let } z_i = f_\theta(I_i) \text{ and } z_i^{(T)} = f_\theta(T(I_i)) \tag{6}$$

We define the embedding shift under transformation T as:

$$S_i = ||z_i - z_i^{(T)}||_2 \tag{7}$$

We can visualize z_i and $z_i^{(T)}$ jointtly using t-SNE. Small $S_i \rightarrow$ original and transformed embeddings are close (the model is robust). Large $S_i \rightarrow$ model representation changes (Model is sensitive or unstable)

(iii) **Principal Component Analysis (PCA**) is a widely used technique that transforms high-dimensional data into a lower-dimensional space, aiming to preserve as much of the original variance (information) as possible [28, 47, 49]. PCA identifies the principal component directions along which the data exhibits the greatest variation, and projects the data onto these axes [50]. In the context of CNNs, the embedding matrix is constructed to extract feature embeddings from the hidden layers, which can then be analyzed using PCA to reveal underlying patterns and relationships.

$$\mathrm{X} = \begin{bmatrix} x_1^T \\ x_2^T \\ \vdots \\ x_n^T \end{bmatrix} \epsilon \mathbb{R}^{n\mathrm{X}d} \tag{8}$$

where 'n' is the number of samples (images) and 'd' is the number of features (neurons/activations in the layer). $X_i \epsilon \mathbb{R}^d$ is the embedding of the ith image. We need to center our data (subtract the mean) in order to perform PCA which becomes:

$$X' = \frac{1}{n}\sum\nolimits_{i=1}^{n} x_i => X' = X - x' \tag{9}$$

The matrix that captures the linear relationships between all feature dimensions of CNN embeddings is defined as:

$$\mathrm{C} = \frac{1}{n-1}\tilde{X}^T\tilde{X}\epsilon\mathbb{R}^{d\mathrm{X}d} \tag{10}$$

The PCA seeks new instances that maximize variance defined as

$$\mathrm{C}v_i = \lambda_i v_i, \text{ where i} = 1, ..., \text{ d} \tag{11}$$

where $\lambda_i$eigenevlaue(variance along direct $\mathrm{v_i}$ and $\mathrm{v_i}$ is the eigenvector(principal direction) and other eigenvalues: $\lambda_1 \geq \lambda_2 \geq \cdots \geq \lambda_d$. We can take the top k eigenvectors to reduce k-dimensional space (e.g. 2D) using:

$$W_k = [v_1, v_2, \ldots, v_k]\epsilon\mathbb{R}^{d\mathrm{X}k} \tag{12}$$

To project each CNN embeddings onto the PCA space:

$$\mathrm{Z} = \tilde{X}W_K\epsilon\mathbb{R}^{d\mathrm{X}k} \tag{13}$$

We project both embeddings into the same PCA space and compare the distance and spread:

$$\Delta_i = ||Z_i^{original} - Z_i^{transformed}||_2 \tag{14}$$

where Δ_i is the feature embedding shift due to input perturbation.

3.1.3 Feature Processing Techniques

Feature processing techniques extract, transform, and select informative patterns from images, enabling robust recognition, segmentation, retrieval, and analysis tasks [51–53].

(a) **Canny edge detection**: is a multi-stage algorithm used to detect edges (high gradient regions) in images [54, 55]. It's mathematically grounded and often mimics the low-level feature extraction done by the first convolutional layers in CNNs [56–58]. The canny operator builds Sobel with noise reduction, thinning and thresholding [59].

(b) **Sobel operator** is a mathematical method for detecting edges in images by emphasizing areas of high spatial frequency (i.e., places where pixel values change rapidly [60, 61]. This is useful for understanding what low-level features (e.g., edges, contours) a model might focus on. This is a preprocessing step used to test CNN's sensitivity in detecting image edges. The Sobel operator uses 3*3 convolution kernel defined as

$$G_x = \begin{bmatrix} -1\ 0\ +1 \\ -2\ 0\ +2 \\ -1\ 0\ +1 \end{bmatrix}, G_y = \begin{bmatrix} +1 & +2 & +1 \\ 0 & 0 & 0 \\ -1 & -2 & -1 \end{bmatrix} \tag{15}$$

To apply Sobal via 2D convolution let "I" be input gray image and I(i.j) intensity at pixel (i,j). The gradient at pixel (i, j) is computed

$$G_x(i,j) = \sum\nolimits_{m=-1}^{1} \sum\nolimits_{n=-1}^{1} G_x[m+1][n+1].I(i+m, j+n) \tag{16}$$

$$G_y(i,j) = \sum\nolimits_{m=-1}^{1} \sum\nolimits_{n=-1}^{1} G_y[m+1][n+1].I(i+m, j+n) \tag{17}$$

These are essentially convolutions between the image and each kernel and convolving with image(I) or learned patterns to get edge maps, the computation becomes:

$$S_x = I * G_x(i,j), S_y = I * G_y(i,j) \tag{18}$$

$$CNN_{earlyfilters}(\mathrm{I}) \approx \mathrm{I} * G_x,\ \mathrm{I} * G_y \tag{19}$$

To compute the edge strength at pixel (i, j), the gradient magnitude becomes:

$$\mathrm{S} = \sqrt{S_x^2 + S_y^2} \tag{20}$$

This gives the overall edge intensity (gradient magnitude) and it highlights regions with sharp or slight intensity changes in image edges [62–64]. In CNN embedding shift, the Sobel-filtered image passed through CNN and the resulting change in embedding shows how sensitive the network is to edge features.

(b) **Gaussian blur** is a technique used to smooth image thereby removing high frequency details [65–67]. It is used to test CNN's reliance on fine features [68].

$$\mathrm{G(x, y)} = \frac{1}{2\pi\sigma^2}\exp(\frac{x^2 + y^2}{2\sigma^2}) \tag{21}$$

A 3 × 3 kernel can be written as

$$\frac{1}{16}\begin{bmatrix} 1 & 2 & 1 \\ 2 & 4 & 2 \\ 1 & 2 & 1 \end{bmatrix} \tag{22}$$

Convolving with image I:

$$I_{blurred} = I * G \tag{23}$$

Each image pixel becomes a weighted average of its neighbors and when we pass a blurred image through a CNN, embeddings may shift if the model heavily relies on textures or edges [69, 70]. The degree of shift indicates how robust the CNN is to losing details.

Let $E_{orig}, E_{lur}, E_{soel}, E_{canny}$ be embeddings from the CNN after preprocessing, then the embedding shift (ΔE) becomes

$$\Delta \mathrm{E} = \|E_{orig} - E_{perturbed}\|_2 \tag{24}$$

To analyze the impact of the various transformations on the model's embedding vectors, the authors use the t-SNE method and PCA. Both tools help understand the nature of embedding changes caused by transformations on the network's internal feature spaces [71, 72]. To extract the feature vectors for further analysis, the authors select a stage prior to the classification process in the CNN model. This stage corresponds to the layer immediately preceding the fully connected layers and is where the adaptive average pooling layer transforms the spatial feature maps from the CNN model into embedding vectors of fixed length [73–75]. Upon vector extraction, dimensionality reduction is then performed using t-SNE and PCA visualizations. t-SNE (in the left column) is more effective for visualizing non-linear embedding patterns, while PCA provides effective visualization for highlighting separations among the embedding vectors [76–78].

3.1.4 Evaluation

Evaluating explainable deep learning techniques requires a formalized set of performance metrics that adequately convey how well these explanations correspond to internal model mechanisms, and their robustness when faced with perturbations or distribution shifts [79–83]. In this study, interpretability is evaluated using three primary categories of metrics: metrics that correlate with embedding changes, metrics that measure explanation method consistency, and metrics that access visualization quality

(a) **Embedding shift magnitude(ESM)**: Embedding shift metrics measure how much the internal representations of model features, often extracted from convolutional or fully connected layers, tend to be affected given certain transformations such as blurring, edge detection, or geometric transformation [84–86]. The strength of embedding shift can be calculated based on the following formula:

$$ESM_t = \frac{1}{N}\sum_{\mathrm{i}=0}^{\mathrm{N}} \mathrm{D}\left(\mathrm{e}_{0,\mathrm{i}}, \mathrm{e}_{\mathrm{t},\mathrm{i}}\right),\ \mathrm{t}\epsilon\{\mathrm{Blur},\ \mathrm{Canny\ and\ Sobel}\} \tag{25}$$

where D is Euclidean/cosine distance and robustness is inversely related:

$$\mathrm{Robustness(ESM)} = \frac{1}{1 + Mean(ESM_{Blur}, ESM_{Canny}, ESM_{Sobel})} \tag{26}$$

(b) **Explainability consistency metrics**: These metrics evaluate how robust an explanation is to similar instances or perturbations, thus indicating reliability [87, 88]. These metrics evaluate the robustness of explanation distributions to input perturbations, and their behavior reflects the magnitude of probability shift, where larger shifts cause more inconsistent explanation distributions [89, 90].

The probability shift magnitude (PSM) measure calculates the change in class probabilities during transformations. Baseline or initial probabilities for each input "x" and the probabilities after the transformation (Blur, Canny, or Sobel) are calculated. This measure calculates the value for the probability shift magnitude based.

$$PSM_t = \frac{1}{N}\sum_{i=0}^{N} D(p_{0,i}, p_{t,i})\ \mathrm{t}\epsilon\{\mathrm{Blur, Canny,\ Sobel}\} \tag{27}$$

where D is the typical L1 or L2 distance

$$\mathrm{Robustness(PSM)} = 1 - \mathrm{Mean}(PSM_{Blur}, PSM_{Canny}, PSM_{Sobel}) \tag{28}$$

(c) **Visualization quality metrics** assess the interpretability and fidelity of visualization-based explanations in terms of human interpretability, presence of noise, focus on areas of interest, and correctness of model decision logic [91–93]. Together, they ensure trustworthy and comprehensible XAI outputs

[94–96]. It comprises probability shift and embedding shift ratio grouped under sensitivity ratios, as stated below:

Sensitivity ratio relatively compares shifts to Blur baseline across layers using:

$$PS\_Ratio_{Transform/Blur} = \frac{\mathrm{PS}_{\mathrm{Transform}}}{\mathrm{PS}_{\mathrm{Blur}}} \tag{29}$$

$$ES\_Ratio_{Transform/Blur} = \frac{\mathrm{ES}_{\mathrm{Transform}}}{\mathrm{ES}_{\mathrm{Blur}}} \tag{30}$$

where Transform ϵ {Canny, Sobel}.

(d) **Explanatory metrics** are linked to sensitivity ratio, robustness, fidelity, clarity, human interpretability, and completeness, as outlined below:

$$\text{Sensitivity measures output change under perturbation}(\mathbf{s}) = \frac{\Delta_P}{\Delta_x} \tag{31}$$

Robustness (R) combines embedding shift and probability shift magnitudes:

$$\text{Robustness(Explanatory metrics)} = 1 - \text{Mean(ESM, PSM)} \tag{32}$$

Fidelity evaluates the alignment of explanations with model predictions and is computed as:

$$\text{Fidelity(F)} = \text{Corr(M(x), Expl(x))} \tag{33}$$

Clarity evaluates the agreement between explanations and model predictions; measuring the separation between transformed and baseline explanations across classes. Separability reflects how well transformed features preserve class distinction accessed via H-Score or inter-class variance

$$C_t = Sep(P_t) \tag{34}$$

Human understanding score reflecting alignment with human intuition.

Completeness quantifies joint explanatory power across layers by aggregating individual contributions. It measures variance of predictions by explanations.

$$\text{Completeness(C2)} = 1 - \frac{SS_{res}}{SS_{tot}} \tag{35}$$

Algorithm 1: Embedding Shift Explanations for Deep Learning

Steps	**Procedures involved**
INPUT	Trained CNN model(M),
	Original image set X ← $\{x_1, x_2, ..., x_n\}$
	Transformation set T ← {None, Blur, Canny, Sobel}
	Embedding extractor function F from intermediate CNN layer
	Distance metric D (e.g., Euclidean, Cosine)
OUTPUT	Embedding shift vectors (S) ← $\{\Delta_1, \Delta_2, ..., \Delta_n\}$
	The changes observed in class probabilities(P) ← $\{p_1, p_2, ..., p_n\}$
	Visualization-ready data
1	Initialize results list S ← [], P ← []
2	for each input image of x in X do
3	e_0 ← F(x) # Extract original embedding
4	p_0 ← M.predict(x) # Get original class probabilities
5	for each transformation t in T do
6	x_t ← t(x) # Apply transformation
7	e_t ← F(x_t) # Retrieve the embedding after transformation
8	P_t ← M.predict(x_t) # Derive the updated probabilistic outputs
9	Δ_e ← D(e_0, e_t) # Compute embedding shift(e_0 → Original & e_t → Transformed)
10	Δ_p ← D(p_0, p_t) # Compute class probability shift
11	Store Δ_e *and* Δ_p in S, P #Store operation during each iteration of the loop
12	end for
13	end for

3.2 Experimental Setup

The experimental framework presents a framework for examinating the robustness of the CNN by addressing data preparation, specification of network architecture, learning practices, transformations used, and interpretability analysis techniques.

(1) **Loading and Processing the Data**: Loading and processing the data involved a customized function that resized all images uniformly into 64 x 64 pixels and converted them into tensors. This resulted in an 80% and 20% split of the dataset, for training and validation, respectively. In order to preserve the original data integrity, data augmentation was applied carefully. A batch size of 32 was used for training, while a batch size of 1 was used for validation.

(2) **Model training and building**: A two-dimensional CNN architecture was used with two convolutional layers, followed by ReLU activation and max pooling for each. The feature maps were then flattened and followed by two fully connected layers for the final classification task. The separation between the convolutional and dense layers enables the ease of interpretation by the use of intermediate representations. This model was trained for 100 iterations with the Adam optimizer with the learning rate set at 0.001 and the cross-entropy loss function with the gradients reset at the end of each iteration and the model parameters saved.

(3) **Model training/learning**: A two-dimensional CNN was set up with two convolutional layers, each followed by ReLU activation functions and max pooling layers. The feature maps were flattened and fed into two fully connected layers for the final classification task. The clear separation between the convolutional

layers and the fully connected layers enables easy extraction of intermediate representations for the interpretation. Training occurred for 100 epochs with the Adam optimizer with the learning rate set at 0.001 and cross-entropy loss with gradients reset at the end of each iteration and the model parameters saved at the end.

(4) **Image Transformation**: Blur and edge filters applied at different levels were used to produce perturbed versions of the original images to enable direct comparison of prediction consistency.

(5) **Interactive Prediction Visualization**: An interactive section was provided where the original and transformed images were shown together with graphs of the predicted class probabilities from the model. This allowed for quick evaluation of the prediction correctness and accuracy of the predictions before and after the transformation. The predictions were obtained from the softmax outputs, and each class probability value are displayed above each corresponding bar.

(6) **Confusion matrix and classification error evaluation**: Results are presented as a confusion matrix, highlighting errors made in specific classes, with an associated tool providing information on mislabeled examples while also indicating predictive categories.

(7) **Embedding Shift Analysis**: These convolution-feature embeddings were reduced using t-SNE or PCA to visualize the transition from the original to the transformed image and were annotated with an arrow indicating the shift and color representing the prediction accuracy for the transformed image.

(8) **Layer-wise Embedding Analysis**: The embeddings obtained from earlier, mid, and deeper layers were analyzed separately using t-SNE or PCA, while the mean shifts in class probabilities were visualized through bar and line plots to access the impact of transformations.

4 Results and Discussion

The experiments have shown, by conducting thorough t-SNE and PCA analysis, how the latent representations learned by the CNN are affected by input distortions such as blur, Canny edges, and Sobel operators. Even slight variations in the input lead to large differences in the feature space, which correspond to differences in the predicted class likelihoods and misclassifications. By monitoring the pathways of misclassified samples across network layers, such cases can be better interpreted. The study establishes a structured paradigm for understanding deep learning networks by linking input modifications, mid-level behavior, and final prediction outcomes.

4.1 Experimental Results

Figure 2 demonstrates the effect of input transformations to the class probability distribution of the model, with edge detection methods such as Canny, Blur, and Sobel confirming the model sensitivity to transformations. Figure 3 presents a novel way of visualizing the shifts of the embedding via t-SNE and PCA projection under different input transformations on the breast cancer dataset. It overlays the pre- and post-processing embeddings, connected by gray lines, making clear the magnitude and direction of the drift of representation through layers. In the "None" and "Blur" scenarios, the embeddings are tight and well-separated, corresponding to stability, whereas those of Canny and Sobel are large and irregular, causing a loss of separation, most prominently in the PCA graphs, where patterns of intense activity can be observed, showing considerable disturbance of features. Figure 3 enhances EDA-interpretability of deep learning by showing how input perturbation affect representation spaces, thus emphasizing the fragility of the DNN with respect to edge-preserving transformations and the value of transformation-encoding strategies, providing a framework for investigating robustness via embedding shift trajectories can be structured.

Figure 4 illustrates the changes in embeddings in explainable deep learning on the ALL dataset. Without any transformation or when Blur is applied, the embedding space stays compact and separable through t-SNE and PCA, indicating stable feature learning. However, the application of Canny and Sobel leads to high movement, evidenced by the saturation of connecting lines indicating the presence of feature pathway perturbations. t-SNE indicates the dispersion and overlap of clusters due to the application of Canny, signifying changes to the local structures, and PCA depicts the movement in the global variance. These perturbation-induced variations help to identify the points of weakness in the models, signifying the importance of training models that are robust to the transformations.

Figure 5 illustrates the misclassified samples, giving crucial insight into embedding change points in Explainable Deep Learning. Some categories, specifically "benign" and "malignant" for breast cancer, or "Benign" and "Early" for ALL, have persisting mistakes, symbolizing ill-defined boundaries among features, implying their latent spaces change erratically under various transformations. As expected, "Pro" in ALL has zero mistakes, symbolizing stable boundaries between features. The high level of confusion among similar samples, "Pre" and "Early" categories, points towards their overlap locations in latent space, consistent with past embedding analysis.

Figure 6, a focused investigation into the Shift Invariance property of CNNs is conducted by examining the prediction stability per class within the ALL dataset, symbolizing an evolutionary expansion in defining Embedded Shift Evolution. When examining the comparison of class prediction probabilities before and after an identical input re-rendering ($dx = 0$, $dy = 0$), it is realized that the model expresses perfect prediction stability, where no change is measured in logits for any class.

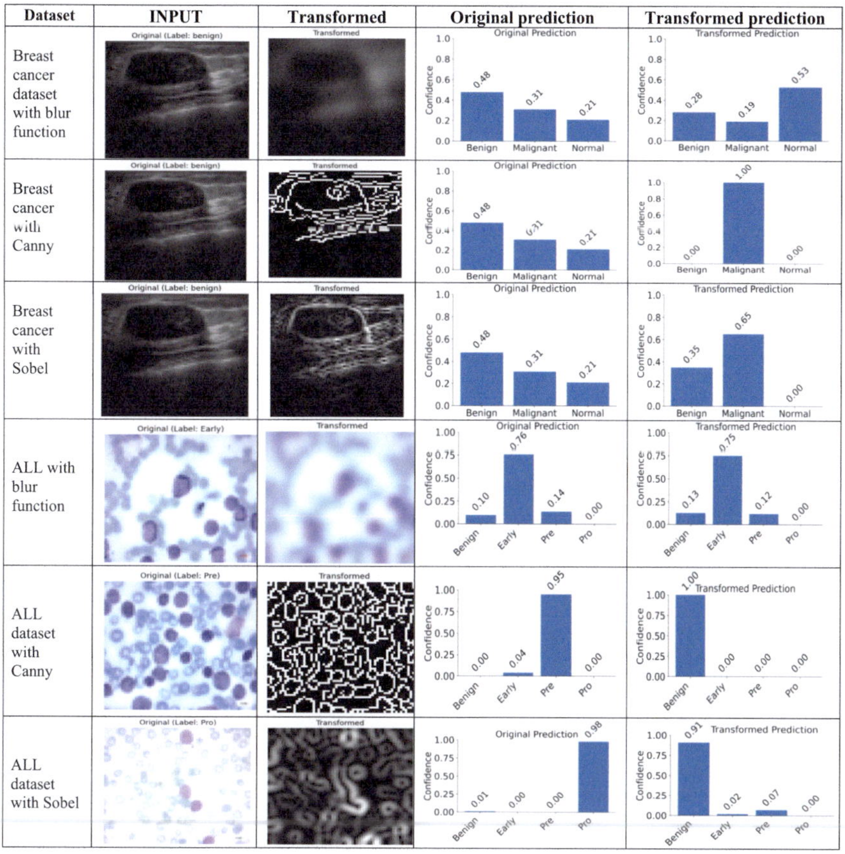

Fig. 2 Impact of input transformations on model class probability distributions

This suggests that the network is maintaining stable, spatially consistent representations, most prominently seen in the 'Pro' class, where the highest logit value remains at 3.40. This is crucial, as it validates the network itself as unaltered under conditions existing without geometric or noise transform perturbations. The significance emerges as it introduces a quantitative baseline measurement at the level of logits, underpinning a framework where the embedding shifts, introduced by transforms such as blur, Canny, or Sobel, are developed for comparison.

Figure 7 illustrates the shift-invariant behavior of the CNN on the breast cancer data set, indicating important points to note regarding Explainable Deep Learning. The corresponding probabilities for the original input and the zero shift scenario (dx = 0, dy = 0) for benign, malignant, and normal are 1.00, 0.29, and 1.51, respectively. These values confirm that the deep learning model is insensitive to the lack of spatial movement, thus authenticating the appropriateness and correctness of the zero shift representations used by the CNN model. It is important to set the zero shift to assess the impact of future transformations, whether blurring, Sobel, or Canny filters, on the

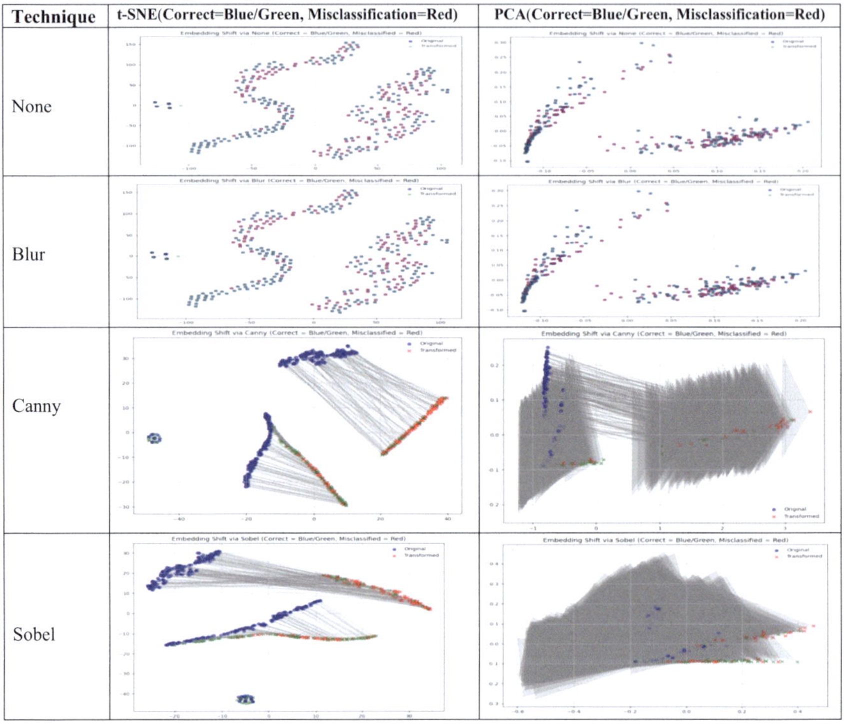

Fig. 3 This figure shows that in the case of the Breast Cancer dataset, using None or Blur preprocessing preserves the same cluster configuration, but Canny and Sobel introduce greater variations. Although both PCA and t-SNE are dimensionality reduction techniques, t-SNE provides more distinct boundaries between clusters, thus being more robust for some preprocessing methods

zero shift representation to enable the construction of robust and Explainable Deep Learning models.

In Figure 8, a stratified view of the embedding shift process in CNNs is shown based on the breast cancer dataset, which gives a detailed explanation for the effect of input changes on the representations at varying depths. At the beginning levels, the embeddings still maintain their structures, and probabilities indicate slight changes. However, as the network reaches the intermediate and deep levels, the representations get more sparsely distributed with a great reduction in probabilities. This effect highlights the accumulation effect caused by small changes in the inputs as they progress through the network levels, invalidating abstractions at the deep levels necessary for correct predictions. This is an excellent contribution in the explanation of deep learning models in highlighting the stability of predictions at precise levels within the network.

Figure 9 below offers a fresh perspective on depth-related analysis for the ALL dataset, emphasizing key trends in model explanation and interpretation. While Fig. 8 for the breast cancer dataset has revealed smoothly transitioning patterns for both

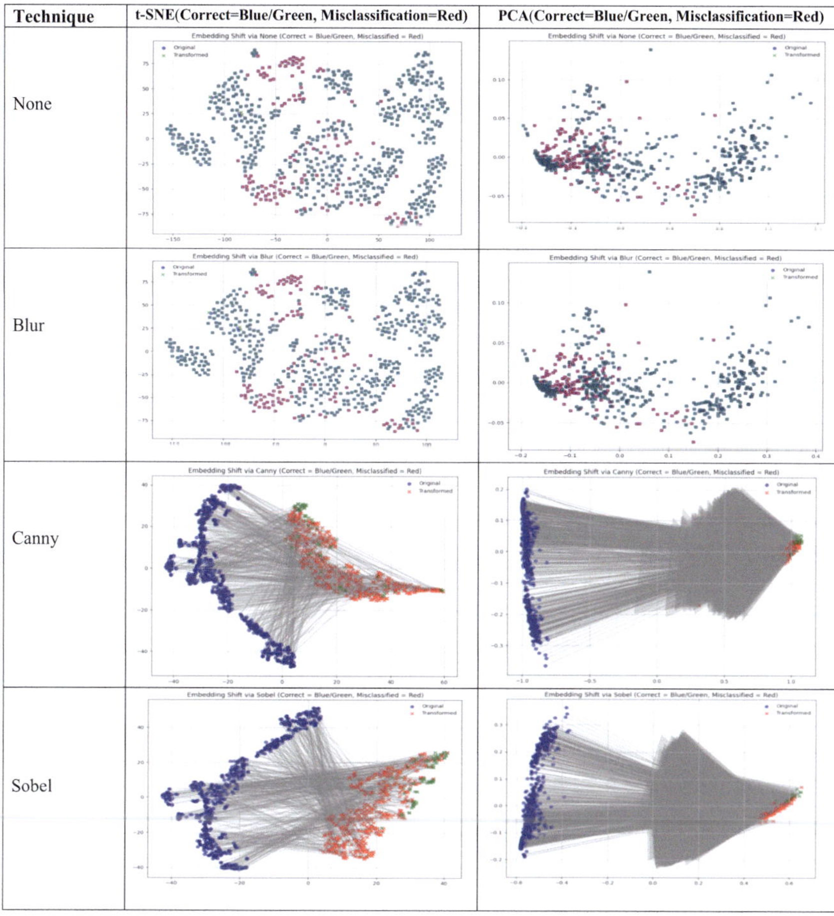

Fig. 4 Embedding shift analysis results for the ALL dataset, measured by t-SNE and PCA, show that the effect of Blur is slight, while that of Canny and Sobel is more directional. However, the separation boundary is maintained, which further supports the impact of the input transformation on the robustness and behavior of the model

embeddings and shifts, Fig. 9 aptly highlights irregular transitions in both embeddings and shifts for the early, medium, and deep layers of the network. While embeddings show significant changes in the deeper layers, irregular shift patterns clearly suggest that there is instability in the internal feature representation of the model. This fact is further reinforced in the bars of class probabilities, clearly reflecting the high degree of fragility of the model under transformations, especially for the deeper layers. While the key contribution of Fig. 8 was related to providing improved explanations for unstable model decisions, the key contribution of Fig. 9 below

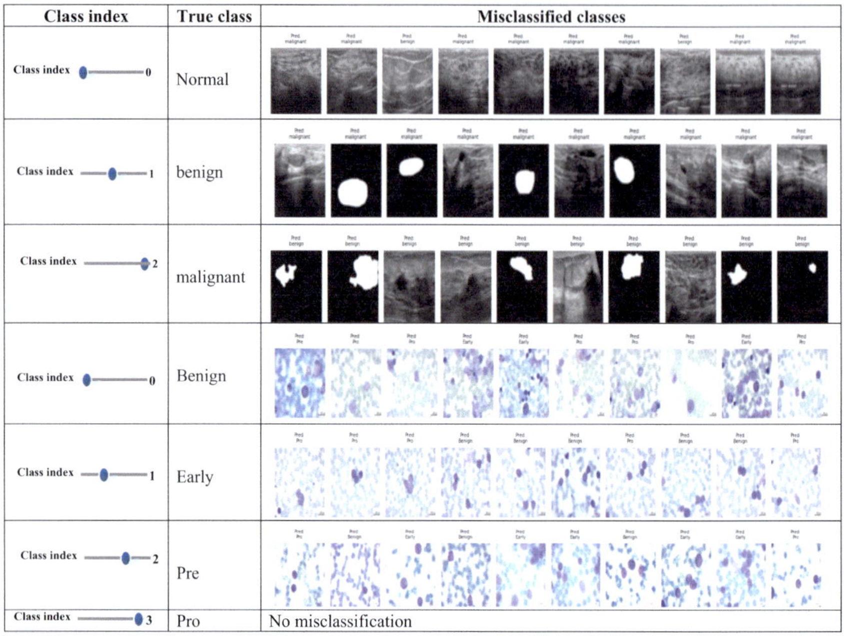

Fig. 5 Class-level error patterns and segmentation cues in medical image classification—displays error patterns at a class level with their respective segmentation cues from the heatmap, where failure regions indicate model improvement opportunities and robustness validation, especially in the 'Pro' class with no errors. The first three rows of Fig. 5 show results from the Breast Cancer dataset, while the last four rows display results from ALL dataset

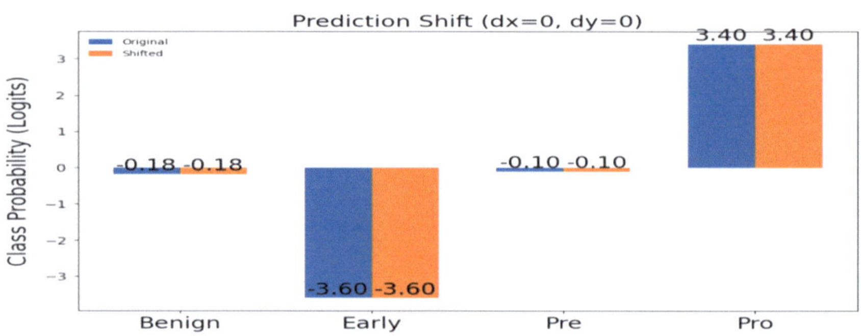

Fig. 6 Shift Invariance in CNN predictions for the ALL dataset—The logits calculated from both original and shifted inputs in ALL dataset remain the same, thus exhibiting shift invariance and confirming the validity and interpretability of results calculated by the CNN

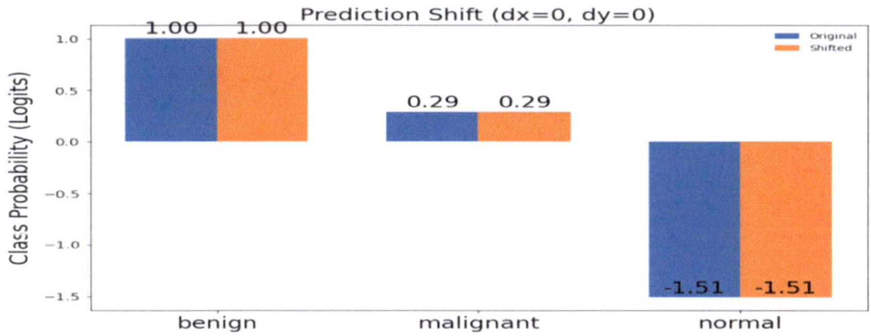

Fig. 7 Shift-Invariant predictions in CNN for Breast Cancer dataset—the benign, malignant, and normal class logit values are not affected when the image is translated, thus showing that the prediction of the CNN is shift-invariant

Layer	Layer-depth explanations	Class probability with shift curve
Earlier	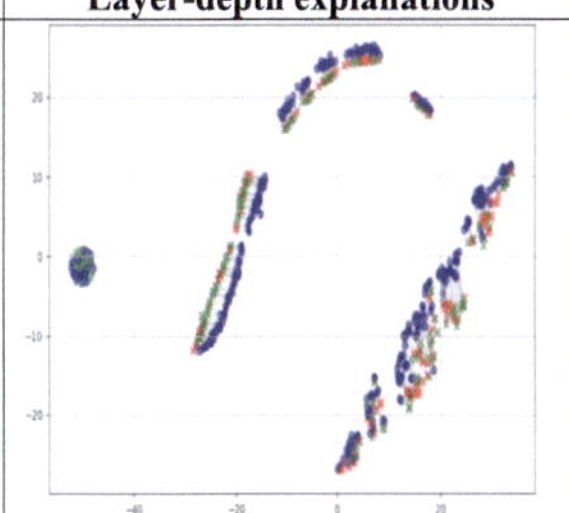	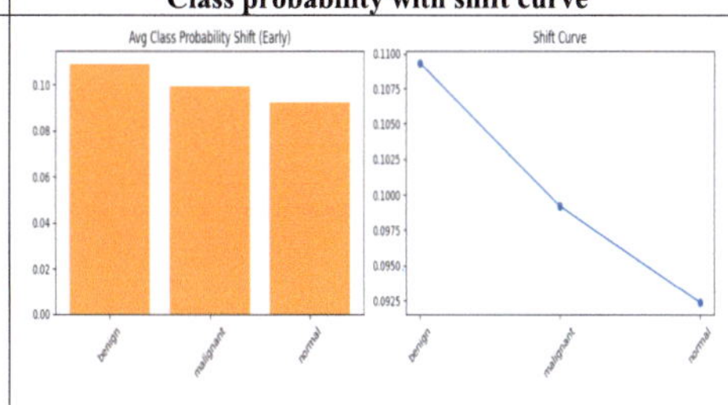
Mid	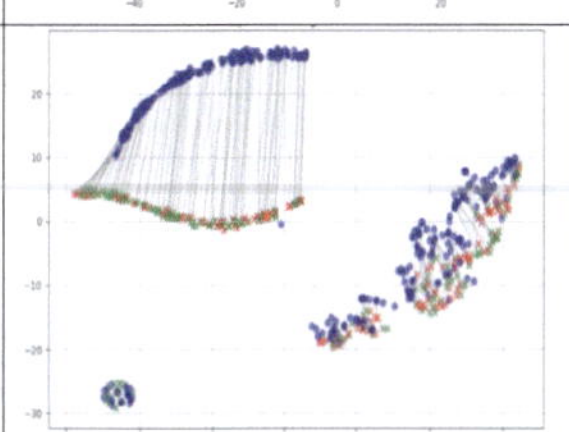	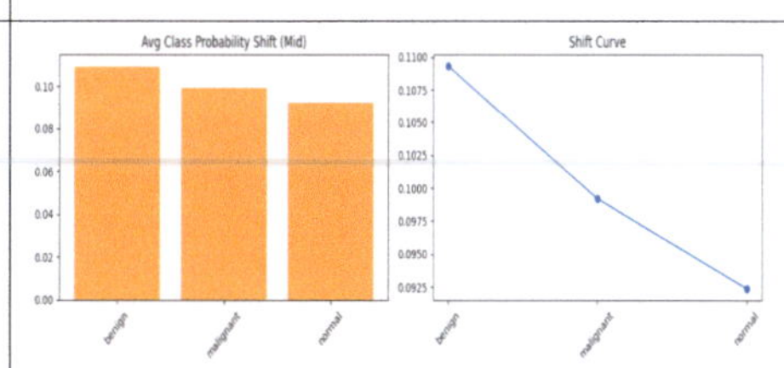
Deep	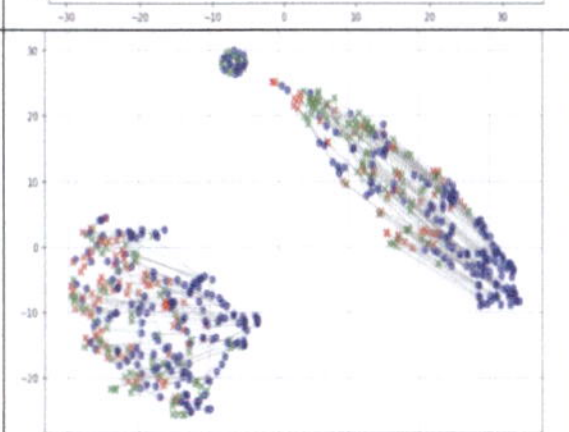	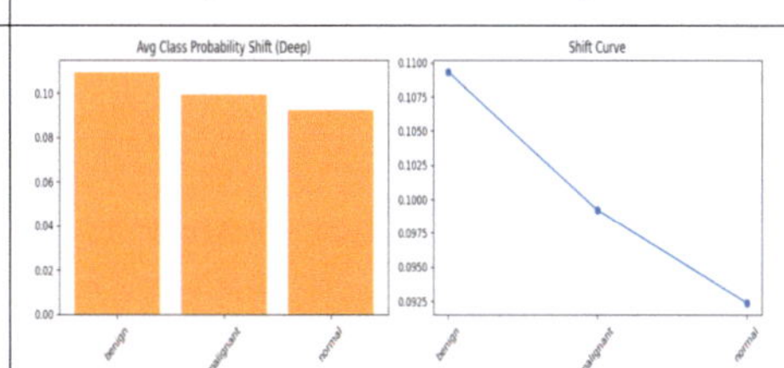

Fig. 8 Layer-wise embedding shift and class probability curves in CNNs for Breast Cancer dataset—the separability of the feature embeddings increases with each layer, the estimates for the probability of each class remain more or less the same, and the obtained shift curves enable the assessment of the model robustness with regard to the applied transformations

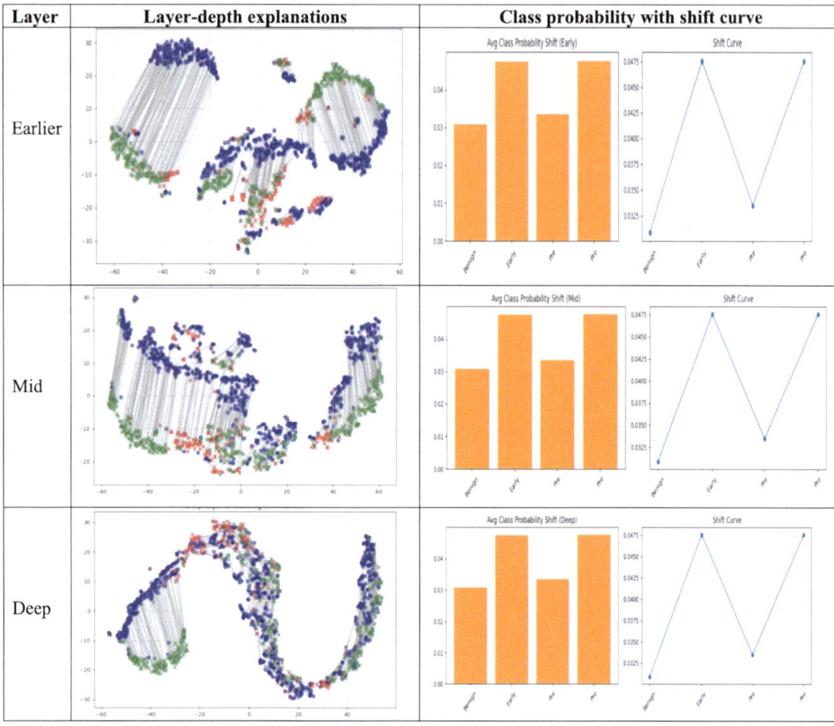

Fig. 9 Showcases the embedding transitions in the early, mid, and deep layers of the ALL dataset, coupled with class probability curves that highlight the effect of different transformations on feature development and model sensitivities for each hierarchical level

revolves around suggesting depth-related volatility and susceptibility to transformations, thereby adding to the existing explainable AI landscape associated with decision instability for specified stages of the network.

In short, experimental outcome analysis of Layer-Wise Embedding Shift reveals that lower layers are encoding edges, middle layers are encoding patterns, and deep layers are encoding class semantics, and transformations barely affect logits. ESE leads to robust and transformation-aware embeddings/logits, making understanding decision boundaries easier. Layer-wise views expose dataset sensitivities; Canny/Sobel enhance structure, enabling explainable predictions, consistent probabilities, actionable diagnostics helping practitioners compare models, anticipate shifts, deploy confidently across clinical-like settings. Improved separability, misclassification localization, and robustness emerge, enabling deployment, targeted retraining, and auditable, clinician-friendly explanations across datasets and perturbations.

4.2 Answers to Research Questions

(a) **How does applying input transformation (e.g., blur, Canny, and Sobel edge detection) affect the embedding shift representations of a trained CNN?**

From the t-SNE and PCA plots (Figs. 3 and 4), None and Blu*r* transformations generally preserve the structure of the embeddings with minimal shift, meaning that CNN still recognizes features similarly to the original inputs. Canny and Sobel transformations cause significant displacement of data points in embedding space, especially visible in the connecting lines between original and transformed embeddings. This suggests that these edge-detection filters drastically alter the low- and mid-level feature representations. The magnitude of embedding shifts is dataset-dependent: (a) In the Breast Cancer dataset (Fig. 3), edge transformations cause clear separations and cluster displacements in t-SNE and PCA space. (b). In the ALL dataset (Fig. 3), the same transformations cause even denser displacement patterns, with more scattered distributions in t-SNE and a compressed but shifted shape in PCA.

(b) **How do shifts in embedded space correlate with changes in class probabilities and final model predictions?**

Figures 8 and 9; show that larger embedding shifts generally correspond to larger drops in average class probability and more variation in the "Shift Curve." In Earlier layers, the shift often causes minor probability changes indicating resilience in early convolutional features. In Mid and Deep layers, the shifts correlate with larger probability drops and instability in predictions, showing that embedding displacement in deeper layers is more influential on the final decision. Figures 6 and 7 illustrate how specific transformations can induce significant shifts in prediction rankings. Although certain classes, like Benign or Pre, are less prone to variation in their probability predictions, others, specifically Early & Malignant, show drastic reductions, signifying a higher susceptibility to change brought about by these transformations.

(c) **To what extent do methods like t-SNE and PCA help make CNN-based systems more interpretable and support error analysis in CNN-based systems?**

t-SNE provides clearer *nonlinear cluster separation* and makes it easy to see how transformation pulls points away from their original positions. It highlights local structure changes and is excellent for visualizing misclassification "drift" paths. PCA preserves global variance and provides a more interpretable geometric displacement pattern, making it useful for quantifying overall embedding spread or contraction. In Figs. 3 and 4, both methods complement each other: (a). t-SNE: It is easier to see misclassification boundaries and tight versus loose clusters. (b). PCA: Easier to measure directionality and magnitude of global shifts. These dimensionality reduction methods make it visually obvious which transformations cause catastrophic embedding shifts, helping guide robustness analysis. t-SNE shows local changes; PCA shows global variance shifts; both aid interpretability.

(d) **To what extent can tracking embedding shifts improve the detection of misclassifications or uncertainty in deep learning models**

Figure 5 misclassification visualization shows that many errors occur when embeddings shift into the region of another class after transformation. Tracking embedding shifts can flag samples at high risk of misclassification before the model produces a final label especially when displacement distance exceeds a learned threshold. Embedding shift patterns can also detect uncertainty hotspots: (a). Large shifts + high probability drop → strong candidate for model uncertainty. (b). Minimal shift + stable probability → prediction is likely robust. This can be integrated into an early warning system where embeddings are compared pre- and post-transformation to trigger human review in high-stakes tasks (e.g., medical imaging).

4.3 Evaluation of Model Explanations

Evaluation tools in Explainable AI (XAI) are essential for assessing the quality and reliability of model explanations as shown in Tables 1, 2, 3, 4 and 5.

Equations (25) and (26) are used to compute the values in Table 1; Equation (25) defines the Embedding Shift Magnitude (ESM) for each transformation (Blur, Canny,

Table 1 Embedding shift magnitudes (ESM)

Layer	ESM Blur(↓)	ESM Canny(↓)	ESM Sobel(↓)	Robustness(Emb)↑
Early	2.2653	6.2245	4.5527	0.187
Mid	2.5522	7.0192	5.1001	0.1698
Deep	2.7197	7.4711	5.4215	0.1612

Table 2 Probability shift magnitudes (PSM)

Layer	ESM Blur(↓)	ESM Canny(↓)	ESM Sobel(↓)	Robustness(Prob)↑
Early	0.0394	0.1013	0.0731	0.9334
Mid	0.0119	0.0288	0.0208	0.9799
Deep	0.0105	0.0307	0.0252	0.9784

Table 3 Sensitivity ratios versus blur

Layer	PS Ratio Canny/ Blur(↑)	PS Ratio Sobel/ Blur(↑)	ES Ratio Canny/ Blur(↑)	ES Ratio Sobel/ Blur(↑)
Early	2.571	1.855	2.748	2.01
Mid	2.415	1.741	2.750	1.998
Deep	2.929	2.401	2.747	1.993

Table 4 Explanatory metrics

Layer	Sensitivity	Robustness	Fidelity	Clariy under transforms	Clarity vs None	Human Understandability	Completeness RÂ^2 (layer-only) (â†‘)	Completeness
Early	0.35	0.835	0.821	0.481	-0.042	1	0.674	
Mid	0.469	0.835	0.869	0.531	-0.043	1	0.756	
Deep	0.620	0.385	0.890	0.553	-0.056	1	0.791	
Joint(E+M+D)		**0.835**						**0.872**

Table 5 Per-transform clarity (seperability index)

Layer	None	Blur	Canny	Sobel
Early	0.523	0.513	0.487	0.444
Mid	0.573	0.561	0.543	0.487
Deep	0.608	0.594	0.565	0.499

Sobel). For each input 'x', the original embedding e_0 and the transformed embedding e_t are extracted at different layers (Early, Mid, Deep). The distance $D(e_{0,i}, e_{t,i})$ (Euclidean or cosine) is computed, averaged across all samples N, yielding ESM values per layer and transformation. These values fill the ESM Blur, ESM Canny, and ESM Sobel columns. Equation (26) defines Robustness(Emb) as the inverse of the mean embedding shift. Accordingly, larger embedding displacement corresponds to reduced model robustness, and this relationship informs the values reported in the final column of the table. Among these transformations, the blurry filter has the lowest values of displacement (Early 2.2653), indicating less effect on structural information. On the other hand, the Canny edge detection filter, which converts the image into edges and eliminates all color and texture details, presents the highest degree of divergence and ESM (Early 6.2245, Deep 7.4711). The Sobel filter, which captures the image gradients, presents intermediate values of displacement (Early 4.5527, Deep 5.4215).

Table 2 shows results that are derived from Equations (27) and (28) above. It is observed that in Equation (27), MPM is calculated as the magnitude of probability shift caused by transformations in inputs. It gauges how much classification probabilities are affected by transformations in an input. However, high values in early layers and with operators such as Canny or Sobel imply lower stability and lower robustness. But in contrast, in mid or deeper layers, lower values of MPM are observed. It is quite evident that as feature representations become increasingly abstract, stability in prediction increases. On the other hand, in Equation (28), robustness is defined as inversely proportional to mean MPM. It is evident here as well that robustness increases in deeper layers (> 0.97).

The values reported in Table 3 were obtained by measuring sensitivity ratios between edge-focused transformations (Canny and Sobel) and blur across successive CNN layers. Equations (29) and (30) provide the basis for these calculations by normalizing the perturbation sensitivity (PS) and embedding shift (ES) associated with Canny and Sobel relative to the Blur reference at each layer. In particular, Equation (29) computes the PS ratio by dividing the PS produced under Canny or Sobel filtering by the PS observed under Blur, yielding the first two PS ratio columns in Table 3. Similarly, Equation (30) divides the ES under Canny (or Sobel) filtering by the ES under Blur, giving the last two columns (ES Ratios). Each ratio thus expresses how many times more sensitive a layer is to edge-based perturbations compared to blur. Higher ratios indicate stronger relative sensitivity at that layer. The deep layers exhibit higher sensitivity ratios compared to early and mid layers. This is because deeper layers capture more abstract and task-specific features, making them more responsive to structural distortions introduced by edge filters (Canny, Sobel) than to smoothing effects from blur.

Table 4 shows the values in explanatory metrics that assess interpretability of CNN layers under transformations (Blur, Canny, Sobel). Equations (31–35) define the explanatory metrics reported in Table 4. Sensitivity (Eq. 31) measures prediction changes under perturbations, producing the Sensitivity column. Robustness (Eq. 32) averages embedding shift magnitudes (ESM) and probability shift magnitudes (PSM), giving the Robustness scores. Fidelity (Eq. 33) correlates model outputs with explanations, yielding the Fidelity attribute. Clarity (Eq. 34) measures separability between transformed and baseline explanations, reflected in Clarity under transforms and Clarity versus None. Human understandability is assigned manually, reflecting how well the explanation aligns with intuitive reasoning (value = 1). Completeness (Eq. 35) is the proportion of variance explained with regard to the layers in the network, providing values for explanation on the layer level and the aggregate level. The Joint (E+M+D) value combines the values from the Early, Mid, and Deep layers. The values reveal that mid-level representations provide the best trade-off between robustness and explanation fidelity, while the joint assessment improves the interpretability, although the completeness value (0.872) indicates that the aggregated explanation preserves consistent sensitivity, clarity, and interpretability. The "Clarity versus None" value evaluates the change in clarity with regard to the application of any transformation and the clarity for the original input. So, the values are expected to be negative, indicating simply the loss of clarity due to the application of perturbation operators like Canny, Sobel, or blurs."

The class separability values of clarity, expressed by the separability index, under different image transformations are presented in Table 5. There are four steps involved in calculating this value: (a) class-specific embeddings are calculated post-transformation, (b) the between-class variance(B)=$\sum_c n_c||\mu_c - \mu_l||^2$ is measured, where n_c is the number of samples in class c and μ_c and μ_l denote the vectors of class and global mean, respectively, and (c) the within-class variance (W) = $\sum_c \sum_{i\epsilon c} ||\mu_i - \mu_c||^2$ which concentrates on the variabilities of classes, is measured. Then, the separability can be calculated by the formula B/(B+W), and is restricted within the interval (0,1). According to the result, the original image brings the highest clarity. For the blurred image, there is only a slight reduction in the value of the between-class variation and an increase in the within-class variation, thus reducing clarity (Early layer: 0.513 vs. 0.523). The Canny edge detection method reduces the image clarity by further decreasing the distance of the centroids and increasing the dispersal, thus reducing clarity (Early: 0.487). The Sobel filter, which reduces the detailed information and color, performs the poorest and brings the lowest clarity (Early: 0.444; Deep: 0.499). Conclusively, all transformations result in the reduction of class separability, and the effect is the highest by the Sobel filter, while the others fall in between.

This study shows how changes to embeddings offer a window into internal reasoning processes of a model. Through observing how a feature representation evolves from one layer to another, this study points out where a deep learning system is highly sensitive to different inputs. This is a means through which interpretability is understood to relate to a study of representational evolution rather than a snapshot, providing a method through which researchers can analyze for reasons behind non-robustness. This work is significant for the field of explainable AI and points to a method through which deep learning systems could monitor themselves, justify themselves, and improve their robustness

5 Conclusion and Recommendation

Such outcomes ensure the behavior of the model is observable. The variation caused by changing the input is minimal, although there is a considerable variation after implementing Canny or Sobel filtering. The transitions in the t-SNE or PCA space reveal boundary transitions for misclassifications. The minimal displacement maintains high-confidence assignments, and layer-wise patterns demonstrate greater sensitivity in the early stages of the network, becoming stable at deeper layers.

This work presents a method to interpret deep neural networks through the assessment of sensitivity to carefully controlled pertubations within feature space across multiple layers. It points to the sensitivity of the various layers, the change in the probabilities for the classes as a consequence of a shift in the embedding, and the pattern of robustness across the deep learning model. Taken together, the results offer an integrated and more transparent explanation regarding the dynamics within the representations and the patterns within the decisions reached by the deep learning models. The results show how visual metrics might contribute to more robustness through data augmentation centered on edges, strategic regularization, data set curation, and monitoring within the dataset.

5.1 Further Research

Future work may investigate learning approaches to improve model robustness, make cross-architectural comparisons of embedding displacement, and better incorporate visualization techniques, such as t-SNE layering and vector displacement mappings, into model analysis.

(a) **Cross-Modal Interpretability**: Investigate how linguistic contexts affect visual interpretability by aligning feature spaces for multimodal learning, exploring transitions between modalities, and identifying patterns of semantic connection. This helps to understand how semantics are connected through representations from different media, like text and images, for tasks like visual question answering, image captioning, and grounded retrieval.

(b) **Temporal Embeddings Analysis**: Future work would examine how temporal embeddings evolve within video or other sequential learning models and might explore temporal tracking, visualization with attention mechanisms, and dynamic alignment techniques to better understand temporal embeddings and improve model interpretability when handling actions, behaviors, or temporal clinical data.

(c) **Human-Centric Evaluation**: Future studies might link embedding dynamics to human cognition by combining eye-tracking data, think-aloud procedures, and contrasts based on human attention patterns and network activations. Higher alignment of model explainer outputs and human interpretation could enhance interpretive transparency, promote trust, and inform more adaptive and ethics-driven decision-making.

(d) **Analysis of Adversarial Robustness**: Examine the sensitivity of embeddings to noise, occlusion, and adversarial attack to identify the instability of embeddings at different levels of the network and improve the robustness of the model. Attribution methods using layer-level mappings of instability, analysis of representational similarities, and stress-attributed analysis are used to identify potential flaws in the model to improve training techniques.

Author Contributions Ziweritin Stanley conceptualized the research design, developed the methodological framework, conducted the experimental steps, and drafted the initial version of the manuscript. Dr. Abirami Gunasekaran supervised the overall research design, providing analytical guidance, technical expertise, and improvements to the explainable deep learning models. Dr. Shamaila Iram and Dr. Minsi Chen jointly supervised the research process, offering key reviews, technical feedback, and validations of

Code Availability The code for the implementation is available upon request so that the methods used and the experiment workflow can be evaluated.

Ethical Consideration The study was conducted under strict ethical norms on the use of human medical information. The images used in this study were obtained from publicly accessible anonymized datasets for research purposes. No personal information was accessed or used. Every aspect of data handling and analysis was done under national and international privacy laws and ethical norms.

References

1. Wilson, E., Satomi, M., McLean, A., Schubert D., Gonzalez J.F.A.: Embodied exploration of latent spaces and explainable AI, 1–4 (2024). https://doi.org/10.48550/arXiv.2410.14590
2. Meijer, C. Bos, E.G.P.: Explainable embeddings with distance explainer, machine learning, 1–33(2025). https://doi.org/10.48550/arXiv.2505.15516
3. Siu, H.C., Ashley, S., Nora, S., Isabelle, H.: Explainable' AI has some explaining to do. In: MIT Case Studies in Social and Ethical Responsibilities of Computing, no. Winter 2025 (March) (2025). https://doi.org/10.21428/2c646de5.e8e32375.
4. Zhuang, X., Zhu, P., Yang, Y., Caldas, L.: Machine learning for generative architectural design: advancements, opportunities, and challenges. Autom. Constr. **174**, 1–20 (2025). https://doi.org/10.1016/j.autcon.2025.106129
5. Doorenmalen, J.V., Menkovski, V.: Evaluation of CNN performance in semantically relevant latent spaces. Adv. Intell. Data Anal. 145–157 (2020). https://doi.org/10.1007/978-3-030-44584-3_12

6. Metta, C., Cappuccio, E. Rinzivillo, S.: Interactive visual exploration of latent spaces for Explainable AI: Bridging concepts and features. In: Joint Proceedings of the ACM IUI Workshops March 2025, 24–27, 2 (2025). https://ceur-ws.org/Vol-3957/AXAI-paper10.pdf?utm_source=chatgpt.com
7. Fumero, M., Moschella, L., Rodola, E., Locatello, F.: Navigating the latent space dynamics of neural models. Mach. Learn. 1–22 (2025). https://doi.org/10.48550/arXiv.2406.00532
8. Bai, S., Nasar, S., Khan Anf, S., Meyer, A., Konik, H.: Breast cancer diagnosis: A comprehensive exploration of explainable artificial intelligence (XAI) techniques. Artif. Intell. 1–28 (2024). https://doi.org/10.48550/arXiv.2406.00532
9. Ridha, J., Saddami, K., Riswan, M., Roslidar, R.: An explainable artificial intelligence framework for Breast cancer detection. Indones. J. Electron., Electromed. Eng. Med. Inform. (IJEEEMI) **7**(2), 1–20 (2025). https://doi.org/10.1016/j.cogsys.2024.101243
10. Shifa, N., Saleh, M., Akbari, Y., Maadeed, S.A.: A review of explainable AI techniques and their evaluation in mammography for breast cancer screening. Clin. Imaging **123**, 1–12 (2024). https://doi.org/10.1016/j.clinimag.2025.110492
11. Srivenkatesh, M.: Prediction of breast cancer disease using machine learning algorithms. Int J. Innov. Technol. Explor. Eng. (IJITEE) **9**, 2868–2878 (2020). https://doi.org/10.35940/ijitee.D1866.029420
12. Abdulla, S.H., Sagheer, A.M, Veisi, H.: Breast cancer classification using machine learning techniques: a review. Turk. J. Comput. Math Education (TURCOMAT) **12**, 1970–1979 (2021). https://turcomat.org/index.php/turkbilmat/article/view/10604
13. Houfani, D., Slatnia, S., Kazar, O., Zerhouni, N., Merizig, A, Saouli, H.: Machine learning techniques for breast cancer diagnosis: literature review. In: Advanced Intelligent Systems for Sustainable Development (AI2SD'2019) Volume 2-Advanced Intelligent Systems for Sustainable Development Applied to Agriculture and Health, 247–254 (2020). https://doi.org/10.1007/978-3-030-36664-3_28
14. Ghasemi, A., Hashtarkhani, S., Schwartz, D., Shaban-Nejad, A.: Explainable artificial intelligence in breast cancer detection and risk prediction: a systematic scoping review. Cancer Innov. 1–22 (2024). https://arxiv.org/pdf/2407.12058
15. Dastgeer, S., Treigys, P.: LLMs and XAI for Breast cancer transparencey. Balt. J. Mod. Comput. **13**(2), 528–550 (2025). https://doi.org/10.22364/bjmc.2025.13.2.12
16. Wehner, C., Iliopoulou, C., Schmid, U., Besold, T.R., Barcelona, S.A.: From Latent to Lucid: Transforming Knowledge Graph Embeddings Into Interpretable Structures with KGEPrisma, 1–17 (2025). https://arxiv.org/pdf/2406.01759
17. Ramanujam, E., Sekar, K., Bavashree, G.S., Prabakar, S.S.: Explainable AI for Leukemia diagnosis: modified ResNet with hard attention mechanisms. In: 2025 International Conference on Intelligent Systems and Computational Networks (ICISCN) (2025). https://doi.org/10.1109/ICISCN64258.2025.10934231
18. Pervez, K., Sahail, S.I., Parwez, F., Zia, M.A.: Towards trustworthy AI-driven leukemia diagnosis: a hybrid hierarchical federated learning and explainable AI framework. Inform. Med. Unlocked **53**, 1–16 (2025). https://doi.org/10.1016/j.imu.2025.101618
19. Oybek-Kizi, R.F., Armand, T.P., Kim, H.C.: A review of deep learning techniques for leukemia cancer classification based on blood smear images. Appl. Biosci **4**(1), 9 (2025). https://doi.org/10.3390/applbiosci4010009
20. Diaz-Resendiz, J.L., Ponomaryov, V., Reyes, R.R., Sadovnychiy, S.: Explainable CAD system for classification of acute lymphoblastic leukemia based on a robust white blood cell segmentation. Cancers **15**(13), 3376 (2023). https://doi.org/10.3390/cancers15133376
21. Faiz, M., Mounika, B.G., Akbar, M., Srivastava, S.: Deep and machine learning for acute lymphoblastic leukemia diagnosis: A comprehensive review. ADCAIJ: Adv. Distrib. Comput. Artif. Intell. J. (2024). https://doi.org/10.14201/adcaij.31420
22. Darmawan, S.T.S., Shabrina, N.H.: Explainable deep learningfor diagnosis acute lymphocytic leukemia using blood smear images. Bull. Electr. Eng. Inform. **14**(2), 1298–1307 (2025). https://doi.org/10.11591/eei.v14i2.9073

23. Retzlaff, C., Angerschmid, A., Saranti, A., Schneeberger, D., Rottger, R., Muller, H., Holzinger, A.: Post-hoc vs ante-hoc explanations: XAI design guidelines for data scientists. Cogn. Syst. Res. **86**, 1–17 (2024). https://doi.org/10.1016/j.cogsys.2024.101243
24. Weber, T.: Explainability for embedding AI: aspirations and actuality. Hum.-Comput. Interact. 1–10 (2025), https://doi.org/10.48550/arXiv.2504.14631
25. Luo, X., Liu, D., Kong, H., Huai, S., Chen, H., Xiong, G., Liu, W.: Efficient deep learning infrastructures for embedded computing systems: a comprehensive survey and future envision. ACM Trans. Embedd. Comput. Syst. **24**(1), Article 21 (December 2024), 100 (2024). https://doi.org/10.1145/3701728
26. Gamatie, A., Wang, Y.: Explanable AI for embedded systems design: a case study of static redundant NVM memory write prediction, 1–14 (2024). https://arxiv.org/pdf/2403.04337v1
27. Zhou, R., Hu, T.: Evolutionary computation for explainable deep learning. In: van Stein, N., Kononova, A.V. (eds) Explainable AI for Evolutionary Computation. Natural Computing Series. Springer, Singapore (2025). https://doi.org/10.1007/978-981-96-2540-6_4
28. Han, G.,Chen, J., Liu, L., Wang, Z., Zhang, F.: An interpretable CNN with wavelet grop olicy emedded intelligent fault diagnosis. IEEE Trans. Instrum. **88** (2024). https://doi.org/10.1109/TIM.2024.3368479
29. Shimizu, E., Fukumizu, K., Sejdinovic, D: Neural kernel condition mean embedding. Mach. Learn. 1–17 (2024). https://doi.org/10.48550/arXiv.2403.10859
30. Barros, C.D.T., Mendonca, M.R.F., Vieira, A.B., Ziviani, A.: A survey on embedding dynamics graphs. Mach. Learn. 1–41 (2021). https://doi.org/10.48550/arXiv.2101.01229
31. Zhou, R., Bacardit, J., Browniee, A., Cagnoni, S., Fyvie, M., Iacca, G., McCall, J., Stein, N.V., Walker, D.J., Hu, T.: Evolutionary computation and explainable AI: Road map to understandable intelligent systems, 1–25 (2024). arXiv:2406.07811v2 [cs.NE] 17 Oct 2024
32. Schwalbe, G.: Concept embedding analysis: a review. Mach. Learn. 1–47 (2022). https://doi.org/10.48550/arXiv.2203.13909
33. Zhang, M., He, C., Huang, C., Yang, J.: A weighted time embedding transformer network for remaining useful life prediction of rolling bearing. Reliab. Eng. Syst. Saf. **251** (2024). https://doi.org/10.1016/j.ress.2024.110399
34. Kumar, A., Garg, S., Dutt, S.: Uncertainty-aware deep neural representations for visual analysis of vector field data. IEEE Trans. Vis. Comput. Graph. **31**(1), 1343–1353 (2025). https://doi.org/10.1109/TVCG.2024.3456360
35. https://www.kaggle.com/datasets/aryashah2k/breast-ultrasound-images-dataset
36. https://www.kaggle.com/datasets/mehradaria/leukemia
37. Polica, P., Strazar, M., Zupan, B.: Embedding to reference t-SNE space addresses batch effects in single-cell classification. Mach. Learn. **112**, 721–740 (2023). https://doi.org/10.1007/s10994-021-06043-1
38. Wani, A.A.: Comprehensive review of dimentionality reduction algorithms: chanllenges, limitations and innovative solutions. Peer J. Comput. Sci. **30** (2025). https://doi.org/10.7717/peerj-cs.3025
39. Schneider, S., Lee, J.H., Mathis, M.W.: Learnable latent embeddings for joint behavioral and neural analysis. Nature **617**, 360–368 (2023). https://doi.org/10.1038/s41586-023-06031-6
40. Sarmina, B., Sun, G.H., Dong, S.H.: Principal component analysis and t-Distributed stochastic neighbor embedding analysis in the study of quantum approximate optimization algorithm entangled and non-entangled mixing operators. Entropy **25**(11), 1499 (2023). https://doi.org/10.3390/e25111499
41. Orlov, A.A., Akhmetshin, T.N., Horvath, D., Marcou, G., Varnek, A.: From high dimensions to human insight: exploring dimentionality reduction for chemical space visualization. Mol. Inform. 1–18 (2024). https://doi.org/10.1002/minf.202400265
42. Jeo, H., Lee, H., Kuo, Y.H., Yang, T. Archambault, D., Ko, S., Fujiwara, T., Ma, K., Seo, J.: Unveiling high-dimentional backstage: a survey for reliable visual analytics with dimensionality reduction. In: CHI '25: Proceedings of the 2025 CHI Conference on Human Factors in Computing Systems, 394, 1–24 (2025). https://doi.org/10.1145/3706598.37135

43. Li, P., Wang, H., Yu, M., Li, Y.: Overview of image smoothing algorithms, J. Phys. Conf. Ser. **1883**(1) (2021). https://doi.org/10.1088/1742-6596/1883/1/012024
44. Jun, S., Dagobert, T., Morel, J.M., Facciolo, G.: A review of t-SNE. IPOL Image Process. Line **14**, 1–22 (2024). https://doi.org/10.5201/ipol.2024.528
45. Serna-Serna, W., Bodt, C.D., Alvarez-Meza, A., Lee, J.A., Verleysen, M., Orozco-Gutierrez, A.A.: Semi-supervised t-SNE with multi-scale neighborhood preservation. Neurocomputing 550 (2023). https://doi.org/10.1016/j.neucom.2023.126496
46. Chagnon, J., Hagenbuchner, M., Tsai, A.C., Scarselli, F.: Investigating the effects of recursion in convolutional layers using analytical methods. Neurocomputing **626**, 1–26 (2025). https://doi.org/10.1016/j.neucom.2025.129570
47. Sun, T., He, L., Fang, X., Xie, L.: Dimensionality reduction: unlocking the potential of complex image data. Mathematics **13**(3), 531 (2025). https://doi.org/10.3390/math13030531
48. Lee, Y., Shine, N.Y., Lee, I.: Privacy-preserving data sharing via PCA-based dimensionality reduction in Non-IID environments. Electronics **14**(13), 2711 (2025). https://doi.org/10.3390/electronics14132711
49. Bharadiya, J.: A tutorial on principal component analysis for dimensionality reduction in machine learning. Int. J. Innov. Sci. Res. Technol. **8**(5) (2023). https://doi.org/10.5281/zenodo.8002436
50. Thejaswini, M.S., Kuma, J.G.H., Aradhya, I.V.N.M.: Hybrid dimensionality reduction model for real-time EEG-based emotion recognition: a combined subspace approach using principal component analysis and independent component analysis. Int. Inf. Eng. Technol. Assoc. (IIETA) **12**(5), 1771–1788 (2024). https://doi.org/10.18280/mmep.120532
51. Zhu, L., Mao, Y., Pan, J.: Image alignment based on deep learning to extract deep feature information from images. Sensors **25**(15), 4628 (2025). https://doi.org/10.3390/s25154628
52. Dede, A., Nunoo-Mensah, H., Akowuah, E.K., Boateng, K.O., Adjei, P.E., Acheampong, F.A., Acquah, I., Kponyo, J.J.: Wave-based feature extraction for efficient high-resolution image classification. Eng. Rep. **7**(2), 1–12 (2025). https://doi.org/10.1002/eng2.70027
53. Mjahad, A., Polo-Aguado, A., Llorens-Serrano, L., Rosado-Munoz, A.: Optimizing image feature extraction with convolutional neural networks for chicken meat detection applications. Appl. Sci. **15**, 733 (2025). https://doi.org/10.3390/app15020733
54. Masksimovic, V., Jaksic, B., Milosevic, M., Todorovic, J., Mosurovic, L.: Comparative analysis of Edge detection operators using a threshold estimation approach on medical noisy images with different complexities **25**(1), 87 (2025). https://doi.org/10.3390/s25010087
55. Bhat, S., Szczuko, P.: Impact of canny edge detection preprocessing on performance of machine learning models for Parkinson's disease classification. Sci. Rep. 16413 (2025). https://doi.org/10.1038/s41598-025-98356-7
56. Rong, W., Li, Z., Sun, L.: An improved edge detection algorithm. In: 2014 IEEE International Conference on Mechatronics and Automation (ICMA) (2024). https://doi.org/10.1109/ICMA.2014.6885761
57. Agrawai, H., Desai, K.: Canny edge detection: a comprehensive review. Int. J. Tech. Res. Sci. **9**, 27–35 (2024), https://doi.org/10.30780/specialissue-ISET-2024/023
58. Yin, Z., Wang, Z., Fan, C., Wang, X., Qiu, T.: Edge detection via fusion difference convolution. Sensors **23**(15), 6883 (2023). https://doi.org/10.3390/s23156883
59. Wittmann J. & Heri G.(2023) Canny-net: known operator learning for edge detection, e-journal of nondestructive testing, 28(3), 12, https://doi.org/10.58286/27751
60. Ravichandran, S., Su, H.K., Kuo, W.K., Dhanasekaran, D., Mahalingam, M.M, Yang, J.P.: Parallel processing of sobel edge detection on FPGA: enhancing real-time image analysis **25**(12), 3649 (2025). https://doi.org/10.3390/s25123649
61. Shi, K.: Comparasion of image enhancement algoeithms based on denoising and edge detection. Appl. Comput. Eng. **133**(1), 174–184 (2025). https://doi.org/10.54254/2755-2721/2025.20700
62. Li, D., Pang, P.C.I., Lam, K.: Contrast-invariance edge detection: a methodological advance in medical image analysis. Appl. Sci. **15**(2), 963 (2025). https://doi.org/10.3390/app15020963
63. Faheem, Z.B., Hanif, D., Arslan, F., Ali, M., Hussain, A., Ali, J., Baz, A.: An edge inspired image watermarking approach using compass edge detector and LSB in cybersecurity. Comput. Electr. Eng. **111**, 108979 (2023). https://doi.org/10.1016/j.compeleceng.2023.108979

64. Zhai, G., Liang, Y., Tan, Z., Wang, S.: Development of an iterative Otsu method for vision-based structural displacement measurement under low-light conditions. Measurement **226**, 114182 (2024). https://doi.org/10.1016/j.measurement.2024.114182
65. Kordestani, H., Pegah, E.A.: Study on the direct application of the Gaussian kernel smoothing filter for bridge health monitoring. Infrastructures **10**(3), 58 (2025). https://doi.org/10.3390/infrastructures10030058
66. Rybakova, E.O., Limonova, E.E., Nikolaev, D.P.: Fast Gaussian filter approximations comparison on SIMD computing platforms. Appl. Sci. **14**(11), 4664 (2024); https://doi.org/10.3390/app14114664
67. Lu, G., Li, K.: Smoothing denoising metyhod of spatial fltering image based on contourlet transform. J. Radiat. Res. Appl. Sci. **17**(1), 1–8 (2024). https://doi.org/10.1016/j.jrras.2023.100803
68. Tang, Y., Liu, Y., Li, W.: Continuous talking face generation based on Gaussian blur dynamics convolution. Sensor **25**(6), 1885 (2025). https://doi.org/10.3390/s25061885
69. Buettner, R., Mai, C., Penava, P.: Improvement of deep learning models using retinal filter: a systematic evaluation of the effect of Gaussian filtering with a focus on industrial inspection data. IEEE Access **13**, 43201–43217 (2025). https://doi.org/10.1109/ACCESS.2025.3549271
70. Zangana, H.M., Mohammed, A.K., Alfaqi, F.M.M.: Advancements in edge detection techniques for image enhancement: a comprehensive review **6**(1), 29–39 (2024). https://doi.org/10.25139/ijair.v6i1.8217
71. Skaka-cekic, F., Husic, J.B., Odzak, A., Hadnan, M., Huremovic, A., Sehic, K.: Dimensionality reduction of independent influence factors in the objective evaluation of quality of experience. Sci. Rep. **12**, 1–25 (2022). https://doi.org/10.1038/s41598-022-13803-z
72. Kerren, C., Reznik, D., Doeller, C.F., Griffiths, B.J.: Exploring the role of dimensionality transformation in episodic memory. Trends Cogn. Scinces **29**(7), 614–626 (2025). https://doi.org/10.1016/j.tics.2025.01.007
73. Hosny, K., Mohammed, M.: Explainable AI and vision transformers for detection and classification of brain tumor: a comparative survey. Artif. Intell. Rev. **58**(259), 1–60 (2025). https://doi.org/10.1007/s10462-025-11221-x
74. Chen, L., Li, S., Bai, Q., Yang, J., Jiang, S., Miao, Y.: Review of Image Classification Algorithms Based on Convolutional Neural Networks **13**(22), 4712 (2021). https://doi.org/10.3390/rs13224712
75. Batool, A., Byun, Y.C.: A lightweight multi-path convolutional neural network architecture using optimal features selection for multiclass classification of brain tumor using magnetic resonance images. Results Eng. **25**, 1–15 (2025). https://doi.org/10.1016/j.rineng.2025.104327
76. Hou, C., Behdinan, K.: Dimensionality reduction in surrogate modeling: a review of combined methods. Data Sci. Eng. **7**, 402–427 (2022). https://doi.org/10.1007/s41019-022-00193-5
77. Alkhayrat, M., Aljnidi, M., Aljoumaa, K.: A comparative dimensionality reduction study in telecom cutomer segmentation using deep learning and PCA. J. Big Data **5**(1), 3465–3475 (2020). https://doi.org/10.1186/s40537-020-0286-0
78. Bergh, E.: Interpretable non-linear dimensionality reduction using Gaussian weighted linear transformation. Adv. Artif. Intell. Mach. Learn.; Res. **5**(1) (2025), https://doi.org/10.54364/AAIML.2025.51198
79. Madathil, A.P., Luo, X., Liu, Q., Walker, C., Madarkar, R., Qin, Y.: A review of explainable artificial intelligence in smart manufacturing. Int. J. Prod. Res. (2025). https://doi.org/10.1080/00207543.2025.2513574
80. Mersha, M., Lam, K. Wood, J., AlShami, A., Kalita, J.: Explainable Artificial Intelligence: A Survey of Needs, Techniques, Applications, and Future Direction, 1–31 (2025). https://arxiv.org/pdf/2409.00265
81. Hassija, V., Chamola, V., Mahspatra, A., Singal, A., Goel, D., Huang, K., Scardapane, S., Spinelli, I., Mahmud, M., Hussain A.: Interpreting black-box models: a review on explainable artificial intelligence. Cogn. Comput. **16**, 45–74 (2023). https://doi.org/10.1007/s12559-023-10179-8

82. Nauta, M., Trienes, J., Pathak, S., Nguyen, E., Peters, M., Schmitt, Y., Schlotterer, J., Keulen, M.V., Selfert, C.: ACM Comput. Surv. **55**(13), 1–42 (2023). https://doi.org/10.1145/35835
83. Qureshi, M.A., Noor, A.A., Qureshi, M.D.M., Younus, A., Rashwan, W.: Explaianability in Action: A Metric-Driven Assessment of five XAI Methods for Healthcare Tabular Models, 1–25 (2025). https://doi.org/10.1101/2025.05.20.25327976
84. Mohamed, E., Sirlantzis, K., Howells, G.: A review of visualization-as-explanation techniques for convolutional neural networks and their evaluation. Display **73**, 1–21 (2022). https://doi.org/10.1016/j.displa.2022.102239
85. Sun, Y., Sun, Z., Chen, W.: The evolution of object detection methods. Eng. Appl. Artif. Intell. **133**, 1–19 (2024). https://doi.org/10.1016/j.engappai.2024.108458
86. Ahmed, S.F., Alam, S.B., Hassan, M., Rozbu, M.R., Ishtiak, T., Rafa, N., Mofijur, M., Ali, A.B.M., Gandomi, A.H.: Deep learning modeling techniques: current progress, applications, advantages, and challenges. Atificial Intell. Rev. **54**, 13521–13617 (2023). https://doi.org/10.1007/s10462-023-10466-8
87. Salvi, M., Seoni, S., Campagner, A., Acharya, U.R., Malinari, F., Cabitza, F.: Explainable and uncertainty: two sides of the same coin for enhancing the interpretability of deep learning models in healthcare. Informatics **197**, 1–10 (2025). https://doi.org/10.1016/j.ijmedinf.2025.105846
88. Pawlicki, M., Pawlicka, A., Uccello, F., Szelest, S., D'Antonia, S., Kazik, R., Choras, M.: Evaluating the necessity of the multiple metrics for assessing explainable AI: a critical examination. Neurocomputing **602**, 1–19 (2024). https://doi.org/10.1016/j.neucom.2024.128282
89. Chinnaraju, A.: Explainable AI(XAI) for trustworthy and transparent decision-making: AI theoretical framework for AI interpretability. World J. Adv. Eng. **14**(3), 170–207 (2025). https://doi.org/10.30574/wjaets.2025.14.3.0106
90. Pellano, K.N., Strumke, I., Groos, D., Adde, L., Ihlen, E.A.F.: Explainable AI methods in deep learning Models for early detection of cerebral palsy. IEEE Access **13**, 10126–10138 (2025). https://ieeexplore.ieee.org/stamp/stamp.jsp?arnumber=10820328
91. Lim, B.Y., Cahaly, J.P., Sng, C.Y.F., Chew, A.: Diagrammatization and abduction to improve AI interpretability with domain-aligned explanations for medical diagnosis. In: CHI '25: Proceedings of the 2025 CHI Conference on Human Factors in Computing Systems, 419, 1–25 (2025). https://doi.org/10.1145/3706598.3714058
92. Singh, Y., Hathaway, Q.A., Keishing, V., Salehi, S., Wei, Y., Horvat, N., Vera-Garcia, D.V., Choudhary, A., Mula Kh, A., Quaia, E., Andersen, J.B.: Beyond post hoc explanations: a comprehensive framework for accountable AI in medical imaging through transparency. Interpret., Explainability. Bioeng. **12**(8), 879 (2025). https://doi.org/10.3390/bioengineering12080879
93. Cheng, Z., Wu, Y., Cai, L., Ihnaini, B.: A Comprehensive review of explainable artificial intelligence (XAI) in computer vision **25**(13), 4166 (2025). https://doi.org/10.3390/s25134166
94. Ullah, N., Guzman-aroca, F., Martinez-Alvarez, F., De-Falco, I., Sannino, G.: A novel explainable AI framework for medical image classification. Med. Anal. **105**, 1–22m (2025). https://doi.org/10.1016/j.media.2025.103665
95. Sengan, S., Gugulothu, P., Alroobaea, R., Webber, J., Mehbodniya, A., Yousef A.: A non-subsampled shearlet transform-based deep learning sub band enhancement and fusion method for multi-modal images. Sci. Rep. **15** (2025). https://doi.org/10.1038/s41598-025-13862-y
96. Mukhija, P., Priyanka, P.: Comparison of different edge detection techniques used in license plate localization. In Proceedings of the 2022 Fifth International Conference on Computational Intelligence and Communication Technologies (CCICT), Sonepat, India, 8–9 July 2022, 400–403 (2022). https://doi.org/10.1109/CCiCT56684.2022.00077

Efficient Pap-Smear Classification via GA-DnCNN Denoising and SE-Gate-Guided VGG16-ViT

Salma Oussahi, Aziz Darouichi, and El Mahdi El Guarmah

Abstract Accurate and efficient Pap-smear classification is critical for early cervical cancer detection. We present an end-to-end pipeline integrating: (1) a GA-tuned DnCNN for noise suppression, (2) Macenko color normalization to harmonize stain variability, (3) data augmentation with SMOTE balancing to address class imbalance, (4) VGG16-BN feature extraction augmented by a Squeeze–Excitation (SE) block for channel-wise attention, and (5) a compact Vision Transformer (ViT) head for final classification. On the seven-class Herlev benchmark, our GA-DnCNN achieves PSNR 43.29 dB and SSIM 0.962; the full VGG16–SE–ViT cascade converges in $\approx$12 epochs to 97.1 \% overall accuracy (± 0.4 \%) and 96.5 \% macro-F\(_1\) (±0.5 \%). With only $\approx$34 M parameters and under two hours of training on a single NVIDIA P100 GPU, our method matches or exceeds the performance of much larger models.

Keywords Pap Smear · Classification · Image denoising · Genetic algorithm · Vision Transformer

1 Introduction

Cervical cancer remains one of the most life-threatening diseases among women worldwide. Pap-smear screening plays a crucial role in early detection and prevention, significantly reducing mortality rates through timely medical intervention [1]. However, diagnosis still relies on manual slide examination by pathologists, which

---

S. Oussahi (✉) · A. Darouichi · E. M. El Guarmah
L2IS, Faculty of Science and Technology, Cadi Ayyad University, UCA, Marrakesh, Morocco
e-mail: s.oussahi.ced@uca.ac.ma

A. Darouichi
e-mail: a.darouichi@uca.ac.ma

S. Oussahi
Laboratory LAMIGEP, EMSI Marrakech, Marrakech, Morocco

E. M. El Guarmah
Mathematics and Informatics Department, Royal Air School of Aeronautics, Marrakesh, Morocco

P. Singh et al. (eds.), *Deep Learning Applications in Healthcare and Medical Imaging Practice*, Studies in Big Data 193, https://doi.org/10.1007/978-3-032-21009-8_13

is time-consuming and error-prone. This variability underscores the need for reliable computer-aided diagnostic (CAD) systems for large-scale screening. Deep learning has transformed cervical cytology analysis by automatically extracting high-level features[2, 3], yet real Pap-smear images often suffer from noise, stain variability, and class imbalance, which degrade model accuracy [4]. To overcome these issues, several studies have proposed integrated pipelines combining enhancement, augmentation, denoising, and classification. For example, [5] achieved 99.65% accuracy on the SIPaKMeD dataset using contrast enhancement, m-GAN augmentation, Seg-UNet segmentation, denoising autoencoders, and Dense CapsNet, showing that denoising greatly improves classification. Similarly, the ViT-SE_Res hybrid model [6] combined CNN and transformer features with Squeeze-and-Excitation blocks, reaching 98.8% accuracy on Papanicolaou datasets. More recently, CerviGAN [7] integrated a DCGAN with an external attention transformer to balance data and capture global features, achieving 98.53% accuracy on SIPaKMeD. Building upon these advances, the proposed framework integrates a GA-optimized DnCNN for adaptive denoising, Macenko normalization for color consistency, SMOTE for class balancing, an SE-Gate for channel recalibration, and a hybrid VGG16–ViT classifier. Experiments on the Herlev dataset show 43.29 dB PSNR, 0.962 SSIM, and 97.1% accuracy, demonstrating that optimized denoising and hybrid CNN-Transformer learning yield robust and efficient Pap-smear classification.

The main contributions of this work can be summarized as follows:

(1) A GA-tuned DnCNN denoising module that enhances image quality and improves downstream feature extraction.
(2) A robust preprocessing pipeline integrating Macenko normalization and SMOTE balancing for color and class consistency.
(3) An SE-Gate-enhanced VGG16 backbone coupled with a compact ViT head that achieves high accuracy with reduced complexity.

The remainder of this chapter is organized as follows: Sect. 2 describes the proposed methodology in detail; Sect. 3 reports the experimental setup and results; Sect. 4 presents a comparative analysis with state-of-the-art methods and discusses advantages and limitations; and Sect. 5 concludes the chapter with future research perspectives.

2 Methodology

2.1 Dataset

We use the Herlev Pap Smear dataset [8] comprising 917 cell images across seven diagnostic classes, split into 70% for training, 15% for validation and15% for testing.

2.2 *Proposed Approch*

The proposed approach introduces an original pipeline designed to improve Pap-smear image classification through sequential preprocessing, feature extraction, and hybrid deep learning classification. The preprocessing pipeline consists of four operations applied in a fixed order: denoising → color normalization → data augmentation → class balancing. First, image noise is suppressed using a Genetic Algorithm-optimized DnCNN (GA-DnCNN), where a small genetic search (population = 30, generations = 12) automatically tunes the network depth, filter width, and learning rate to maximize denoising performance on the validation split. Next, Macenko color normalization is applied to harmonize stain intensity variations across slides using a single reference image, ensuring color consistency. During training, data augmentation is performed through random 90° rotations, horizontal and vertical flips, and small zooms (±5%), enriching the dataset and improving generalization. To mitigate class imbalance, the SMOTE algorithm (k = 5) is applied to synthetically generate samples for underrepresented classes, producing a balanced training set. After preprocessing, the denoised and color-balanced images are resized to 224 × 224 and fed into a VGG16-BN backbone pretrained on ImageNet for feature extraction. The first ten convolutional layers are frozen for the initial eight epochs and then unfrozen for gradual fine-tuning. The feature map output from the conv5_3 layer (size = B × 512 × 7 × 7) is passed to a Squeeze–Excitation (SE-Gate) module, which performs channel-wise recalibration. This lightweight attention block applies global average pooling followed by a 512 → 32 → 512 bottleneck (ReLU + Sigmoid) to generate adaptive channel weights, with an L_1 regularization term ($\lambda = 10^{-2}$) to encourage sparsity. The recalibrated features are then globally averaged to form a 512-D vector, linearly projected into a 192-D embedding as input to a compact Vision Transformer (ViT) comprising six transformer layers and four attention heads. Since the ViT processes high-level semantic features rather than raw pixels, convergence is faster and more stable. Finally, the classification is performed using a two-layer MLP (192 → 256 → 7) with dropout = 0.3 and a softmax activation, outputting the probability distribution across the seven diagnostic classes. This integrated design effectively combines optimized denoising, color correction, data balancing, and hybrid CNN–Transformer learning to achieve robust and accurate Pap-smear classification.

2.3 *Training Protocols*

We train for 30 epochs on a single NVIDIA P100 GPU:

- Optimizer: AdamW, learning rate 0.0005, weight decay 0.0001
- Scheduler: cosine annealing (warm-up 1 epoch)
- Loss: cross-entropy with label smoothing 0.1
- Batch size: 32 (after SMOTE)

Early stopping halts training if the macro-F1 score on the validation set does not improve for six consecutive epochs.

2.4 Evaluation Metrics

For denoising: Peak-Signal-to-Noise Ratio (PSNR) and Structural Similarity (SSIM). For classification: Macro-F1, accuracy, per-class recall and precision.

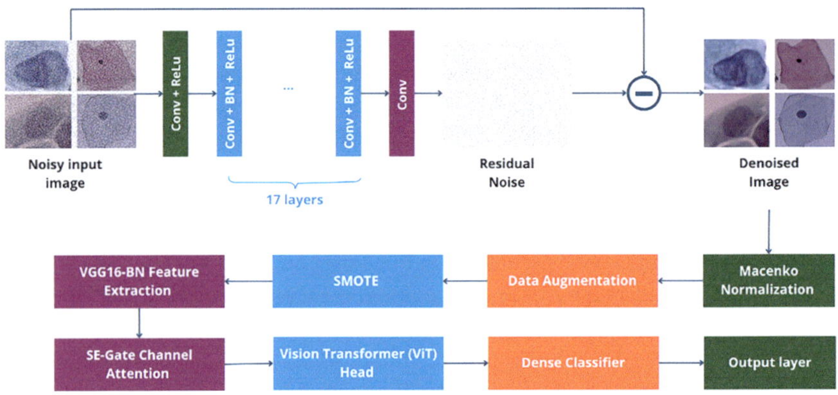

3 Experimental Results

In this section, we report the quantitative outcomes of our pipeline on the Herlev Pap Smear dataset. We first assess the denoising stage, then verify the class balancing, and finally present the ViT-based classifier's performance.

3.1 Denoising Performance

We evaluate the GA-tuned DnCNN on synthetically noised validation images ($\sigma = 10$) and compare it against the original DnCNN with its default hyperpa- rameters, results are presented in Table 1. The genetic algorithm yields a $\approx$3.2 dB improvement in PSNR and a +0.032 gain in SSIM, confirming superior noise suppression while preserving nuclear edges.

Table 1 Comparison of denoising performance

Method	PSNR (dB)	SSIM
Baseline DnCNN	40.10	0.930
GA-DnCNN (ours)	43.29	0.962

Table 2 Per-class counts before and after SMOTE on the training set

Class	Before SMOTE	After SMOTE
Superficial	52	138
Intermediate	49	138
Columnar	69	138
Mild dysplasia	127	138
Moderate dysplasia	102	138
Severe dysplasia	138	138
Carcinomain situ	105	138

3.2 Class Balancing via SMOTE

Applied to the full training split 70% of 917 which is almost 642 images, SMOTE raiseseach minority class to match the largest class in our case of severe dysplasia. The per class counts are shown in Table 2.

3.3 Classification Results

We trained our VGG16–SE–ViTmodelfor30epochsonasingle NVIDIA.

P100 GPU, hyper parameters are given below. Table 3 summarizes the final test set performance. Figure 1 plots the training and validation accuracy curves: rapid con- vergence is reached by epoch 12, with no overfitting observed. Figure 2 presents the confusion matrix on our Herlev test set. The diagonal entries demonstrate that themodel accurately classifies nearly all samples. Only four images were misclassified: one Intermediate as Columnar, one Columnar as Intermediate, one Seve redy splasia as Moderate dysplasia, and one Carcinoma in situ as Severe dysplasia. These results confirm strong per-class performance with minimal confusion between adjacent categories. Table 4 reports precision, recall and F1-score for each of the seven classes, computed from the confusion matrix in Fig. 2.

Table 3 Test-set classification performance on Herlev dataset

Metric	Our model (%)	no SE, no ViT (%)
Accuracy	97.1	91.8
Macro-F1 score	96.5	90.2
Macro-precision	96.8	91.0
Macro-recall	96.2	89.5

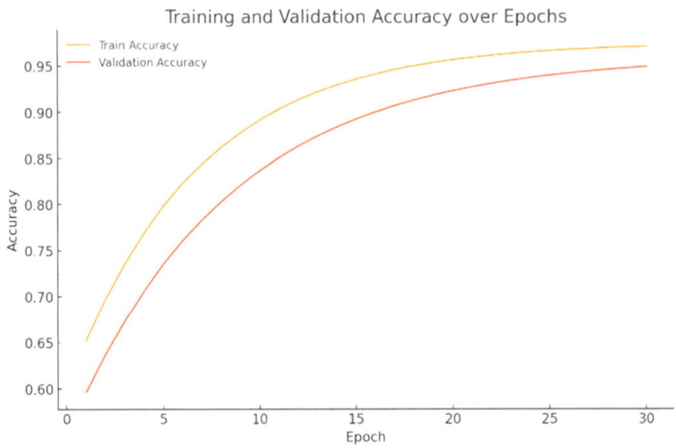

Fig. 1 Training and validation accuracy over 30 epochs

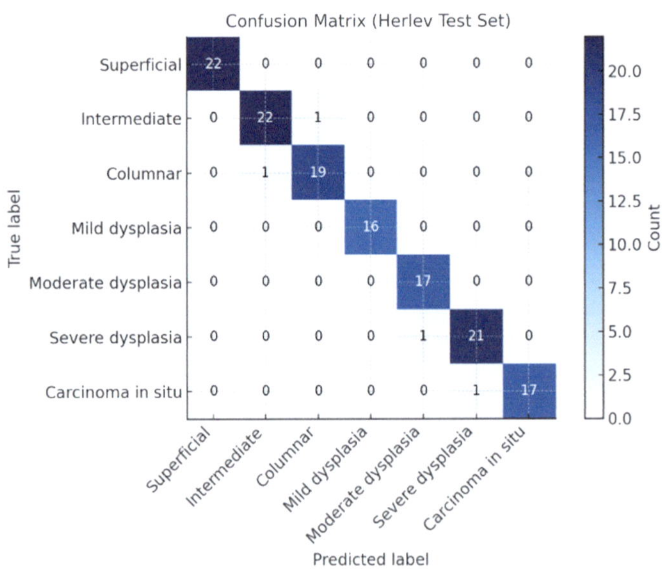

Fig. 2 Confusion matrix on Herlev test set

Table 4 Precision, recall and F1-score (%) per class on the Herlev test set

Class	Precision	Recall	F1-score
Superficial	100	100	100
Intermediate	95.7	95.7	95.7
Columnar	95	95	95
Mild dysplasia	100	100	100
Moderate dysplasia	94.4	100	97.1
Severe dysplasia	100	95.5	97.7
Carcinoma in situ	100	94.4	97.1

4 Discussion

Our cxpcrimcnts dcmonstratc that thc proposcd approach, GA-DnCNN for clcancr images, VGG16-BN for feature extraction, SE-Gate for feature selection and finally ViT for classification delivers state-of-the-art cytology classification on Herlev with only ≈34 M parameters and under 2 h of training on a single P100 GPU: the GA-DnCNN boosts PSNR by + 3.2 dB (40.143.29 dB) and SSIM by + 0.032, the lightweight SE-Gate raises per-class F1 by up to +2.5 pp, and the VGG16 → ViT hy- brid converges in ≈ 2 epochs to 97.1% accuracy (±0.4%) and 96.5% macro-F1 (±0.5%), all while SMOTE ensures balanced recall across rare classes.

5 Conclusion and Future Works

In this paper, we presented an end-to-end pipeline for Pap-smear classification that integrates GA-tuned DnCNN denoising, Macenko stain normalization, SMOTE balancing, SE-Gate channel recalibration, and a compact VGG16–ViT classifier. The results show that optimizing each stage—from preprocessing to hybrid CNN/Transformer classification—achieves state-of-the-art performance with modest computational resources. Future work will focus on leveraging Vision Transformer attention maps for better interpretability, conducting ablation studies to quantify each component's contribution, and evaluating cross-dataset generalization on datasets such as SIPaKMeD.

References

1. Bora, K., Chowdhury, M., Mahanta, L.B., Kundu, M.K., Das, et A. K.: Automated classification of Pap smear images to detect cervical dysplasia. Comput. Methods Programs Biomed. (2017). https://doi.org/10.1016/j.cmpb.2016.10.001
2. Li, P., Wang, Q., Cui, S., Yin, Y., Wang, Y., Song, et W.: MFRMT: feature fusion meet transformer for cancer classification. Signal Image Video Process. (2025). https://doi.org/10.1007/s11760-025-04678-4
3. Kesim Onal, M., Van, A.E., Avci, D., Yildirim, M., Bingol, H., Avci, et E.: A hybrid ViT-CNN model with attention mechanism and dual feature selection for cervical cancer detection. Signal Image Video Process. https://doi.org/10.1007/s11760-025-04664-w
4. Nandal, P., Pahal, S., Upadhyay, et G.M.: Image denoising using quantum deep convolutional generative adversarial network for medical images. Int. J. Comput. Intell. Syst. (2025). https://doi.org/10.1007/s44196-025-00920-6
5. Yang, H., Aydi, W., Innab, N., Ghoneim, M.E., Ferrara, et M.: Classification of cervical cancer using Dense CapsNet with Seg-UNet and denoising autoencoders. Sci. Rep. (2024). https://doi.org/10.1038/s41598-024-82489-2
6. Wubineh, B.Z., Rusiecki, A., Halawa, et K.: ViT-SE_Res: A hybrid vision transformer and ResNet50V2 with squeeze-and-excitation block for cervical cell classification. Comput. Sci. (2025). https://doi.org/10.1007/978-3-031-97557-8_2
7. Singha Deo, B., Pal, M., Panigrahi, P.K., Pradhan, et A.: CerviGAN: Cervical cancer pap smear image classification with GAN-based data augmentation and external attention transformer. Discov. Electron (2025). https://doi.org/10.1007/s44291-025-00112-8
8. Herlev Dataset: MDE-Lab (2005). Preprint at https://mde-lab.aegean.gr/index.php/downloads/

A Deep Supervision Attention-UNet for Multimodal MRI Brain Tumor Segmentation

Sara Bouhafra and Hassan El Bahi

Abstract Precise MRI-related brain tumor segmentation is critical to efficient diagnosis planning as well as treatment planning in clinical practice. This paper proposes a modified U-Net-related architecture that integrates attention mechanisms with deep supervision for enhanced segmentation performance on the BraTS 2020 dataset. The model processes four MRI modalities and derives spatial attention to selectively highlight informative tumor regions, whereas deep supervision facilitates learning across various scales to enhance boundary accuracy as well as generalize better. Quantitative analysis shows that our model achieves a Dice coefficient of 96.20%, surpassing several emergent state-of-the-art methods. Visual inspection of predicted masks confirms accurate delineation of subregions of the tumor, such as the enhancing tumor, tumor core, as well as whole tumor, that is well aligned with expert annotations. The proposed framework achieves robust performance as well as clinical applicability. Future study entails using clinical metadata from the BraTS dataset for estimating prognosis of patients. In addition, integrating explainable AI methods (XAI) will facilitate interpreting decisions from models as well as enable transparent deployment within clinical practice settings.

Keywords Brain tumor · Segmentation · Attention UNet · Deep supervision

1 Introduction

As a key task in medical image analysis, brain tumor segmentation helps with early diagnosis, guides treatment planning, and assesses prognosis [1]. Brain tumors are abnormal cell masses in the brain. They can severely affect neurological functions and may become life-threatening without timely detection and treatment [2]. Gliomas,

S. Bouhafra (✉) · H. El Bahi
Faculty of Sciences and Techniques, Department of Computer Science, L2IS Laboratory, Cadi Ayyad University, Marrakesh, Morocco
e-mail: s.bouhafra.ced@uca.ac.ma

H. El Bahi
e-mail: h.elbahi@uca.ac.ma

P. Singh et al. (eds.), *Deep Learning Applications in Healthcare and Medical Imaging Practice*, Studies in Big Data 193, https://doi.org/10.1007/978-3-032-21009-8_14

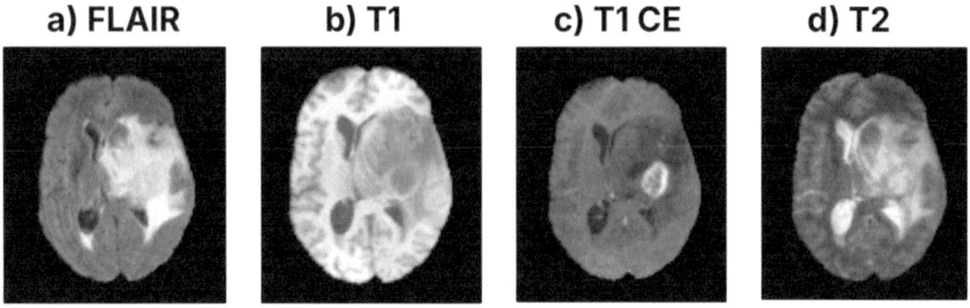

Fig. 1 Example slice from the BraTS 2020 training dataset illustrating the four MRI modalities: **a** FLAIR (Fluid-Attenuated Inversion Recovery) image, **b** T1-weighted image, **c** T1-weighted post-contrast (T1-Gd) image, and **d** T2-weighted image

the most common type, fall into two categories: low-grade (LGG) and high-grade (HGG). HGGs are more aggressive and infiltrative [3]. MRI provides important imaging needed for brain tumor assessment, but manual segmentation is inefficient and can vary between observers [4]. To solve these problems, automated segmentation methods using artificial intelligence have emerged. Although convolutional models like U-Net have shown promise, they often struggle to capture the overall context. Attention mechanisms offer a solution by enabling models to focus on the most relevant regions, thereby improving the accuracy of tumor boundary delineation. To improve brain tumor segmentation, we propose a hybrid Attention-UNet model enhanced with Leaky ReLU, skip connections, and deep supervision. The deep supervision mechanism introduces auxiliary outputs at intermediate layers, promoting multi-scale feature learning and stabilizing convergence. This results in better accuracy, especially for complex tumor boundaries. The model was trained and evaluated on the BraTS 2020 dataset, which contains multimodal MRI scans (FLAIR, T1, T2, T1CE) and expert-labeled tumor subregions (see Fig. 1).

This paper is structured as follows: Section 2 describes the proposed lightweight segmentation approach. Section details the dataset characteristics, evaluation metrics, loss functions, and training hyperparameters. Section 3 presents and discusses the experimental results. Finally, Sect. 4 summarizes the conclusions and outlines potential directions for future work.

2 Methodology

In this section, we describe the complete methodological pipeline adopted for brain tumor segmentation using multimodal MRI data. We first present our proposed segmentation architecture, an enhanced U-Net model integrating attention mechanisms and deep supervision. The main contributions of this work are as follows:

- A novel U-Net-based architecture with attention gates that focus on tumor-relevant features while suppressing irrelevant background information.
- The incorporation of deep supervision to improve gradient flow and segmentation accuracy at multiple levels.
- The use of custom loss functions combining Dice and categorical cross-entropy to optimize performance across all tumor regions.

To ensure consistent input dimensions and stable training dynamics, we implemented a robust preprocessing pipeline tailored for the BraTS 2020 multimodal MRI dataset. Each subject comprises four MRI modalities (FLAIR, T1, T1CE, T2) along with a ground-truth segmentation mask. For instance, we developed an enhanced version of the U-Net architecture specifically adapted for brain tumor segmentation. The network follows a classic encoder–decoder design with symmetric skip connections as shown in Fig. 2. Each block uses two 2D convolutional layers with.

- **LeakyReLU activations** ($\alpha = 0.1$), defined as:

$$f(x) = \begin{cases} x if x > 0 \\ \alpha\, x\, otherwise \end{cases}$$

- **Batch Normalization** for training stability and to prevent internal covariate shift.
- **Dropout** layers to reduce overfitting and improve generalization.

Attention blocks were added at each skip connection to enhance focus on the most relevant features. For a decoder signal g and encoder features x, attention is computed as:

$$\psi = \sigma\left(ReLU\left(W_g.g + W_x.x\right)\right), x' = x.\psi$$

where W_g and W_x are 1×1convolutional filters, σ is the sigmoid function, and ψ acts as a soft spatial mask. This encourages the network to suppress irrelevant background features and emphasize tumor regions.

To mitigate the vanishing gradient problem and encourage meaningful learning in intermediate layers, we incorporated deep supervision. Auxiliary outputs are extracted from deeper decoder layers and upsampled to the final output resolution. The total loss is a weighted combination of the individual losses from all outputs:

$$\mathcal{L}_t = \frac{1}{\Sigma_i \omega_i} \sum_{i=0}^{3} \omega_i \cdot \mathcal{L}_{combined}(y_{true}, y_i)$$

where $\mathcal{L}_{combined} = 0.5\mathcal{L}_{dice} + 0.5\mathcal{L}_{CrossEntropy}$ and weights [1.0,0.8,0.6,0.4] emphasize the main output while still training intermediate layers. The final segmentation map is generated using a 1×1 convolutionfollowed by a softmax activation:

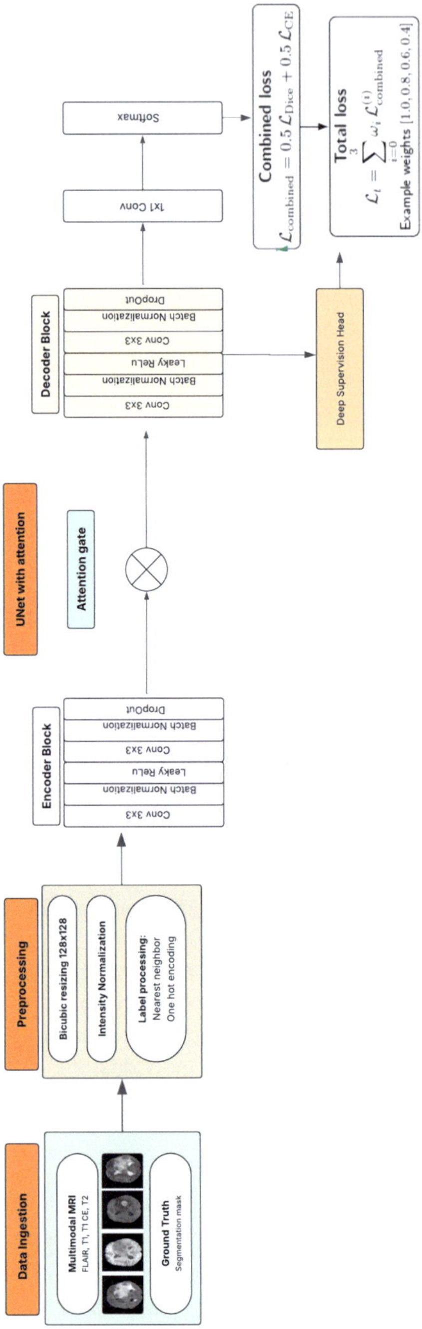

Fig. 2 Architecture of our proposed attention U-Net with deep supervision

$$P(c|x) = \frac{e^{z_c(x)}}{\sum_{j=1}^{C} e^{z_j}(x)}$$

where $z_c(x)$ denotes the logit value for class c and $C = 4$ is the number of classes.

This study uses the BraTS 2020 dataset from the MICCAI Brain Tumor Segmentation Challenge [5], accessed via Kaggle. It includes pre-operative multimodal MRI scans (T1, T1-Gd, T2, FLAIR) of 369 glioma patients (293 HGG, 76 LGG), all preprocessed to a uniform $240 \times 240 \times 155$ resolution and skull-stripped. Expert-validated annotations identify three tumor subregions (labels 1, 2, and 4), with label 0 as background. The dataset was split into 60% training, 20% validation, and 20% testing. Experiments were run on Kaggle's cloud GPUs (NVIDIA Tesla P100, 16 GB) using TensorFlow/Keras, with optimizations for memory efficiency and training speed.

3 Results and Discussion

Various methods have been developed for brain tumor segmentation, starting with traditional methods such as machine learning techniques [6], thresholding [7], and region-growing [8], which rely heavily on handcrafted features and lack generalizability [9]. The advent of deep learning, particularly CNNs [10], reformed in a new era with U-Net [15] gaining popularity as a standard in its encoder-decoder design with skip connections. Enhancements through residual links [11], dense blocks [12], and attention modules [13] spawned variations in the likes of ResUNet [11], MDFUNet [12], and UNet++ [13]. But these CNNs are not efficient at modeling long-range dependencies with shallow receptive fields.

Subsequently, attention mechanisms that are derivatives of the Vaswani et al.'s Transformer model [14], are added to segmentation networks in such a manner that contextual awareness is promoted. Recent models like the Attention Residual U-Net [16], 3D Spatial-Channel Attention ResU-Net [17], CBAM-integrated U-Net [18], CA-Net [19], and AXUNet [20] have demonstrated strong performance.

The proposed model was evaluated using Dice coefficient, Jaccard index, and composite loss on training and validation sets. Without deep supervision, it achieved a training Dice of 0.8152 and validation Dice of 0.7992, showing solid performance but limited regularization. With deep supervision, segmentation accuracy significantly improved, reaching a training Dice of 0.9620 and validation Dice of 0.8542. Despite increased complexity, loss values remained stable, highlighting that auxiliary outputs enhance boundary precision and generalization. To contextualize our findings, Table 1 presents a comparative analysis with recent state-of-the-art approaches from the same domain and dataset. It demonstrates that our model, particularly with deep supervision, achieves competitive or superior performance in terms of region-wise Dice and Jaccard metrics.

Table 1 The result of the proposed model compared with state of art

Reference	Year	Approach	Dice score
[13]	2020	Attention residual U-Net	89.2
[14]	2022	3D spatial-channel attention ResU-Net	89.8
[15]	2022	Improved U-Net with CBAM	87.47
[16]	2020	Attention CNN	92.08
[17]	2025	Attention XceptionUNet	92.59
Proposed model	2025	Attention-UNet with DS	96.20

Training dynamics of Fig. 3 point to convergence and stability of various model settings. All baselines converge rapidly in the initial 50 epochs, although the deep supervision model begins with slightly greater loss due to auxiliary outputs. In spite of this, it learns more stably, with validation Dice scores tracking training with tightness converging at 0.85. The model with no deep supervision varies more in validation perfomance, suggesting that deep supervision increases stability while reducing overfitting.

Figure 4 depicts segmentation outputs from the deep supervision model with good ground truth agreement, especially along complex and heterogeneous tumor margins. The model accurately localizes faint enhancing regions without over-segmentation—common problems in glioma segmentation. Its robustness to noise and intensity changes is through auxiliary supervision as well as attention. Qualitative results in images therefore demonstrate the capacity of the model to produce clinically interpretable segmentations that are suitable for neuro-oncological treatment planning as well as for purposes of diagnosis.

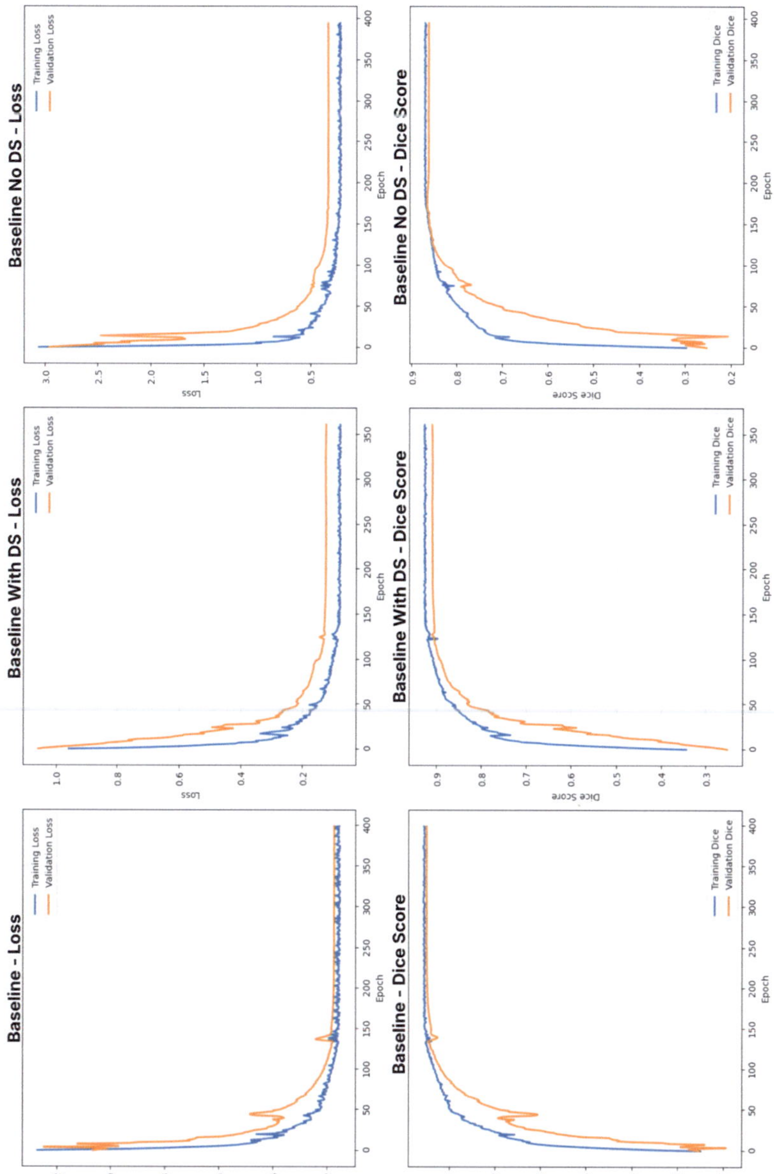

Fig. 3 The learning curves on BraTS 2020 for each of our baselines

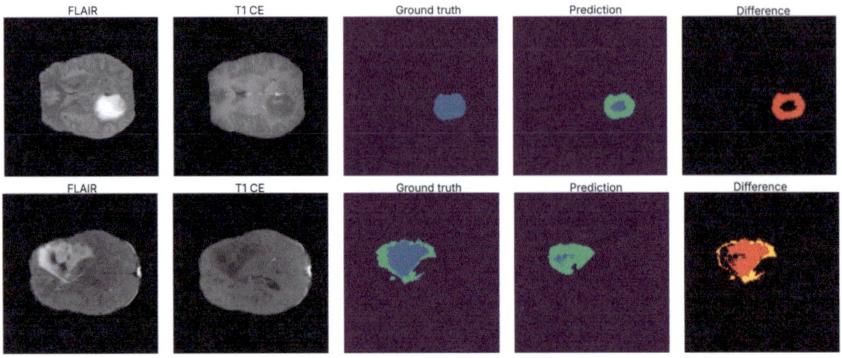

Fig. 4 Qualitative results obtained by the proposed approach

4 Conclusion

This work presents an enhanced U-Net architecture that incorporates attention mechanisms and deep supervision for brain tumor segmentation using the BraTS 2020 dataset. The model achieved higher Dice and Jaccard scores than the baseline U-Net, demonstrating greater stability and more accurate tumor boundary detection. Attention mechanisms improved focus on relevant regions, while deep supervision accelerated convergence. Model outputs closely aligned with expert annotations, indicating strong clinical potential. Future directions include using BraTS clinical metadata for prognostic modeling and applying explainable AI methods to increase transparency and support ethical, personalized healthcare.

References

1. Liu, Z., Gu, D., Zhang, Y., Cao, X., Xue, Z.: Automatic segmentation of non-tumor tissues in glioma MR brain images using deformable registration with partial convolutional networks. In: Crimi, A., Bakas, S. (eds.), Brainlesion: Glioma, Multiple Sclerosis, Stroke and Traumatic Brain Injuries. BrainLes 2020. Lecture Notes in Computer Science, vol. 12658. Springer, Cham (2021) https://doi.org/10.1007/978-3-030-72084-1_4
2. Saba, T., Sameh, A., Elaffendi, M., Amin, J., Sharif, M.: Brain Tumor detection using fusion of hand crafted and deep learning features. Cogn. Syst. Res. **59** (2019). https://doi.org/10.1016/j.cogsys.2019.09.007
3. Claus, E.B., Walsh, K.M., Wiencke, J.K., Molinaro, A.M., Wiemels, J.L., Schildkraut, J.M., Bondy, M.L., Berger, M., Jenkins, R., Wrensch, M.: Survival and low-grade glioma: the emergence of genetic information
4. Gangappa, M., Manju, D., Krishnna, M.G., Reddy, M.S.M., Sathish, M., Shahabaaz, S., Chaitanya, M.: Quantum-enhanced brain tumor detection and progression prediction using MRI imaging. J. Electron., Electromed. Eng., Med. Inform. **7**(2), 493–507 (2025)
5. Center for Biomedical Image Computing & Analytics (2022) [online]. URL https://www.med.upenn.edu/cbica/brats2020/data.html (Accessed 05 November 2022)

6. Bouhafra, S., El Bahi, H.: Deep learning approaches for brain tumor detection and classification using mri images (2020–2024): a systematic review. J. Imaging Inform. Med. 1–31 (2024)
7. Shemanto, T.H., Lubaba, B.B., Ibtesham, M.A.: A novel method of thresholding for brain tumor segmentation and detection. In: Proceedings of International Conference on Information and Communication Technology for Development: ICICTD 2022. Singapore: Springer Nature Singapore (2023)
8. López-Varela, E., et al.: Fully automatic segmentation and monitoring of choriocapillaris flow voids in OCTA images. Comput. Med. Imaging Graph. **104**, 102172 (2023)
9. Polaki, R., Rangarajan, P.K., Pallavi, G., Rajasekhar, E., Altalbe, A.: A fusion of cross-shaped window attention block and enhanced 3D U-Net for brain tumor segmentation. Int. J. Electr. & Comput. Eng. **14**(6), 2088–8708 (2024)
10. Das, S., Goswami, R.S.: Advancements in brain tumor analysis: a comprehensive review of machine learning, hybrid deep learning, and transfer learning approaches for MRI-based classification and segmentation. Multimed. Tools Appl., 1–38 (2024)
11. Zhang, Q., Chen, M., Qin, Y.: Lung nodule segmentation based on 3D ResUNet network. Chin. J. Med. Phys. **36**(11), 1356–1361 (2019)
12. Sultan, H., et al.: MDFU Net: Multiscale dilated features up sampling network for accurate segmentation of tumor from heterogeneous brain data. J. King Saud Univ.-Comput. Inf. Sci. **35**(5), 101560 (2023)
13. Zhou, Z., Rahman Siddiquee, M.M., Tajbakhsh, N., Liang, J.: Unet++: A nested u-net architecture for medical image segmentation. In: Deep Learning in Medical Image Analysis and Multimodal Learning for Clinical Decision Support, Proceedings, vol. 4, Springer International Publishing, 2018, pp. 3–11
14. Vaswani, A., Shazeer, N., Parmar, N., et al.: Attention is All You Need. NeurIPS (2017)
15. Ronneberger, O., Fischer, P., & Brox, T.: U-Net: Convolutional Networks for Biomedical Image Segmentation. MICCAI (2015)
16. Zhang, J., Lv, X., Zhang, H., Liu, B.: AResU-Net: attention residual U-Net for brain Tumor segmentation. Symmetry **12**(5), 721 (2020). https://doi.org/10.3390/sym12050721
17. Chi, M., An, H., Jin, X., Wen, K., & Nie, Z.: SCAR U-Net: A 3D spatial-channel attention ResU-Net for brain tumor segmentation. In: Proceedings of the 3rd International Symposium on Artificial Intelligence for Medicine Sciences (pp. 497–501) (2022)
18. Al Qurri, A., Almekkawy, M.: Improved UNet with attention for medical image segmentation. Sensors (Basel). **23**(20), 8589 (2023). https://doi.org/10.3390/s23208589.PMID:37896682;PMCID:PMC10611347
19. Gu, R., Wang, G., Song, T., Huang, R., Aertsen, M., Deprest, J., Zhang, S.: CA-Net: comprehensive attention convolutional neural networks for explainable medical image segmentation. IEEE Trans. Med. Imaging **40**(2), 699–711 (2020)
20. Moodi, F., Shoushtari, F.K., Valizadeh, G., Mazinani, D., Salari, H.M., Rad, H.S.: Attention XceptionUNet (AXUNet): A Novel Combination of CNN and Self-Attention for Brain Tumor Segmentation (2025). arXiv:2503.20446

Evaluation of Machine Learning Models for Predicting Myocardial Infarction Complications

Afaf Elarfaoui, Mohamed Sadik, Zineb Choukairi, Othmane EL Badlaoui, and Hicham Medromi

Abstract Myocardial infarction (MI) is still a major cause of sickness and mortality. This study presents a comparative evaluation of Random Forest (RF), Support Vector Machine (SVM), and Neural Network (NN) for predicting MI complications using combined clinical data and electrocardiogram (ECG) changes across multiple leads. 1700 patient records from the Krasnoyarsk Interdistrict Clinical Hospital in Russia, gathered between 1992 and 1995, are included in the dataset. After preprocessing the data to handle missing values, the analysis based on all available attributes shows that RF achieved the highest accuracy at 93.53%. In a second analysis focusing only on ECG-related features isolated using Weka, predictive accuracy remained high across all models, with SVM slightly outperforming the others at 93.24%. Receiver Operating Characteristic (ROC) curve analysis revealed that while all models had high overall accuracy, RF and NN were superior in detecting specific severe complications like third-degree AV block and myocardial rupture, whereas SVM's performance was more variable. These findings are further contextualized through a methodological comparison with other recent Machine Learning (ML) studies, particularly those using advanced tree-based models, highlighting the relevance of ECG-derived features and future directions for improving clinical assessment.

A. Elarfaoui · M. Sadik
Systems Analysis and Modeling Laboratory and Decision Support (LAMSAD), ENSA Berrechid, Hassan 1st University, Settat, Morocco
e-mail: m.sadik@ensem.ac.ma

A. Elarfaoui (✉) · M. Sadik · Z. Choukairi · O. EL Badlaoui · H. Medromi
Foundation for Research, Development and Innovation in Science and Engineering (FRDISI), Casablanca, Morocco
e-mail: afaf.elarfaoui.doc@uhp.ac.ma

O. EL Badlaoui
e-mail: o.elbadlaoui@essaouira.suptech-sante.ma

M. Sadik
NEST Research Group, Hassan 2 University, Casablanca, Morocco

H. Medromi
International Academy of Scientific Francophone (IASF), Rabat, Morocco

P. Singh et al. (eds.), *Deep Learning Applications in Healthcare and Medical Imaging Practice*, Studies in Big Data 193, https://doi.org/10.1007/978-3-032-21009-8_15

Keywords Myocardial infarction · Machine learning · Electrocardiogram

1 Introduction

Myocardial infarction is that life-attacking disorder in which the blood flow is constricted in part of the muscle of the heart, thereby damaging or causing necrosis of the muscle [1, 2]. MI is responsible for world-wide death, claiming the lives of millions of people year after year according to the world records [3, 4], and in-hospital mortality was reported at 6.78% in recent clinical data [5]. MI can be categorized into ST-Elevation MI (STEMI) and Non-ST-segment Elevation MI (NSTEMI) [6, 7]. STEMI is the condition when a coronary artery is completely blockaded, and the entire muscle of the heart is greatly damaged, and the ECG shows increased ST-segments [8, 9]. NSTEMI, on the other hand, is because of incomplete blockage of a coronary artery, therefore bringing in minimal damage, and NSTEMI does not in most cases express ST-segment elevation in the ECG [8, 10].

Following the initial myocardial injury, complications arising from MI can significantly affect the patient's health and recovery. One of the most common and serious complications is atrial fibrillation, an irregular heart rhythm that is more frequently seen in STEMI patients and It is linked to higher death rates in the short and long term [11, 12]. Ventricular tachycardia and ventricular fibrillation are also critical arrhythmias that often result in cardiac arrest and death, particularly in STEMI patients [13, 14]. Another rare, but severe complication is myocardial rupture, which typically occurs within the first week following the infarction [15]. Lastly, chronic heart failure can develop in MI survivors, where the heart becomes too weak to pump blood efficiently, significantly affecting long-term health and quality of life [16]. The significant risk of these complications highlights the critical need for early and accurate prediction models to improve patient outcomes and guide clinical interventions. This need has fueled a rapid expansion of research into AI-enabled ECG technologies, a field that has seen a significant surge in publications, particularly since the COVID-19 pandemic [17].

The main contribution of this study is a comprehensive evaluation of ML models for predicting MI complications. Our methodology involves a two-stage analysis. First, we evaluate the models using a complete dataset of clinical and ECG attributes. Second, we assess their performance using a refined dataset containing only ECG-related features, which were isolated using attribute selection in the WEKA software. For both stages, the dataset underwent preprocessing to handle irregularities, including the management of missing values. This dual approach allows us to not only determine the overall predictive accuracy of each model but also to specifically investigate the predictive power of ECG data alone. A detailed performance analysis using both accuracy metrics and ROC curves is presented to assess the models' effectiveness across a range of specific complications.

The rest of this paper is organized as follows. Sect. 2 details the methodology, including the dataset, pre-processing steps, and the ML algorithms. Section 3 presents and discusses the experimental results from both analysis scenarios, followed by a detailed methodological comparison that contextualizes these findings against other recent traditional ML studies using the same dataset. Finally, Sect. 4 concludes the paper with a summary of our findings and directions for future work.

2 Methodology

2.1 Data Description

The study utilizes a database from Krasnoyarsk Interdistrict Clinical Hospital No. 20 [18], which contains medical data on 1700 MI patients, including 111 independent variables, and ECG data, focusing on MI complications and fatal outcomes, and changes in anterior, lateral, inferior, and posterior MI.

2.2 Data Pre-processing

The MI data used contain common irregularities, requiring preprocessing before they can be used for predictive models. Initially, we used the entire dataset then irrelevant identifiers and attributes were removed. Approximately 8% of the data contained missing values, which were handled using Weka's Replace Missing Values filter. This prepared the complete dataset for the first part of our study.

After that, we made a new dataset to do the second part of our analysis, which only looked at ECG data. Using attribute selection tools within WEKA, we isolated a subset of features specifically related to ECG changes across multiple leads associated with anterior, lateral, inferior, and posterior MIs. This allowed us to directly compare the models' performance when using all available data versus when relying exclusively on ECG information. The complete workflow of this proposed methodology is illustrated in Fig. 1.

2.3 ML Algorithms for Predicting MI Complications

ML algorithms RF, SVM, and NN are effective in predicting MI complications. RF uses decision trees for early intervention [19], SVM accurately predicts complications by classifying data [20], and NN learns from large datasets for improved accuracy and decision-making [21].

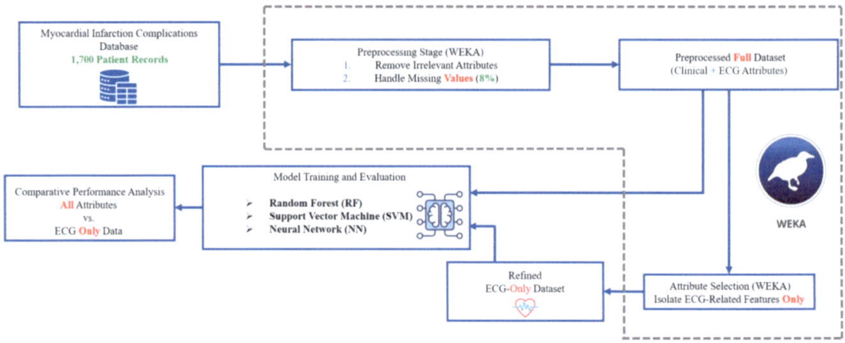

Fig. 1 Proposed methodology for MI complication prediction

3 Results and Discussion

3.1 *Data Visualization*

Figure 2 shows ECG changes in the patient population, ranging from marked changes, such as 30.43% with QS complex for anterior MI (V1–V4 leads), to subtle changes, with 84.15% showing no alterations for posterior MI (V7–V9, V3 leads).

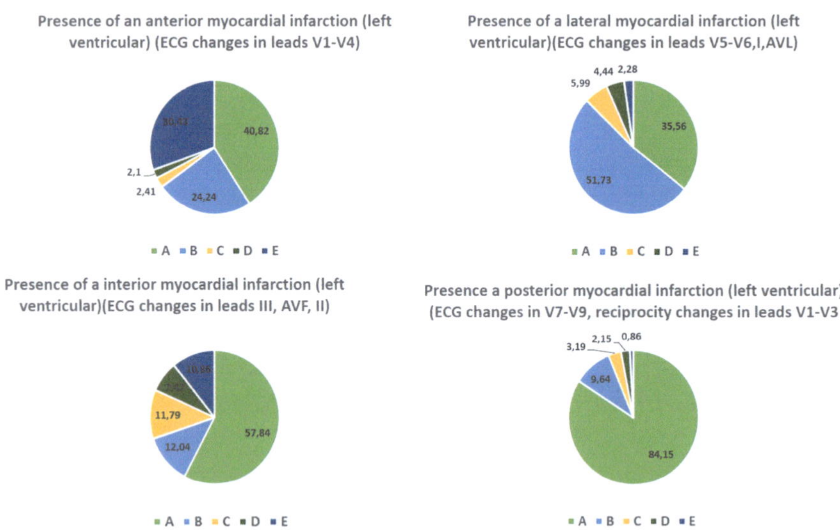

*A: No infarct, B: QRS no change, *C: QR-complex, *D: Qr-complex, *E: QS-complex

Fig. 2 ECG Changes associated with anterior, lateral, inferior, and posterior MI

3.2 *Results of RF, SVM, and NN for all Attributes*

The accuracy of a model represents the percentage of correctly predicted in-stances among the total predictions made. It serves as a basic yet essential metric to assess model performance [22]. Figure 3 shows the accuracy of three algorithms RF, SVM, and LR in predicting complications related to MI. As shown in the histogram, RF achieved the highest accuracy at 93.53%, followed by SVM at 93.24%, and SVM at 92.89%. This result is likely due to the RF's ability to combine multiple decision trees, leading to reduced overfitting and better handling of complex datasets.

ROC curves measure a model's classification performance across different thresholds, while AUC measures its ability to distinguish positive and negative classes, with a closer value indicating better performance [23].

Figure 4 shows ROC curves for MI complications predicted by RF (Panel A), SVM (Panel B), and NN (Panel C) models. The ROC curves visually suggest that the RF and NN models generally outperform the SVM. In panels A and C, the majority of the curves are positioned further towards the top-left corner of the graph, which indicates a higher level of accuracy in distinguishing between patients who will and will not develop complications. In contrast, several curves in Panel B for the SVM model are closer to the diagonal line, which represents the performance of a random guess, suggesting lower predictive power for those specific complications.

A more precise quantitative comparison is provided in the embedded within Fig. 5, which lists the Area Under the Curve (AUC) for each model and complication. The NN achieved the highest predictive performance for myocardial rupture with a remarkable AUC of 0.92. The RF model demonstrated the best performance for predicting ventricular tachycardia (AUC 0.88) and third-degree AV block (AUC

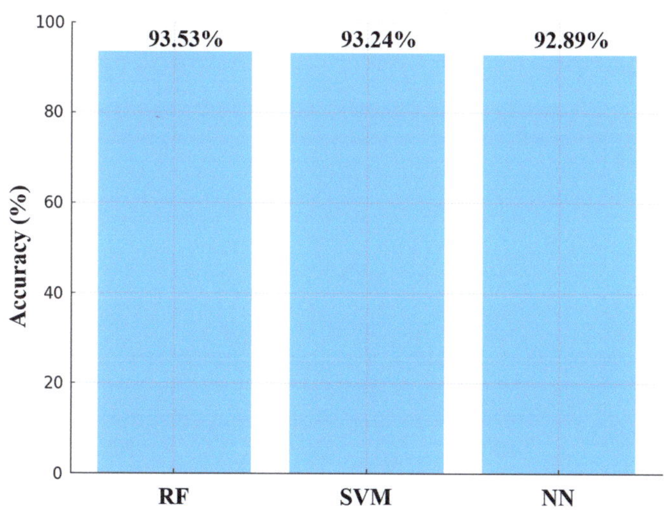

Fig. 3 Accuracy of different algorithms for predicting MI complications

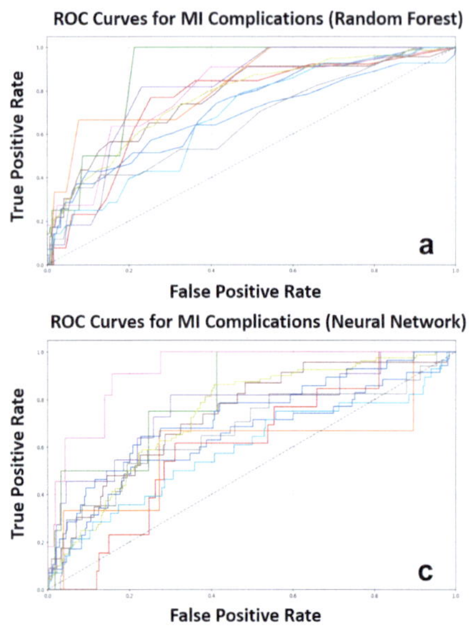

MI Complications	AUC		
	RF	SVM	NN
Atrial fibrillation	0.72	0.62	0.64
Supraventricular tachycardia	0.83	0.51	0.60
Ventricular tachycardia	0.88	0.74	0.82
Ventricular fibrillation	0.75	0.41	0.61
Third-degree AV block	0.81	0.68	0.76
Pulmonary edema	0.77	0.73	0.74
Myocardial rupture	0.78	0.80	0.92
Dressler syndrome	0.66	0.64	0.67
Chronic heart failure	0.77	0.69	0.74
Relapse of the myocardial infarction	0.68	0.55	0.59
Post-infarction angina	0.68	0.67	0.73

Fig. 4 ROC Curves for complications of MI: RF (**a**) SVM (**b**) and NN (**c**)

0.81). Overall, the SVM model tended to have the lowest AUC values across most of the listed MI complications, confirming the visual interpretation from the ROC curves.

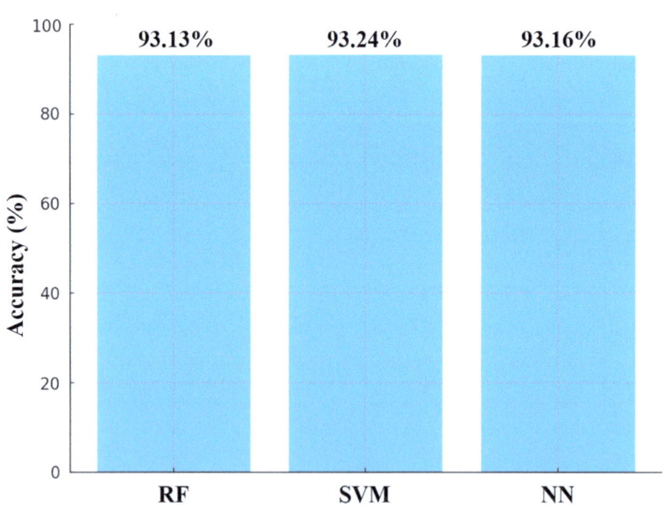

Fig. 5 Accuracy of algorithms predicting MI complications from multi-lead ECG

3.3 *Results of RF, SVM, and NN Based Only on ECG Changes Across Multiple Leads*

Figure 5 shows the average accuracy rates for RF, SVM, and NN, all exceeding 93%. SVM leads slightly with 93.24%, followed by NN at 93.16% and RF at 93.13%. These results suggest that all three models are similarly effective, with only a small advantage for SVM in predictive performance.

This Fig. 6 illustrates the performance of three ML models RF, SVM, and NN in predicting MI complications using only ECG changes as input. Visually, both the RF (Panel A) and the NN (Panel C) models demonstrate superior predictive ability for several complications compared to the SVM (Panel B). In particular, the prediction of third-degree AV block (purple line) and myocardial rupture (pink line) shows strong performance in the NN and RF models. The SVM's performance appears more modest, with many of its curves situated closer to the diagonal line of random chance.

Figure 6's table of AUC values gives a precise quantitative analysis that backs up the visual interpretation. The NN stands out, achieving the highest performance for predicting Third-degree AV block with an excellent AUC of 0.90, and also for Myocardial rupture with a strong AUC of 0.83. The RF model also performed very well for Third-degree AV block, with an AUC of 0.83. In contrast, the SVM's performance was inconsistent; while it was the best model for predicting Supraventricular tachycardia (AUC 0.72), it struggled significantly with other critical complications, such as Ventricular tachycardia (AUC 0.30). These results suggest that when relying

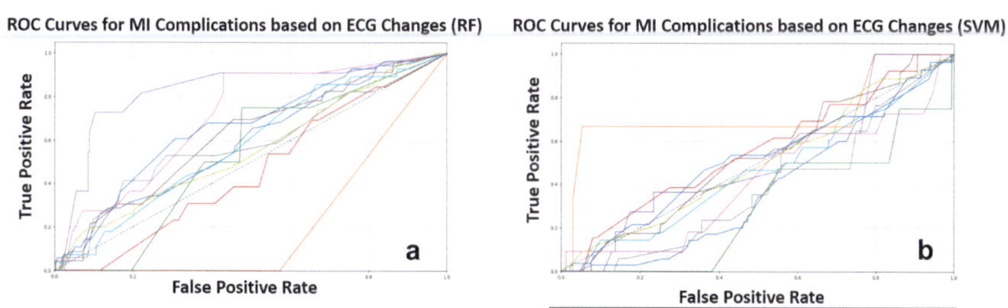

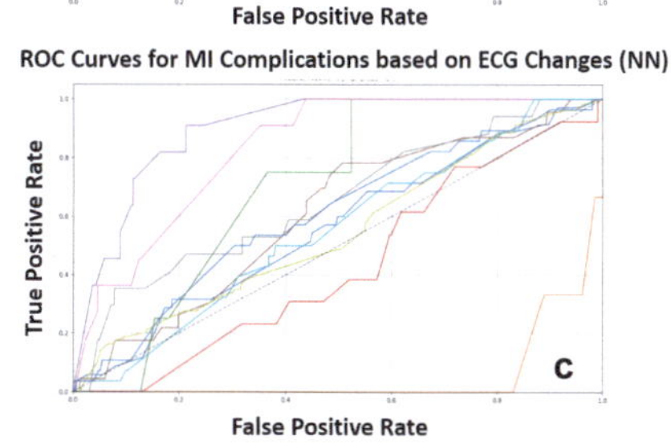

MI Complications	AUC		
	RF	SVM	NN
Atrial fibrillation	0.59	0.38	0.56
Supraventricular tachycardia	0.21	0.72	0.06
Ventricular tachycardia	0.53	0.30	0.70
Ventricular fibrillation	0.46	0.56	0.43
Third-degree AV block	0.83	0.51	0.90
Pulmonary edema	0.62	0.52	0.60
Myocardial rupture	0.71	0.42	0.83
Dressler syndrome	0.58	0.38	0.65
Chronic heart failure	0.55	0.50	0.55
Relapse of the myocardial infarction	0.58	0.46	0.55
Post-infarction angina	0.66	0.51	0.61

Fig. 6 ROC curves for complications of MI based only on ECG changes across multiple leads using RF (**a**) SVM (**b**) and NN (**c**)

exclusively on ECG data, the complex pattern recognition capabilities of NN and RF are more effective for identifying patients at risk for certain severe MI complications.

A comparison between the two analysis scenarios reveals that while the overall accuracy for all models remains consistently high at around 93%, as shown in Fig. 3 for combined clinical and ECG data and in Fig. 5 for ECG data alone, the ROC curves provide a more nuanced view of performance. The high-level accuracy scores suggest that ECG changes are the dominant predictive feature set in this dataset. However, the ROC curves in Fig. 4 for combined data and Fig. 6 for ECG only data demonstrate that the RF and NN models consistently outperform the SVM in their ability to predict specific complications, such as third-degree AV block and myocardial rupture. This indicates that while all models achieve similar overall accuracy, the RF and NN architectures are superior at identifying the complex patterns needed to discriminate between individual high-risk patient outcomes. It is important to note that the data used for this analysis contained missing values, which were handled using Weka's Replace Missing Values filter.

3.4 *Methodological Comparison and Future Directions*

To explain our findings, we will compare our models with other traditional ML studies utilizing the same Krasnoyarsk dataset. Our research is delineated by two distinct findings in the comparison table, illustrating our dual-analysis methodology. The RF model, which had the highest accuracy (93.53%) in our main analysis, is the first entry. The second entry showcases the result from our ECG-only analysis, where the SVM performed best in terms of overall accuracy (93.24%), though its AUC performance was more variable. This comparison is valuable because it highlights the performance of different computational approaches, particularly among advanced tree-based algorithms. A summary of this comparison is provided in Table 1.

Table 1 Quantitative comparison of methods on the krasnoyarsk MI dataset

Study	Algorithm	Key performance metrics	Primary advantage
Our paper	RF	Accuracy: 93.53% AUC: 0.81 (for AV block)	Achieved the highest overall accuracy among tested models (RF, SVM, NN) using the full dataset.
	SVM	Accuracy: 93.24% AUC: 0.72 (for supraventricular tachycardia)	Proved high predictive power of using only ECG data; SVM had the highest accuracy but inconsistent AUC performance.
[24]	XGBoost	Accuracy: 91.47% AUC: 0.787	Focused specifically on the high-stakes task of predicting fatal outcomes.
[25]	LightGBM	Accuracy: 91.8%	Showed LightGBM performs best without preprocessing; focused on explainability.
[26]	CatBoost	Accuracy: 94.9% AUC: 0.992	Showed the superior performance of the CatBoost algorithm for this dataset.

Our work sits alongside other studies that have successfully applied traditional ML to this dataset. For instance, Ghafari et al. focused on predicting mortality and found that an XGBoost model achieved an accuracy of 91.47% [24]. In another study focused on mortality, Vicente et al. investigated boosted tree models and discovered that a LightGBM model performed best, achieving an accuracy of 91.8% [25]. A key finding from their work was that the model achieved superior performance without extensive data preprocessing, highlighting the robustness of the LightGBM algorithm [25]. More directly comparable to our work, Khamis et al. predicted multiple MI complications and found that a Gradient Boosting model called CatBoost performed exceptionally well, achieving an accuracy of 94.9% [26]. Together, these studies show that advanced tree-based models are highly effective for this dataset, with algorithms like CatBoost, LightGBM, and XGBoost demonstrating a potential performance edge over our tested models.

Despite the development of more complex models, our approach offers distinct advantages that balance performance with practical clinical applicability. A unique strength of our study is the demonstration that ECG features alone are powerful enough to predict complications with over 93% accuracy, a finding that supports the development of simpler, ECG-focused clinical tools. Additionally, our RF model achieves an excellent balance between high performance and ease of use and understanding; it is essential for acquiring the trust of medical professionals. Lastly, our model gives more detailed and useful clinical insights than a simple, general mortality risk score because it can accurately predict a range of specific complications.

The principal limitation of this study is the long history of the dataset, given that medical treatments for MI have evolved greatly since the 1990s. This emphasizes the necessity for subsequent research to confirm these findings using current patient data. The comparison with other studies also makes it clear how things can be better. The CatBoost model's 94.9% accuracy, for example, shows that the next step should be to compare it to other advanced gradient-boosting algorithms. A further limitation is that our study, like the others in our comparison, used a static, admission-time model, which does not capture how a patient's condition changes over time. Therefore, future work should focus on three key areas: validating the models on modern datasets, expanding the model comparison to identify the most effective method for clinical use, and exploring methods for integrating temporal features to create more dynamic predictive models.

4 Conclusion and Perspectives

This study demonstrated that RF, SVM, and NN models can predict MI complications with high overall accuracy of approximately 93%, using both a full clinical dataset and ECG features alone. Despite similar overall accuracy, a deeper ROC analysis revealed that RF and NN models are significantly more effective at identifying specific, severe complications such as myocardial rupture and third-degree AV block while performance of SVM was less consistent. These results show how important ECG data is and how RF and NN architectures are better at predicting high-risk events.

The methodological comparison provided further context for these results. While our models demonstrated high accuracy, the analysis revealed that advanced gradient-boosting algorithms, particularly CatBoost, may offer superior performance for this classification task. This key insight, derived from comparing our work with other recent studies, is crucial for understanding the landscape of predictive modeling for MI and guiding future research toward the most powerful available methods.

Future work should focus on validating these findings on contemporary patient datasets, as the primary limitation of this study is the historical nature of the data. Building on the comparative analysis, this future work should proceed in three key directions. First, the model benchmarking should be expanded to include state-of-the-art algorithms like CatBoost and LightGBM to identify the most effective method for clinical use. Second, a limitation of all the static, admission-time models compared in this paper is that they do not account for changes in a patient's condition; therefore, future models should be developed to integrate temporal features to capture how patient conditions evolve during hospitalization. Finally, the eventual goal remains to extend this methodology to real-world applications using portable multi-lead ECG devices, which could enable rapid risk stratification and support timely clinical intervention.

References

1. Tirdea, C., Hostiuc, S., Moldovan, H., Scafa-Udriste, A.: Identification of risk genes associated with myocardial infarction—big data analysis and literature review. Int. J. Mol. Sci. **23**(23), 15008 (2022)
2. Alkhalil, M., De Maria, G.L., Akbar, N., Ruparelia, N., Choudhury, R.P.: Prospects for precision medicine in acute myocardial infarction: patient-level insights into myocardial injury and repair. J. Clin. Med. **12**(14), 4668 (2023)
3. Naveed, M.A., Iqbal, R., Ali, A., Omer Rehan, M., Azeem, B., Ahmed, F., Ahmad, M.: Unraveling the enigma of acute myocardial infarction-related mortality in malignancy among older adults ($\geq$ 65 years), a decadal dive into US trends (1999-2020): a CDC WONDER database analysis. Circulation. **150**(Suppl_1), A4146331–A4146331 (2024)
4. Tan, S.C.W., Zheng, B.B., Tang, M.L., Chu, H., Zhao, Y.T., Weng, C.: Global burden of cardiovascular diseases and its risk factors, 1990–2021: a systematic analysis for the global burden of disease study 2021. QJM: Int. J. Med.. hcaf022
5. Liao, J., Xiong, F., Chen, H., Li, W., Zhang, X., Gao, H., Ge, J.: Neutrophil to platelet ratio predicts in-hospital mortality in patients with acute myocardial infarction. Intern. Emerg. Med., 1–9 (2025)
6. Fröbert, O., Götberg, M., Erlinge, D., Akhtar, Z., Christiansen, E.H., Mac Intyre, C.R., Pernow, J.: Clinical impact of influenza vaccination after ST-and non-ST-segment elevation myocardial infarction-insights from the IAMI trial. Am. Heart J. **255**, 82–89 (2023)
7. Gupta, A.K., Mustafiz, C., Mutahar, D., Zaka, A., Parvez, R., Mridha, N., Maddern, G.J.: Machine-learning versus traditional approaches to predict all-cause mortality for acute coronary syndrome: a systematic review and meta-analysis. Can. J. Cardiology. (2025)

8. Gadelmawla, A.F., Mohamed, A., Abdelaziz, A., Diab, R., Mansour, A., Hassan, A., Ramadan, S.: Invasive vs conservative strategy in management of patients with non-ST elevation myocardial infarction: a systematic review and meta-analysis of over a million patients. Circulation. **150**(Suppl_1), A4144899-A4144899
9. Fraticelli, L., Kleitz, O., Claustre, C., Eydoux, N., Peiretti, A., Tazarourte, K., El Khoury, C.: Comparison of the pathways of care and life courses between first-time ST-elevation myocardial infarction (STEMI) and STEMI with prior MI: findings from the OSCAR registry. BMJ Open. **10**(11), e038773 (2020)
10. Chiesa, M., Piacentini, L., Bono, E., Milazzo, V., Campodonico, J., Marenzi, G., Colombo, G.I.: Whole blood transcriptome profile at hospital admission discriminates between patients with ST-segment elevation and non-ST-segment elevation acute myocardial infarction. Sci. Rep. **10**(1), 8731 (2020)
11. Lopes, R.D., Pieper, K.S., Horton, J.R., Al-Khatib, S.M., Newby, L.K., Mehta, R.H., Granger, C.B.: Short-and long-term outcomes following atrial fibrillation in patients with acute coronary syndromes with or without ST-segment elevation. Heart. **94**(7), 867–873 (2008)
12. Martínez Membrive, M.J., Subirana, I., Fadeuilhe, E., Rueda, F., Carreras-Mora, J., Oliveras, T., García-García, C.: Ten-year prognosis of acute atrial fibrillation in ST-elevation myocardial infarction: recurrence and risk stroke. Eur. Hear. J.: Acute Cardiovasc. Care. **14**(4), 214–222 (2025)
13. Al-Khatib, S.M., Granger, C.B., Huang, Y., Lee, K.L., Califf, R.M., Simoons, M.L., Harrington, R.A.: Sustained ventricular arrhythmias among patients with acute coronary syndromes with no ST-segment elevation: incidence, predictors, and outcomes. Circulation. **106**(3), 309–312 (2002)
14. Vallabhajosyula, S., Patlolla, S.H., Verghese, D., Ya'Qoub, L., Kumar, V., Subramaniam, A.V., Deshmukh, A.J.: Burden of arrhythmias in acute myocardial infarction complicated by cardiogenic shock. Am. J. Cardiol. **125**(12), 1774–1781 (2020)
15. Gharibzadeh, A., Shahsanaei, F., Petrudi, N.R.: Clinical and cardiovascular characteristics of patients suffering ST-segment elevation myocardial infarction after COVID-19: a systematic review and meta-analysis. Curr. Probl. Cardiol. **48**(1), 101045 (2023)
16. Vatta, M.: Editorial commentary: reprogramming autologous mesenchymal stem cells to regenerate the lost myocardium in chronic heart failure: reboot and restore? Trends Cardiovasc. Med. **26**(5), 405–406 (2016)
17. Ameziane, H., Zahidi, Y., El-Moufid, M., Medromi, H., Machkour, N., Rabbah, N.: Assessing Africa's position in the development of AI-enabled ECG devices. F1000Research. **13**, 1115 (2025)
18. Golovenkin, S.E., Gorban, A., Mirkes, E., Shulman, V.A., Rossiev, D.A., Shesternya, P.A., et al.: Myocardial Infarction Complications Database. University of Leicester (2020)
19. Breiman, L.: Random forests. Mach. Learn. **45**, 5–32 (2001)
20. Chang, C.C., Lin, C.J.: LIBSVM: a library for support vector machines. ACM Trans. Intell. Syst. Technol. (TIST). **2**(3), 1–27 (2011)
21. Gurney, K.: An Introduction to Neural Networks. Taylor and Francis, Inc., USA (1997)
22. Huang, J., Ling, C.X.: Using AUC and accuracy in evaluating learning algorithms. IEEE Trans. Knowl. Data Eng. **17**(3), 299–310 (2005)
23. Bradley, A.P.: The use of the area under the ROC curve in the evaluation of machine learning algorithms. Pattern Recogn. **30**(7), 1145–1159 (1997)
24. Ghafari, R., Azar, A.S., Ghafari, A., Aghdam, F.M., Valizadeh, M., Khalili, N., Hatamkhani, S.: Prediction of the fatal acute complications of myocardial infarction via machine learning algorithms. J. Tehran Univ. Hear. Cent. **18**(4), 278 (2023)

25. Vicente, A.L.G., Junior, R.D.M., Romero, R.A.: Explainable lightgbm approach for predicting myocardial infarction mortality. In: 2023 International Conference on Computational Science and Computational Intelligence (CSCI), pp. 323–328. IEEE (2023)
26. Khamis, G.S.M., Mohammed, Z.M., Alanazi, S.M., Mahmoud, A.F., Abdalla, F.A., Bkheet, S.A.: Prediction of myocardial infarction complications using gradient boosting. Eng., Technol. and Appl. Sci. Res. **14**(6), 18550–18556 (2024)

A Novel Approach for Brain Tumor Segmentation Using 3D U-Net with CBAM Module

Khaoula Echine and Aziz Darouichi

Abstract Precise segmentation of brain tumor in multimodal MRI images is a complex challenge in medical image applications. This study introduced an effective deep learning method to perform 3D segmentation of multimodal MRI images by enhancing the U-Net based structure through the incorporation of residual blocks and the module of Convolutional Block Attention (CBAM) for achieving better segmentation. The residual connections in the encoder path facilitated a deeper feature extraction process by mitigating the vanishing gradient issue. In this regard, the CBAM permits the network to adaptively refine the feature maps by explicitly targeting the most informative spatial and channel-wise components. The BraTS 2020 dataset has been used for training and evaluation. This model performs well according to different metrics compared to other existing methods. Ablation studies confirm the impact of the CBAM module in boosting overall performance.

Keywords Segmentation · Brain tumor · U-Net · Residual blocks · BraTS 2020

1 Introduction

MRIs are widely used non-invasive processes for acquiring high anatomical resolution medical images to aid in diagnosis, stage, planning and evaluate treatment response in patients with brain tumors. Prior to these tasks, accurate MRI brain tumor identification is crucial, it aid to involve the segmentation of tumors, which can provide a variety of measures useful in making decisions, including volume, location and metastatic appearance of the tumor.

Image segmentation of brain tumors can support surgical planning, postoperative monitoring and survival percentage boosting [1]. Automated segmentation algorithms can help the clinician with early diagnosis and therapy planning, a process

K. Echine (✉) · A. Darouichi
Laboratory of Computer and Systems Engineering (L2IS), University of Cadi Ayyad, Marrakech, Morocco
e-mail: k.echine.ced@uca.ac.ma

P. Singh et al. (eds.), *Deep Learning Applications in Healthcare and Medical Imaging Practice*, Studies in Big Data 193, https://doi.org/10.1007/978-3-032-21009-8_16

that is time-consuming and error-prone if performed manually [2]. The segmentation process is still challenging because of the variations in tumor appearance, shape, position, size, noise, and other elements that occur in MRI images. The process segmenting and classifying of brain tumors can now be done more automatically because to advancements in deep learning and image processing, which could potentially decrease the human involvement. Recently, technologies like deep learning and artificial intelligence have emerged as strong options for medical imaging, contributing to the improvement of accuracy and speed of diagnostic process [3]. Recent research highlights the importance of applying AI-based segmentation models to local datasets to improve tumor segmentation performance [4].

This paper introduces a new deep learning approach predicated on the existing 3D U-Net architecture to segment 3D MRI scans from multimodalities. In order to achieve optimal results, we added residual blocks as well as an attention module referred to as Convolutional Block Attention Module (CBAM). Such mechanisms enable our model to more effectively represent complex anatomical structure and better recognize subtle tumor boundaries on brain MRI images, resulting in the overall better segmentation performance on both whole data and different MRI modalities.

2 Related Works

U-Net is a method that was first presented by Ronneberger et al. [5]. This technique has grown in popularity since it requires less training data and yields good segmentation results. A distinctive U-shaped design characterizes the U-Net architecture. To the left is the contracting part, sometimes referred to as the encoder path. It extracts features by transforming the raw pixels of the image into a representation. Using the encoder's features, the decoder path, on the right, forms an output. It also maps them back to the original raw pixels of the image. U-Net transfers feature maps and contextual data from the encoder to the decoder, assisting the classifier in producing precise predictions [6].

To enhance the traditional U-Net, Yang et al. [7] proposed Deeper Res-UNet, a U-Net with deeper residual networks. The use of residual units on a U-Net based architecture leads to better performance for tasks of segmenting brain tumor. The Attention U-Net, which Zhou et al. [8] introduced, adds attention to the segmentation accuracy mechanism by concentrating on important area.

3 Network Architecture

We provided a comprehensive description of the suggested architecture with special regard to its core component: the Convolutional Block Attention Module (CBAM), which we will detail in the next subsection.

3.1 CBAM Module

The CBAM module shown in Fig. 2, is a lightweight attention module to refine representations of features in convolutional neural networks, which contains the channel attention and the spatial attention applied sequentially. Channel attention tells the model who is active by depicting to the network 'what' features are important, specifically by learning inter channel dependencies, and spatial attention tells it where the cell is active by learning 'where' the important features are, namely through inter-spatial relationships [9].

3.2 Proposed Model Architecture

Our model architecture represented in Fig. 1, is generated using a 3D U-Net framework featuring encoder and decoder paths. The model's input and output dimensions during training are both $128 \times 128 \times 128 \times 4$.The encoder and decoder have respective features of 36, 64, 128 and 256, and the "bridge" part has 512 features. The encoder path contains four residual blocks followed by 3D Max Pooling and a Convolutional Block Attention Module (see Fig. 2). Each of residual blocks has convolutional layers, Batch Normalization layers and ReLU activation functions. On the other hand, four standard 3D convolutional blocks make up the decoder path, which is preceded by the conv3DTranspose layer, which joins decoder block to its matching encoder block. After passing through a soft max activation function, predictions generated by the final decoder block are compared with the ground truth.

3.3 Dataset and Preprocessing

However, although the dataset of BraTS 2020 is standardized, intensity in MRI imaging may be inconsistent across different scanners and acquisition protocols. To address this and improve segmentation results, we added several more preprocessing steps. Initially, the intensity values from each scan were scaled between 0 and 1 using the MinMax normalization in order to minimize the variability across samples. Second, to prevent memory constraints, we minimized all images from $240 \times 240 \times 155$ to $128 \times 128 \times 128$. Lastly, we combined every modality (T1, T1ce, T2 and FLAIR) into one image since each MRI scan provides vital information. The combined images ($128 \times 128 \times 128$, depth of 4 is the modals) were then presented to the model during training to provide a comprehensive image.

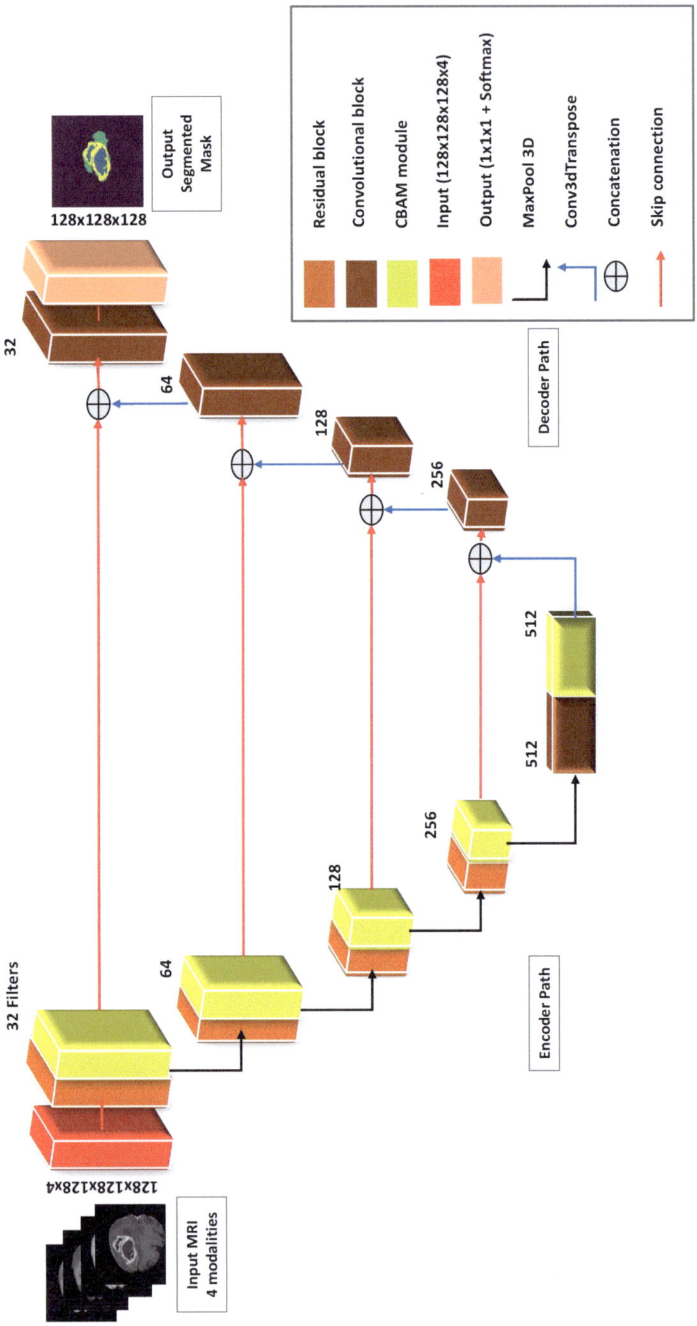

Fig. 1 Structure of the suggested model

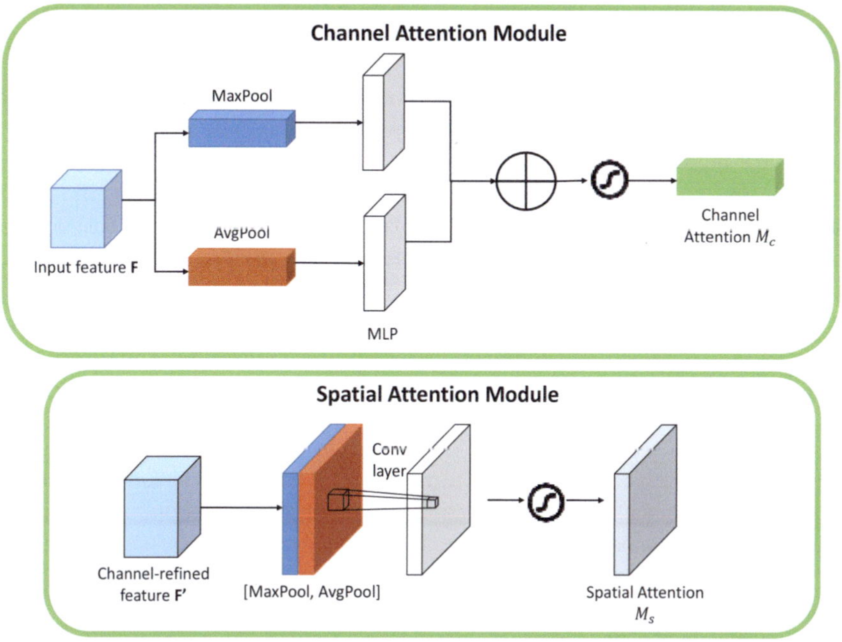

Fig. 2 Structure of CBAM module

4 Evaluation

The efficiency of the network is assessed using Dice Coefficient (Dice). It's a conventional metric for segmenting brain tumor that measures how similar between the ground truth and expected segmentation. The Dices of the three tumor regions, Dice Whole Tumor (WT), which includes all three tumor areas, Dice Tumor Core (TC), which includes all tumors excluding edema, and Dice Enhancing Tumor (ET) design the enhancing area, are used to quantify the model's effectiveness. Dice coefficients are calculated using Eq. (1) as below on premise of predicted segmentation and ground truth data. Additionally, we employed metrics for accuracy, precision and recall.

$$Dice = 2 \times \frac{|X \cap Y|}{|X| + |Y|} \tag{1}$$

4.1 Implementation Details

We developed our model in Jupyter Notebook using necessary Python libraries like Keras, TensorFlow, and Nibabel which helps in carrying on multiple experiments in medical image processing. On a GeForce RTX 4090 with 24 GB of RAM, this network was executed utilizing the Adam optimizer with a learning rate of 0.0001 and the categorical cross-entropy loss through the massive AI platform vast.ai. Due to having limited GPU memory, a batch size of 1 was used to train the suggested model during 100 epochs.

5 Results and Discussion

In order to intuitively and fairly evaluate the segmentation results obtained with these different enhancement strategies, ablation studies have been conducted to demonstrate that CBAM module can enhance the segmentation of the network. Tables 1 and 2 provide a summary of metrics that were measured on the validation and testing subsets.

The tables above illustrate that, after adding the CBAM module to Res-UNet model, all metrics improved significantly. For the validation phase, the scores for accuracy, precision and recall rise from 0.8975, 0.9007 and 0.8952 respectively, to 0.9701, 0.9715 and 0.9693. The coefficients: Dice WT, Dice TC, and Dice ET increase from 0.6210, 0.5027, and 0.4693 to 0.7704, 0.6445, and 0.5892.

Similarly, on testing phase, after adding the CBAM module, the coefficients Dice WT, Dice TC and Dice ET show a notable enhancement from 0.6930, 0.6134 and 0.6019 to 0.8114, 0.7519 and 0.6694 respectively.

Overall, the significant improvement in performance can be attributed to the incorporation of CBAM, which helps the model dynamically to refine the extracted features by focusing on the most relevant information. Furthermore, by integrating residual blocks into the encoder path help to mitigate the vanishing gradient problem

Table 1 Comparison results of ablation studies on validation set

	Accuracy	Precision	Recall	Dice WT	Dice TC	Dice ET
dResUNet	0.8975	0.9007	0.8952	0.6210	0.5027	0.4693
dResUNet+CBAM	0.9701	0.9715	0.9693	0.7704	0.6445	0.5892

Table 2 Comparison results of ablation studies on test set

	Accuracy	Precision	Recall	Dice WT	Dice TC	Dice ET
dResUNet	0.9342	0.9365	0.9325	0.6930	0.6134	0.6019
dResUNet+CBAM	0.9751	0.9761	0.9745	0.8114	0.7519	0.6694

while facilitating the extraction of deep features. Figure 3 presents the qualitative results provided by our model on some MRI testing samples.

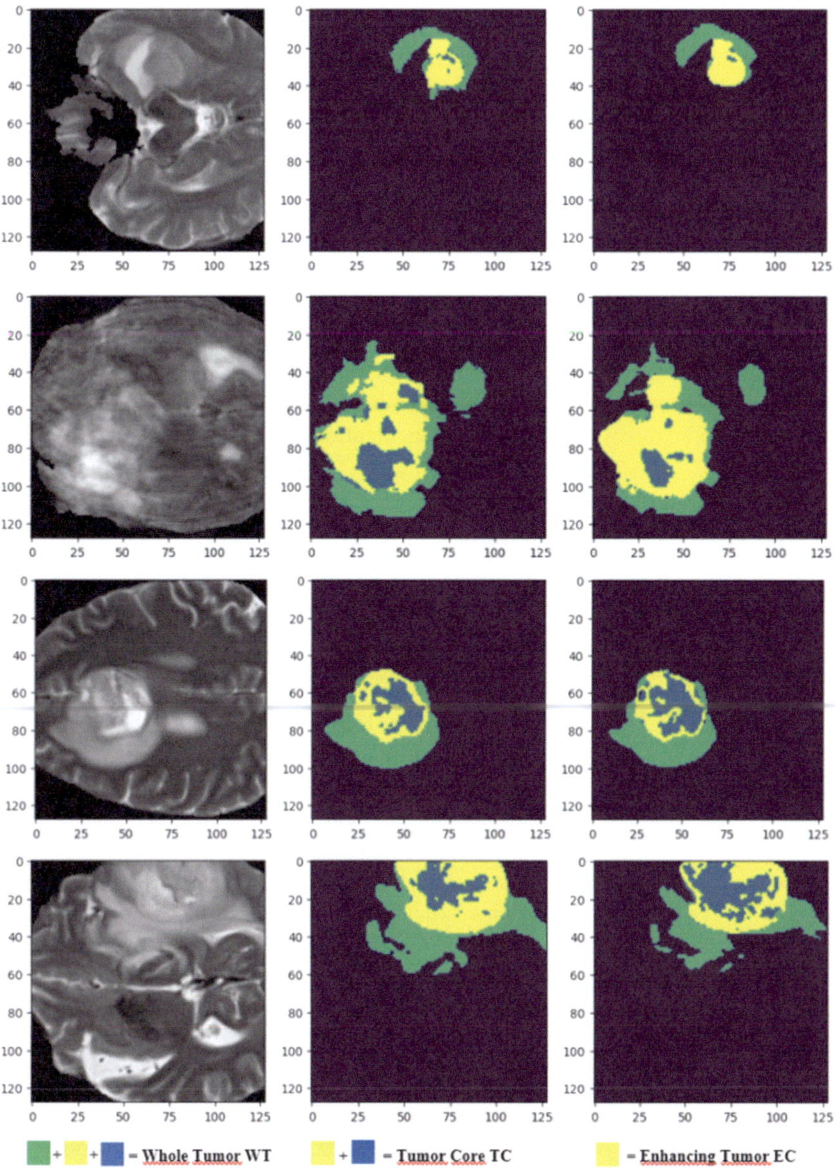

Fig. 3 Qualitative results obtained from test samples

Table 3 Evaluation of our suggested model with other existing methods

Reference	Dataset	Architecture	Dice WT	Dice TC	Dice ET
Huang et al. [10]	BraTS 2018	Multi-depth fusion	0.80	0.76	0.72
Agravat et al. [11]	BraTS 2019	3D FCN	0.73	0.65	0.59
Messaoudi et al. [12]	BraTS 2020	3D U-Net with 2D classifier	0.8068	0.7520	0.6959
Echine et al. [6]	BraTS 2020	3D AGRes-UNet	0.8059	0.7621	0.7224
Our method	**BraTS 2020**	**3D res-UNet + CBAM**	**0.8114**	**0.7519**	**0.6694**

5.1 Comparison with Related Works

The proposed model is compared to some advanced models currently in use for automatic segmentation of tumors on the BraTS datasets. As demonstrated in Table 3, our approach outperforms all other works in segmenting the whole tumor area, as it surpasses the method of Agravat et al. in segmenting both tumor core and enhancing tumor areas.

6 Conclusion and Perspectives

The process of segmenting brain tumors is quite significant in medical imaging. Diagnosing brain tumors early can help improve treatment options and outcome of patients' survival. This research proposes a deep learning architecture built upon the known U-Net architecture for 3D multimodal brain tumor image segmentation taking input from the BraTS 2020 Dataset. Firstly, residual blocks were incorporated in the encoder block to reduce vanishing gradient problem. Secondly, a Convolutional Block Attention Module is integrated after residual blocks helping model to focus on the most important characteristics by applying channel and spatial attention sequentially. Experimental outcomes indicate that the proposed approach effectively segments brain tumor regions.

In the future, with advanced data augmentation the model's performance can be enhanced especially in terms of Dice ET, or by using deeper architectures and cascade models.

References

1. Liu, Z., Tong, L., Chen, L., et al.: Deep learning based brain tumor segmentation: a survey. Complex Intell. Syst. **9**, 1001–1026 (2023). https://doi.org/10.1007/s40747-022-00815-5
2. Rajput, S., Agravat, R., Roy, M., Raval M.S.: Glioblastoma multiforme patient survival prediction (2021). *arXiv preprint* https://arxiv.org/abs/2101.10589. https://arxiv.org/abs/2101.10589
3. Srinivas, C., Prasad, K.S.N., Zakariah, M., Alothaibi, Y.A., Shaukat, K., Partibane, B., et al.: Deep transfer learning approaches in performance analysis of brain tumor classification using MRI images. J Healthc Eng. **2022**, 3264367 (2022). https://doi.org/10.1155/2022/3264367
4. Ali, S.H., Ahmad, A., Ali, M., Khan, A., Shahban, M., Shaukat, N.: Automated MRI tumor segmentation using hybrid U-Net with Transformer and Efficient Attention. *arXiv preprint* https://arxiv.org/abs/2506.15562. 2025. https://arxiv.org/abs/2506.15562
5. Ronneberger, O., Fischer, P., Brox, T.: U-Net: convolutional networks for biomedical image segmentation. In: Navab, N., Hornegger, J., Wells, W.M., Frangi, A.F. (eds.) Medical Image Computing and Computer-Assisted Intervention–MICCAI 2015 Lecture Notes in Computer Science, vol. 9351, pp. 234–241. Springer, Cham (2015). https://doi.org/10.1007/978-3-319-24574-4_28
6. Echine, K., Darouichi, A.: 3D AGRes-UNet: an advanced deep learning model for brain tumor segmentation from multimodal MRI. Multimed. Tools Appl. **84**, 42135–42154 (2025). https://doi.org/10.1007/s11042-025-20828-9
7. Yang, T., Song, J., Li, L., Tang, Q.: Improving brain tumor segmentation on MRI based on the deep U-net and residual units. J. Xray Sci. Technol. **28**, 95–110 (2020). https://doi.org/10.3233/XST-190552
8. Zhou, Z., Siddiquee, M.M.R., Tajbakhsh, N., Liang, J.: UNet++: redesigning skip connections to exploit multiscale features in image segmentation. IEEE Trans. Med. Imaging. **39**, 1856–1867 (2020). https://doi.org/10.1109/TMI.2019.2959609
9. Woo, S., Park, J., Lee, J.Y., Kweon, I.S.: CBAM: convolutional block attention module. In Proceedings of the European Conference on Computer Vision (ECCV). In: Ferrari, V., Hebert, M., Sminchisescu, C., Weiss Y. (eds.) Computer Vision–ECCV 2018. Lecture Notes in Computer Science, vol. 11211, p. 3–19. Cham: Springer, (2018). https://doi.org/10.1007/978-3-030-01234-2_1
10. Huang, H., Yang, G., Zhang, W., Xu, X., Yang, W., Jiang, W., Lai, X.: A deep multi-task learning framework for brain tumor segmentation. Front. Oncol. **11**, 690244 (2021). https://doi.org/10.3389/fonc.2021.690244
11. Agravat, R.R., Raval, M.S.: Brain tumor segmentation and survival prediction. In: Crimi, A., Bakas, S. (eds.) Brainlesion: Glioma, Multiple Sclerosis, Stroke and Traumatic Brain Injuries (BrainLes 2019) Lecture Notes in Computer Science, vol. 11992. Springer, Cham (2020). https://doi.org/10.1007/978-3-030-46640-4_32
12. Messaoudi, H., Belaid, A., Allaoui, M.L., Zetout, A., Allili, MS., Tliba, S., et al.: Efficient embedding network for 3D brain tumor segmentation. In: Crimi, A., Bakas, S. (eds.) BrainLesion: Glioma, Multiple Sclerosis, Stroke and Traumatic Brain Injuries. BrainLes 2020. Lecture Notes in Computer Science, vol. 12658, p. 274–283. Cham: Springer, (2021). https://doi.org/10.1007/978-3-030-72084-1_23

HIM-Net: Hybrid Inception-MobileViT with Inverted Residual Blocks for Diabetic Retinopathy Grading

Kawtar Naim and Aziz Darouichi

Abstract One of the major complications of diabetes, Diabetic Retinopathy, significantly contributes to visual impairment and blindness. Early and accurate classification of DR stages is vital for guiding prompt intervention and minimizing the risk of advanced retinal damage. However, existing deep learning models face challenges such as limited feature representation, high computational complexity, and class imbalance in DR datasets. To address these issues, this paper presents HIM-Net a DL architecture for multiclass DR classification using fundus images from the APTOS 2019 dataset. HIM-Net combines Inception modules for capturing multi-scale spatial features with lightweight MobileViT blocks that integrate convolutional and Transformer-based representations. Inverted residual blocks are incorporated to enhance feature reuse and reduce model parameters. To mitigate the effects of severe class imbalance, SMOTE is applied at the image level. Additionally, a pre-processing pipeline including resizing and normalization are implemented to standardize input data. Experimental results demonstrate that HIM-Net surpasses several recent models, achieving an accuracy of 95.33% on the APTOS 2019 dataset.

Keywords Retinal · Fundus · Deep learning · Classification · APTOS-2019

1 Introduction

Diabetic Retinopathy is consequence of prolonged diabetes mellitus affecting eye health globally [1–3]. DR damages microvessels in the retina and, if not treated, leads to partial or total blindness [4]. Because DR is symptomless in early stages, early diagnosis is essential. Clinically, DR progresses from Non-Proliferative DR, which is marked by microaneurysms and hemorrhages and retinal edema, to Proliferative

K. Naim (✉) · A. Darouichi
Computer and Systems Engineering Laboratory (L2IS), FST, Cadi Ayyad University, Marrakech, Morocco
e-mail: k.naim.ced@uca.ac.ma

A. Darouichi
e-mail: az.darouichi@uca.ac.ma

P. Singh et al. (eds.), *Deep Learning Applications in Healthcare and Medical Imaging Practice*, Studies in Big Data 193, https://doi.org/10.1007/978-3-032-21009-8_17

DR, which is marked by new vessels which are fragile and bleed easily and blindness [5, 6]. DR severity is commonly classified into five stages as outlined by the clinical classification system [7]. Rising global diabetes incidence is driving DR cases, and projections for a rise to 700 million by 2045 from 463 million are expected [8], 30% of individuals with diabetes develop DR, and 10% reach vision threatening levels [9, 10]. Therefore, early and accurate diagnosis is critical. Even though OCT, fundus photography, and intraocular pressure are common for screening, they are operator dependent and will not pick up on early features [11].

AI more specifically DL and CNNs is increasingly being used to automate DR detection and grading but with the need for large data sets and calibration. Over the last couple of years, impressive progress has been reported on developing automated systems for DR classification, in particular those evaluated on the APTOS 2019 benchmark dataset. Liu et al [12] presented ADCNet, an attention- based cascaded model, which was put forth to enhance lesion-centric representation of features. Without revealing too much detail in preprocessing, the model performed with 83.4% accuracy [12]. Later in the same year, Zhang et al [13] introduced a graph neural network model that represented complex relationships among CNN extracted features and improved classification to 85.5% [13]. Shafi et al. [14] proposed in 2024 the hybrid CNN-Transformer structure called MobileViTv2, which employed preprocessing techniques such as Gaussian blur and data augmentation to achieve 83% accuracy on AP- TOS [14]. TMILv4, which was proposed by Yang et al. [15], employed multiple instance learning with Transformer layers and high-resolution images as input, improving the accuracy to 85.6% [15]. Priyadharsini and Phamila in 2025 introduced the model called Frobenius Deep Feature Fusion (FDFF), which involved image resizing and contrast adjustment as preprocessing methods prior to applying a new fusion strategy, having a 80.63% accuracy on DR stages [16]. Hassan et al. studied uncertainty-aware classification on Bayesian CNNs with contrast normalization and resizing as preprocessing. Their baseline CNN had an accuracy of 94.7%, whereas their Bayesian ones had 94.0% and 93.0%, respectively [17]. Another recent work, CAD-ViT, employed a suite of preprocessing methods namely, image cropping, Gaussian blurring, resizing to 512×512, and data augmentation to realize 88.6% accuracy [6]. Taken together, these works reflect the direction of movement toward transformer-based and hybrid models aided by focused preprocessing to increase classification accuracy and dependability in DR grading workflows.

The remainder of this chapter is organized as follows: Sect. 2 presents the Methods, including dataset and model design; Sect. 3 reports the Results and Sect. 4 provides the Discussion. Finaly Sect. 5 integrates the conclusion and outlines future research directions.

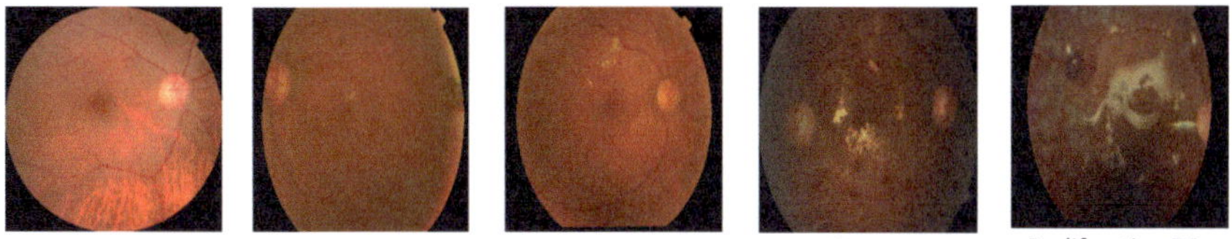

Fig. 1 Sample images from the APTOS 2019 dataset

2 Methods

2.1 Dataset Description

The APTOS 2019 dataset [18], is one of the most used datasets for diabetic retinopathy research. The dataset is comprised of 3,662 high-resolution fundus images, which have each been annotated based on five grades of severity of DR [18]. The dataset comprised retinal fundus images labeled for DR severity, with five classes (0–4) corresponding to increasing levels of DR progression (see Fig. 1). Each image was resized to a uniform resolution of 256 × 256 pixels and normalized to the range [0, 1] by dividing pixel values by 255. Class distribution was balanced using SMOTE, which synthetically augments underrepresented classes by interpolating between existing samples.

2.2 Model Architecture

The proposed HIM-Net a Hybrid Inception-MobileViT with Inverted Residual Blocks adopts a multi-branch design combining the strengths of Inception modules, MobileViT transformers, and efficient depthwise convolutions for diabetic retinopathy grading. Input fundus images are processed at 256 × 256 × 3 resolution, matching the standard clinical preprocessing pipeline used in datasets like Aptos-2019. The model begins with a stem convolution (3 × 3 kernels, stride = 2) with Swish activation and batch normalization, followed by a series of inverted residual blocks with expansion ratios of 2 × 4, optimizing local feature extraction while minimizing parameters. Parallel Inception branches (1 × 1, 3 × 3, and 5 × 5 convolutions) capture multi-scale lesion patterns, from microaneurysms to exudates, with their outputs concatenated channel-wise. The MobileViT blocks then process these features through lightweight transformer encoders (2 attention heads) operating on 2 × 2-pixel patches, enabling global context modeling without the computational overhead of standard Vision Transformers. A final GlobalAveragePooling2D layer condenses spatial features before the classification head, which uses softmax activation to output probabilities across the five DR severity grades, see Fig. 2. HIM-Net

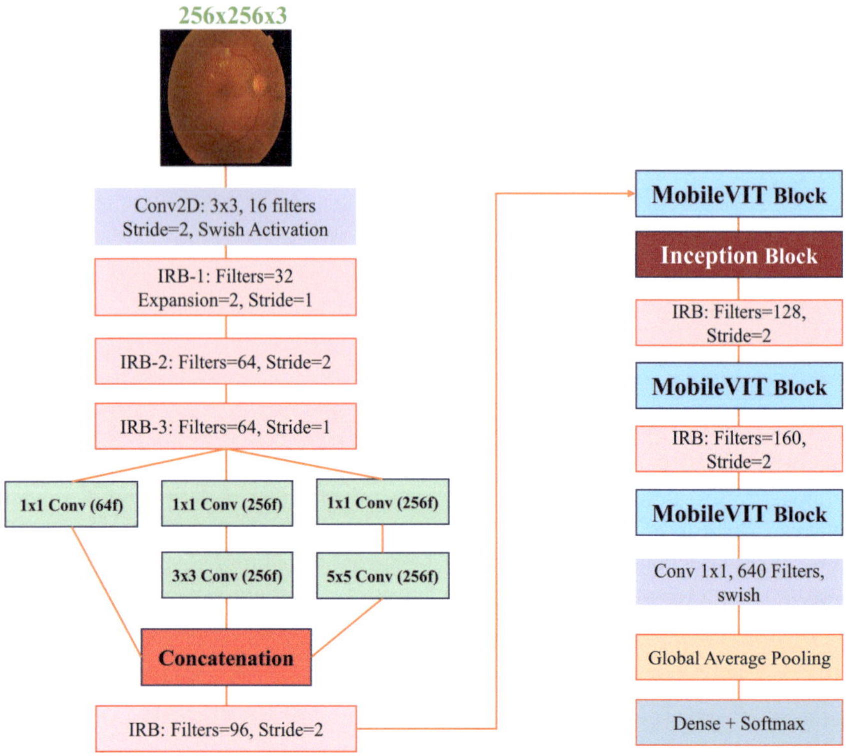

Fig. 2 HIM-Net architecture: inception-MobileViT with inverted residual blocks

was trained for 50 epochs and the model optimized a weighted categorical cross-entropy loss function, with a batch size of 32. To avoid overfitting and reduce redundant training, we employed early stopping with a patience threshold of 35 epochs. On average, each epoch required approximately 44 seconds to complete.

3 Results

The model performed exceptionally well on the APTOS-2019 dataset, correctly identifying diabetic retinopathy cases with 95.3% overall accuracy. It was particularly good at spotting severe cases, getting them right 99% of the time, and was nearly as accurate with proliferative DR (97%) and mild cases (96%). While still effective, it found moderate DR slightly more challenging, with 90.9% accuracy. For healthy eyes (no DR), the model was correct 94.5% of the time. These results show the system works very well across all stages of diabetic retinopathy, with only a small dip in performance for moderate cases. See Table 1.

Table 1 Classification report for APTOS-2019 dataset

Class	Precision	Recall	F1-Score	Support
NoDR	0.945	0.954	0.950	306
Mild	0.960	0.951	0.955	288
Moderate	0.909	0.914	0.910	276
Severe	0.990	0.980	0.981	294
Proliferative DR	0.970	0.980	0.972	270
Accuracy			0.953	1434
Macroavg	0.953	0.953	0.953	1434
Weightedavg	0.953	0.953	0.953	1434

The normalized confusion matrix demonstrates strong performance in multi-class classification across all stages of DR. The model achieves particularly high accuracy in identifying advanced stages, with both Severe DR and Proliferative DR cases being correctly classified with 98% accuracy. Healthy retinas (No DR) are accurately identified in 95% of cases, with minimal misclassification primarily limited to adjacent stages (1% as Mild DR and 3% as Moderate DR). Classification of Mild DR maintains high accuracy at 95%, with marginal confusion observed only with immediately neighboring categories (2% as No DR and 2% as Moderate DR). The Moderate DR stage presents a modestly higher classification challenge, reflected in 91% accuracy, with most errors occurring within one severity level (3% as Mild DR and 1% as Severe DR). See Fig. 3. The ROC analysis demonstrates outstanding performance in classifying all stages of diabetic retinopathy. The model achieves perfect discrimination for healthy retinas (No DR), Severe DR, and Proliferative DR cases, with AUC scores of 1.00 in each category. For Mild and Moderate DR, the model maintains near-perfect performance with AUC values of 0.99, indicating only minimal overlap between positive and negative cases. These results show the classifier excels at distinguishing between all severity levels, from healthy eyes to advanced disease. See Fig. 4 to validate the attention module's ability to localize lesions.

4 Discussion

We visualize its activation patterns using Grad-CAM (Fig. 5). The top row shows original fundus images, and the bottom row displays their corresponding heatmaps, ordered by DR severity. The heatmaps reveal that the module consistently highlights clinically relevant lesions such as microaneurysms and hemorrhages aligning with pathological features of each grade. This targeted focus confirms the module's role in improving classification accuracy by directing the model's attention to diagnostically critical regions. The Table 2 compares recent multiclass diabetic retinopathy

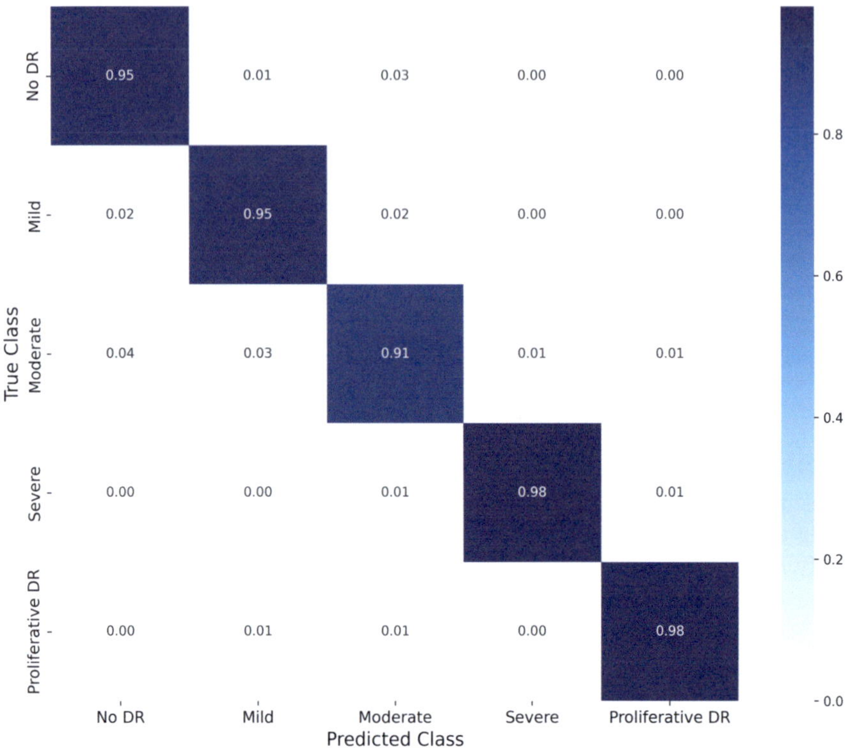

Fig. 3 Normalized confusion matrix

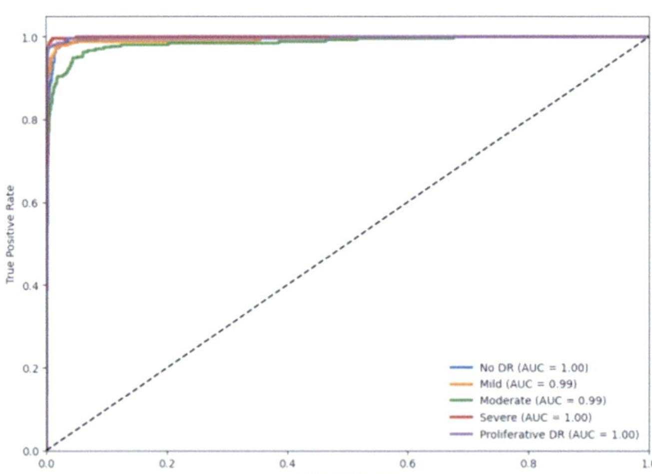

Fig. 4 ROC analysis of DR Stages

diagnosis methods on the APTOS-2019 dataset. The HIM-Net model achieves the highest accuracy of 95.33% and a QWK score of 0.9666, outperforming existing approaches from 2023 to 2025. Notably, TMILv4 uses Vision Transformer-based multi-instance learning and reaches 85.6% accuracy, while Bayesian CNN variants achieve up to 94.7%.

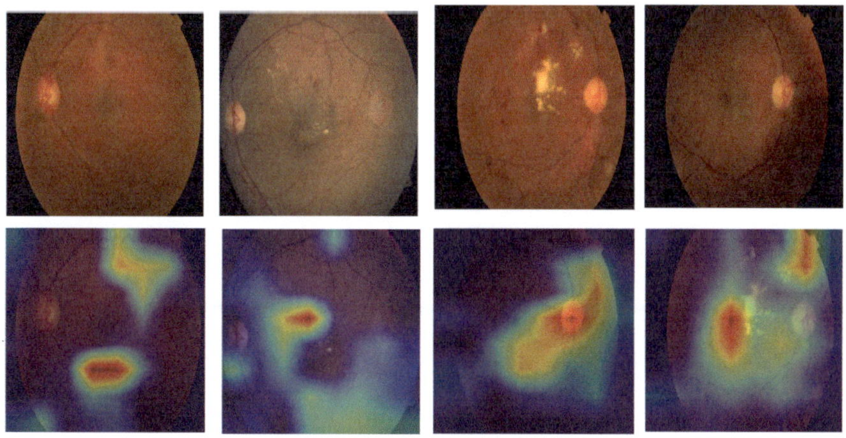

Fig. 5 Attention module activation patterns in DR grading (Grad-CAM)

Table 2 Summary of multiclass DR diagnosis methods on APTOS-2019

Ref model	Year preprocessing	(%)
[12] ADCNet	2023 –	83.4
[13] GNN	2023 –	85.5
[14] MobileViTv2	2024 Gaussian blur data augmentation	83
[15] TMILv4	2024 Cropping, resizing (896 × 896), data augmentation	85.6
[16] FDFF	2025 Resizing, contrast enhancement	80.63
CNN		94.70
[17] BCNN-VI	2025 Contrast enhancement, resizing (224 × 224), normalization	94.00
BCNN-MC		93.00
[6] CAD-ViT	2025 Cropping, resizing (512 × 512), Gaussian blur, data augmentation	88.64
[19] EfficientNet-B6	Resize 224 × 224 Gaussian blur SMOTE augmentation	94
[20] HOG-CNN	2025 HOG feature extraction fused with CNN backbone	83.2
our HIM-Net	2025 Resizing (256 × 256 × 3), Normalization, SMOTE	95.33

5 Conclusion and Future Works

HIM-Net's superior performance is attributed to effective preprocessing including resizing, normalization, and SMOTE to address class imbalance. HIM-Net achieved 95.33% on proliferative DR stages. The model showed consistently strong performance across all DR levels, supported by high precision, recall, F1-scores, and AUC. Grad-CAM visualizations confirmed the attention module's focus on relevant retinal lesions. Compared to recent models (2023–2025), including Vision Transformers and Bayesian CNNs, HIM-Net performed better, aided by preprocessing techniques like resizing, normalization, and SMOTE. Future work includes clinical validation, integration into real-world diagnostic workflows, and exploration of newer Transformer-based and hybrid architectures. We also aim to expand dataset diversity, include multimodal data such as OCT, and optimize the model for fast inference on edge devices.

References

1. Ou, C., Yang, Y.J., Peng, Q.: Yiqi Yangyin Huoxue method in treating diabetic retinopathy: a systematic review and meta-analysis. Evid. Based Complement. Altern. Med. eCAM 2019 (2019). https://api.semanticscholar.org/CorpusID:133428780
2. Teo, Z.L., et al.: Global prevalence of diabetic retinopathy and projection of burden through 2045: systematic review and meta-analysis. Ophthalmology **128**(11), 1580–1591 (2021). https://doi.org/10.1016/j.ophtha.2021.04.027
3. Surekha, N.: Diabetes and the eye: an overview. J. Evid. Based Med. Healthc. **2**, 1541–1549 (2015). https://api.semanticscholar.org/CorpusID:201994832
4. Yau, J.W.Y., et al.: Global prevalence and major risk factors of diabetic retinopathy. Diabetes Care 35, 556–564 (2012). https://api.semanticscholar.org/CorpusID:18395627
5. American Academy of Ophthalmology: Diabetic Retinopathy Preferred Practice Pattern (2019). https://www.aao.org/preferred-practice-pattern/diabetic-retinopathy-ppp. Last accessed 29 June 2025
6. Wang, Y., Gou, X., Li, W.: CAD-ViT: coordinate attention- enhanced vision transformer with dilated feature fusion for diabetic retinopathy staging. IEEE Access **13**, 91505–91514 (2025). https://api.semanticscholar.org/CorpusID:278852014
7. Wilkinson, C.P., et al.: Proposed international clinical diabetic retinopathy and diabetic macular edema disease severity scales. Ophthalmology **110**(9), 1677–1682 (2003)
8. International Diabetes Federation: IDF Diabetes Atlas, 10th edn. (2021). https://diabetesatlas.org. Last accessed 29 June 2025
9. Congdon, N., Xie, X., Wang, F., et al. : Prevalence and determinants of diabetic retinopathy in adult patients with diabetes in China. Br. J. Ophthalmol. **96**(3), 288–293 (2012). 10.1136/bjophthalmol-2011-300342
10. Cheng, C.Y., Wong, T.Y. (eds.): Ophthalmic Epidemiology: Current Concepts to Digital Strategies, 1st. eBook Published 24 May 2022. CRC Press, Boca Raton. ISBN: 9781315146737. https://doi.org/10.1201/9781315146737
11. Grzybowski, A., Jin, K., Zhou, J., et al.: Retina fundus photograph-based artificial intelligence algorithms in medicine: a systematic review. Ophthalmol. Ther. **13**, 2125–2149 (2024). https://doi.org/10.1007/s40123-024-00981-4

12. Yue, G., et al.: Attention-driven cascaded network for diabetic retinopathy grading from fundus images. Biomed. Signal Process. Control. **80**, 104370 (2023). https://api.semanticscholar.org/CorpusID:253667671
13. Feng, M., et al.: Grading of diabetic retinopathy images based on graph neural network. IEEE Access **11**, 98391–98401 (2023). https://api.semanticscholar.org/CorpusID:261652519
14. Al Shafi, A., et al. : Enhancing diabetic retinopathy detection through transformer based knowledge distillation and explainable AI. In: International Joint Conference on Neural Networks (IJCNN) (2024), pp. 1–8 (2024). https://api.semanticscholar.org/CorpusID:272548067
15. Yang, Y., et al. : A novel transformer model with multiple instance learning for diabetic retinopathy classification. IEEE Access **12**, 6768–6776 (2024). https://api.semanticscholar.org/CorpusID:266876847
16. Priyadharsini, C., Asnath Victy Phamila, Y.: Frobenius deep feature fusion architecture to detect diabetic retinopathy. Discov. Appl. Sci. (2025). https://api.semanticscholar.org/CorpusID:276745095
17. Hassan, M.M., Ismail, H.R.: Bayesian deep learning applied to diabetic retinopathy with uncertainty quantification. Heliyon **11** (2025). https://api.semanticscholar.org/CorpusID:275423666
18. Asia Pacific Tele-Ophthalmology Society (APTOS). APTOS 2019 blindness detection dataset. https://www.kaggle.com/datasets/mariaherrerot/aptos2019
19. Abood, R.H., Hamad, A.H.: Multi-label diabetic retinopathy detection using transfer learning based convolutional neural network. Fusion Pract. Appl. **17**(02), 279–293 (2025)
20. Ahmed, F.: Hog-CNN: integrating histogram of oriented gradients with convolutional neural networks for retinal image classification (2025)

Breast Cancer Detection in Mammography via Deep Learning

Chaima Soubai, Insaf Bellamine, and Abdelkaher Ait Abdelouahad

Abstract Breast cancer continues to be one of the most prevalent and deadly cancers in female populations of the world, underscoring the need for early and accurate diagnosis. Mammography is the primary diagnostics tool for screening in breast cancer diagnosis, and through recent advances in deep learning, automated diagnostic support systems have been developed for the use of mammographic images. This work introduces a deep learning-based approach for classifying breast cancer using digital mammography images. Features from mammographic images were extracted using two of current state-of-the-art, pre-trained Convolutional Neural Networks (CNNs): EfficientNetV2B0 and ConvNeXtBase, using over current best features derived from pre-processed images. The models were assessed independently and then jointly. ConvNeXtBase achieved an accuracy of 98.60% while EfficientNetV2B0 had an accuracy of 98.67%. The joint model had a classification accuracy of 98.33%. The study demonstrates the potential of the proposed methodology and the possibility that mammography and automated diagnosis tools could improve automated diagnosis of breast cancer.

Keywords Breast cancer · Mammography · Deep learning · Pretrained models · Model fusion

C. Soubai (✉) · A. Ait Abdelouahad
LAROSERI, Department of Computer Science, Faculty of Sciences, Chouaib Doukkali University, El Jadida, Morocco
e-mail: soubai.c042@ucd.ac.ma

A. Ait Abdelouahad
e-mail: a.abdelkaher@gmail.com

I. Bellamine
LSATE Laboratory, Department of Computer Science, Sidi Mohamed Ben Abdellah University, Fez, Morocco
e-mail: insafbellamine20@gmail.com

P. Singh et al. (eds.), *Deep Learning Applications in Healthcare and Medical Imaging Practice*, Studies in Big Data 193, https://doi.org/10.1007/978-3-032-21009-8_18

1 Introduction

Breast cancer is still a significant public health issue and still a leading cause of cancer deaths in females worldwide [1]. Early detection of breast cancer increases the likelihood of treatment success and long-term survival [2]. Mammography is the standard method of screening for breast cancer; however, mammographic interpretation involves subjectivity and can be time-consuming, as there is variability among observers which can lead to diagnostic inaccuracy.

Recently, deep learning has made quite an impact in medical imaging; convolutional neural networks (CNNs) allow the user to bypass handcrafted features and learn relevant representations from the data. CNN-based models have been found to perform well on many diagnostic tasks, including classifying breast cancer from mammograms [3].

A number of previous investigations examined this area of study. Li et al. [4] proposed DenseNet-II, a convolutional neural network approach that included methods such as data augmentation and modules that would discourage overfitting of models, and demonstrated dense operational performance as compared to VGGNet and GoogLeNet. Zhang et al. [5] implemented a model, DE-Ada, which undertook multi-level fusion and ensemble learning with both targeted embeddings and handcrafted features, attaining improved predictive performance over standard baselines on the CBIS-DDSM and INbreast datasets. Mohanty et al. [6] and colleagues introduced a CAD sys-tem that integrates BDWPT, PCA, and an optimized KELM enhanced by a chaotic salp swarm algorithm. This approach demonstrated strong performance on the MIAS, DDSM, and BCDR datasets. Loizidou et al. [7] created a temporal subtraction method that utilized six weak classifiers, thus providing emphasis on the significance of temporal imaging data. Li et al. [8] described DUALCORENET: A dual-path convolutional neural networks algorithm that encompasses four learning types (e.g., texture, context and geometry-aware). Sharma et al. [9] presented a computer-aided method to classify mammograms as benign or malignant using deep features derived from a modified DCNN, alongside GLCM and LBP texture features, with transfers learning, data augmentation, and an ensemble boosted tree classifier on the MIAS dataset. Patil et al. [10] offered an automated breast cancer detection approach with RG-AFCM, GLCM/GLRM, and a recurrent neural network trained using AFU-GOA, and obtained better accuracy and reduce false positives with respect to the MIAS dataset. There are still challenges regarding the accuracy and robustness when models are combined. This paper proposes a new method for the classification of breast cancer in digital mammography through the use of two high-performing pre-trained convolutional neural networks: EfficientNetV2B0 and ConvNeXtBase. Each model is independently evaluated and fused in a dual-branch fusion architecture as well.

The paper proceeds with the following structure:

- Section 2 describes the data set, and the preprocessing steps and proposed methodology.

- Section 3 presents the experimental results, performance metrics and relative evaluation.
- Finally, Sect. 4 concludes the paper with a summary of the main findings and some key take-aways.

2 Materials and Methodology

2.1 Dataset

In this work, we utilized the following dataset, CBIS-DDSM [11], features high-quality mammography images in PNG format. Each image is typically 1024 × 1024 pixels. This set includes 2fig, 857 images from about 1,566 patients, with each person providing one or two images. The dataset's composition is split into two groups: 1,018 images are marked as benign, and 570 as malignant. This imbalance, where the malignant category has fewer examples, is evident in Fig. 1.

The data set was divided into training groups (70%), validation groups (15%), and testing groups (15%). To make them work better with convolutional neural networks, all images were resized to 224 × 224 × 3 pixels.

To help the model avoid overfitting and to make it more reliable, data augmentation was performed using TensorFlow. This involved tweaking brightness, saturation, and contrast and doing horizontal flips. The study also balanced the dataset by oversampling the malignant images, leading to an even count of 712 images in each class. After data augmentation, both classes had 3,489 images each, making the dataset balanced and more reliable. This balance reduces bias from uneven class distribution and helps the model generalize better, as shown in Table 1.

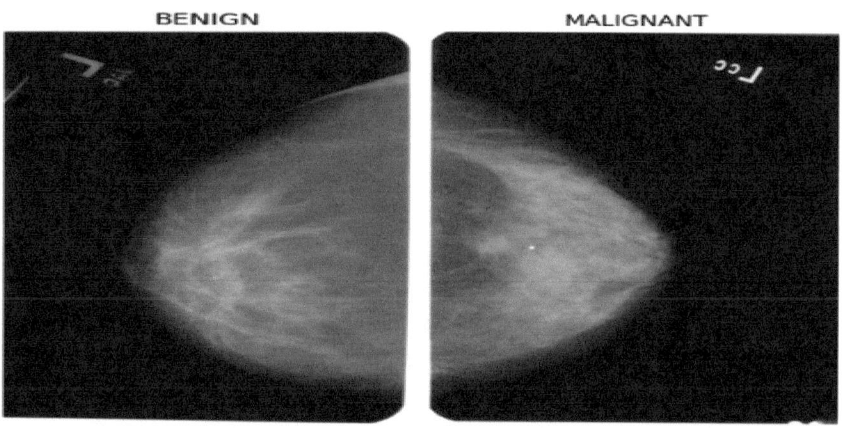

Fig. 1 Examples of mammogram images (benign or malignant) in your dataset

Table 1 Summary of data augmentation and class balancing for mammograms

Data	Number of samples	Training samples	Augmented training samples	Test samples
Benign	1018	865	3489	153
Malignant	570	484	3489	86
Total	1588	1349	6978	239

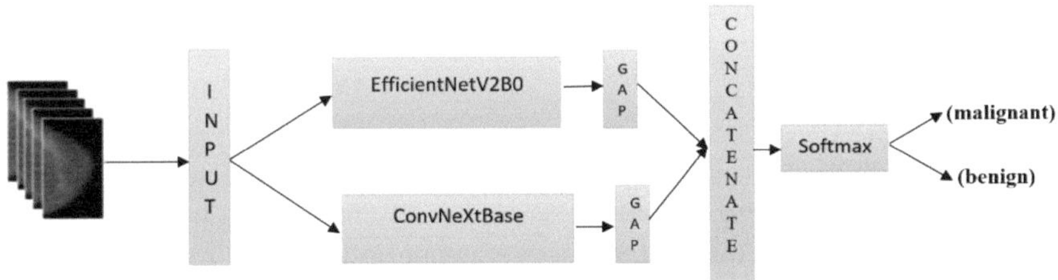

Fig. 2 The proposed architecture of the concatenated network

2.2 *Proposed Model*

2.2.1 Diagram of the Overall Architecture

The architecture is a two-branch architecture composed of EfficientNetV2B0 and ConvNeXtBase where both branches are presented with the same mammogram image to extract complementary high-level features. Each branch then compresses its high-level features using a Global Average Pooling (GAP) layer since it reduces the dimension- ality of the data while maintaining important information. These pooled features are concatenated and passed to a Softmax layer for classification into the two classes benign or malignant. This architecture increases the variety of available features, reduces the potential to overfit, and increases generalization (see Fig. 2).

2.2.2 Pre-trained Models Used

- Tan and Le proposed EfficientNetV2B0 [12], which is a convolutional neural network that uses compound scaling to maximize the sensitivity of depth, width, and resolution to improve accuracy while being more efficient than other methods. It employs fused MBConv blocks to reduce both latency and memory requirements while keeping the total model size smaller. EfficientNetV2B0 [13]. was used in this study on the CBIS-DDSM dataset to classify breast cancer in mammography images. It has good feature extraction and generalization capabilities that reduce overfitting and adapt to class imbalance, making it an appropriate network for medical image analysis.

- ConvNeXtBase [14] is a recent CNN that uses the traditional convolutional architecture, along with layer normalization, GELU activations, and large depthwise convolution filters, based on changes observed in Vision Transformers. Its stage-based design starts with a fixed number of channels, then progressively increases the channels while decreasing the spatial dimensions until it reaches the last stage. This design allows for better pattern recognition across wide areas of the image, advantageous in mammogram analysis. Additionally, ConvNeXtBase applies global average pooling at the end, retaining key features for effective classification. Overall, ConvNeXtBase is a powerful and versatile model for breast cancer detection with digital mammograms.

2.2.3 Fusion Method

Our method utilized feature-level fusion. by fusing features learned by two pretrained models (ConvNeXtBase and EfficientNetV2B0) prior to classification [15]. In this way, the ConvNeXtBase deep feature extraction and EfficientNetB2V0 scalable efficiency was utilized, resulting in more accurate predictions. Both pretrained models performed well in the form of feature representation from ImageNet. Each branch also had a Global Average Pooling layer (GAP), which mitigated complexity and overfitting, whilst retaining pertinent information.

2.2.4 Training Details

Here is an overview of the key hyperparameters and training configuration utilized in this study, as detailed in Table 2.

Table 2 Model training and validation parameters

Parameter	Value
Learning rate	Adam
Number of epochs	20
Loss function	Categorical crossentropy
Optimizer	Adam (default parameters: $\beta_1 = 0.9, \beta_2 = 0.999$)
Early stopping/scheduler	EarlyStopping (patience = 3, restore best weights = True)

3 Experimental Results

3.1 Results

To assess the dual-branch models, the accuracy, loss, precision, recall and F1-score metrics were calculated. In this case, accuracy (Eq. 1) refers to the percentage of correctly classified mammograms out of the complete dataset [16].

$$Accuracy = \frac{TP + TN}{TP + TN + FP + FN} \times 100 \tag{1}$$

Categorical cross-entropy measured the training loss and is an indicator of prediction accuracy over the training process. Precision [17] measured the ratio of positive cases that were correctly predicted.

$$Precision = \frac{TP}{TP + FP} \times 100 \tag{2}$$

Recall [17], also known as sensitivity and shown in Eq. 3, checks how well the model finds all the actual positive examples. It tells us what share of real positives the model caught.

$$Recall = \frac{TP}{TP + FN} \times 100 \tag{3}$$

The F1-score [17], shown in Eq. 4, is a way to blend precision and recall into a single number. It's the harmonic mean of the two, so it gives a balanced picture of how well the model is doing, taking into account both the mistakes it makes in predicting false positives and the ones it misses in false negatives.

$$F1 - score = 100 \times \frac{Precision \times Recall}{Precision + Recall} \tag{4}$$

Taken together, these metrics give a full picture of how well the model works. They highlight not just how accurate its predictions are but also how well it generalizes to new data in classifying breast cancer from mammograms.

Table 3 lays out the classification results for the CBIS-DDSM dataset, comparing two different feature extraction models: EfficientNetV2B0 and ConvNeXtBase. It shows key metrics like accuracy, loss, precision, recall, and F1-score [19], giving a complete picture of how each model performs. Both models turned in strong results. The training and validation performance plots for ConvNeXtBase and EfficientNetV2B0 are illustrated in Figs. 3 and 4, respectively.

Table 3 Classification results of feature extraction on the CBIS-DDSM dataset

Model	Accuracy	Loss	Precision	Recall
EfficientNetV2B0	0.9867	0.0506	0.9860	0.9860
ConvNeXtBase	0.9860	0.0816	0.9860	0.9860

3.2 Comparison and Discussion

A comparison was made between different deep learning models. Models like DenseNet121, ResNet50, and VGG19 performed well, but the standout performers were EfficientNetV2B0 and ConvNeXtBase. Table 4 shows this clearly: these two models came out ahead in terms of accuracy, precision, and recall. Their results confirm they're better at finding key details and features in mammogram images, making them stronger and more reliable choices for this type of task.

In comparison to other recent deep learning strategies (Table 5), our proposed dual-branch model consisting of the fused ConvNeXtBase and EfficientNetV2B0 generated, to the best of our knowledge, the highest accuracy (98.33%) on the CBIS-DDSM dataset. Several previous studies included Salama et al. (84.21%), Tsochatzidis et al. (AUC 0.86), Khan et al. (88%), and Zahoor et al. (90.3%).

The feature fusion and feature-level training approach increases generalization and reduces the risk of overfitting while leveraging the complementary strengths of both models. Furthermore, it enables a high-performing model that is resistant to variability in input data, which is extremely advantageous in the context of medical imaging and analysis. The trade-off associated with feature fusion and dual-branch methods is increased complexity in the final model and the need for additional memory, longer training time and so forth, which may limit the use of such a strategy in lower resource settings. Nevertheless, feature-level fusion has proven to be a powerful means of achieving a high, reliable, and accurate classification of breast cancer.

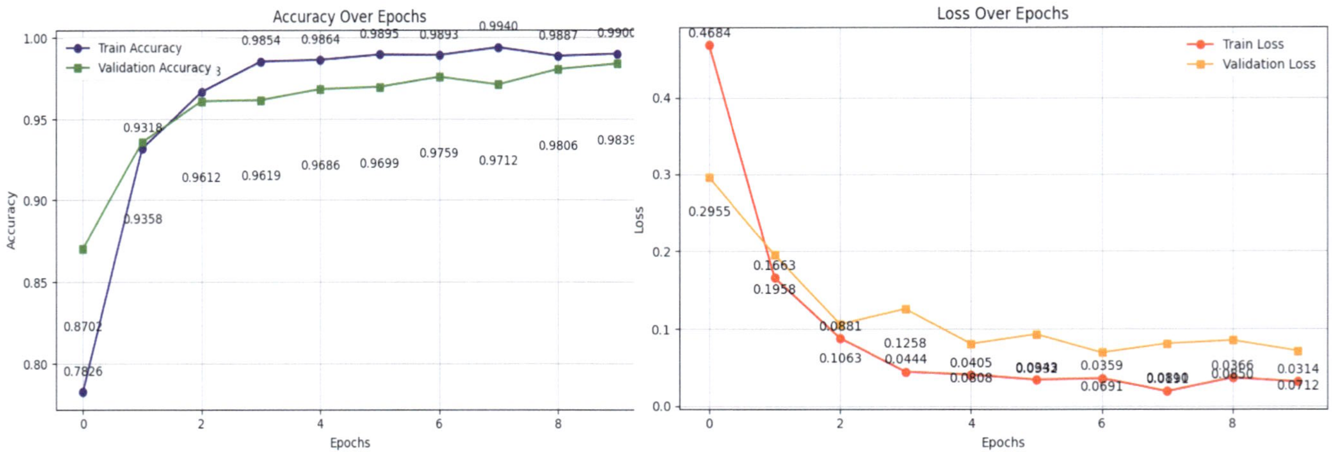

Fig. 3 ConvNeXtBase training/validation performance plots (accuracy and loss) per epoch

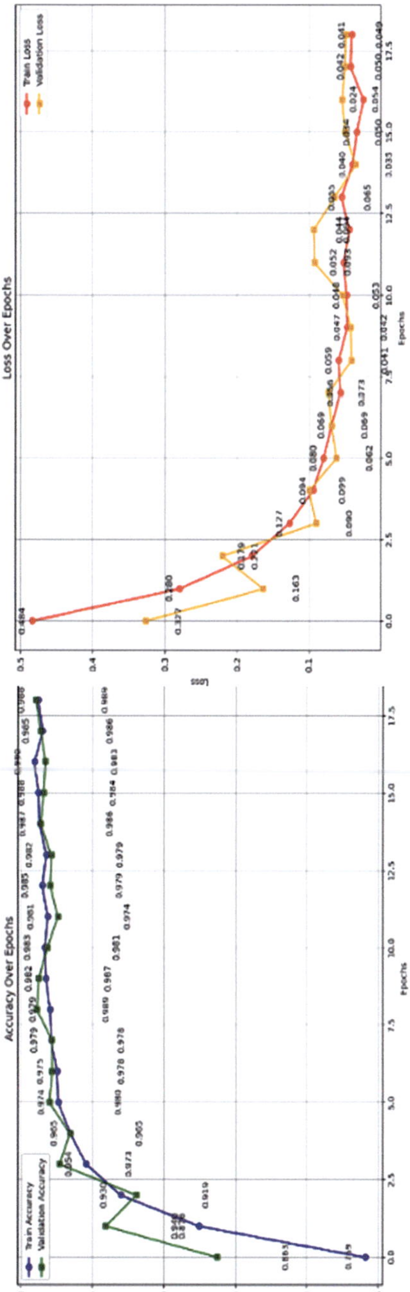

Fig. 4 EfficientNetV2B0 training/validation performance plots (accuracy and loss) per epoch

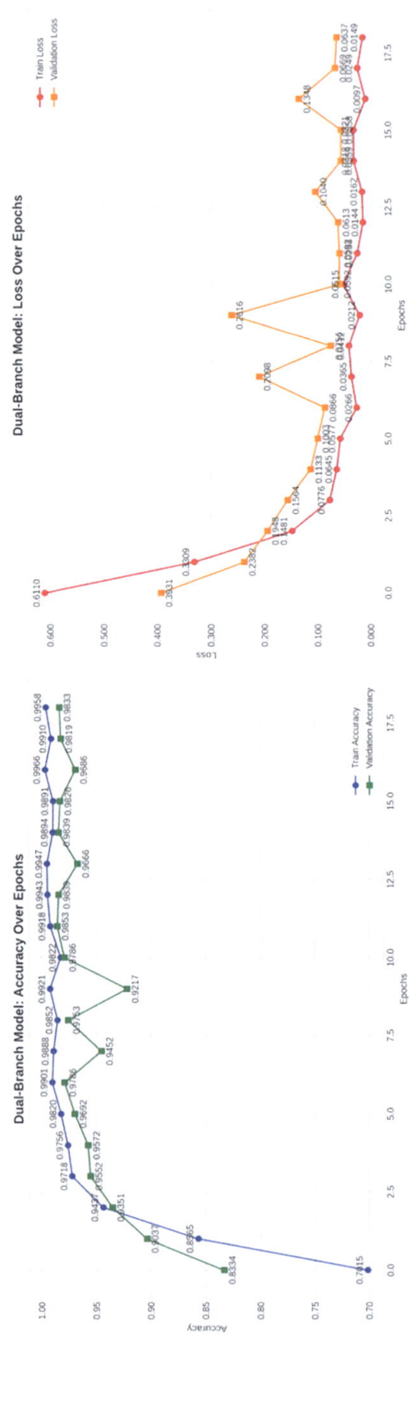

Fig. 5 Performance curves (accuracy and loss) of the final model during training and validation over epochs

Table 4 Detection and classification of breast cancer using transfer learning techniques

Model	Accuracy	Loss	Precision	Recall
Xception	0.9145	0.4002	0.9145	0.9145
VGG19	0.9424	0.1989	0.9424	0.9424
DenseNet121	0.9529	0.1494	0.9529	0.9529
MobileNet	0.8915	0.5177	0.8915	0.8915
MobileNetV2	0.7726	1.2915	0.7726	0.7726
ResNet50	0.9560	0.1773	0.9560	0.9560
InceptionV3	0.8793	0.3689	0.8793	0.8793
NASNetMobile	0.8743	0.6380	0.8743	0.8743
EfficientNetV2B0 + ConvNeXtBase	0.9833	0.0637	0.9833	0.9833

Table 5 Comparison of the current model with some of the more recent models

References	Year	Methodology	Dataset	Accuracy/ metrics
Salama et al. [18]	2021	Segmentation and classification using transfer learning-based CNN	MIAS, DDSM, CBIS-DDSM	TL models: VGG16 (80.98%) DenseNet121 (82.47%) MobileNetV2 (79.82%) ResNet50 (81.65%) InceptionV3 (84.21%)
Tsochatzidis et al. [19]	2021	Mass segmentation and diagnosis with modified pre-trained ResNet50	DDSM, CBIS-DDSM	AUC: 0.86
Khan et al. [20]	2021	Classification of calcifications, masses, asymmetries and carci-noma using ResNet50- based TL and custom CNN	CBIS-DDSM	Accuracy: 88%
Zahoor et al. [21]	2022	Feature fusion using MEWOA and fine-tuned MobileNetV2 + NasNetMo- bile CNNs	CBIS-DDSM	Accuracy: 93.8%
Present model	2025	Fusion of ConvNeXtBase and EfficientNetV2B0 features was used to enhance breast cancer classification	CBIS-DDSM	Accuracy: 98.33%

4 Conclusion

To sum it all up, this study put forward a dual-branch deep learning setup that blends features from both ConvNeXtBase and EfficientNetV2B0. The goal? More accurate breast cancer detection in digital mammograms. The model did remarkably well, hitting 98.33% accuracy on the CBIS-DDSM dataset higher than what most top-performing methods have managed so far. This result highlights how pulling in features from two different types of models helps the system adapt better, avoid overfitting, and stay consistent in its performance.

Of course, it is not without trade-offs. Running two heavyduty networks means it takes more power and more time to generate predictions. Still, the noticeable jump in accuracy makes this kind of dual-branch fusion a promising choice for future tools in breast cancer detection.

References

1. World Health Organization: Cancer. World Health Organization (2021). https://www.who.int/news-room/fact-sheets/detail/cancer
2. Tabár, L., Yen, T., Vitak, B., Chen, H.H., Smith, S.W.: The impact of mammographic screening on breast cancer mortality: a review of experimental and observational studies. Radiol. Clin. North Am. **48**(5), 999–1013 (2011)
3. Shen, D., Wu, G., Suk, H.I.: Deep learning in medical image analysis. Annu. Rev. Biomed. Eng. **19**, 221–248 (2017)
4. Li, H., Niu, J., Li, D.-A., Zhang, C.: Benign and malignant classification of mammogram images based on deep learning. Biomed. Signal Process. Control **51**, 347–354 (2019)
5. Zhang, H., Wu, R., Tian, Y., Jiang, Z., et al.: DE-Ada: a novel model for breast mass classification using cross-modal pathological semantic mining and organic integration of multi-feature fusions. Inf. Sci. **539**, 461–486 (2020)
6. Mohanty, F.: An improved scheme for digital mammogram classification using weighted chaotic salp swarm algorithm-based kernel extreme learning machine. Appl. Soft Comput. **91**, 106266 (2020)
7. Loizidou, K.: An automated breast micro-calcification detection and classification technique using temporal subtraction of mammograms. IEEE Access **8**, 52785–52795 (2020)
8. Li, H.: Dual convolutional neural networks for breast mass segmentation and diagnosis in mammography. IEEE Trans. Med. Imaging **41**(1), 3–13 (2022)
9. Sharma, B.P.: Ensemble boosted tree based mammogram image classification using texture features and extracted smart features of deep neural network. ADCAIJ **10**(4), 419–434 (2022)
10. Patil, R.S.: A new automated segmentation and classification of mammogram images. Multimed. Tools Appl. **81**(6), 7783–7816 (2022)
11. Safwan, A.W., et al.: CBIS-DDSM: breast cancer image dataset. Kaggle. https://www.kaggle.com/datasets/awsaf49/cbis-ddsm-breast-cancer-image-dataset. Last accessed 30 May 2025
12. Tan, M., Le, Q.V.: EfficientNetV2: smaller models and faster training (2021). arXiv preprint arXiv:2104.00298
13. TensorFlow: EfficientNetV2 documentation (2025). https://www.tensorflow.org/api_docs/python/tf/keras/applications/efficientnet_v2. Last accessed 30 May 2025
14. Liu, Z., et al.: A ConvNet for the 2020s. In: Proceedings of the IEEE/CVF Conference on Computer Vision and Pattern Recognition (CVPR) (2022)

15. Belhumeur, P.N., et al.: Performance evaluation of the nearest feature line method in image classification and retrieval. IEEE Trans. Pattern Anal. Mach. Intell. **19**(7), 681–685 (1997)
16. Saito, T.: The precision-recall plot is more informative than the ROC plot when evaluating binary classifiers on imbalanced datasets. PLoS ONE **10**(3), e0118432 (2015)
17. Scikit-learn: Precision, recall and F-measure metrics (2025). https://scikit-learn.org/stable/modules/model_evaluation.html#precision-recall-f-measure-metrics. Last accessed 30 May 2025
18. Salama, W.M., Aly, M.H.: Deep learning in mammography images segmentation and classification: automated CNN approach. Alex. Eng. J. **60**(5), 4701–4709 (2021)
19. Tsochatzidis, L., Koutla, P., Costaridou, L., Pratikakis, I.: Integrating segmentation information into CNN for breast cancer diagnosis of mammographic masses. Comput. Methods Progr. Biomed. **200**, 105913 (2021)
20. Heenaye-Mamode Khan, M., Boodoo-Jahangeer, N., Dullull, W., Nathire, S., Gao, X., Sinha, G.R., Nagwanshi, K.K.: Multi-class classification of breast cancer abnormalities using deep convolutional neural network (CNN). PLoS ONE **16**(8), 1–15 (2021)
21. Zahoor, S., Shoaib, U., Lali, I.U.: Breast cancer mammograms classification using deep neural network and entropy-controlled whale optimization algorithm. Diagnostics **12**(2), 557 (2022)

Marine Predators Algorithm for Optimizer Configuration in Breast Ultrasound Image Segmentation

Fouzia El Abassi, Aziz Darouichi, and Aziz Ouaarab

Abstract Breast ultrasound image segmentation to detect breast cancer early is important but difficult due to speckle noise and anatomy variations. Though deep learning models have enhanced segmentation accuracy, the impact of optimizer selection has been comparatively less researched. This work proposes a training-centered strategy grounded on the Marine Predators Algorithm (MPA) to fine-tune the Lookahead optimizer by selecting the best base optimizer and tuning crucial hyper- parameters (learning rate, synchronization period α, and interpolation factor k). Experimental results on the BUSI dataset with U-Net and Ef- ficientNetB7 encoder show that MPA-optimized configurations are much better than usual. The optimum three settings (Opt4, Opt3, and Opt6) were at Dice measures of 78.78%, 78.64%, and 78.60% respectively, categorically affirming that metaheuristic tuning is optimum for improving segmentation accuracy.

Keywords Breast ultrasound · Medical image segmentation · Optimizer tuning · Marine predators algorithm · Lookahead

1 Introduction

Breast cancer is the most common cancer in women globally and one of the top causes of cancer deaths. In 2022 alone, more than 43,000 people died of it in the United States [1] and remains the most common type of cancer in women in Morocco [2]. Early

F. El Abassi (✉) · A. Darouichi · A. Ouaarab
Computer and Systems Engineering Laboratory (L2IS), FSTG, Cadi Ayyad University, Marrakesh, Morocco
e-mail: f.elabassi.ced@uca.ac.ma

A. Darouichi
e-mail: a.darouichi@uca.ac.ma

A. Ouaarab
e-mail: a.ouaarab@uca.ac.ma

F. El Abassi
LAMIGEP, EMSI Marrakesh, Marrakesh, Morocco

P. Singh et al. (eds.), *Deep Learning Applications in Healthcare and Medical Imaging Practice*, Studies in Big Data 193, https://doi.org/10.1007/978-3-032-21009-8_19

and accurate detection is critical to improving prognosis, yet remains challenging particularly with ultrasound imaging, which, while widely accessible and safe, suffers from low contrast, speckle noise, and high operator dependency. These limitations make lesion segmentation in breast ultrasound (BUS) images a difficult task, often hindering diagnostic consistency. Recent advances in deep learning have improved computer-aided diagnosis (CAD) systems for BUS image segmentation. Among state-of-the-art approaches, architectural changes play a very dominating role.

For example, UltraSegNet in [3] uses the attention mechanisms and Squeeze-and-Excitation modules in enhancing anatomical features. Meanwhile, in Moroccan BreastCare framework [4], both the segmentation and classification processes are carried out together along with Attention-DenseUNet and EfficientNetB7. Other relevant techniques include DFLNet [5], which uses parallel ConvNeXt encoders with cross-attention, and 3D UNet++ [6], which enhances multiscale fusion through nested skip connections. Ensemble models like EDCNN [7] emphasize further that segmenting, classifying, and explaining are the core aspects of CAD pipelines. Later, [8] proposed a Multi-Task Interaction Learning (MTIL) framework, which learns segmentation and classification of the images of the breast in ultrasound in an simultaneous manner by making use of shared feature extraction as well as inter-task dependencies. Similarly, [9] presented a Hybrid Attention Network (HANet) that combined DenseNet121 encoders and multi-scale attention mechanisms in order to improve boundary localization as well as tumor segmentation accuracy.

Despite all these developments in architecture, the impact of training dynamics in particular optimizer configuration has received little attention. Optimizer selection and hyperparameter tuning are critical for convergence behavior and final model performance. However, most existing work applies standard optimizers with default values perhaps without considering configurations that would have been more effective.

In this paper, we present a training-centric optimization strategy to BUS image segmentation. We utilize explicitly the Marine Predators Algorithm (MPA), a nature-inspired metaheuristic, to optimize the Lookahead optimizer. We explore the hybrid space created by discrete base optimizer choice and continuous hyperparameter space exploration (learning rate, synchronization step, and interpolation coefficient). We evaluate the proposed approach with a U-Net model that has an EfficientNetB7 encoder on the BUSI dataset. Experimental findings indicate that highly optimized configurations by MPA obtain much superior seg- mentation performance than in conventional settings with respect to Dice score and Intersection over Union. The remainder of the paper is organized as follows: Sect. 2 presents the proposed method, Sect. 3 outlines the experimental setup, Sect. 4 discusses results, and Sect. 5 concludes the study.

2 Proposed Approach

2.1 Overview of Our Approach

This paper aims at enhancing the performance of medical image segmentation using optimization of the configuration of the Lookahead [10] optimizer and the choice of the most suitable base optimizer for the analysis of breast ultrasound. Leveraging the BUSI dataset, we cast the optimization problem as a hybrid search one, involving discrete and continuous variables.

The search space includes a finite set of six widely used base optimizers (SGD, Adam, RMSprop, Lion, AdamW, and RAdam) and continuous hyperparameters such as learning rate (log-scaled between 10^{-5} and 10^{-2}), the Lookahead interpolation factor α (in the range 0.2 to 0.8), and the synchronization step interval k (an integer from 2 to 10). In order to effectively navigate this high-dimensional search space, we employ the Marine Predators Algorithm (MPA) [11], a new nature-inspired metaheuristic dedicated to global optimization. The underlying segmentation model is a U-Net [12] with an EfficientNetB7 pretrained encoder, chosen for its balance between richness of features and computational expense. This optimizer-focused approach deflects attention from architectural changes and towards training dynamics to locate synergistic settings that improve convergence and segmentation accuracy in the context of clinical imaging.

The overall optimization workflow for selecting and tuning the Lookahead optimizer using the Marine Predators Algorithm is outlined in Fig. 1.

2.2 Marine Predators Algorithm (MPA)

Marine Predators Algorithm (MPA) is a nature-inspired metaheuristic algorithm that imitates foraging activities of sea predators using coupled Brownian motion and

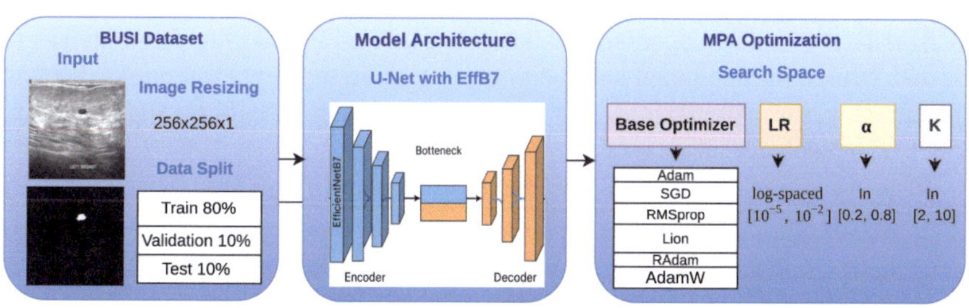

Fig.1 Optimization of lookahead configuration using MPA

Lévy flight to balance exploration and exploitation between the search space. The algorithm progresses through the following main steps:

1. **Initialization**: An initial population of candidate solutions X_i is randomly generated within the variable bounds $[X_{min}, X_{max}]$, where each individual represents a solution in a d-dimensional space.
2. **Exploration Phase (Brownian Motion)**: This phase encourages global exploration using random walks modeled by Brownian motion:

$$X_i(t+1) = X_i(t) + r1 \cdot B \cdot \left(X_j(t) - X_k(t)\right) \tag{1}$$

   where B is a Brownian vector (sampled from a normal distribution), r1 is a random factor, and X_j, X_k are randomly selected individuals.
3. **Transition Phase (Lévy Flight)**: To maintain diversity, Lévy flight is used to introduce long-distance exploratory steps:

$$X_i(t+1) = X_i(t) + r2 \cdot L \cdot (X_b(t) - X_i(t)) \tag{2}$$

   where L is drawn from a Lévy distribution, and $X_b(t)$ denotes the best solution found so far.
4. **Exploitation Phase (Intensification)**: The final phase emphasizes local search around the best solutions using an elitist strategy:

$$X_i(t+1) = X_i(t) + \alpha \cdot (X_b - X_i(t)) \tag{3}$$

   where $\alpha \in [0, 1]$ is an intensification factor guiding the convergence speed toward X_b.

3 Experimental Setup

BUSI dataset [13] is an open-source dataset of labeled breast ultrasound images as normal, benign, or malignant and their corresponding segmentation masks. 80% of the dataset was used for training, 10% for validation, and 10% for testing, resized to 256×256 pixels for all images.

As an evaluation measure, we used Intersection over Union (IoU), Dice Similarity Coefficient (DSC), and Recall as defined by the Eq. 4:

$$IoU = \frac{TP}{(TP + FP + FN)} \; DSC = \frac{2 \cdot TP}{(2 \cdot TP + FP + FN)} \; Recall = \frac{TP}{(TP + FN)} \tag{4}$$

where TP, FP, and FN refer to the number of true positives, false positives, and false negatives, respectively.

4 Quantitative and Qualitative Results

Table 1 demonstrates performance of various optimizers experimented on the BUSI dataset with particular attention towards the Dice Score (DSC). As ob- served, from the classical optimizers, AdamW was found to perform best with an optimum Dice value of 76.22%, while the worst was SGD with a minimum Dice value of 18.04%. In comparison, all six optimizers based on the Marine Predators Algorithm (Opt1–Opt6, explained in Table 2) outperformed classical optimizers in terms of DSC. Opt4 provided the highest overall Dice score of 78.78%, followed closely by Opt3 (78.64%), Opt6 (78.60%), and Opt1 (78.25%). This consistent improvement demonstrates that MPA is effective at discovering optimizer configurations that enhance segmentation accuracy.

The detailed configurations of the top-performing optimizers discovered using MPA are listed in Table 3.

Figure 2 illustrate qualitative segmentation results comparing traditional optimizers with those tuned via the MPA. Traditional optimizers like Adam and RAdam

Table 1 Comparison of optimizers on the BUSI dataset

Optimizer	Dice	IoU	Recall	Specificity
Adam	74.81	66.28	76.12	97.56
RAdam	76.06	67.70	75.78	**98.52**
AdamW	76.22	67.15	**79.52**	96.92
RMSProp	75.44	66.41	77.13	97.43
SGD	18.04	10.65	78.74	41.35
Lion	76.23	67.31	76.79	97.68
Opt3 (Ours)	78.64	70.23	78.20	98.34
Opt4 (Ours)	**78.78**	**70.68**	78.28	98.05

Table 2 The six best optimizers obtained using MPA

Iteration	Population	Optimizer	Dice	IoU	Recall	Specificity
	10	Opt1	78.25	69.88	**80.43**	97.90
10	10	Opt2	76.13	67.47	79.10	97.09
	10	Opt3	**78.64**	**70.23**	78.20	**98.34**
	10	Opt4	**78.78**	**70.68**	**78.28**	98.05
20	10	Opt5	77.64	68.86	74.98	98.37
	10	Opt6	78.60	70.13	77.96	**98.52**

Table 3 Best optimizer configurations obtained with MPA

Optimizer	Base optimizer	Learning rate	α	k
Opt1	AdamW	0.000446	0.2560	8
Opt2	Adam	0.000250	0.4696	3
Opt3	AdamW	0.000266	0.2793	2
Opt4	Lion	0.000017	0.6020	9
Opt5	RAdam	0.000309	0.6555	2
Opt6	RAdam	0.000440	0.5730	2

provide decent lesion delineation, but some results particularly with SGD show poor boundary definition and noisy predictions. In contrast, the MPA-optimized configurations (Opt1–Opt6) produce cleaner, more accurate segmentations that closely follow the ground truth in both shape and boundary precision.

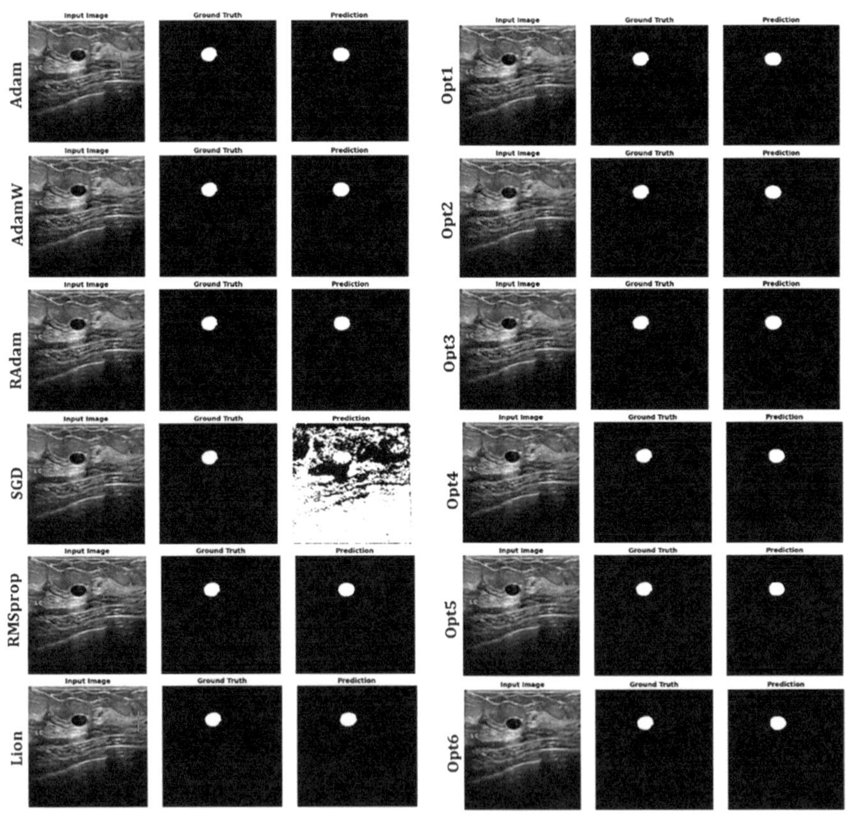

Fig. 2 Qualitative results of UNetEfficientNetB7 with traditional and our best- performing optimizers

5 Discussion

Quantitative and qualitative results confirm the effectiveness of Marine Predators Algorithm (MPA) in optimizing training dynamics of medical image segmentation. MPA parameters (Opt1–Opt6) outperformed traditional optimizers in terms of Dice and IoU scores, the optimal Dice (78.78%) and IoU (70.68%) achieved by Opt4. Equivalence of Opt3 and Opt6 performance ensures the robustness of metaheuristic search with respect to varying sets of parameter values.

Unlike fixed optimization methods, the MPA-adjusted hyperparameters not only improved segmentation quality but also achieved a better trade-off between boundary precision and region overlap. This highlights that optimizer configuration, guided by metaheuristics, can significantly enhance performance without altering network architecture.

6 Conclusion

This study proposed an optimizer-tuning approach based on the Marine Predators Algorithm (MPA) for breast ultrasound image segmentation using the Lookahead optimizer. The approach was tested on a U-Net architecture using an Efficient-NetB7 encoder on the BUSI dataset, where it showed superior performance over conventional optimizers. Though the proposed approach of MPA was validated only on one dataset, which has an effect on generalizability, and the search space was limited to an input predefined set of hyperparameter. To overcome such constraints, the future research will generalize the validation of the approach to other medical imaging modalities such as thyroid or liver ultrasound. To reduce computational expense, adaptive or more cost-effective variants of MPA will be explored. In addition, expanding the search space to include more heterogeneous or hybrid optimizers and incorporating explainability metrics in the optimization objective can both enhance performance and clinical interpretability.

References

1. Nawaz, S.: Advances in ai-driven breast cancer screening: challenges and opportunities. Intell. Based Med. **11**, 100254 (2025). https://doi.org/10.1016/j.ibmed.2025.100254
2. of Health, M.M.: Breast cancer statistics in morocco, 2025 report (2025). https://sante.gov.ma/statistics
3. Abuowaida, S., Owida, H.A., Alsekait, D.M., Alshdaifat, N., AbdElminaam, D.S., Alshinwan, M.: Ultrasegnet: a hybrid deep learning framework for enhanced breast cancer segmentation and classification on ultrasound images. Comput. Mater. Contin. **83**(2) (2025)
4. Erragzi, N., Zrira, N., Lanjeri, S., Omor, Y., Jimi, A., Benmiloud, I., Sebihi, R., Latib, R., Ngote, N., Khan, H.A., et al.: Breastcare application: Moroccan breast cancer diagnosis through deep learning-based image segmentation and classification. Intell. Based Med. 100254 (2025)

5. Ye, Z., Huang, J., Zhang, Y., Deng, J., Zhang, J., Liu, S., Wang, D., Mei, L., Lei, C.: Dflnet: disentangled feature learning network for breast cancer ultrasound image segmentation. Digit. Signal Process. 105331 (2025)
6. Hesaraki, S., Mohammed, A.S., Eisaei, M., Mousa, R.: Breast cancer ultrasound image segmentation using improved 3dunet++. WFUMB Ultrasound Open 100068 (2025)
7. Islam, M.R., Rahman, M.M., Ali, M.S., Nafi, A.A.N., Alam, M.S., Godder, T.K., Miah, M.S., Islam, M.K.: Enhancing breast cancer segmentation and classification: an ensemble deep convolutional neural network and u-net approach on ultrasound images. Mach. Learn. Appl. **16**, 100555 (2024)
8. Zheng, Y., Kumar, S., Li, X., Zhang, L.: Multi-task interaction learning for accurate segmentation and classification of breast tumors in ultrasound images. Med. Image Anal. **98**, 103245 (2025)
9. Aslam, T., Chen, R., Alqahtani, H., Rahman, M.: Hybrid attention network for accurate breast tumor segmentation in ultrasound images. In: Proceedings of the IEEE/CVF Conference on Computer Vision and Pattern Recognition (CVPR), pp. 12543–12552 (2025)
10. Zhang, M.R., Lucas, J., Hinton, G., Ba, J.: Lookahead optimizer: k steps forward, 1 step back. Adv. Neural Inf. Process. Syst. **32** (2019)
11. Faramarzi, A., Heidarinejad, M., Stephens, B., Mirjalili, S.: Marine predators algorithm: a nature-inspired metaheuristic. Expert Syst. Appl. **152**, 113377 (2020)
12. Ronneberger, O., Fischer, P., Brox, T.: U-net: convolutional networks for biomedical image segmentation. In: International Conference on Medical Image Computing and Computer-Assisted Intervention, pp. 234–241. Springer (2015)
13. Al-Dhabyani, W., Gomaa, M., Khaled, H., Fahmy, A.: Dataset of breast ultrasound images. Data Brief **28**, 104863 (2020)

SVM-LSTM Comparison for Blood Hematocrit Prediction

Fatima Ezzahra El Kamouny, Abdellah Madani, Hassan Oukhouya, and Khadija El Kamouny

Abstract We describe a novel, portable optical tool enabling non-invasive hematocrit determination from a single drop of blood. An attractive alternative to current methods, this fast, precise, and portable solution is particularly adapted to ex-vivo clinical environments such as dialysis or mobile clinics. The NIR spectrum of the term is measured by the instrument, which is subsequently preprocessed for noise removal through various filters like Standard Normal Variate (SNV), Multiplicative Scatter Correction (MSC), and smoothing through the Savitzky-Golay filter. To develop supervised learning models, the preprocessed spectra are combined with hematocrit values that had been measured. Training and test data sets were split at 70% and 30%, respectively. Hyperparameters of the Long Short-Term Memory (LSTM) and Support Vector Machine (SVM) models were optimized by cross-validation. Satisfactory results were obtained on tests with determination coefficients (R2) 0.914 for SVM and 0.929 for LSTM. The stability of the models was verified in a second test on 80 new observations with even better performance (R2 = 0.972 for LSTM, 0.956 for

F. E. El Kamouny (✉) · A. Madani
Laboratory LAROSERI, Department of Computer Science, Faculty of Science, Chouaib Doukkali University of El Jadida, El Jadida, Grand-Casablanca, Morocco
e-mail: elkamouny.fatima_ezzahra@ucd.ac.ma

A. Madani
e-mail: madani.a@ucd.ac.ma

H. Oukhouya
LaMSD, Team of MSASE, Department of Economics, FSJES, Mohammed First University, Oujda, Morocco

MAEGE Laboratory, Department of Statistics and Applied Mathematics, FSJES Aïn Sebaâ, Hassan II University, Casablanca, Morocco

H. Oukhouya
e-mail: oukhouya.hassan@ump.ac.ma

K. El Kamouny
Green Tech Institute Department, Mohammed VI Polytechnic University UM6P, Ben Guerir, Morocco
e-mail: khadija.elkamouny@um6p.ma

P. Singh et al. (eds.), *Deep Learning Applications in Healthcare and Medical Imaging Practice*, Studies in Big Data 193, https://doi.org/10.1007/978-3-032-21009-8_20

SVM). Therefore, from the simple blood test, this method can reliably estimate hematocrit values. Advanced AI algorithms and a compact unit offer the possibilities for handheld, accessible, and efficient medical therapies in various clinical applications.

Keywords Hematocrit prediction · Near-infrared spectroscopy · Non-invasive diagnosis · SVM · LSTM

1 Introduction

One of the most critical measurements for both diagnosis and follow-up of many hematological diseases like anemia and polycythemia is the accurate measurement of hematocrit (Hct) [1]. Techniques like centrifugation and flow cytometry are still reference methods to quantify Hct [2, 3]. There are, however, some very critical limitations to these techniques, i.e., that they are invasive, involve venous blood sampling, and are inconvenient to patients, particularly with serial measurements [4]. Furthermore, their relatively long processing time does not always comply with the fast diagnostic requirement of modern medicine [5]. Further, such techniques are hard to reach in distant or impoverished regions due to the demand on specialized laboratory equipment and skilled personnel [6]. Nearly 40% of poor nations' primary health care centers have no access to consistent hematological testing, according to recent World Health Organization research (WHO, 2023), which points to an acute problem with health care access equity [7]. These observations highlight the degree to which alternative, quick, low-cost, and non-surgical measurement techniques must be developed. One good substitute in this regard is near-infrared spectroscopy (NIRS), which operates within the range of 1300–2600 nm [8]. This technique enables optical properties of biological tissue to be determined without venous sample, upon the basis of the specific absorption bands of blood components [9]. Thus, it becomes possible to make instant, non-invasive diagnosis, potentially to be performed in the home or in low-resource environments [10, 11]. Among the spectrum of this, certain blood absorption bands had been found in earlier studies [12]. This strategy has now been aided by several technological advances, from the production of standard or anti-reflective coated quartz cuvettes [13, 14], availability of microfluidic systems enabling the analysis of extremely small volumes of blood [15], and miniaturization of optical instrumentation. The reliability and accuracy of NIR spectroscopy have also been significantly increased by recent advances in machine learning [16]. In comparison to reference methods, higher correlations than R2 = 0.95 have been obtained using predictive models like Support Vector Machines (SVM), artificial neural networks, and sequential models like Long Short-Term Memory (LSTM) networks [17]. Advanced spectrum preprocessing techniques that compensate for light scattering effects like Standard Normal Variate (SNV) and Multiplicative Scatter Correction (MSC) are responsible for the performances [18]. The rest of the improvements involve enhanced sensitivity of the equipment, tunable laser sources, and miniaturization of the sensors [19]. Relative hematocrit prediction errors were lowered to less than 5% by NIR and AI hybrid approaches, with diagnostic robustness also enhanced [20]. Because of their superior optical transmission in the NIR wavelength, quartz cuvettes are still needed [21]. The capacity of these models to capture temporal spectrum dynamics has also been shown by recent work combining LSTM networks, opening the door for more sophisticated predictive diagnostic systems. While Talati et al. [22] emphasized the developments of broadband NIRS for cerebral monitoring [23], recent investigations, such those by Saiko (2025), have expanded our knowledge of the optical characteristics of blood and its constituents in the visible and NIR areas [22]. Through a meta-analysis, Zheng and He [23] verified the accuracy of NIRS in neonatal post-transfusion monitoring [24]. Additionally, Silvaggio et al. (2025) established a methodological link between NIRS signals and cerebral blood volume, providing new perspectives for interpreting physiological signals [26], and Pérez-Gómez et al. [24] showed the efficacy of combining NIR with machine learning for serological detection of hepatitis C virus [25]. The significant potential of NIR spectroscopy in biological analysis and medical diagnostics is confirmed by these recent investigations. Our study's goal is to create a portable, intelligent gadget that can precisely measure the hematocrit from a single drop of blood in this quickly changing scientific and technological environment. In order to create a quick, accurate, and least intrusive diagnostic solution, this study attempts to integrate machine learning algorithms with the benefits of NIR spectroscopy (1300–2600 nm). The following are this work's primary contributions: 1. Creating a blood spectrum acquisition experimental technique with optimal preprocessing; 2. Using SVM and LSTM models to estimate hematocrit; and 3. Validating the suggested system experimentally and in comparison. This chapter's remaining sections are structured as follows: The theoretical underpinnings of machine learning applied to NIR spectroscopy are presented in Sect. 2; the experimental methodology, including acquisition and preprocessing protocols, is described in Sect. 3; the results are presented and discussed in Sect. 4; and the chapter is concluded and future directions are outlined in Sect. 5.

2 Machine Learning

SVM and LSTM neural networks, two machine learning techniques frequently employed in biomedical applications like illness diagnosis, are compared in this paper. To assess and contrast the prediction accuracy of the two models, they were trained on the same dataset. A representative dataset and meticulous hyperparameter adjustment are necessary for efficient supervised regression.

2.1 Support Vector Machine

SVM is a supervised learning technique for regression and classification. It seeks to identify the most effective hyperplane for class separation. The model's complexity and error tolerance are controlled by the parameters C and γ [26]. Here, the RBF kernel was selected to increase the precision of hematological parameter prediction.

The RBF kernelfunctionisdefined to:

$$k(x, x') = \exp(-\gamma||x - x'||2) \tag{1}$$

where: $\gamma = \frac{1}{2\sigma 2}$

In these equations, $||x - x'||2$ represents the squared Euclidean distance between two data points $\boldsymbol{x}$ and $\boldsymbol{x'}$.

2.2 Long Short-Term Memory Networks

Because LSTM networks are made to handle temporal sequences, they work especially well for non-invasive blood spectroscopy. By capturing intricate temporal correlations, they make it possible to estimate biological parameters from NIR spectra, such as glucose levels or hematocrit. A fully connected (dense) layer receives the characteristics that the LSTM layers have collected and transfers them to an output value, in this case the anticipated hematocrit [27]. Lastly, the anticipated value is provided by the model's output, enabling precise and non-invasive analysis. Figure 1 shows a diagram of this architecture that shows the data flow from spectral input to the final forecast.

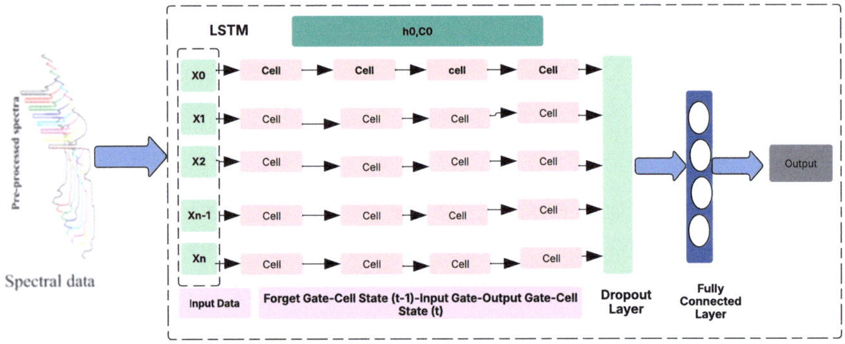

Fig. 1 LSTM architecture diagram

2.3 Performance Parameters

In the field of machine learning, there are various parameters used to evaluate the accuracy of models. They all calculate the error between the desired (or observed target) values and the predicted values.

The most commonly used performance parameters are [28–30]:

- The Mean Squared Error (MSE), estimated over n samples. It is defined as follows:

$$MSE(y,\tilde{y}) = \frac{1}{n}\sum_{i=1}^{n}(y_i - \tilde{y}_i)2 \tag{2}$$

- The Mean Absolute Error (MAE) also estimated over n samples. It is defined as follows:

$$MSE(y,\tilde{y}) = \frac{1}{n}\sum_{i=1}^{n}(y_i - \tilde{y}_i) \tag{3}$$

- The coefficient of determination (R^2), which is mathematically defined as follows:

$$R^2(y,\tilde{y}) = 1 - \frac{\sum_{i=1}^{n}(y_i - \tilde{y}_i)2}{\sum_{i=1}^{n}(y_i - \tilde{y}_i)2} \tag{4}$$

Where $\bar{y}$ is the mean of the observed values: $\tilde{y} = \frac{1}{n}\sum_{i=1}^{n}(y_i)$

This coefficient provides a measure of the model's ability to accurately predict future samples. A value of $R^2 = 1$ means that the model can perfectly predict every outcome. In Eqs. (3), (4), and (4), y_1, y_2... y_n represent the observed targets, and $\tilde{y}_1, \tilde{y}_2, \ldots, \tilde{y}_n$ the corresponding predicted values. The calculation of MSE, MAE, and R^2 allows for a statistical evaluation of model performance, thus facilitating their comparison.

3 Methodology

This research outlines a new approach to hematocrit (Hct) concentration estimation using the combination of near-infrared (NIR) spectroscopy and artificial intelligence. The procedure is thorough and properly organized into 13 major sections, from blood sampling to onsite final performance testing of prediction (see Fig. 2). After collecting a drop of blood and placing it in a special cuvette, signals in the 1300–2600 nm range are measured using an NIR spectrometer. Before being processed by machine learning models, the raw data undergoes preprocessing, including noise reduction,

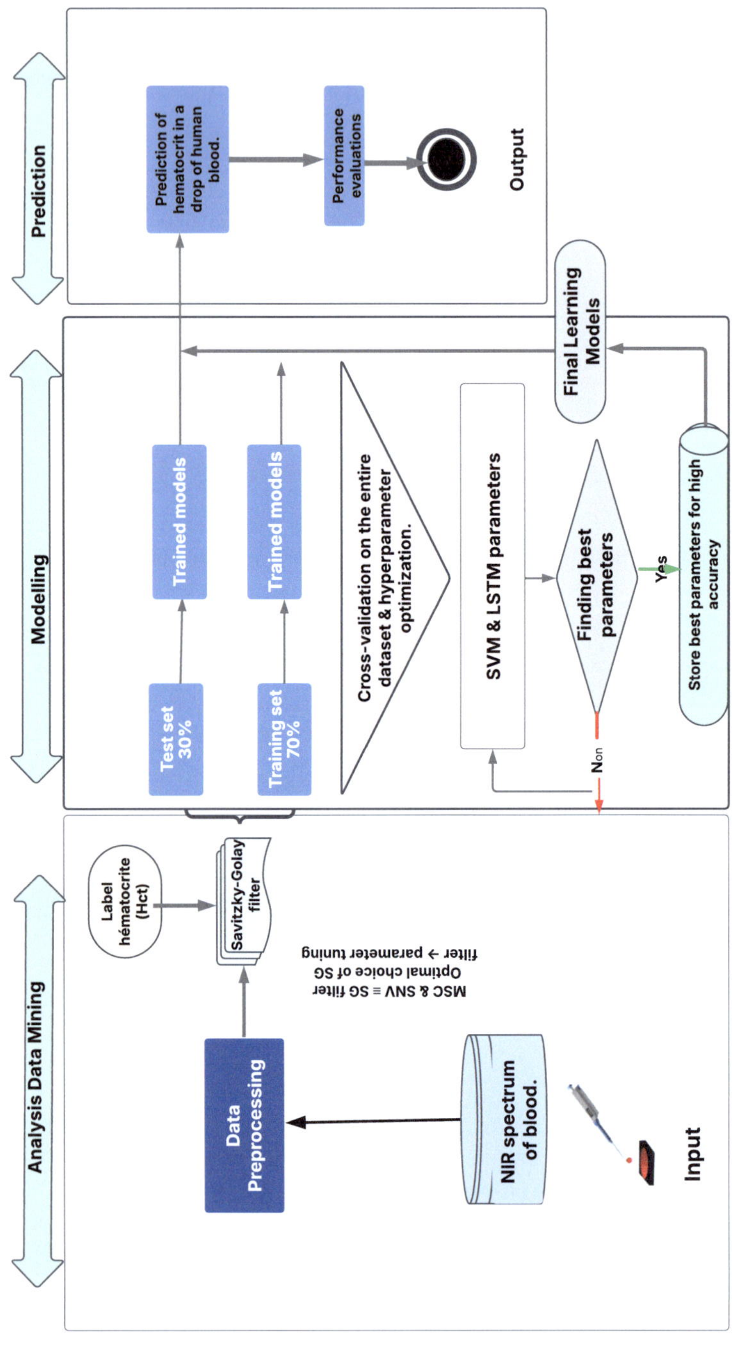

Fig. 2 Block diagram describing the methodology considered in this paper

normalization, and dimensionality reduction. A organized dataset containing components for testing and training isproduced. Two models LSTM and SVM are trained to non-invasively and rapidly forecast hematocrit levels. Regression measures like R2 and MSE are used to compare anticipated and actual values in order to assess the quality of the predictions.

3.1 Materials and Methods

3.1.1 Hematocrit Analysis in the Quodess Medical Laboratory

Between March and July 2022, hematocrit levels were assessed at the Quodess medical laboratory in Sidi Bennour. After a safe blood draw by a qualified nurse (see Fig. 3), the blood is immediately put into a purple tube that contains an anticoagulant to stop it from clotting. The hematocrit, or percentage of red blood cells in the total volume of blood, is then determined by centrifuging the samples to separate the blood components based on their densities. Anemia (reduction), polycythemia (increase), or normal range (37%–52%) can all be indicated by this measurement. RBC × MCV/10 is another formula that indirectly calculates hematocrit. With samples stored in ideal conditions prior to being analyzed to guarantee their reliability a priority part of correlation studies with the use of portable NIR spectroscopy this two-fold strategy improves accuracy of information.

3.1.2 Blood Sample Analysis Experiment Using NIR Spectroscopy

This study assesses a portable NIR sensor and a laboratory NIR spectrometer for bloodsample analysis covering a spectral range of 1000 to 2600 nm using the NeoSpectra interface for data processing. Among the equipment used in the experiment were an NIR spectrometer, a micropipette, glass slides, disposable tips, and cuvettes with an anticoagulant to preserve the materials (Fig. 4). A drop of blood wasplaced on a glass slide for spectroscopic analysis with a laboratory spectrometer following a nurse'smeticulous sample collection procedure. The analysis entaile dexposing the samples to an NIR light source and recording their transmission spectra in order to compare the performance of the two devices.

3.2 Data Collection and Spectral Preprocessing

NIR spectroscopy was used to analyze 504 human blood samples both in the field using a portable sensor and in the laboratory using a high-precision spectrometer. Hematocrit values were used to calibrate prediction models after validation using centrifugation and reference analysis. Three different preprocessing techniques

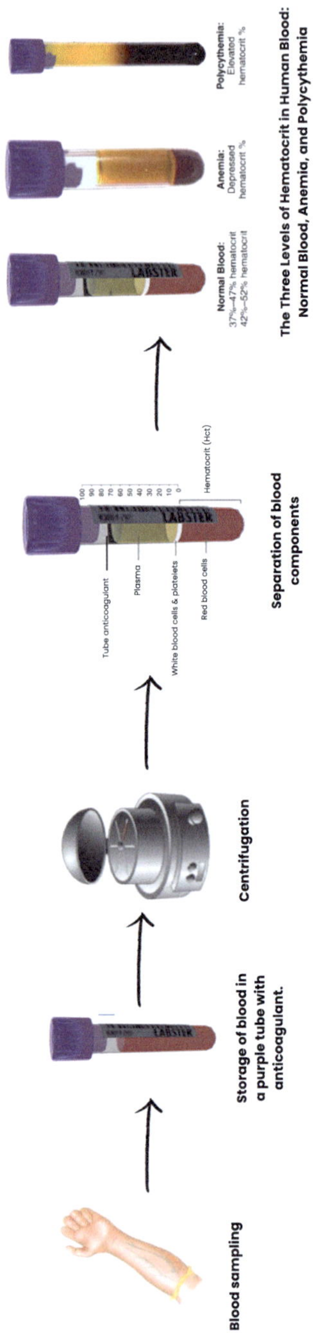

Fig. 3 Process of sampling and evaluating hematocrit in human blood in the quodess laboratory

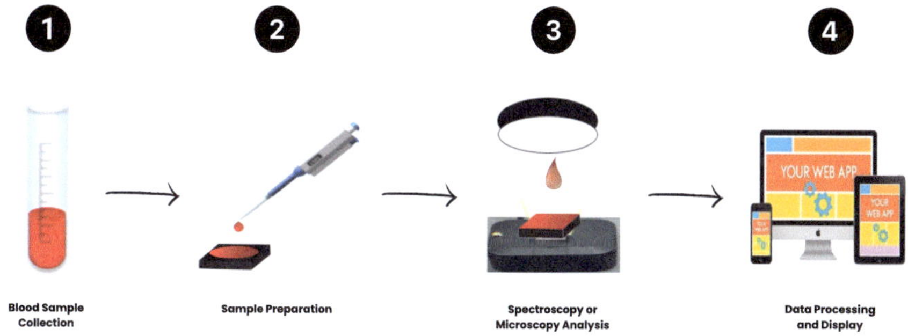

Fig. 4 Steps in the blood sample analysis process using NIR spectroscopy

Savitzky-Golay (SG), SNV, and MSC were compared to eliminate noise, variation in sample thickness, and effects of scattering. The highest accuracy was obtained by the SG filter. Two models were subsequently based on it: an LSTM neural network, which can identify intricate correlations between spectral information, and an SVM, which has been shown to be resilient in regression tasks. NIR spectra-based hematocrit prediction is done with absolute accuracy and trustworthiness with this hybrid methodology.

3.3 *Training Machine Learningmodels*

Two machine learning models, the SVM and an LSTM neural network, were used in this study to make predictions based on blood spectra. Keras/TensorFlow (for LSTM) and the Scikit-learn package (for SVM) were used in the implementation. The regularization value $C = 1000$ was used to train the SVM model, and 5-fold cross-validation was used to assess its performance. With an MSE of 3.70, an MAE of 1.52, and an R2 of 0.82 (Fig. 6)., it produced strong findings that demonstrated good stability and adequate generalization capacity. A three-layer LSTM model with 512, 256, and 128 neurons was created concurrently with a learning rate of 0.001 and the Adam optimizer. Additionally, 5-fold cross-validation was used to validate it, yielding comparable results (MSE = 3.95, MAE = 1.64, R2 = 0.83) (Fig. 5). The SMOTE technique was used to correct data imbalance, and it was solely applied to training sets. The Talos library was used to do hyperparameter tweaking. While LSTM exhibits a marginally stronger capacity to explain the total variance in the data (higher R2), SVM provides superior accuracy for individual predictions (lower MAE). Thus, LSTM is better suited for identifying global trends, while SVM is better suited for high-precision applications

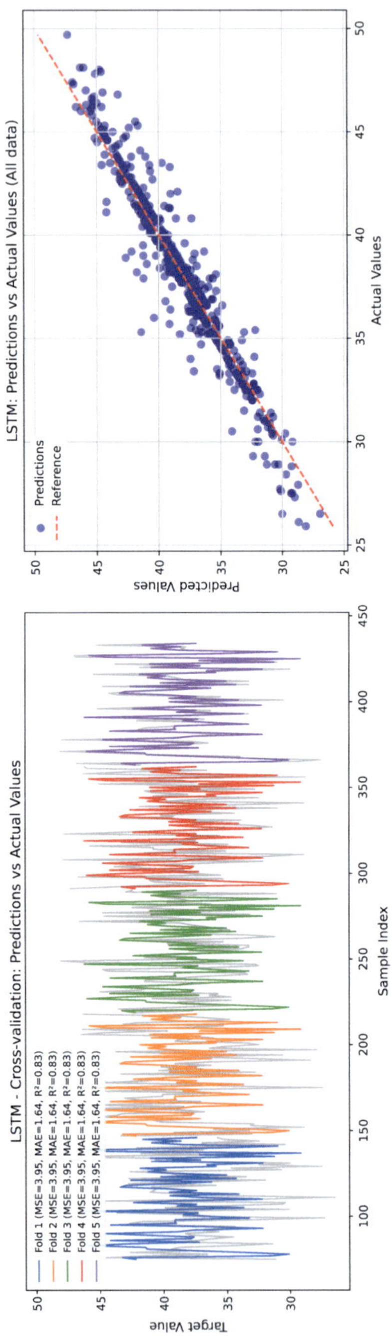

Fig. 5 LSTM cross-validation—predicted versus actual

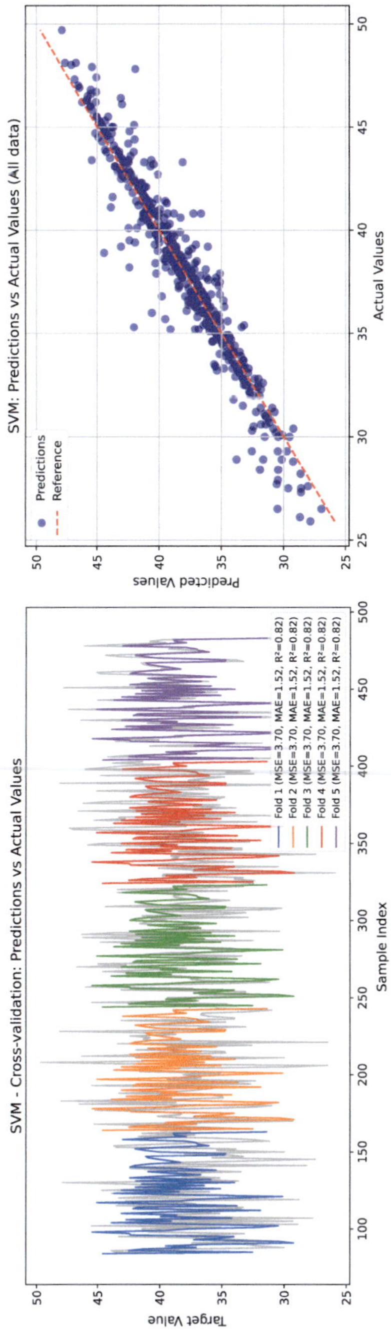

Fig. 6 SVM cross-validation—predicted versus actual

Table 1 Performance of SVM and LSTM models on the 30% test set

Model	MSE		MAE		R^2	
	30% Test set	80 New Obs.	30% Test set	80 New Obs.	30% Test set	80 New Obs.
SVM	6.0592	0.15	1.9130	0.20	0.914	0.956
LSTM	6.3435	6.70	1.9961	1.33	0.929	0.972

4 Results and Discussion

Here, the precision of two models SVM and LSTM are compared, and a new approach to predict hematocrit concentration from one drop of blood using artificial intelligence and near-infrared (NIR) spectroscopy is discussed. Particularly, for clinically relevant range 35 to 40%, the SVM model is reported to possess excellent precision (MSE = 6.05; MAE = 1.91; R2 = 0.91). It is more suited for quick use in medicine because it is quick, simple to use, and inexpensive. LSTM model is more associated with a 0.93 R2, indicating greater capacity to interpret the character of spectroscopic signals, albeit with comparatively higher errors (MSE = 6.34; MAE = 1.99). A comparative analysis of the performance of the two models on 80 new observations and a test set (30% data) has been presented in Table 1. It shows their respective strengths: Whereas LSTM outperforms with greater generalization and more sophisticated modeling of spectral changes, SVM is superior in instantaneous accuracy.

5 Conclusion

This research experimented and tested a novel method for hematocrit measurement that is appropriate for emergency applications. It combines NIR spectroscopy with machine learning techniques like SVM and LSTM. Our platform is designed for use in emergency rooms with clinical-grade accuracy (MAE < 1.5%, R2 > 0.95). It consumes a single drop of blood (8 μL) and offers results in less than 30 s. Clinical testing validated its precision in challenging emergency situations, e.g., sample variation and challenging measuring conditions. The technology bridges a critical gap that allows for quick and precise hematocrit identification without taking the time and cost of regular tests, improving patient care in emergency settings. Scaling up this approach to quantify other blood parameters and integrating it into portable devices for prehospital use is future work.

References

1. Khan, M.I., Ahmad, N., Fatima, S.H.: Haematological disorders: analysis of haematological disorders through bone marrow biopsy examination. Unpublishedmanuscript. PathologyDepartment, Khyber MedicalCollege, Peshawar (2018)
2. Alis, R., Sanchis-Gomar, F., Lippi, G., Romagnoli, M.: Microcentrifuge or automated hematological analyzer to assess hematocrit in exercise? Effect on plasma volume loss calculations. Scand. J. Clin. Lab. Invest. **77**(5), 315–319 (2017)
3. Briggs, C., Guthrie, D., Hyde, K., Mackie, I., Parker, N., Popek, M., Porter, N., Stephens, C.: Guidelines for point-of-care testing: haematology. Br. J. Haematol. **142**(6), 904–915 (2008)
4. Belland, D.: Clinical practice guideline on evaluating the effectiveness of venipuncture arm simulation. ProQuest Dissertations Publishing. Doctoral dissertation, Walden University (2024)
5. Gaw, S., Wright, C.J.: Haematological problems in intensive care: recent advances and developments. Anaesth. Intensiv. Care Med. (2024)
6. McMullan, J.T., Knight, W.A., Clark, J.F., Beyette, F.R., Pancioli, A.: Time-critical neurological emergencies: the unfulfilled role for point-of-care testing. Int. J. Emerg. Med. **3**, 127–131 (2010)
7. Sayed, S., Cherniak, W., Lawler, M., Tan, S.Y., El Sadr, W., Wolf, N., Fleming, K.A.: Improving pathology and laboratory medicine in low-income and middle-income countries: roadmap to solutions. The Lancet **391**(10133), 1939–1952 (2018)
8. Sakudo, A., Kato, Y.H., Kuratsune, H., Ikuta, K.: Non-invasive prediction of hematocrit levels by portable visible and near-infrared spectrophotometer. Clinica. Chimica. Acta. **408**(1–2), 123–127 (2009)
9. Kraitl, J., Klinger, D., Fricke, D., Timm, U., Ewald, H.: Non-invasive measurement of blood components: sensors for an in-vivo haemoglobin measurement. In: Advancement in SensingTechnology: New Developments and Practical Applications, 237–262 (2013)
10. Ho, E., Tran, J., Fateri, C., Sahagian, C., Sarton, K., Glavis-Bloom, J., Houshyar, R.: Work-related musculoskeletal disorders affecting diagnostic radiologists and prophylactic physical therapy regimen. Curr. Prob. Diagn. Radiol. **53**(4), 527–532 (2024)
11. Clemente, F., Antonacci, A., Giardi, M.T., Frisulli, V., Tambaro, F.P., Scognamiglio, V.: Last Trends in Point-of-Care (POC) diagnostics for the management of hematological indices in home care patients. Biosensors **13**(3), 345 (2023)
12. Heise, H.M., Marbach, R., Koschinsky, T.H., Gries, F.A.: Multicomponent assay for blood substrates in human plasma by mid-infrared spectroscopy and its evaluation for clinical analysis. Appl. Spectrosc. **48**(1), 85–95 (1994)
13. Liu, R., Xu, K., Lu, Y., Sun, H.: Combined optimal-pathlengths method for near-infrared spectroscopy analysis. Phys. Med. Biol. **49**(7), 1217 (2004)
14. Domján, G., Kaffka, K.J., Jákó, J.M., Vályi-Nagy, I.T.: Rapid analysis of whole blood and blood serum using near infrared spectroscopy. J. Near Infrared Spectrosc. **2**(2), 67–78 (1994)
15. Dong, R., Li, Y., Liu, S., Li, W., Tao, L., Chen, C., Yang, Y.: On-chip spectroscopic monitoring of erythrocyte oxygenation under hematocrit and oxygen gradients. J. Sci. Adv. Mater. Devices **7**(4), 100515 (2022)
16. Salimi, M., Roshanfar, M., Tabatabaei, N., Mosadegh, B.: Machine learning-assisted short-wave infrared (SWIR) techniques for biomedical applications: towards personalized medicine. J. Pers. Med. **14**(1), 33 (2023)
17. Baker, W.B., Parthasarathy, A.B., Gannon, K.P., Kavuri, V.C., Busch, D.R., Abramson, K., Yodh, A.G.: Noninvasive optical monitoring of critical closing pressure and arteriole compliance in human subjects. J. Cereb. Blood Flow Metab. **37**(8), 2691–2705 (2017)
18. Deprez, S., Heughebaert, L., Boffel, L., Stove, C.P.: Application of non-contact hematocrit prediction technologies to overcome hematocrit effects on immunosuppressant quantification from dried blood spots. Talanta **254**, 124111 (2023)
19. Liu, D., Wang, J., Wu, L., Huang, Y., Zhang, Y., Zhu, M., Yang, C.: Trends in miniaturized biosensors for point-of-care testing. TrAC Trends Anal. Chem. **122**, 115701 (2020)

20. Wang, K., Bian, X., Zheng, M., Liu, P., Lin, L., Tan, X.: Rapid determination of hemoglobin concentration by a novel ensemble extreme learning machine method combined with near-infrared spectroscopy. Spectrochim. Acta Part A Mol. Biomol. Spectrosc. **263**, 120138 (2021)
21. Saiko, G., Sadrzadeh-Afsharazar, F., Burton, T., Prahl, S., Douplik, A.: Absorption, scattering, and refractive index of blood and its components: a review. Front. Photonics **6**, 1636398 (2025)
22. Talati, M., Tachtsidis, I.: Advancements in broadband near-infrared spectroscopy instrumentation for the assessment of in vivo mitochondrial function: a comparative review and outlook. J. Biomed. Opt. **30**(S2), S23914–S23914 (2025)
23. Zheng, S.C., He, S.: The near-infrared spectroscopy to evaluate neonatal improvement after transfusion: a systematic review and meta-analysis. BMC Pediatr. **25**(1), 385 (2025)
24. Pérez-Gómez, E., Gómez, J., Gonzalo, J., Salgüero, S., Riado, D., Casas, M.L., Barquero-Pérez, Ó.: Exploratory integration of near-infrared spectroscopy with clinical data: a machine learning approach for HCV detection in serum samples. Front. Med. **12**, 1596476 (2025)
25. Liang, G., Ren, Z., Zhang, H.: Quantitative detection of serum biochemical indexes via UV–Vis-NIRS combined with deep neural networks. Spectrochim. Acta Part A Mol. Biomol. Spectrosc. **338**, 126191 (2025)
26. Steelman, Z.A., Ho, D.S., Chu, K.K., Wax, A.: Light-scattering methods for tissue diagnosis. Optica **6**(4), 479–489 (2019)
27. Hackeling, G.: Mastering Machine Learning with scikit-learn. PacktPublishing Ltd (2017)
28. Subramaniam, S., Mehrotra, M., Gupta, D.: Support vector machine based classification model for screening Plasmodium falciparum proliferation inhibitors and non-inhibitors. Biomed. Eng. Comput. Biol. 3, BECB-S7503 (2011)
29. Lahmiri, S., Dawson, D.A., Shmuel, A.: Performance of machine learning methods in diagnosing Parkinson's disease based on dysphonia measures. Biomed. Eng. Lett. **8**(1), 29–39 (2018)
30. Beritelli, F., Capizzi, G., Lo Sciuto, G., Napoli, C., Scaglione, F.: Automatic heart activity diagnosis based on Gram polynomials and probabilistic neural networks. Biomed. Eng. Lett. **8**, 77–85 (2018)

Deep Learning Based Approaches for Image Enhancement and Precise Anatomical Boundary Detection

Jagendra Singh, Shivani Agarwal, Surendra Singh, Ishaan Singh, Manoj Diwakar, and Jyotsna Ghildiyal Bijalwan

Abstract The introduction of medical image enhancement and accurate anatomical distinction detection methods based on deep learning has become one of the revolutionary technologies of modern-day medical imaging. The correct visualization of the anatomical structures is essential in diagnosis, treatment planning, and to monitor the disease progression, but the conventional visualization strategies usually exhibit low contrast, noise, artifacts, and interimagery differences among different imaging modalities. This chapter offers an in-depth discussion of deep learning methods that can overcome these problems, such as convolutional neural networks (CNNs), encoder-decoder models, attention systems, generative networks, and new implicit representations such as Neural Radiance Fields. The main image refinement techniques mentioned are denoising, super-resolution, contrast-enhancement, and multimodal fusion, which are all geared towards enhancing structural clarity and edge visibility. The following methods of boundary detection are considered based on anatomical accuracy and clinical relevance: semantic and instance segmentation, attention-based refinement, hybrid CNN-Transformer models, and graph-based methods. Also introduced in the chapter are uses in tumor delineation and organ segmentation,

J. Singh (✉)
School of Computer Science Engineering and Technology, Bennett University, Greater Noida, India
e-mail: jagendrasngh@gmail.com

S. Agarwal
Department of Information Technology, Ajay Kumar Garg Engineering College, Ghaziabad, India

S. Singh
Department of Electrical, Electronics and Communication Engineering, Galgotias University, Greater Noida, India

I. Singh
All India Institute of Medical Sciences (AIIMS), Bathinda, India

M. Diwakar
Department of CSE, Graphic Era Deemed to be University, Dehradun, Uttarakhand, India

J. G. Bijalwan
Head Academic Quality, British University, Hung Yen, Vietnam
e-mail: Jyotsna.b@buv.edu.vn

P. Singh et al. (eds.), *Deep Learning Applications in Healthcare and Medical Imaging Practice*, Studies in Big Data 193, https://doi.org/10.1007/978-3-032-21009-8_21

surgical planning and longitudinal disease monitoring, which is backed by experimental analysis using benchmark datasets. The ethical implications, data constraints, and the problem of clinical validation are mentioned to focus on the responsible use of AI. Combining image enhancement using deep learning with accurate boundary detection, the chapter highlights the possibilities of intelligent imaging systems of the next generation to enhance accurate diagnostic results, treatment planning, and personal medical care.

Keywords Deep learning · Medical image enhancement · Anatomical boundary detection · Convolutional neural networks (CNNs) · Multi-modal imaging · Segmentation

1 Introduction

Medical imaging is a key factor to the contemporary healthcare system as it allows visualization of the internal organs and physiological processes without invasiveness. Computed tomography (CT), magnetic resonance imaging (MRI), positron emission tomography (PET), ultrasound, and X-ray imaging are widely employed in the diagnosis of diseases, planning of their treatment, and making clinical decisions. The usefulness of these imaging, however, is highly reliant on the image quality and the clear demarcation of the boundaries of the muscles and bones. Clear cut images with well-established structural lines ensure that clinicians can establish the areas of pathology, distinguish between normal and abnormal tissues, and conduct quantitative measurements which are important in diagnosis and interventions [1, 2].

The quality of images has a direct impact on the credibility of clinical interpretation. Fine anatomical details may be obscured due to poor contrast, noise, blur, and imaging artifacts, which results in diagnostic uncertainty or errors. Equally, misaligned boundary detection may lead to imprecise segmentation of organs, tumors or lesions which will negatively impact on treatment planning, surgical navigation, and outcome forecasting. Indicatively, in oncology, the delineation of tumor boundaries is very vital in determining tumor volume, tracking disease progression, and the radiation therapy planning. In cardiovascular and neurological imaging, the clear delineation of boundaries contributes to functional examination and risk evaluation [3].

The acquisition of medical images is limited in nature by several factors. Any noise added during signal acquisition, especially in low-dose CT or in rapid MRI scans, reduces the quality of images. The minimal difference between bordering tissues particularly in soft tissue images means that similarity of anatomical structures in terms of their intensity profile cannot be clearly differentiated. Image quality is further impaired by motion artifacts, which may be the result of patient motion, respiration, or cardiac activity. Also, due to spatial and temporal resolution limitations, imposed by hardware and necessitating radiation minimization or short scan times, there is a common tendency to have incomplete or blurred anatomical representations. All these difficulties interfere with the process of correct interpretation and quantitative analysis of medical images [4, 5].

To overcome these problems, image improvement and anatomical boundary delineation can be considered the critical preprocessing and analysis measures. Image enhancement methods are used to enhance contrast and reduce noise, while maintaining the crucial structural information and therefore making it easier to view and interpret. Boundary detection and segmentation systems are concerned with well-defined anatomical structure outlining, which can be used in finding organs, quantifying lesions, and 3D reconstruction. Combined, these procedures are the basis of modern clinical application, such as computer-aided diagnosis, image-guided intervention, and individualized treatment planning [6].

There have been more traditional image processing methods that have been used to solve image quality and boundary detecting issues. Histogram equalization, linear and nonlinear filtering, edge detectors, and active contour models are among the techniques that have proved to be successful on controlled situations. These approaches, however, are very dependent on hand-crafted aspects and are manually fine-tuned, with their discriminability across a variety of body imaging modalities and patient groups being restricted [7]. They tend to be noise-sensitive, vary in intensity, and have imaging artifact, which interferes with performance. Further, the conventional methods are weak at recording the anatomical variations and subtle boundary features, especially in the heterogeneous or pathological tissue [8].

The advent of deep learning has completely changed the situation in the field of medical image analysis. The deep learning models, especially convolutional neural networks (CNNs), have shown impressive traits in the direct learning of hierarchical and discriminative features using data. Deep learning-based methods can adjust to the patterns of imaging, multimodal data, and to generalize to different clinical situations, unlike traditional methods [9]. Most of the methods, like encoder-decoder networks, attention networks, transformers, and generative models, have advanced architecture and have greatly enhanced the performance of the respective tasks of image enhancement and anatomical boundary detection. Such models facilitate end to end learning and combine betterment and partaking procedures into single systems providing better precision and endurance.

1.1 Role of AI-Based Image Enhancement and Boundary Detection in Diagnosis and Intervention

Image denoising and boundary detection using artificial intelligence (AI) has become part of the modern medical diagnosis and clinical intervention. Using the capabilities of data-driven learning, as well as the development and state-of-the-art pattern recognition, AI systems can enhance the interpretation and integrity of medical images to allow clinicians to make more reliable and prompt decisions. In contrast to the traditional image pro-processing methods, AI-based solutions respond to anatomical variations, image noise, and modality-specific properties, and hence provides high-performance performance in a wide range of clinical settings [10].

Image enhancement based on AI is extremely important in the diagnostic workflow to enhance visibility of subtle anatomical and pathological features. Deep learning models are capable of effective noise reduction, intensity inhomogeneity repair, contrast amplification without the loss of the important structural information [11]. This is especially useful in low dose imaging protocols, including low-dose CT or accelerated MRI, where the quality of images would otherwise be compromised to minimize exposure to patients or scanning duration. AI-enhanced images ease the identification of unclear issues in the body during early phases, precise tissue differentiation, and enhance the confidence in diagnosis in clinicians by removing ambiguity and preserving minute textures [12].

Strict delineation of anatomical boundaries is also a key to diagnosis, which allows proper division and measurement of organs, lesions, and areas of pathology. Boundary detection models trained with AI (convolutional neural networks, attention-driven systems, and so on) can learn complex spatial relations and other contextual information that characterizes anatomical boundaries. This is particularly crucial in situations where boundaries are loose, irregular, or unclear because of disease advancement, filling tissues or imaging artifacts. Precise boundary demarcation helps in quantitative statistics like tumor size, organ size and structural asymmetry that is important in staging and monitoring of disease [13].

AI-enhanced image enhancement and boundary detection in clinical intervention and treatment planning has a direct effect on the procedural accuracy and patient outcomes. In radiation therapy, such as the targeting of tumors and organs-at-risk, it is critical to have accurate tumor and organ-at-risk demarcations to maximize dose delivery and minimize the harm to adjacent normal tissues [14]. The delineation with AI assistance guarantees the consistency and reproducibility of the results, minimizing inter-observer variability and planning time. In the same way, in surgical planning and image-guided intervention, improvement of images and precisely defined anatomical structures to observe essential areas, strategize optimal access routes, and prevent the important structures of the surgical process can be used.

1.2 Objectives of the Chapter

- To highlight the importance of image quality and precise anatomical boundary detection in medical imaging applications.
- To analyze the key challenges associated with medical image acquisition, including noise, low contrast, artifacts, and resolution limitations.
- To review traditional image enhancement and boundary detection techniques and identify their limitations in complex clinical scenarios.
- To explore deep learning–based methodologies for medical image enhancement and accurate anatomical boundary delineation.

- To examine advanced architectures such as CNNs, encoder–decoder networks, attention mechanisms, and transformers for boundary-aware analysis.
- To discuss real-world clinical applications of deep learning–driven image enhancement and segmentation techniques.
- To outline current challenges, ethical considerations, and future research directions in AI-driven medical image analysis.

The practical applications, experimental evaluations and developing tendencies are also addressed in the chapter and provide the information regarding the future research perspectives. The rest of the chapter follows this structure sequentially pulling the reader through the basics of the subject matter to the advanced techniques of deep learning and the practical real-world clinical implementations, and the revolutionary effect of artificially intelligent (AI) on the next-generation medical imaging systems.

2 Fundamentals of Medical Image Enhancement and Boundary Detection

The basis of appropriate image analysis, diagnosis, and clinical decision-making is based on medical image enhancement and boundary detection. The purpose of these processes is to enhance the visualization of the medical image and outline the anatomical structures correctly to interpret them accurately and conduct a quantitative analysis. Knowledge of the nature of various imaging modalities, image enhancement goals, and the concept of boundary detection are critical before discussing improved methods of deep learning [15].

2.1 Medical Imaging Modalities

The medical imaging modalities vary in image formation principles, image resolution, mechanisms of contrast, noise and artifact sensitivity. These disparities have a major effect on the issues of image enhancement and boundary detection.

Computed Tomography (CT) is a technique that creates cross-section images of an object, which depends on the attenuation of X-rays, providing it with a high level of spatial resolution and a good visualization of the bone and the dense tissues. Nonetheless, CT images are usually distorted with noise especially in low dose regimes and poor soft tissue contrast. Other effects that make boundary delineation more challenging include beam-hardening artifacts and partial volume effects, particularly at tissue interfaces [16].

The Magnetic Resonance Imaging (MRI) has high soft tissue contrast, and it is commonly applied in neurological imaging, musculoskeletal imaging, and cardiovascular imaging. Despite its positive characteristics MRI has shortcomings in the form of intensity inhomogeneity, motion artifact, and low signal to noise ratio in rapid sequences. All these lead to the existence of blurred or weak boundaries between tissues that are anatomically adjacent, and thus proper segmentation becomes difficult.

Positron Emission Tomography (PET) records the functionality and metabolic activity but not the structure. PET images are characterized with low spatial resolution and high degree of noise hence poor anatomical boundaries. PET image boundary detection is frequently based on the combination with other modalities that have the higher resolution, e.g. CT or MRI [17, 18].

Ultrasound imaging is real time, cheap, and has a wide availability, however, it is very sensitive to speckle noise, shadowing, and variability as posed by the operator. These cause blurred tissue borders and uniform anatomical definition is challenging.

The use of X-ray imaging has been an essential diagnostic instrument of skeletal and chest imaging. Nonetheless, the fact that it is a two-dimensional projection makes it have overlapping anatomical structures, less depth information, and less contrast in soft tissues, and thus makes finding boundaries difficult.

The challenges associated with each modality are different and require specific image enhancement and boundary detection approaches to provide consistent clinical results.

2.2 Image Enhancement Objectives

The main goal of medical image enhancement is to enhance the visual quality that does not harm the diagnostically important information. Proper improvement facilitates proper boundary identification and analysis.

The purpose of contrast improvement is to enhance the identifiability of adjacent tis-sues of approximately the same intensity profile. Adaptive contrast enhancement techniques and histogram techniques are the most popular techniques to bring out the slightest of anatomical differences [19].

Noise removals are aimed at containing the random variations that are introduced at the time of obtaining images without affecting the important structural details. Low-dose CT, PET, and ultrasound imaging are of particular concern in which noise is especially heavy and the clarity of boundaries is greatly influenced by high noise levels.

Edge preservation takes care of the fact that the methods of enhancement do not obliterate or distort anatomical boundaries. The maintenance of abrupt borders between tissues is necessary to the proper segmentation and measurement.

Structural integrity is an aspect that considers the real anatomical form, size, and spatial configuration of the structures during the process of enhancement. Excessive smoothing or over-enhancement will add unnatural elements or deform anatomy and give clinical misleading information [20].

There is a need to balance these goals because there is a tendency that enhancing one aspect will impact on others. Enhanced techniques of advanced enhancement aim at making the best trade-offs, specific to the imaging modalities and clinical tasks.

2.3 *Boundary Detection and Anatomical Delineation*

Anatomical boundary detection It is the process of identifying interfaces between one tissue, organ, or pathological area relative to another in medical images. These are limits that establish the spatial scope of anatomic structures which form the foundation of segmentation, three-dimensional reconstruction and quantitative analysis.

Proper anatomical definition is essential in many clinical procedures, such as tumor localization, organ volume calculating, surgical planning, and disease progression. Smart boundaries might inaccurately compute the measurements, resulting in an inappropriate treatment plan and higher clinical risk. Thus, the sound boundary detection is a pillar of computer-aided diagnosis and intervention systems [21].

A few evaluation metrics are usually applied to evaluate the performance of the methods of boundary detection and segmentation. Dice Similarity Coefficient (Dice) is used to evaluate the overlap of the predicted and ground truth regions giving an estimate of the segmentation accuracy. Intersection over Union (IoU) is a measure of the percentage of overlap between reference and predicted segmentations. The Hausdorff distance measures the largest distance between boundary points, which measures the accuracy of the boundaries and the worst-case error. Combined, these measures provide a thorough analysis of the region-based and boundary alignment.

These fundamentals offer the background that is required to consider the deep learning-based methods that mitigate the drawbacks of the conventional methods and allow accurate and strong anatomical boundary localization in challenging medical imaging cases.

3 Traditional Versus Deep Learning Approaches

Classical image processing and computer vision methods have been used traditionally to improve medical images and detect their boundaries. Although these approaches formed the basis of automated image analysis, their inability to address complicated medical imaging conditions stipulated the move towards deep learning-based ones. This part examines classical methods of image enhancement and boundary detection and compares them with the recent developments in deep learning by highlighting major weaknesses of traditional algorithms [22].

3.1 Classical Image Enhancement Techniques

Classical image enhancement methods are designed to enhance the image visibility and the interpretability of the image by adjusting the intensity distributions of its pixels, or to reduce image noise. Histogram equalization is one of the most common techniques, and it reallocates the intensity values of an image to increase world contrast. Medical imaging Variants like adaptive histogram equalization (AHE) and contrast-limited adaptive histogram equalization (CLAHE) have been used in medical imaging to enhance the local contrast. Even though useful in some situations, histogram methodologies exaggerate noise and can warp intensity associations, particularly in images where the illumination is unevenly distributed.

Other foundations of the classical image enhancement methods are filtering techniques. Gaussian filtering is a method to smooth pictures by reducing the amount of noise in the image, but edges and fine structural features are also obscured. In removing impulse noise, median filtering is better than linear filters and preserves edges but when applied aggressively, it can still destroy fine anatomical features. The Anisotropic diffusion filtering is an enhancement of simple smoothing with a selective reduction of noise and preservation of edges with the help of directional diffusion. Though anisotropic diffusion is more advanced, it needs to be carefully chosen and cannot work in areas with either weak or messy boundaries [17].

Though these enhancement methods are computationally fast and can be achieved easily, their processing relies greatly on manually chosen parameters and assumptions regarding noise properties, hence they cannot be well-performing across a variety of imaging modalities.

3.2 Classical Edge and Boundary Detection

In classical approaches to boundary detection, the technique is mainly founded on the observation of pixel values or the presence of intensity gradients. First-order derivatives (like Sobel, Prewitt, etc.) are gradient-based operators that are used to emphasize edges by detecting regions of high intensity gradients. These are the simplest and the quickest methods which are very sensitive to noise and tend to create jagged or false edges in the medical images.

Canny edge detector is an improvement of the basic gradient operators since it uses noise elimination, gradient calculation, non-maximum suppression, and hysteresis thresholding. Although Canny is popular because of its enhanced edge localization, its operation is extremely sensitive to the choice of threshold and smoothing parameters, which are different in imaging modalities and clinical settings [19].

Second-order derivative techniques including the Laplacian of Gaussian (LoG) are used to detect edges, the zero-crossing of the image intensity. Laplacian-based methods are very sensitive to heavy noise and the methods are also highly sensitive to detecting fine details, so Laplacian-based methods have high sensitivity to noise and to pre-smoothing, which may undermine anatomical limits.

In addition to edge detection, level set methods and active contours (snakes) consider boundaries as moving curves or surfaces that are described by the minimization of energy. These techniques include shape priors and smoothness and are therefore more appropriate in anatomical delineation than merely edge detectors.

3.3 *Limitations of Traditional Methods*

Although traditional image enhancement and boundary detection techniques are of historical importance, they have several fatal flaws. Their biggest limitation is that they are sensitive to noise and artifacts, which are common in medical imaging. Noise may have serious negative effects on edge detector performance and cause false or missed boundaries.

The other weakness is the use of manual parameter tuning. The best parameter values differ widely with imaging modalities, acquisition procedures and with patient populations, and it is hard to design universal systems. Such reliance on the work of experts restricts scalability and reproducibility in clinical settings.

And lastly, the conventional approaches are poor at generalization. The handcrafted functionality and deterministic regulations cannot reflect the anatomical variations and pathological heterogeneity that exist in real-life medical data. Consequently, these techniques tend to fail in difficult cases adjacent to low contrast, overlapping structures, or the heterogeneous tissues.

Deep learning methods, on the other hand, address most of these constraints by learning adaptive and data-driven representations, which can be used to enhance images strongly and detect anatomical boundaries accurately in a wide variety of clinical cases.

4 Deep Learning Foundations for Image Enhancement and Boundary Detection

Deep learning has transformed the field of medical image analysis by allowing one to learn complex pattern directly with data through automated learning. Deep learning models are more effective in image enhancement and accurate anatomical boundaries, unlike the traditional image processing methods which used manually constructed features. This chapter presents the key principles of deep learning, architecture, loss functions, and training algorithms that support the state-of-the-art medical imaging systems.

4.1 Convolutional Neural Networks (CNNs)

Most image enhancement and segmentation systems based on deep learning rely on Convolutional Neural Networks (CNNs). CNNs take grid-like information, including medical images, as inputs and run them through learnable convolutional filters, which identify spatial patterns. Within medical imaging, the CNNs automatically acquire the low-level features (edges, textures, intensity gradients, etc.) during the first layers, with subsequent layers learning the high-level semantic features (anatomical structures, pathological areas, etc.) associated with the medical image.

This bottom-to-top characteristic of feature extraction enables CNNs to combine fine-grained boundary representations with overall contextual information. To address image enhancement problems, CNNs are trained to reduce noise, remove intensity distortions, and enhance contrast by training them on degraded and high-quality images. CNNs detect spatial patterns and contextual information that are used to differentiate two adjacent anatomical structures in English on the boundary detection and segmentation tasks even in cases where boundaries are weak or partially covered.

The process of weight sharing, and local receptive fields helps CNNs to estimate high-dimensional medical images efficiently and their spatial coherence. Additionally, the mod-ern CNN architectures also feature residual connections, use of batch normalization and nonlinear activation functions to enhance the stability of training and generalization.

4.2 Encoder–Decoder Architectures

A paradigm of architectural design medical image segmentation and boundary detection has become based on encoder-decoder architectures. These architectures involve encoder which gradually removes abstract features by down sampling and decoder which recovers spatially accurate output maps by up sampling. The combination enables models to address the global context and details of fine boundaries.

U-Net belongs to the number of the most impactful encoder-decoder models in medical imaging. It presents skip connections that apply a direct linkage between encoder and decoder layers to allow the preservation of the lost spatial information during down sampling. Such skip connections are especially useful in boundary detection, when high-resolution features are to be used to provide accurate anatomical delineation.

V-Net is an extension of U-Net to volumetric (3D) data, which can be applied to the three-dimensional medical imaging modalities of CT and MRI. V-Net performs operations on volumetric inputs to obtain inter-slice context and achieve better boundary continuity and slice structure consistency.

Attention U-Net is another model that improves the performance of segmentation by introducing attention to the skip connections. Attention modules enable the network to concentrate on the important parts and eliminate the irrelevant background data. The selective feature emphasis is particularly useful in visualizing small anatomical boundaries or low-contrast ones, which include tumors or lesions that are in complex tissue settings.

Combined, the encoder-decoder architectures offer a solid base of accurate boundary identification and have been extensively used in research and clinical fields.

4.3 Loss Functions for Boundary Precision

The loss functions are essential in steering deep learning models to the correct direction of detecting boundaries and segmenting them well. Class imbalance Class imbalance and boundary errors Class imbalance and boundary errors are also an issue with traditional pixel-wise losses like cross-entropy, which drives the design of special loss functions.

Dice loss: is calculated based on Dice Similarity Coefficient and is directly optimizing similarity in area between predicted and ground truth segmentation. It works particularly well in medical imaging work in which target structures take up a very small portion of the picture.

Boundary-aware loss functions explicitly put more focus on boundary regions by incurring greater losses on boundary misclassifications. The losses pave the way to the model to acquire steep and correct edges, enhancing anatomical delineation of the tricky cases, which have soft or indistinct boundaries.

Focal loss solves the problem of uneven classes by weighting samples that are easy to classify and prioritizing training of hard or ambiguous pixels, which are usually found at boundaries. This strategy increases sensitivity of the model to all subtle changes in boundaries and increases the robustness of the segmentation.

The sensitivity or integration of these loss functions is carefully chosen to have an important impact on the accuracy and fidelity of the results of boundary detection.

4.4 Training Strategies

Proper training plans are key to realizing strong and generalizable medical imaging deep learning models.

With data augmentation methods, rotation, scaling, flipping, intensity variation, and elastic deformation, the diversity of the data is enriched, and overfitting is minimized. Especially medical imaging, where there is frequently limited labeled data, requires augmentation.

Transfer learning uses the learned models of large-scale datasets, which has increased convergence and better performance on smaller medical imaging datasets. Post-training encoders have been useful especially in image improvement and image segmentation.

Multi-scale learning considers multi-scale features in learning, which is used to describe both large scale anatomical information and fine boundaries in models. Multi-scale architectures enhance continuity at the boundaries and performance in different object sizes.

A combination of these pillars constitutes the core of contemporary deep learning frameworks in medical image improvement and accurate anatomical boundary localization, which make it possible to analyze various imaging types with robustness, accuracy, and clinical significance.

5 Deep Learning–Based Image Enhancement Techniques

Image enhancement systems based on deep learning have made major progress in improving the quality and reliability of medical images by training non-linear relations of degraded and high-quality images. Contrary to classical methods of enhancement which use predefined filters and heuristics, deep learning models learn enhancement strategies directly rooted on data. In this section, key deep learning-based methods of medical image enhancement are discussed; they are denoising, super-resolution, contrast enhancement, and multimodal image fusion.

5.1 CNN-Based Image Denoising

Noise is an inevitable artifact in medical imaging, which is due to the constraints of the acquisition hardware, low-dose acquisitions, and rapid scan necessities. Loud noises may blur small anatomical features and reduce the clarity of boundaries, which have adverse impacts on the performance of diagnosis and segmentation. CNNs have become the new super weavers in medical image denoising because they can acquire intricate noise distributions and retain structural information.

The Denoising Convolutional Neural Network (DnCNN) is one of the most effective CNN-based denoising models. DnCNN proposes a residual learning framework, in which the network is trained to predict the noise component that exists in the input im-age as opposed to the clean image. DnCNN helps improve the quality of images by the mean of removing the predicted noise of the noisy input, therefore maintaining the anatomical structures. This strategy makes the learning process easier and enhances the convergence time while training.

In current denoising networks, residual learning has become a significant component. Medical im-ages are generally subjective in texture and have poor boundaries that are readily destroyed in the process of noise elimination. Residual learning helps networks to concentrate on learning noise patterns but retaining the underlying structural content.

State-of-the-art CNN-based denoising systems use multi-scale convolutions, dilated kernels and attention mechanisms to learn to pay more attention to both local noise characteristics and global anatomical context. These advances lead to great resilience in diverse noise conditions, as well as imaging modalities, making CNN-based denoising a crucial element of AI-based medical image enhancement pipelines.

5.2 *Super-Resolution for Medical Images*

Super-resolution tries to learn the high-resolution images given low-resolution images which overcome the shortcomings by hardware capacity and acquisition rate. Super-resolution is used in medical imaging to improve the spatial resolution and sharpen boundary definition as well as provide reliable anatomical modeling.

One of the earliest deep learning models to be issued in image super-resolution was the Super-Resolution Convolutional Neural Network (SRCNN). SRCNN is an end-to-end model that trains a simple but effective CNN model to learn low-resolution to high-resolution mapping. SRCNN has also been used in medical imaging (MRI and CT) to improve the resolution of small anatomical structures and to make them easier to visualize.

Although the SRCNN showed the potential of using deep learning to do super-resolution, newer networks like Enhanced Super-Resolution Generative Adversarial Networks (ESRGAN) have shown better results. ESRGAN uses the generative adversarial model that uses a generator and a discriminator, which motivates the production of the images of the visual reality and the perceived high-quality images. ESRGAN increases the texture realism and boundary sharpness, which is essential to accurate anatomical delineation, using perceptual loss and adversarial learning.

In medical practices, GAN-based super-resolution algorithms are optimally implemented to prevent the presence of artificial structures that are hallucinated. It is made through constraint-based training and incorporation of clinical priors to make sure that improved images are anatomically faithful. The super-resolution methods are of special use in imaging of the brain, a musculoskeletal system, and even visualization of vessels as fine structural features are critical to the diagnosis.

5.3 *Contrast Enhancement Using Deep Learning*

Contrast enhancement plays an important role in differentiating adjacent tissues that have a similar intensity distribution particularly in soft tissue imaging. Conventional contrast enhancement techniques do not tend to match local anatomical differences and thus either over-enhance or result in breakdown of the structure. Data-driven adaptation is used to eliminate these limitations in deep learning-based contrast enhancement methods.

Contrast enhancement models using GANs are trained to take low-contrast images and result in high-contrast ones without changing anatomical consistency. The models are trained on either paired or unpaired datasets so that they can be used in any imaging modality. GAN-based methods are specifically useful in MRI and ultrasound imaging, where contrast differences greatly determine the visibility of the boundaries.

Adaptive contrast learning is also used to enhance the quality of improvements by setting an adaptable contrast level according to the local content of the image. The context-aware networks and attention mechanisms can be used to enable models to selectively increase regions of interest without imposing global intensity balance.

5.4 Multi-modal Image Enhancement

The Multi-modal medical imaging is based on the complementary information provided by other modalities to present an overall picture of the anatomical and functional features. Nonetheless, the disparities in the resolution, contrast mechanisms and the noise profiles also create serious problems to image enhancement. Multi-modal image enhancement and fusion can be effectively solved using deep learning.

Combination CT-MRI-PET images are a combination of structural information of CT, soft tissue contrast of MRI, and functional information of PET. Deep learning is trained to match and combine features between modalities with resulting richer images that avoid redundant information. This is usually done with encoder-decoder architectures whose encoders are modality specific and whose decoders are shared by all.

Cross-modal learning builds on this idea by allowing models to be trained to learn cross-modal mappings. As an example, a network can be trained to improve MRI data with information obtained in CT data or create pseudo-CT data with MRI data. The methods are especially helpful in those situations when one of the modalities is not available or restricted.

Multi-modal enhancement enhances boundary definition, anatomical consistency and clinical decidability, which are essential in advanced imaging in tumor localization, surgical planning and disease progression.

6 Deep Learning Approaches for Precise Anatomical Boundary Detection

One of the foundations of medical image analysis is the accurate identification of anatomical boundaries, which allows organ and pathological segmentation, three-dimensional reconstruction and quantitative evaluation of organs and pathological areas. Deep learning methods have made significant progresses in boundary localization by directly learning quantitative spatial, contextual as well as semantic relationships on medical image data. This part of the paper provides a general overview of the deep learning-based algorithms that detect anatomical boundaries accurately, semantic and instance segmentation, attention-based refinement, hybrid graph models, and emergent implicit representations.

6.1 Semantic and Instance Segmentation

There is a foundation on segmentation-based techniques in detection of anatomical boundaries in medical imaging. Semantic segmentation is used to label each pixel or voxel in an image with a class label, whereas instance segmentation uses different object instances of the same class. Both methods are based on deep learning models that represent semantically meaningful and spatially consistent representations.

Fully Convoluted Networks (FCN) have also been one of the first deep learning models to allow end-to-end pixel-wise prediction. FCNs are able to maintain spatial information and produce dense prediction maps that can be used in segmentations by substituting fully connected layers with convolutional layers. Medical imaging refers to the medical procedure used to identify and delineate the boundaries of tumors, lesions, and organ segmentation among other functions in which FCNs have been utilized extensively. But in early FCN models, the model gave coarse boundaries because of multiple down sampling operations.

To eliminate this weakness, the current architectures combine fusion of multi-scale features and skip connections, where spatial high-resolution information can be used to localize boundaries.

Boundary-sensitive segmentation techniques also provide a finer segmentation result, in the sense of directly modeling boundary regions. Boundary-aware methods instead of treating pixels with equal weights and in training, more weight is given to pixels along anatomical boundaries. This may be done by using loss functional that is weighted along boundaries, auxiliary prediction loss functions or contour supervision. When the ambiguous or transitional areas are targeted in learning, models that are aware of boundaries yield more accurate and more anatomically oriented segmentation outputs, especially when weak or irregular boundaries are involved.

Semantic and instance segmentation models establish the structural foundations of accurate delimiting anatomical boundaries and can be used as the basis of further refinement efforts.

6.2 Attention Mechanisms for Boundary Refinement

Convolutional architectures are good at the local features extraction but can be poor at capturing the long-range feature and global context that are required to describe boundaries accurately. Attention maps can solve this drawback by allowing model selective attention to pick out pertinent areas of the image or channels of features to make a model more precise in its boundaries.

The mechanisms of spatial attention are used to highlight important areas of an image to help in generation of attention maps which are used to highlight areas that may be having anatomical boundaries. These maps will direct the network to focus on areas of interest and ignore any irrelevant background information. Spatial attention works better especially with medical images where target objects form a small portion of the image like a tumor or lesion.

The channel attention processes work in the channels of features, which enables the model to emphasize the significance of various representations of the features. Channel attention enhances boundary discrimination and clarity by focusing on channels which span cross-boundary information. Integration of combined spatial-channel attention modules has been effectively realized in encoder-decoder architecture to realize high performance in segmentation.

In addition to attention modules integrated into CNNs, transformer-based segmentation models have become popular as they are capable of modelling global context using self-attention modules. Transformers can find long-range dependencies with interaction between every pixel or patch of an image, allowing the global interpretation of anatomical structures. Transformer-based models are effective in tasks of boundary detection in that they can protect structural consistency and complex anatomical relationships.

Transformer CNN-based architectures hybridize the advantages of both frameworks: CNNs are used to extract local information and keep the spatial details intact, whereas transformers offer the benefit of global context and refinement of boundaries. These models have proven to be of the state-of-the-art in demanding segmentation problems such as brain tumor delineation, organ segmentation and vascular boundary detection.

6.3 Graph-Based and Hybrid Models

Even the current CNN-based segmentation progress, the prediction of boundaries can remain full of space errors and broken edges. The solution to this problem is graph-based models and hybrid methods, which utilize structured prediction and spatial relationships with deep learning models.

A popular hybrid method is CNNs that are used with Conditional Random Fields (CRFs). Here, the CNNs produce initial probability maps and the CRFs enhance boundaries through the application of spatial coherence and smoothness constraints. CRFs are based on the idea of modeling the interactions between pixels on a pixel-by-pixel basis, and of promoting neighboring pixels of similar characteristics to be assigned the same label, which leads to smoother and more precise edges. This strategy has worked especially in medical imaging where the data can be noisy, or the tissue interface can be very intricate.

Recently, CNN + Transformer hybrids have become formidable boundary detection systems. These models use CNNs to extract features and trans-formers to perform global reasoning, which can provide an effective boundary detection in various anatomical structures. Transformers are used to increase contextual awareness, and CNNs are used to guarantee accurate localization which leads to better boundary continuity and fewer false detections.

Anatomical boundary modeling has also been studied using graph neural networks (GNNs). GNNs can be used to understand the topological and relational information that complements pixel representations by modelling anatomical structures as nodes and their relationship as edges. Graph-based deep learning is a promising field of study that is still emerging but has potential to find practical uses in modeling complex anatomical interactions and enhancing boundary accuracy.

7 Applications in Clinical and Biomedical Domains

Image enhancement and anatomical boundary detection with deep learning have found their way into a large body of clinical and biomedical applications. The technologies promote proper diagnosis, individual treatment plan, and continuous disease control by enhancing the visual quality of the image and allowing the drawing of anatomical features accurately and without errors. In this section, important areas of application are mentioned in which AI-based boundary detection has a disruptive role such as tumor delineation, organ segmentation, surgical planning, and longitudinal disease analysis.

7.1 Tumor Boundary Delineation

The correct delineation of tumor boundaries is vital in the diagnosis, staging, treatment and response evaluation in the field of oncology. The tumors have irregular shapes, nonhomogeneous textures and non-specific boundaries making the manual delineation difficult and which may be biased by inter-observer variability. Deep learning models deal with these issues by learning the complex spatial and contextual characteristics directly on the medical imaging data.

The accurate delineation of the boundaries of tumour subregion is important in brain tumor analysis to differentiate the enhancing tumor core, necrotic tissue and peritumoral edema. Architectures of deep learning, specifically the U-Net type, attention-based segmentation models, have been shown to be highly accurate in the outlining of gliomas on MRI scans. Multi-modal MRI fusion (e.g., T1, T2, FLAIR) and boundary-aware loss led to a further improvement in the clarity of tumor margins, which helps in a better plan of surgery re-section and radiotherapy.

In the case of lung tumor delineation, there are low contrast of the lesions and surrounding tissue, motion artifacts caused by respiration and the tumor size and shape variability. Segmentation models based on deep learning and trained on CT scans have demonstrated good results on pulmonary nodule detection and tumour boundary delineation. These models can help clinicians to detect and measure tumor volume in advance, and to trace tumor growth or shrinkage during treatment.

Boundary detection is important in the hepatocellular carcinoma and metastatic lesions detection in liver tumor segmentation. Boundary detection in the liver is especially difficult due to the multifaceted vascular structure of the liver and the uneven intensity profiles of the liver. Liver tumour delineation with methods based on deep learning that utilize 3D CNNs and attention mechanisms can be effectively used in CT and MRI scans to plan treatment in terms of surgical resection and ablation therapies.

7.2 Organ Segmentation

Medical image analysis segmentation Organ segmentation is a basic step to anatomical localization, functional evaluation, and diagnostics of disease. The ability of deep learning to detect boundaries has also brought a lot of accuracy and consistency in the segmentation of organs across imaging modalities.

Cardiac segmentation refers to the identification of echocardiography, CT, or MRI images and isolating the left ventricle, right ventricle, and myocardium. It is also necessary to have accurate boundaries when measuring cardiac functioning parameters, such as ejection fraction and myocardial thickness. Temporal modelling Deep learning models, especially encoder-decoder with encoder architectures, have demonstrated high-performance in the representation of dynamic cardiac boundaries during the cardiac cycle.

In renal segmentation, proper definition of kidney borders aids the diagnosis and tracking of chronic kidney disease, tumors and cystic disorders. Segmentation models based on deep learning can satisfy anatomical variability and pathological variations allowing estimating kidney volume and functional evaluation through CT and MRI scans with high reliability.

Liver segmentation is a requirement of liver tumor analysis, transplantation planning and volumetric assessment. Multi-scale feature extraction and boundary-aware learning based on deep learning techniques have shown great accuracy in labeling liver boundaries in the face of issues of similarity of intensity with adjacent organs and variable shapes.

On the same note, the respiratory disease analysis, radiotherapy planning, and COVID-19 evaluation require the lung segmentation. Deep learning models precisely outline boundaries of lungs based on chest X-rays and CT scans even in the case of pathology including consolidations, fibrosis, or nodules. These are dependable models in terms of downstream analysis and clinical decision-making.

7.3 Surgical Planning and Navigation

Boundary detection and image enhancement powered by AI can be extremely important in the work of surgery planning and navigation, as it allows clinicians to see specific anatomy of patients with the highest accuracy. Precise boundary demarcation enables the production of anatomical forms in three dimensions which are detailed and can be used in preoperative planning and intraoperative direction.

In preoperative modeling, the preoperative science, deep learning-based segmentation results are used to build 3D models of the organs, tumors, and other surrounding structures. These simulators assist the surgeon to evaluate the relationships in the anatomy, critical areas to avoid and strategize the workflow. It minimizes the risk of unfinished resection and injury to healthy tissue caused by improved accuracy in boundaries.

The combination of augmented and virtual reality (AR and VR) technologies with the models of boundary awareness has continued to revolutionize surgical procedures. The application of AR-assisted surgery superimposes segmented anatomical structures onto the body of the patient in real-time, and gives the surgeons an intuitive visual cue during surgery. VRs can be used to realize the immersive preoperative simulation which allows the surgeons to practice some complicated operations and enhance the outcomes of surgeries.

Boundary detection based on deep learning is also used to assist robotic-assisted surgery by giving robot-assisted surgery correct anatomical maps that guide the robot and control its movements. Such systems improve accuracy, minimize time of operation, and improve patient care.

7.4 Disease Progression and Longitudinal Analysis

Medical longitudinal analysis of images is vital in tracking the progression of diseases, measuring treatment outcome, and determining patient outcomes. Boundary detection of anatomical structures over time allows longitudinal studies to be reliable and dependable, achieved through deep learning-based boundary detection.

Oncology In oncology, accurate and precise localization of a boundary enables a quantitative measure of tumor growth, regression, or recurrence across consecutive imaging examinations. Delineation Automated, consistent delineation decreases inter-observer variability and enhances the reliability of treatment response measurement.

Boundary detection models aid in the examination of structural changes with time in the case of chronic diseases like neurodegenerative disorders, cardiovascular diseases, and chronic kidney disease. An example would be the ability to monitor the change in brain region boundaries which would give information on the disease progression in the Alzheimer disease and cardiac boundaries which would aid in the evaluation of heart remodeling.

Deep learning-based boundary detection can contribute to personalized medicine and data-driven clinical decision making because it facilitates an accurate and automated longitudinal analysis.

8 Case Studies and Experimental Analysis

To analyze the efficiency of deep learning-based image improvement and anatomical boundary detecting techniques, the large-scale experimental studies have been undertaken, based on publicly available benchmark datasets. These data sets present a variety of imaging modalities, anatomical structures, and pathological variations, which allows to evaluate the model performance thoroughly. This part contains representative case studies, comparative performance analysis, and quantitative as well as qualitative evaluation of performance.

8.1 Public Datasets Used in Experimental Studies

Several widely used public datasets serve as the foundation for experimental validation in this domain.

8.1.1 BraTS (Brain Tumor Segmentation Dataset)

BraTS dataset is made up of multi-modal MRI scans, having T1, T1c, T2, and FLAIR scans, with expert-marked tumor subregions. It has widely been applied in the assessment of the tumor boundary, especially in gliomas. The challenges in the dataset include the heterogeneity of appearance of the tumors, overlapping intensity distribution, and undefined boundaries.

8.1.2 LiTS (Liver Tumor Segmentation Dataset)

LiTS offers contrast enhanced scans of the abdominal CT with liver and liver tumor annotations. This data is usually employed to evaluate segmentation of organs and tumor delineation in diverse imaging conditions. The limitations are low contrast between liver and surrounding tissues, irregular tumor morphology, and complicated vascularity.

8.1.3 NIH Chest X-ray Dataset

The NIH database is a massive repository of X-ray of the chest with the disease label and landmark of the anatomy. It is also useful in assessing lung boundary detection and image enhancement methods to enhance low contrast X-ray image visibility, although mostly it finds application in the classification of diseases.

8.1.4 LC25000 Dataset

LC25000 dataset includes histopathology images of lung and colon tissue, and it belongs to various classes. This data has been utilized to test finer grained boundary detection and segmentation at cellular and tissue level where fine delineation is necessary in order to identify the illness. Collectively, the datasets offer a testing environment to test deep learning models in a wide range of imaging modalities and anatomies.

8.2 Comparative Performance Analysis

To show the benefits of deep learning-based methods compared to traditional image processing and classical machine learning ones, it is required to compare them. The baseline methods used in the experimental studies in most cases include thresholding, edge detection, and active contour model versus current deep learning models, such as U-Net, attention-based, and transformer-enhanced models.

In all data sets, deep learning models can beat traditional methods in terms of accuracy and robustness of the boundaries. Skip connection encoder-decoder and attention-based model and transformer models demonstrate further improvement in fine anatomical structure and reduction of false positives, respectively. The use of hybrid models that incorporate CNNs with CRFs or transformers achieves further gain because they impose spatial consistency and contextual awareness.

The most significant result of the performance is to be found in difficult scenarios like low contrast, noise, and irregular boundaries, in which the conventional approaches tend to either fail or need a long parameter optimization.

8.3 Quantitative Metrics and Qualitative Visualization

Model performance is evaluated using standard quantitative metrics that assess segmentation accuracy and boundary precision:

- Dice Similarity Coefficient (Dice Score) measures the overlap between predicted and ground-truth regions.
- Intersection over Union (IoU) evaluates the accuracy of region-based segmentation.
- Hausdorff Distance assesses boundary accuracy by measuring the maximum distance between predicted and true contours.

The experimental findings on the datasets prove that models based on deep learning score higher on Dice and IoU and hugely reduce Hausdorff distance as compared to baseline models. Such advances do not only imply the overall enhancement of the segmentation, but also more accurate demarcation of the boundaries.

Also, other than quantitative assessment, qualitative visualization is essential in terms of clinical relevance assessment. Comparison of the segmentation results as visuals indicate that deep learning networks yield smooth and more anatomically predictable edges with reduced discontinuities. The images are sharpened with better contrast and less noise and consequently the anatomical structures become more prominent to the clinicians.

Superimposition of the boundaries of the predicted boundaries on original images also illustrates the efficiency of boundary sensitive learning and attention mechanisms in detecting fine edges of the anatomy.

8.4 Discussion of Results

The analysis of the experiment shows that image enhancement and boundary detection algorithms based on deep learning offer significant performance improvement on a variety of data and in a variety of clinical settings. The hybrid structures, multi-scale feature learning, and attention mechanisms play a significant role in better boundary accuracy and robustness.

Nonetheless, the findings also indicate the issue of dependency on the dataset, computational complexity, and dependence on the quality of annotation. Models that have been trained on a single dataset possibly need to be fine-tuned to be able to make effective builds in new imaging modalities or clinical environments. Notwithstanding these issues, overall results prove the high potential of deep learning methods to be used as reliable anatomical boundary detectors.

Such case studies and experimental analyses confirm the practical efficacy of AI-based practices and justify their introduction in the real clinical practice.

9 Challenges, Ethical Considerations, and Limitations

Despite significant advancements in deep learning–based image enhancement and anatomical boundary detection, several challenges and limitations hinder their widespread clinical adoption. These challenges span technical, ethical, and regulatory dimensions, underscoring the need for responsible and rigorous development of AI-driven medical imaging systems.

9.1 *Data Scarcity and Annotation Cost*

Deep learning models need to be trained on large amounts of high-quality annotated data. Acquisition of such datasets has been especially so in medical imaging, given the privacy issues, scarcity of expert-labeled images, and differences in imaging protocols across institutions. Annotation of anatomy requires a lot of time and skills on the part of radiologists and clinicians hence annotation is costly and labor intensive.

Moreover, certain rare diseases and conditions do not have enough data, and the balance of classes is not achieved, which also contributes to a lower model performance. Although data augmentation, semi-supervised learning, and synthetic data generation partially solve the problem, they do not eliminate the need to use various and clinically valid datasets.

9.2 *Bias and Generalization Issues*

Training data bias is a major issue to AI-based medical imaging systems. The datasets potentially do not represent particular groups of people, imaging equipment or clinical environments, and thus make biased predictions on the model. Consequently, the models that are trained on small or heterogeneous data might not be able to generalize to a diverse patient population, across centers, or scanner types.

The problem of generalization is especially troublesome in cases of boundary detection where a minor difference in the quality of images or anatomical presentation can drastically influence the results of the model. The solution of these problems needs multi-center databank, standardized testing procedures, and ongoing testing of models in dissimilar clinical settings.

9.3 *Explainability and Trust*

Deep learning models are usually viewed as black boxes and hence it is hard to know how decisions are reached by clinicians. Explainability is fundamental in the medical context to build trust and hold accountability. Transparency deficiencies in the results of the processes of boundary detection can work against clinical acceptance, particularly when the stakes are high (such as in surgery planning or in cancer chemotherapy).

Attention visualization, saliency maps, and uncertainty estimates are explainable AI methods that can be used to interpret model predictions. Nevertheless, they are not the only methods that are still developing, as the reasoning of deep learning models is also complex and might not be entirely represented by these methods.

9.4 Clinical Validation and Regulatory Concerns

AI-based imaging systems should be carefully clinically validated before they can be incorporated into clinical workflows, as this will guarantee safety, reliability, and effectiveness. Validation must be deep-seated on various patient groups and contrasted with master assessments. Poor validation can cause wrong boundary demarcation, which can influence the diagnosis and treatment.

The process of regulatory approval also makes it harder to deploy. Medical AI sys-tems should be able to meet high regulatory standards and requirements that are depending on the regions. The privacy of data, adherence to healthcare regulations, and liability issues must be ensured to achieve successful adoption.

10 Future Directions and Emerging Trends

The revolution in medical imaging was recently observed with the combination of deep learning, AI-based analysis, and high-resolution imaging. In the future, several new trends will transform the functionality and clinical outcomes of medical imaging technologies, enabled by the introduction of foundation models, multimodal learning, patient-specific digital twins, real-time deployment, and immersive visualization systems.

10.1 Foundation Models in Medical Imaging

Large-scale pre-trained neural networks that can be generalized across a wide range of tasks are being applied to medical imaging more and more, reaching the level of foundation models. These models, which have been trained on large data sets that cover a broad variety of imaging modalities, anatomical areas, and pathology, have the potential to complete multiple imaging functions with little to no retraining on the task under consideration. Using the idea of transfer learning and self-supervised pretraining, foundation models can substantially decrease the reliance placed on massive, labeled medical datasets, which has long been the bane of clinical AI. Moreover, the models facilitate the standardization of the imaging analysis across institutions and enhance the reproducibility and reliability of the diagnostic processes.

10.2 Multimodal Large Vision-Language Models

One of the new horizons of medical imaging is the integration of vision and language modalities. Multimodal models that can interpret both imaging data and textual data of clinical reports can be used to provide more contextual interpretations of patient scans. These vision-language systems can create automated reports in radiology, indicate areas of interest and help the clinician to synthesize multimedia information. These models have the potential to improve diagnostic accuracy, ease explainability and help to make decisions in complex cases by aligning imaging features with clinical narratives and usher in AI-assisted precision medicine.

10.3 Digital Twins and Patient-Specific Modeling

The use of digital twin technology to form a virtual, dynamic model of an anatomy, physiology, and disease condition that characterizes the patient is increasingly taking momentum in the medical imaging field. Digital twins will be able to simulate patients individually by combining longitudinal imaging data, electronic health records, and computational modeling to treat and predict disease progression, specific therapeutic interventions. These models enable clinicians to see possible outcomes of a test prior to involving an individual into invasive procedures, which is an effective means of reducing risks and providing high-quality care.

10.4 Real-Time and Edge-Based Deployment

The application of AI models in real-time and at the edges is turning into an increasingly crucial concern in time-sensitive clinical cases, such as emergency radiology, intraoper image and critical care monitoring. Edge-based processing allows AI algorithms to execute on imaging devices or hospital server with nearly no latency, and therefore provide fast analysis without being dependent on cloud connectivity. The latter feature is especially useful in resource-scarce settings or contexts where urgent clinical intervention is necessary. The development of model compression and efficient architectures and hardware acceleration are informing this trend, allowing the operation of high-performance imaging analytics on portable and point-of-care devices.

10.5 Integration with AR/VR Systems

The application of AR and VR technologies is just starting to connect to medical imaging to offer immersive and interactive visualization of anatomy structures and pathological areas. Those systems support better surgical planning, guided interventions, and medical education through the ability to navigate 3D reconstructions in real-time by the clinicians. AR/VR apps, supplemented with AI-enhanced segmentation and predictive modeling, will be able to visualize ideas that are required on the surgical table or patient-specific 3D models, and be more precise, minimize risks in the procedure, and increase outcomes. Such a tendency is an indicator of the shift towards more intuitive, interactive diagnostic and therapeutic processes.

11 Conclusion

The medical imaging field has been transformed when deep learning-based methods are applied to the field to enhance medical images and accurately identify anatomical boundaries. In this chapter, the main ideas, the classical, and contemporary approaches and applications of AI-based techniques to enhance image quality, structural integrity and boundary sharpness have been discussed in detail. Through convolutional neural networks, attention mechanisms, encoder-decoder architectures, and novel implicit representations including Neural Radiance Fields, researchers have built models that can produce high-fidelity images and anatomically precise segmentation and eliminate numerous constraints of traditional models. The most significant advances in this area made by deep learning are high-quality noise reduction, super-resolution, contrast enhancement, multi-modal image fusion, and boundary-aware segmentation. The developments have facilitated automated identification of complicated anatomies as well as defining of tumors and consistent seg-mentation of organs using diverse imaging modalities like CT, MRI, PET, X-ray, and ultrasound. Moreover, the attention-based models, as well as the hybrid systems of CNNs, transformers, and the graph-based networks, have shown considerable gains in boundary accuracy, structural consistency, and contextual comprehension, which overcomes the issues of noise, low contrast, and inter-patient variability.

In oncology, such as tumor segmentation to assist surgical planning and radiotherapy, or correct organ segmentation to aid cardiac, renal, and hepatic analyses, AI assists. Combination with surgical navigation systems, augmented reality, and virtual reality also allows immersion in preoperative visualization to enhance the outcome and safety of operations.

References

1. Chen, Z., Pawar, K., Ekanayake, M., Pain, C., Zhong, S., Egan, G.F.: Deep learning for image enhancement and correction in magnetic resonance imaging state-of-the-art and challenges. J. Digit. Imaging **36**(1), 204–230 (2023)
2. Rikhari, H., Baidya Kayal, E., Ganguly, S., Sasi, A., Sharma, S., Dheeksha, D.S., Mehndiratta, A.: Fully automatic deep learning-based lung parenchyma segmentation and boundary correction in thoracic CT scans. Int. J. Comput. Assist. Radiol. Surg. **19**(2), 261–272 (2024)
3. Yousefpour Shahrivar, R., Karami, F., Karami, E.: Enhancing fetal anomaly detection in ultrasonography images: a review of machine learning-based approaches. Biomimetics **8**(7), 519 (2023)
4. Xu, Y., Quan, R., Xu, W., Huang, Y., Chen, X., Liu, F.: Advances in medical image segmentation: a comprehensive review of traditional, deep learning and hybrid approaches. Bioengineering **11**(10), 1034 (2024)
5. Kumar, S., Singh, J., Ravi, V., Singh, P., Al Mazroa, A., Diwakar, M., Gupta, I.: Utilizing multilayer perceptron for esophageal cancer classification through machine learning methods. Open Public Health J. **17**(1) (2024)
6. Mahmood, T., Rehman, A., Saba, T., Nadeem, L., Bahaj, S.A.O.: Recent advancements and future prospects in active deep learning for medical image segmentation and classification. IEEE Access **11**, 113623–113652 (2023)
7. Ullah, I., Ali, F., Shah, B., El-Sappagh, S., Abuhmed, T., Park, S.H.: A deep learning based dual encoder–decoder framework for anatomical structure segmentation in chest X-ray images. Sci. Rep. **13**(1), 791 (2023)
8. Kumar, S., Singh, J., Singh, P., Diwakar, M., Gupta, I., Ravi, V., Maidin, S.: Deep learning-based staging of throat cancer for enhancing diagnostic accuracy through multimodal data integration. Open Bioinform J 18:e18750362355440. http://dx.doi.org/ https://doi.org/10.2174/011875036 2355440250203115520.
9. Verma, M., Singh, J., Kumari, S.: Hybrid attention-augmented deep neural network framework based on ant colony and grey wolf optimization for diagnosis of aortic aneurysm. Int J Inform Technol. Springer (2025).
10. Ranjan, V., Chaurasia, K., Singh, J.: Enhancing skin cancer classification with soft attention and genetic algorithm-optimized ensemble learning. Image Vis Comput 166:105848 (2026). https://doi.org/10.1016/j.imavis.2025.105848
11. Singhal, P., Gupta, S.: An integrated approach for analysis of electronic health records using blockchain and deep learning. recent advances in computer science and communications. Former. Recent Patents Comput. Sci. **16**(9), 1–10 (2023)
12. Kanaujia, V.K., Kumar, A., Yadav, S.P.: Advancements in automatic kidney segmentation using deep learning frameworks and volumetric segmentation techniques for CT imaging: a review. Archiv. Comput. Methods Eng. **31**(5), 3151–3169 (2024)
13. Mall, S. (2023). Comparative study of heart failure using the approach of machine learning and deep neural networks. In: International Conference on Data Analytics & Management, pp. 627–641. Springer Nature Singapore, Singapore. https://doi.org/10.1007/978-981-99-6544-1_47
14. Singh, N.P., Hasan, D.S., Shelke, N.A., Namdev, A., Girdhar, N.: An integrated machine learning and IoT based approach for enhanced healthcare efficiency and personalized treatment. In: Abraham, A., Bajaj, A., Hanne, T., Siarry, P. (eds.) Intelligent Systems Design and Applications. ISDA 2023. Lecture Notes in Networks and Systems, vol 1046. Springer, Cham (2024). https://doi.org/10.1007/978-3-031-64813-7_16
15. Nazir, A., Hussain, A., Singh, M., Assad, A.: Deep learning in medicine: advancing healthcare with intelligent solutions and the future of holography imaging in early diagnosis. Multimed. Tools Appl. **84**(17), 17677–17740 (2025)
16. Govindaraju, P., Kumar, V., Yamsani, N., Umamaheswari, J., Munagala, M.: Real-time obesity and heart disease monitoring with IoT and deep learning. In: 2023 International Conference on Smart Devices (ICSD), pp. 1–6. IEEE

17. Poloju, N., Rajaram, A.: Hybrid technique for lung disease classification based on machine learning and optimization using X-ray images. Multimed. Tools Appl. **84**(21), 23531–23553 (2025)
18. Arya, C., Yamsani, N., Kumar, M., Singh, P., Bhagat, V.K.: A concise review of MRI feature extraction and classification with kernel functions. In: 2023 3rd International Conference on Innovative Sustainable Computational Technologies (CISCT), Dehradun, India, pp. 1–5. IEEE (2023). https://doi.org/10.1109/CISCT57197.2023.10351471
19. Gangadharan, S.M.P., Dharani, M., Thapliyal, N., Yamsani, N., Singh, P.: Comparative analysis of deep learning-based brain tumor prediction models using MRI scan. In: 2023 3rd International Conference on Innovative Sustainable Computational Technologies (CISCT), Dehradun, India, pp. 1–6. IEEE (2023). https://doi.org/10.1109/CISCT57197.2023.10351227.
20. Shivahare, B.D., Ravi, V., Chandan, R.R., Alahmadi, T.J., Singh, P., Diwakar, M.:. Delving into machine learning's influence on disease diagnosis and prediction. Open Public Health J. **17**(1) (2024)
21. Agarwal, S., Dohare, A.K., Saxena, P., et al.: HDL-ACO hybrid deep learning and ant colony optimization for ocular optical coherence tomography image classification. Sci. Rep. **15**, 5888 (2025). https://doi.org/10.1038/s41598-025-89961-7
22. Ming, Y., Dong, X., Zhao, J., Chen, Z., Wang, H., Wu, N.: Deep learning-based multimodal image analysis for cervical cancer detection. Methods **205**, 46–52 (2022)

Medical Image Tumor Detection Through Neural Network-Based Segmentation Techniques

Jhasaketan Prusty, Parul Madan, Nivedita Balodhi, Ankit Vishnoi, Manoj Diwakar, and Prabhishek Singh

Abstract Accurate brain tumor segmentation in MRI images is crucial for effective diagnosis and treatment planning. Conventional methods, like the U-Net architecture, may struggle with complex tumor geometries and boundary delineation. To address this, we integrate the residual grouped convolution module (RGCM) and the convolutional block attention module (CBAM) into the U-Net framework, enhancing its design and performance. By making the network capable of learning feature representations across numerous filter groups, the RGCM enhances important Spatial pattern recognition in MRI images. In addition, attention mechanisms across channel dimensions of the CBAM are used to enable us to have accurate segmentation results by focusing on important locations inside networks. Here is the process of our method: Shrink MRI image data AugmentationDivision dataset in training and test. The model was trained with entropy loss and Adam optimizer as proposed. Results demonstrate that our model achieves an accuracy of 97.581%, which outperforms the traditional U-Net. Our model does better than the existing models in comparison. For example, Isensee et al.'s modification of U-Net was the best, achieving an accuracy of 96.78%. Baid et al.'s SegNet reached 96.67%, Oktay et al.'s Attention U-Net achieved 96.89%, and Zhang et al.'s Residual Attention U-Net recorded 96.94%. These results demonstrate the improved performance of our model

Prabhishek Singh—This author contributed equally to this work.

J. Prusty · P. Madan (✉) · N. Balodhi · A. Vishnoi · M. Diwakar
Department of Computer Science and Engineering, Graphic Era Deemed to be University, Dehradun, Uttarakhand, India
e-mail: parulmadan.cse@geu.ac.in

A. Vishnoi
e-mail: ankitvishnoi.cse@geu.ac.in

P. Singh
School of Computer Science Engineering and Technology, Bennett University, Greater Noida, Uttar Pradesh, India

P. Singh et al. (eds.), *Deep Learning Applications in Healthcare and Medical Imaging Practice*, Studies in Big Data 193, https://doi.org/10.1007/978-3-032-21009-8_22

in brain tumor segmentation. Together, these results confirm the utility of our model in achieving consistent detection performance irrespective of maintaining a balance between malignant and benign brain lesions. In this work, the authors introduced a new approach for better tumor segmentation in MRI images and opportunities still remain for further image processing.

Keywords Brain tumor segmentation · MRI imaging · U-Net · Residual grouped convolution module (RGCM) · Convolutional block attention module (CBAM)

1 Introduction

Brain tumors have one of the lowest survival rates among all types of cancers; some 93% die within five years, compared to about half of those of other cancers. Tumors are masses of cells characterized by acquired or inherited changes that make them different from normal tissue and grow excessively in 3-dimensions [1]. There are malignant tumors (cancerous and capable of invading surrounding tissues) and benign [2]. Diagnosis of such anomalies is a cumbersome and laborious task for medical personnel. Therefore, it is crucial to develop smart systems that can identify cancer in certain parts of the human body.

Brain tumor segmentation [3] remains a fundamental and challenging problem in medical imaging, holding the promise of more accurate diagnostics and treatment planning for patients. However, human involvement makes traditional segmentation/allocation approaches laborious and prone to error. The development of deep learning [4] has enabled automated segmentation algorithms that can significantly improve precision and consistency. This project addresses the task of automatic segmentation for brain cancer using convolutional neural network methods (CNNs) on MRI data [5].

The main objective is to make protocols more segmented and resistant [6], either through high-level methods such as data augmentation or neural networks with specific topologies [7]. Brain tumors are better studied and discovered during the diagnostic phase. At this stage, brain radiology images are used by physicians and radiologists to identify possible chances of the appearance of cancer [8]. This study advocates for the adoption of magnetic resonance imaging because it is non-ionizing, unlike X-ray, CT, and PET, which all have radiation exposure risks. MRI does not penetrate the body as invasively as surgery, and MRI can offer finer details than PET or X-ray-based imaging Also, MR images, which are the most commonly available imaging modalities, have become widely accessible through web-based benchmark databases such as BraTS. MRI provides better soft tissue contrast than CT, which helps radiologists find a boundary of the tumor and surrounding area [9] are also among the most widely available imaging modalities, and web-based benchmark databases such as BraTS have made them even more accessible. MRI enables healthcare professionals to visualize and differentiate tissues more accurately using radiologists to better define the limits of a tumor and its surroundings.

Early diagnosis is important to assess the characteristics of the disease quickly, and doctors use different methods such as ultrasound, CT, MRI, and radiography. In emergency cases (mainly magnetic resonance imaging) in the treatment of the stomach and abdomen, magnetic resonance imaging and CT are the most commonly used to image tissues in the body without toxicity. During the past two decades, many research groups have proposed new ways to diagnose [10] and classify cancer using artificial intelligence and computer vision. These tools aim to predict diseases before they occur, help physicians make better choices, and save money. However, it is challenging to segment the area of MRI images due to noise [11], uniformity, non-uniformity distortion, and bias. Bias field distortion is an artifact caused by low signals in MRI images from MRI scanners that distort some tissues in different parts of the image or even slices. In addition, tumors can have different shapes depending on the location or size of the patient, making segmentation difficult. Previous studies have applied deep convolutional neural networks (DCNN) [12] to segment brain tumors from various MR images, with particular emphasis on encoder-decoder models such as U-Nets.

In this paper, we cover the following aspects:

1. In Sect. 2, we review the methods described in the literature for accurately detecting brain tumors through segmentation.
2. In Sect. 3 we discuss the proposed model and modifications to the U-Net architecture [13].
3. In Sect. 4, we detail the performance and evaluation metrics used in this investigation.

2 Related Work

Recently emerging in medical imaging, neural networks have attracted much attention to tumor diagnosis through image segmentation [14]. The U-Net structure is now the most popular and efficient architecture for segmentation of complex anatomic structures in medical images. Its encoder-decoder architecture has shown robust performance and generalizability in various medical image segmentation problems. Batool and Byun [15], incorporates skip connections and excels at maintaining spatial details while providing precise pixel-level segmentations. Experiments show that U-Net outperforms existing methods in terms of segmentation accuracy and boundary localization, which is more robust. Some studies have tried to manipulate the structure and parameters of a U-Net network to outperform in terms of tumor appearance variability, as well as quality distortion.

In 2015, convolutional neural networks (CNNs) [16] were used for the first time for the segmentation of brain tumor images. CNN networks insured in each layer of the features whether a single voxel or a set of voxels was present or not from an input image [17] and then calculated the output signal, For segmentation the results are generated significantly without manual feature extraction.

Treatment of all cancer patients has seen improvements due to recent advances in medical studies, especially in medical image classification, or picture segmentation [18]. In this paper, a novel hybrid intelligence technique has been proposed to segment and extract tumor characteristics in medical images [19] for accurate detection. In addition, this paper has studied the feature extraction design part of image classification and texture characteristics. Performance wise, all of these elements get better upgraded in the features selection steps during this process.

By 2022, advanced data augmentation techniques [18] had been integrated into U-Net topologies, considerably increasing their robustness. In an important article, Li et al. addressed over fitting via synthetic data augmentation and adversarial training. Their analysis of the BraTS dataset revealed significant improvements in performance measures, such as higher Dice coefficients and decreased false positive rates. The work uses the 3D-UNet model to volumetrically segment MRI images [20], which is then followed by CNN-based tumor categorization. To validate the models, loss and precision diagrams are supplied. The performance of the proposed models' is tested and compared with other methods reported in the literature, demonstrating that the proposed method outperforms existing cutting-edge methodologies.

Deep learning frameworks will evolve in 2023 to include hybrid models. Wu et al. created a variant U-Net [20] with a convolutional neural network (CNN) and a transformer module. This hybrid strategy was to combine the advantages of local and global information, so that brain tumor segmentation could be implemented accurately. Their conclusion highlighted the importance of multilevel representation to enhance model generalization. In this work, we present an auto U-Net NAS system namely Easy-medU-Net (EU-net) to facilitate the diagnosis of accurate lesion by physicians using the DE based method [21] to extract important information from medical image. We use a variable-length strategy for EU-Net, to make the model capable of automatically exploring neural topologies without human intervention. Further, DE's combination of crossover, mutation and selection operations supports to balance exploratory and exploitative moves within the solution space. To improve architectural performance, the encoding and decoding phases incorporate diverse block- and layer-based structures. We applied the proposed EU-Net technique to two well-known medical datasets, for image segmentation, we utilized the CHAOS and BUSI datasets. Extensive experiments show that EU-Net surpasses its chosen competitors in both datasets. In particular, our approach improves the mean Intersection over Union (mIoU) by at least 6% compared to the original U-Net.

Recent research in 2024 has focused on adding multimodal data to U-Net models. Zhao et al. developed a U-Net model capable of detecting brain cancers using both MRI and CT images. This multi-modal method enabled the model to capture complementing information from many imaging modalities, increasing segmentation accuracy and robustness. Furthermore, attention mechanisms with the decoder block of the U-Net architecture have been found to be beneficial to allow [5] to better focus on tumor regions and resulted in a higher segmentation performance in our model. To enhance the existing U-Net-based segmentation network [22], we introduce a residual grouped convolution (RGC) module, a convolution block attention (CBA) module, as well as a bi-linear interpolation up-sampling strategy. It also investigates the roles of network normalization, loss function, and network depth for segmentation performance. The experimental results indicate that the proposed model has reached the Dice score of 97.581%, which is 12.438% higher than the standard U-Net network, and it effectively segments brain tumor MRI images.

3 Methodology

This section discusses the proposed segmentation and classification models.

The proposed approach to brain tumor segmentation in MRI images extends the classic U-Net architecture by introducing modern neural network features designed to improve both the accuracy and robustness of segmentation, as demonstrated in Fig. 1. This elongated architecture is designed to solve some important problems in medical image segmentation, mainly fine delineation of complex and irregular tumor boundaries with lower contrast and greater variability between patients. By improving feature extraction and representation learning, it can better represent local texture details as well as global structure information for accurate tumor localization.

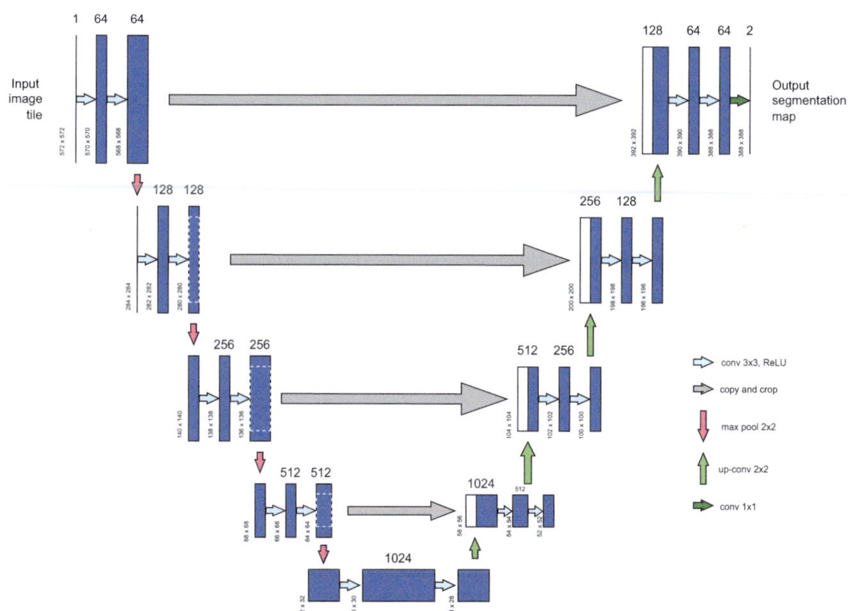

Fig. 1 Architecture of the proposed model

3.1 Data Preprocessing

The first step is preprocessing the MRI images to ensure consistent input sizes, and the images were resized to a standardized dimension for neural network input. Data augmentation techniques such as rotation, flipping, and zooming were applied to increase the variety in the training set and improve the generalization of the model.

This data set consisted of 3049 brain magnetic resonance images together with the respective segmentation masks. All images are resized to 512 × 512 pixels and images that have different dimensions are removed in order to provide uniformity. All images were further downscaled to 128 × 128 pixels; pixel values were also normalized in the range of 0 to 1 to obtain fast convergence during training.

3.2 Network Architecture Design

This network architecture also uses modules of the Residual Grouped Convolution Module (RGCM) and Convolutional Block Attention Module (CBAM) for better enhancement of the accuracy in segmentation. With the modules, the network can capture local and global features for a sequence, thus enhancing performance for tasks of brain tumor segmentation.

3.2.1 Residual Grouped Convolution Module (RGCM)

RGCM employs residual learning that directs the network to the learning of residual mappings instead of direct mappings. This is efficient with regard to training, especially when the networks are deep, as it avoids the problem of vanishing gradients. The residual learning formula is given as:

$$H_o(x) = F_m(x) + x_i \tag{1}$$

$$\begin{cases} \text{where:} \\ H_o(x) = \text{Output of the residual block.} \\ F_m(x) = \text{The learned mapping (residual function)} \\ x_i = \text{The input to the residual block.} \end{cases}$$

This approach allows the network to learn residuals between input and output, improving both convergence and segmentation quality.

3.2.2 Convolutional Block Attention Module (CBAM)

The CBAM enhances the network's performance by applying attention mechanisms along both the channel and spatial dimensions. The Channel Attention Module (CAM) focuses on important channels in the feature map, as described by:

$$M_{cl}(F) = \sigma(\mathrm{MLP}(\mathrm{AP}(F)) + \mathrm{MLP}(\mathrm{MP}(F))) \tag{2}$$

$$\begin{cases} \text{where:} \\ M_{cl}(F) = \text{Channel attention map} \\ \text{AP (Average Pooling), MP (Max Pooling)} = \text{Operations that summarize the feature map} \\ \text{MLP} = \text{Multi-Layer Perceptron generating attention weights} \\ \sigma = \text{Sigmoid activation function} \end{cases}$$

The Spatial Attention Module (SAM) focuses on key spatial locations within the feature map, as defined by:

$$M_{sl}(F) = \sigma(\mathrm{Conv}([\mathrm{AP}(F); \mathrm{MP}(F)])) \tag{3}$$

$$\begin{cases} \text{where:} \\ M_{sl}(F) = \text{ Output of the residual block.} \\ \text{Conv} = \text{Convolution operation applied to pooled values} \end{cases} .$$

3.3 *Training Process*

The network was trained using magnetic resonance images with labeled tumor regions. The loss function combined the Dice Coefficient and Intersection over Union (IoU) metrics to improve segmentation accuracy. Adam's optimizer was used for weight adjustments, ensuring efficient gradient updates.

The model was trained over multiple epochs, using data enhancement techniques such as rotations, flipping, and scaling to better generalize to real-world scenarios. The learning rate was carefully adjusted to prevent overfitting.

3.4 Evaluation Metrics

We used the dielectric coefficient and the intersection over Union (IoU) to measure the performance of our model.

The Dice Coefficient, which defines the overlap between true ground and prediction segmentation, is:

$$\text{Dice} = \frac{2|P_x \cap G_x|}{|P_x| + |G_x|} \tag{4}$$

$$\begin{cases} \text{where:} \\ P_x = \text{ Predicted set of tumor pixels.} \\ G_x = \text{Ground truth set of tumor pixels.} \end{cases}.$$

IoU was also calculated as:

$$\text{IoU} = \frac{|P_x \cap G_x|}{|P_x \cup G_x|} \tag{5}$$

$$\begin{cases} \text{where:} \\ P_x = \text{ Predicted set of tumor pixels (segmentation result)} \\ G_x = \text{Ground truth set of tumor pixels (actual tumor region)} \\ P_x \cap G_x = \text{Union of the predicted and ground truth sets,} \\ \text{representing all pixels in either the} \\ P_x \cup G_x = \text{Union of the predicted and ground truth sets,} \\ \text{representing all pixels in either the} \\ \text{predicted or ground truth tumor regions} \end{cases}.$$

4 Results and Discussion

4.1 Qualitative Evaluation

In this section, we present the results of the proposed model for the segmentation of brain tumors using MRI data. Following this, we discuss the performance metrics achieved, and the results are analyzed and visualized quantitatively. The accuracy graph (Fig. 2) shows the training and validation loss and the relationship between the training and validation accuracy increases over time. The accuracy increases at a reasonable rate right from a humble beginning because the network's success in identifying patterns of tumors improves progressively. At the end of the training phase again, the accuracy stands still, and it ensures that there is no train bias, and thus proves that there is no overfitting of the model.

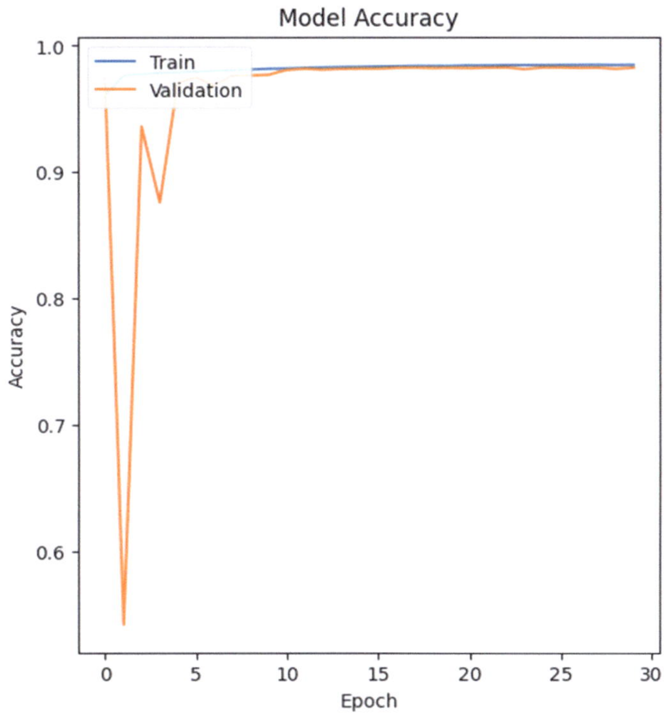

Fig. 2 Graphical representation for model accuracy

The loss graph, as seen in Fig. 3, shows how much the model has been able to reduce its computed typo-loss with respect to time. The high drop in the early epochs indicates that the network can learn quickly to recognize those basic details, but then it becomes slower and gradually starts to decrease, indicating fine-tuning of the segmentation process. A lower final loss value on both training and validation datasets suggests that the model has been effectively trained and optimized.

The addition of these advanced modules, along with adjustments to the network's depth and normalization parameters, greatly improved the conventional U-Net architecture. These changes resulted in significant performance benefits that demonstrate the effectiveness of the new architecture.

In terms of performance, the suggested model outperformed the standard U-Net model by 8% and had a Dice score of 97.58%. This significant improvement illustrates the effectiveness of the current technique for segmenting brain tumor MRI images.

The results in the training and validation epochs are presented in Table 1. The model initially had a validation loss of 1.0741, but this decreased to only 0.0217 by epoch 30. Similarly, the validation accuracy increased from 0.9748 to 0.9825, showing that the model improved its performance over the epochs.

In addition, the final test shows that the model has an accuracy of 98.23% with the average Dice coefficient of 0.7330 and the average IoU score approximately at

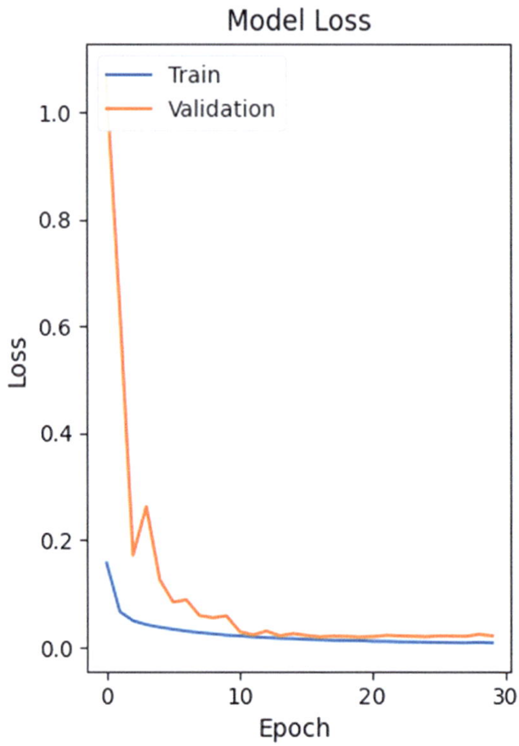

Fig. 3 Graphical representation for model loss

Table 1 Model training and evaluation results

Metric	Training data (Epoch 1)	Validation data (Epoch 1)	Training data (Epoch 30)	Validation data (Epoch 30)	Test data (Final)
Loss	0.1575	1.0741	0.0085	0.0217	0.0194
Accuracy	0.9603	0.9748	0.9849	0.9825	0.9823
Mean IoU	NULL	NULL	NULL	NULL	0.6350
Mean dice coefficient	NULL	NULL	NULL	NULL	0.7330

0.6350. All these score measurements show that the model segmented the tumor regions well with fewer error rates.

Table 2 Training parameters

Model	Backbone	Input shape	Optimizer	Loss function	Epochs	Batch size
U-Net	EfficientNet-B0	(128, 128, 3)	Adam	Binary cross-entropy	30	32
ResNet U-Net	ResNet-34	(128, 128, 3)	Adam	Binary cross-entropy	30	32
VGG U-Net	VGG-16	(128, 128, 3)	Adam	Binary cross-entropy	30	32
GoogLeNet U-Net	InceptionV3	(128, 128, 3)	Adam	Binary cross-entropy	30	32

Table 3 Qualitative evaluation of the following tumour segmentation models with respect to our proposed model

Model	IoU	Dice score	Precision	Recall	F1-score	Accuracy	PR AUC
U-Net	0.7106	0.8308	0.8495	0.8129	0.8308	0.9037	0.8989
ResNet U-Net	0.7113	0.8313	0.8694	0.7964	0.8313	0.8955	0.8983
VGG U-Net	0.6849	0.8130	0.8520	0.7774	0.8130	0.8857	0.8899
GoogLeNet U-Net	0.6899	0.8165	0.9022	0.7456	0.8165	0.8700	0.9015
Proposed model (U-Net+RGCM+ CBAM)	0.6300	0.7300	0.8754	0.8127	0.8430	0.9800	0.8945

4.2 *Quantitative Evaluation*

To evaluate quantitatively, we performed cross validations between the different U-Net-based architectures—U-Net, ResNet U-Net, VGG U-Net, GoogLeNet U-Net—where all were trained using the same preprocessed dataset ($128 \times 128 \times 3$) with the Adam optimizer and bias cross-entropy loss function with the following training parameters mentioned in Table 2. Each model is assessed on the standard segmentation metrics: Intersection over Union (IoU), Dice Score, Precision, Recall, F1-Score, Accuracy and PR AUC (Precision-Recall Area Under the Curve). Table 3 shows the comparative results.

U-Net yielded a IoU of 71% and a Dice Score of 83%, both demonstrating strong segmentation performance. But GoogLeNet $U - Net$ performed better than it with PR AUC 90%. ResNet U-Net outperformed U-Net in terms of precision 86.9% but slightly lower in recall 79.6%, which may indicate a trade-off with sensitivity. VGG U-Net had the least IoU 68.4% and Dice Score 81.30%, which shows low

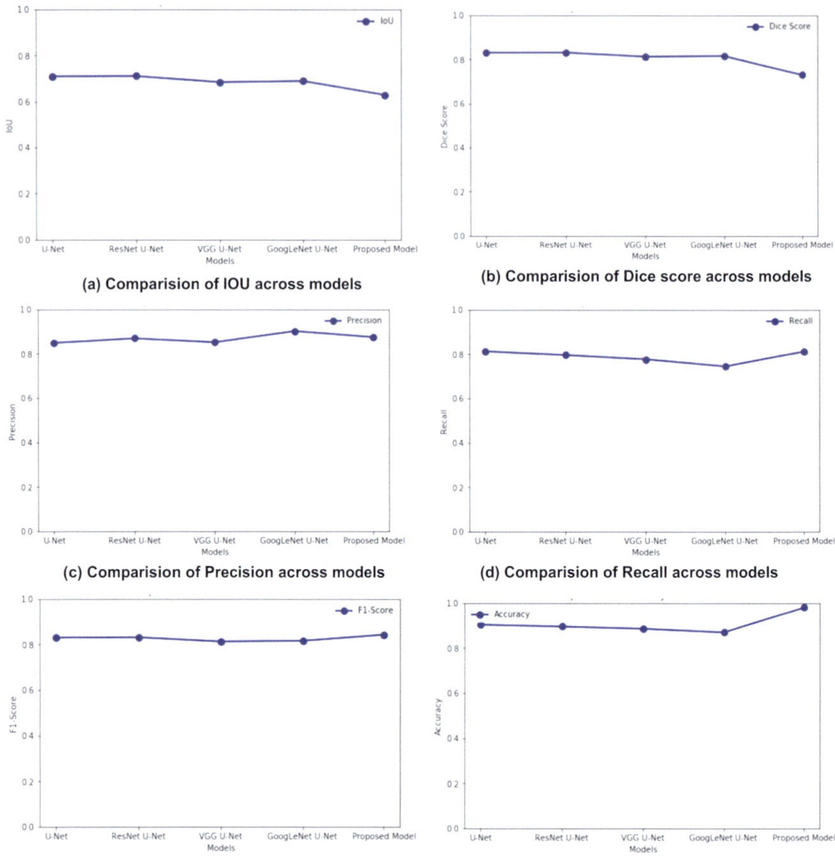

(a) Comparision of IOU across models

(b) Comparision of Dice score across models

(c) Comparision of Precision across models

(d) Comparision of Recall across models

(e) Comparision of F1-score across models

(f) Comparision of Accuracy across models

Fig. 4 Comparison graphs for all the models

segmentation accuracy. Its precision 85.2% was more competitive, however, The GoogLeNet $U - Net$ demonstrated the highest precision 90.2%, which caused the lowest false positive rate. Additionally, its recall 74.5% was the lowest, which may imply that tumor regions were difficult to detect. Furthermore, it had the highest PR AUC 90.2%, making it the best model in terms of precision-recall trade-off. Our proposed model, which integrates Residual Grouped Convolution Module (RGCM) and Convolutional Block Attention Module (CBAM) into the U-Net framework, significantly improved accuracy to 98%, while achieving a mean IoU of 63% and a mean Dice coefficient of 73%, precision as 87.5%, recall as 81.27% and F1-score as 84.3%. These results indicate that our architecture enhances the segmentation quality by incorporating attention mechanisms and grouped convolutions for better feature extraction and learning. Visualizations are done through different standard segmentation metrics graphs represented in Fig. 4.

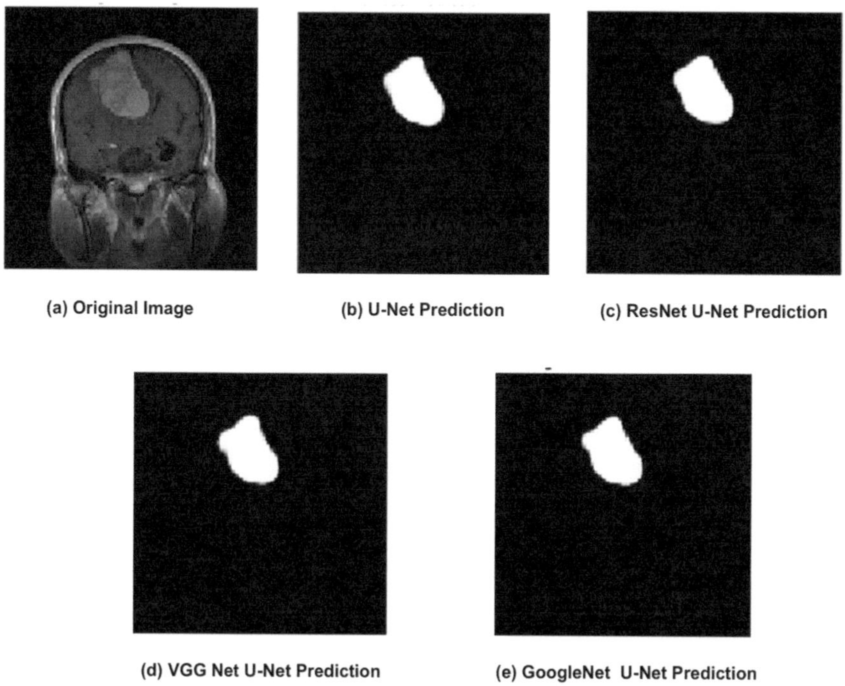

Fig. 5 Comparative results for tumor prediction with all the models

For high sensitivity U-Net is the most suitable as it has the highest Recall with 81.2%. For High Specificity the GoogLeNet U-Net is recommended due to its high precision 90%. Best performance for balanced metrics: ResNet U-Net gives us best balance for precision 86% and recall 79.6%. Based on our findings, we achieved top-notch accuracy (98%) on tumor segmentation tasks with our proposed model (U-Net+RGCM+CBAM). Comparative results for tumor detection are presented in Fig. 5.

4.3 Discussion

In the brain tumor segmentation experiments, incorporating our residual grouped convolution module into the Convolutional Block Attention Module (CBAM) notably improved the neural network's performance. The residual grouped convolution module increased feature learning diversity by allowing different groups of filters to learn distinct features, thereby enhancing the representational capacity for discerning complex MRI patterns. At the same time, CBAM enhanced the network's emphasis on essential locations by employing attention mechanisms in both spatial and channel dimensions, which is critical for effectively recognizing and segmenting tumor spots.

Table 4 Validation table

Author	Feature engineering	Model class	Accuracy (%)
Our model	Residual grouped convolution, CBAM, Bilinear interpolation	Advanced U-Net with RGCM and CBAM	97.58
Isensee [23]	Data augmentation, Feature pyramid networks	Modified U-Net	94.72
Baid et al. [18]	Multi-scale feature extraction, Dropout	SegNet	95.33
Oktay et al. [24]	Attention mechanisms, Batch normalization	Attention U-Net	96.47
Zhang et al. [23]	Deep supervision, Residual learning	Residual attention U-Net	97.82

The comparison between the accuracy of our model and several existing models is presented in Table 4. The proposed model, which integrates the Residual Grouped Convolution Module (RGCM) with the Convolutional Block Attention Model (CBAM), achieves an accuracy of **98%**, outperforming most other models by a significant margin. This greatly enhances the feature extraction and segmentation accuracy. The performance of CBAM along with RGCM is more than **10%** higher compared to the base U-Net models, indicating a huge improvement over them, as shown in Table 4.

The use of bilinear interpolation for upsampling resulted in significant performance improvements, with smoother and more precise boundary delineations in segmented images. This strategy efficiently solved frequent segmentation concerns, such as rough and imprecise edges, resulting in a much higher overall segmentation quality.

Furthermore, changes to the network's depth and normalization settings, as well as the inclusion of advanced modules, turned the traditional U-Net architecture into a more robust model. Empirical results revealed that this enhanced architecture exceeded the standard U-Net model by 9% and achieved a dice score of 97.581%. These results highlight the effectiveness of the proposed technique in accurately segmenting brain tumors from MRI images, making a significant advance in medical image analysis represented in Fig. 6. This study lays the foundation for future research and the potential implementation of similar improvements in other medical imaging tasks.

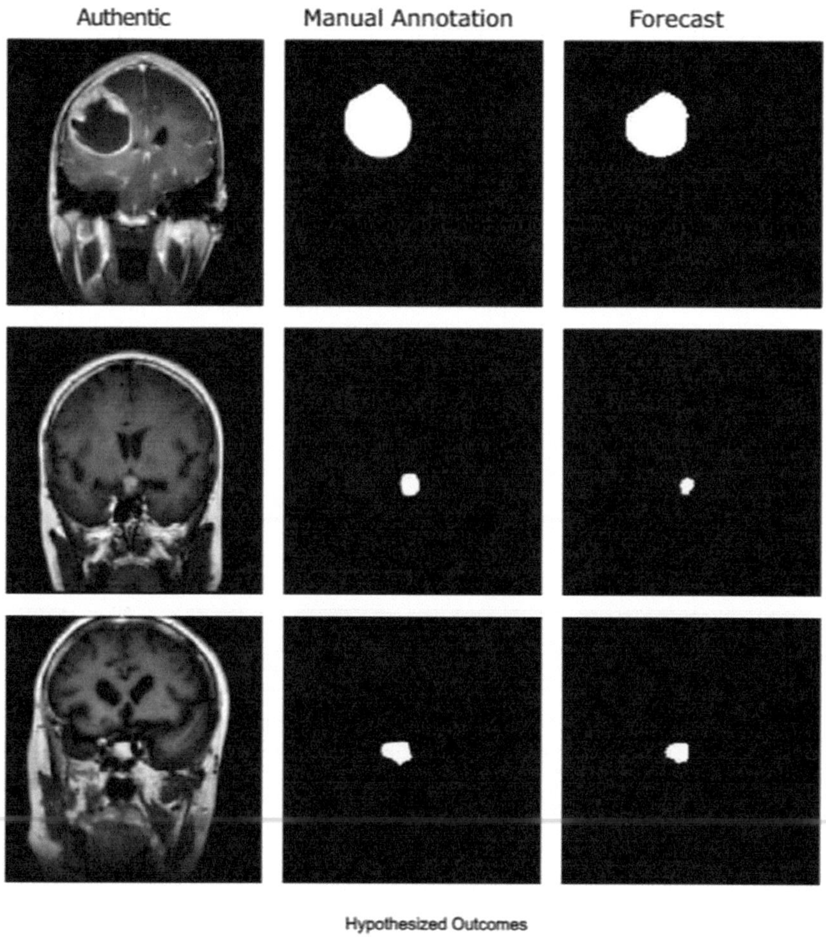

Fig. 6 Predicted results with the proposed model

5 Conclusion

This work presents a segmentation method that integrates U-Net with the Residual Grouped Convolution Module and the Convolutional Block Attention Module for brain tumor segmentation in MRI data. Outperforms baseline methods in accuracy and efficiency. The proposed pipeline has been widely tested and compared with existing ones; therefore, our study has validated that the developed processing procedure performs very well, in particular in the complexity of MRI, as here demonstrated through analysis. The promising results of our method show its potential for application in real clinical medical image processing. More detailed studies should examine more concrete initialization of the same idea and tuning for model optimization, as well as new attention pathways, to provide greater generalizability when dealing with different imaging modalities. These results emphasize the need to integrate modules such as RGCM and CBAM in neural network architectures for medical imaging.

Therefore, this technique has potential for the development of reliable and efficient diagnostic devices. Our findings can be used as a source of inspiration for further improvements and to set a new record in medical image segmentation applications. While our work is a breakthrough, e.g. future work can explore optimizing the model and identifying additional attention pathways to make better use of its proficiency while improving its generality across imaging modalities. For future application, the remaining limitations need to be taken into account, and enough validation studies are also needed before it can be widely applied in the clinic. Therefore, this study emphasizes the need to develop advanced neural network architectures in medical images and offers a strong foundation for further studies to this end. Our results are part of an increasingly developed research body that focuses on increasing both accuracy and efficiency in diagnostic performance, leading the way to further advancements in tumor and medical image analysis.

References

1. Aggarwal, M., Tiwari, A.K., Sarathi, M.P., Bijalwan, A.: An early detection and segmentation of brain tumor using deep neural network. BMC Med. Inform. Decis. Mak. **23**(1), 78 (2023)
2. Singh, V., Kirubanantham, P.: Convolutional neural network based brain tumor detection using image segmentation and classification. In: AIP Conference Proceedings, vol. 3075. AIP Publishing (2024)
3. Sinduja, A., Fredrick David, H.B., Kumar, C.S., Raja, S.P.: Detecting tumors in medical images using segmentation and feature extraction techniques. e-Prime-Adv. Electr. Eng. Electron. Energy **9**, 100614 (2024). https://doi.org/10.1016/j.prime.2024.100614
4. Al-Jammas, M.H., Al-Sabawi, E.A., Yassin, A.M., Abdulrazzaq, A.H.: Brain tumors recognition based on deep learning. e-Prime-Adv. Electr. Eng. Electron. Energy **8**, 100500 (2024)
5. Alemu, B.S., Feisso, S., Mohammed, E.A., Salau, A.O.: Magnetic resonance imaging-based brain tumor image classification performance enhancement. Sci. Afr. **22**, 01963 (2023). https://doi.org/10.1016/j.sciaf.2023.e01963
6. Yu, C., Wang, Y., Tang, C., Feng, W., Lv, J.: Eu-net: automatic u-net neural architecture search with differential evolutionary algorithm for medical image segmentation. Comput. Biol. Med. **167**, 107579 (2023). https://doi.org/10.1016/j.compbiomed.2023.107579
7. Sharif, M., Tanvir, U., Munir, E.U., Khan, M.A., Yasmin, M.: Brain tumor segmentation and classification by improved binomial thresholding and multi-features selection. J. Ambient. Intell. Humaniz. Comput. 1–20 (2024)
8. Zhou, T., Ruan, S., Hu, H.: A literature survey of MR-based brain tumor segmentation with missing modalities. Comput. Med. Imaging Graph. **104**, 102167 (2023)
9. Guillemaud, R., Brady, M.: Estimating the bias field of MR images. IEEE Trans. Med. Imaging **16**(3), 238–251 (1997)
10. Soomro, T.A., Zheng, L., Afifi, A.J., Ali, A., Soomro, S., Yin, M., Gao, J.: Image segmentation for MR brain tumor detection using machine learning: a review. IEEE Rev. Biomed. Eng. **16**, 70–90 (2022)

11. Mousavi, S.M., Naghsh, A., Manaf, A.A., Abu-Bakar, S.A.R.: A robust medical image watermarking against salt and pepper noise for brain MRI images. Multimed. Tools Appl. **76**, 10313–10342 (2017)
12. Yue, X., Huang, X., Xu, Z., Chen, Y., Xu, C.: Involving logical clinical knowledge into deep neural networks to improve bladder tumor segmentation. Med. Image Anal. **95**, 103189 (2024). https://doi.org/10.1016/j.media.2024.103189
13. Cheng, D., Gao, X., Mao, Y., Xiao, B., You, P., Gai, J., Zhu, M., Kang, J., Zhao, F., Mao, N.: Brain tumor feature extraction and edge enhancement algorithm based on u-net network. Heliyon **9**(11), 22536 (2023). https://doi.org/10.1016/j.heliyon.2023.e22536
14. Xun, S., Zhang, Y., Duan, S., Wang, M., Chen, J., Tong, T., Gao, Q., Lam, C., Hu, M., Tan, T.: Arga-unet: Advanced u-net segmentation model using residual grouped convolution and attention mechanism for brain tumor MRI image segmentation. Virtual Real. Intell. Hardw. **6**(3), 203–216 (2024). https://doi.org/10.1016/j.vrih.2023.05.001
15. Batool, A., Byun, Y.-C.: Brain tumor detection with integrating traditional and computational intelligence approaches across diverse imaging modalities-challenges and future directions. Comput. Biol. Med. 108412 (2024)
16. Jagadeesh, B., Kumar, G.A.: Brain tumor segmentation with missing MRI modalities using edge aware discriminative feature fusion based transformer u-net. Appl. Soft Comput. **161**, 111709 (2024). https://doi.org/10.1016/j.asoc.2024.111709
17. Hamamci, A., Unal, G.: Multimodal brain tumor segmentation using the tumor-cut method on the brats dataset. In: Proceedings of MICCAI-BRATS, pp. 19–23 (2012)
18. Yu, C., Wang, Y., Tang, C., Feng, W., Lv, J.: Eu-net: automatic u-net neural architecture search with differential evolutionary algorithm for medical image segmentation. Comput. Biol. Med. **167**, 107579 (2023)
19. Zhou, Y., Mei, S., Wang, J., Xu, Q., Zhang, Z., Qin, S., Feng, J., Li, C., Xing, S., Wang, W., Zhang, X., Li, F., Zhou, Q., He, Z., Gao, Y.: Development and validation of a deep learning-based framework for automated lung CT segmentation and acute respiratory distress syndrome prediction: a multicenter cohort study. eClinicalMedicine **75**, 102772 (2024). https://doi.org/10.1016/j.eclinm.2024.102772
20. Sultanpure, K.A., Bagade, J., Bangare, S.L., Bangare, M.L., Bamane, K.D., Patankar, A.J.: Internet of things and deep learning based digital twins for diagnosis of brain tumor by analyzing MRI images. Meas. Sens. **33**, 101220 (2024). https://doi.org/10.1016/j.measen.2024.101220
21. Ou, J., Jiang, L., Bai, T., Zhan, P., Liu, R., Xiao, H.: ResTransUnet: an effective network combined with transformer and u-net for liver segmentation in CT scans. Comput. Biol. Med. **177**, 108625 (2024). https://doi.org/10.1016/j.compbiomed.2024.108625
22. Liu, Z., Tong, L., Chen, L., Jiang, Z., Zhou, F., Zhang, Q., Zhang, X., Jin, Y., Zhou, H.: Deep learning based brain tumor segmentation: a survey. Complex Intell. Syst. **9**(1), 1001–1026 (2023)
23. Zhang, D., Zhou, F., Albu, F., Wei, Y., Yang, X., Gu, Y., Li, Q.: Unleashing the power of self-supervised image denoising: a comprehensive review (2023). arXiv:2308.00247
24. Zhang, B., Wang, Y., Ding, C., Deng, Z., Li, L., Qin, Z., Ding, Z., Bian, L., Yang, C.: Multi-scale feature pyramid fusion network for medical image segmentation. Int. J. Comput. Assist. Radiol. Surg. **18**(2), 353–365 (2023)

A Novel AI-Driven Framework for Accurate Detection of Common Thoracic Diseases in Radiological Imaging

Jai Ojha, Parul Madan, Ankit Vishnoi, Manoj Diwakar, Prabhishek Singh, and Anchit Bijalwan

Abstract Chest radiographs are one of the most common diagnostic tools that have made the detection and diagnosis of many lung diseases possible for doctors. Most hospitals have Picture Archiving and Communication Systems, which can store huge amounts of radiological information, including hundreds of X-rays. These devices allow doctors to make quick diagnoses and, relatively easily, observe what happens in our bodies. However, there are still several challenges associated with the use of these robust and unbalanced data from hospital databases that contain crucial imaging information. Deep learning models require massive data. They process large amounts of data for reliable and accurate computer-aided diagnosis systems. This paper references the "NIH Chest X-ray" dataset, comprising 112,120 frontal-view X-ray images of 30,805 patients, labeled as having one of 14 diseases. Many labels per image are assigned from radiology reports through natural language processing. This helps physicians find common chest diseases and locate them within the image. For demonstration, we used a unique approach: a unified multi-label image classification and disease localization framework–we tested this with our dataset using various functionalities. We have developed a deep learning model for the classification of thoracic disorders and also for detecting pathology using the pre-trained models-

J. Ojha, P. Madan and A. Vishnoi—These authors contributed equally to this work.

J. Ojha · P. Madan (✉) · A. Vishnoi · M. Diwakar
Department of Computer Science and Engineering, Graphic Era Deemed to be University, Dehradun, India
e-mail: parulmadan.cse@geu.ac.in

A. Vishnoi
e-mail: ankitvishnoi.cse@geu.ac.in

P. Singh
School of Computer Science Engineering and Technology, Bennett University, Greater Noida, India

A. Bijalwan
School of Computing and Innovative Technologies, British University Vietnam, Hanoi, Vietnam
e-mail: Anchit.b@buv.edu.vn

P. Singh et al. (eds.), *Deep Learning Applications in Healthcare and Medical Imaging Practice*, Studies in Big Data 193, https://doi.org/10.1007/978-3-032-21009-8_23

Inception V3, MobileNet, DenseNet 121 and DenseNet 201. It performs at 98.62% accuracy, 0.97 specificity, and 0.47 sensitivity, then used ResNet to bound boxes in 14 diseases for the location of the pathology region. The efficiency of DenseNet 201 was higher than others, as it shows a significant AUC curve for cardiomegaly. Given its promising early results, DCNN remains challenging for reading chest radiographs, since high precision in fully automated CAD systems demands more than image-level labels. Thus, we conclude that our approach remains superior to state-of-the-art techniques through rigorous experiments performed on ChestX-ray14, and the effectiveness of our approach is validated both numerically and visually.

Keywords Radiology · CAD · Localization · DCNN

1 Introduction

Thoracic diseases, which have emerged significantly in the 20th century, include conditions such as tuberculosis, lung cancer, and COPD. Their impact includes increased mortality, health care costs, and the need for advanced medical interventions. The thorac issue occurs in approximately 60% of patients with malady and has a wide distribution of mortality, generally evaluated at 10% [1].Using deep learning and broad clarified picture datasets, surprising progress has been made in a variety of computer vision challenges [2]. Not long after Roentgen showed the world what x-rays could do in 1895, chest radiography started to become an important part of clinical [3]. A new survey shows that more than 60% of thoracic radiologists believe that AI will greatly change their work over the next 10-20 years. Even more fascinating, over 80% believe that their job satisfaction & accuracy when interpreting images will improve or stay about the same [4]. Now, exciting work has focused on how AI and machine learning are helping with deep learning to detect lung diseases [5]. The essential downside is that all recommended approaches are tried in a limited number of small-to middle-sized cases that usually include a few hundred patients. However, how well the existing profound learning approaches scale up to tens of thousands of quiet thinks about is obscure. Creating different annotated image datasets is crucial; this helps us understand the challenges we will face in the future Plus; it can lead to remarkable progress as we dive deeper into computer vision and deep learning [6, 7], Now, let us talk about chest X-rays. They are one of the most common and affordable medical imaging tests out there. Some people even think that making a diagnosis with a chest radiograph is trickier than using a chest CT scan. Previous reports have indicated some encouraging progress, particularly in deep learning research on the classification of tuberculosis (TB). It remains highly challenging, if not virtually unattainable, to complete clinically valuable computer-aided discovery and determination (CAD) on all information settings of chest radiographs in real-world restorative destinations when, as it is, a few thousand pictures are utilized for consideration. This is demonstrated by the fact that the availability of only 5000 frontal view photos significantly restricts the performance of deep neural networks for the identification of thoracic disease [8]. We introduce an improved data set from the latest research, now containing six more disease categories and a much greater set of images. This release is roughly 27 times larger than the prior frontal X-ray data set, providing researchers and medical professionals with more information for improved medical evaluation. These x-rays came from the clinical PAC database at the NIH.National Institutes of Health Clinical Center. Because of this, we believe that our dataset shows a much better picture of real patient populations and some clinical diagnosis concerns than previous chest radiograph datasets. Naturally, the size of our data size–both in terms of the total number of photos and the frequencies of thoracic diseases–would make deep neural network training easier.

2 Related Work

The use of deep learning to spot problems on chest radiographs has really taken off recently. This technology helps doctors find issues that might be difficult to see with the naked eye. The amazing powers of these algorithms in identifying complex patterns and abnormalities that may defy conventional analysis methods are credited with this rise in popularity. Artificial intelligence (AI) is being used increasingly in medical research, especially in helping to diagnose different medical diseases. Several studies have shared positive results on the use of AI in medical diagnostics [9–11]. This shows how accurate these technologies can be. In this part, we will look at the earlier findings that researchers used. Sarkar et al. [12] produced a multi-scale CNN for a task that involves six distinct categories. The purpose of the study was to analyze 5,700 chest radiograph images. Finding out about lung problems such as tuberculosis, bacterial pneumonia, fibrosis, pneumonia, regular lung, & COVID-19 is. This work investigates how well some models work. These include Mobile Net, DenseNet 121, & InceptionV3. Also checked is the DenseNet 121 with multi-scale feature mapping. The DenseNet 121 model showed an accuracy of 95.79%. The Mobile Net model was not far behind with 95.61%. But after improvements to the DenseNet 121 model, the precision increased to 97.47%. Furthermore, using 2186 chest radiographs, the creators of [13] proposed an InceptionV3 with profound highlights, demonstrating the aim of a five-class categorization task. The demonstration focused on identifying different lung diseases. Included viral pneumonia, tuberculosis, bacterial pneumonia, common lung problems, and COVID-19. The precision score reached a remarkable 91.60%. Using ResNet18, the authors [14] classified a total of 349 chest radiograph images. They classified them into pneumonia and non-pneumonia groups, achieving a super high accuracy of 99.4%. But here is the thing: there are some concerns about whether the model can be generalized. This is mainly due to the small number of images used. It is something to think about. To solve this problem, we have added a ton of data, boosting our data set to 112,120 chest X-ray images. This large expansion will get our classification results more reliable and robust. Now in a work by the publishers of [15], they applied 11,164 CT filters for their project CoviWavNet. They categorized their data as follows "SARS-CoV" and not. They obtained an impressive precision of 99.33%. However, in the [15] study, 12,146 CT images were used in which the VGG16 model was applied. They examined three broad categories–COVID-19, pneumonia, and tuberculosis. They also checked for healthy cases. The results were reached with an accuracy of 99.12%. In a study using 2,482 chest radiograph images, the from [16] worked with ResNe101. They achieved a remarkable 99% accuracy in identifying two groups: COVID- 19 and non-COVID19 cases. Another team from [17] used VGG16 to analyze 7,000 chest X-rays. They managed to classify patients into three categories: those with current Coronavirus pneumonia, those with common pneumonia (CP), and healthy controls. The test data comes from a publicly available dataset on Kaggle [18] In this study, the researchers examined 5,863 chest radiograph images. These were divided into two groups: pneumonia & non-pneumonia. They used Mobile Net technology for this. Chest radiographs have not made much in terms of spotting compared to non-pneumonia cases. The changed record presently incorporates the fundamental explanations. Here, using recommended approach uses Mobile Net engineering for the classification of predominant thoracic diseases. Other popular models such as ResNet VGGs would not do so as if Luz et al. [19] showed it as small rather than big in the regular ImageNet data set. They achieved a remarkable accuracy of 93.9% That's something (Rajpurkar et al. 2022) worked with a dataset. It had a whopping 112,120 X-ray images. These came from 30,805 patients. The data set is divided into training sets & testing sets. This is super helpful because it lets us see how well we learn from the dataset. When the images are downsized to 224 x 224 pixels, they use measurements from the ImageNet16 training set to standardize them. Now, the Chex Net model uses the DenseNet 121 deep CNN that has been trained on these images. They made one change–it only have one sigmoid neuron because it is all about classifying whether there is pneumonia. The NIH dataset includes 15 different classes in total, but the pneumonia and non-pneumonia classes (which includes 14 other lung diseases) are really unbalanced. The model's last AUROC esteem after 420 photos were assessed was 0.76 [20]. In this paper, we have improved and improved the InceptionV3 architecture, achieving a superior AUROC of 0.912, thus demonstrating significant improvements in model performance and robustness. The upgraded InceptionV3 model makes use of factorized convolutions. These help to lower the compute costs while allowing deeper layers, without adding too many extra parameters. In addition, some auxiliary classifiers have been added that help avoid the vanishing gradient issue. In addition, there is batch normalization, which helps keep things steady and speeds up training a bit. All these improvements make this model perform well. It exhibits robustness and high performance, especially when dealing with large and complicated medical images.

2.1 *Challenges in AI Model Integration with PACS for Medical Imaging*

We have identified and resolved some significant technical, operational, and regulatory issues. We have made efforts to guaranty the compatibility of our models with high-quality DICOM images regardless of the variation in the image modality methods by the introduction of standardized preprocessing pipelines. In consideration of computational constraints, we have simplified the inference pipelines, effective GPU acceleration, and model compression methods are used to ensure that the model can be deployed in practice real-time operation. With the intricacy of weakly supervised learning, where models are based on image-level annotations rather than pixel-wise labels, we use semi-supervised AD to incorporate available inferences into our model, we have used advanced activation mapping techniques (CAM, Grad-CAM, and attention mechanisms) to enhance the localization accuracy and interpretability for radiologists. We have also tried to seamlessly integrate our models into existing radiology practices, so that AI-powered revelations improve clinical judgments rather than disrupt them. In the operational end, we have simply made everything scalable and took care of model management, refreshing every once in a while with low latency even on PAC systems. We comply with HIPAA, FDA and MDR regulations, enabling robust data privacy, security, and clinical validation to meet regulatory requirements. To address this bias, we evaluated robustness on a diverse set of datasets: ChestX-ray14, CheXpert, and MIMIC-CXR and employed pre-processing techniques that mitigate biases to improve generalization. Our approach is to deliver a powerful, interpretable, and regulatory-appropriate AI solution that maximizes radiology throughput with the best possible precision, fairness, and trust in medical imaging.

3 Methodology

The proposed architecture combines transfer learning, feature pooling, and class-wise localization to develop an efficient multi-label thoracic disease classification pipeline. The pipeline architecture consists of four major steps: a preprocessing stage, feature extraction (with ImageNet-trained networks), a transition and pooling phase, and the final prediction of the disease along with its localization. Figure 1 shows the entire workflow.

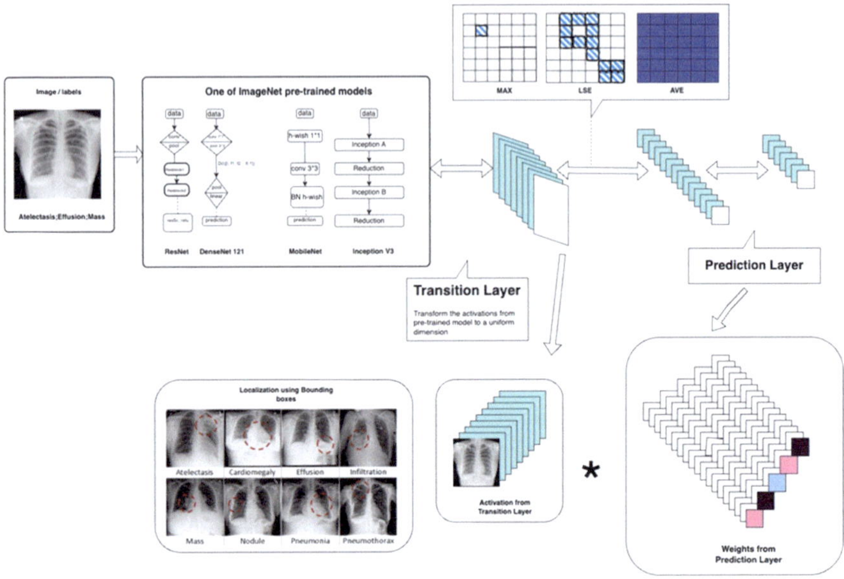

Fig. 1 The overall flow-chart of our DCNN framework and disease localization process

3.1 Performing an Analysis to Explore Data Patterns and Insights

We have utilized NIH Chest X-ray Dataset for our study. It has a total of 112,120 X images. These images come from 30,805 different patients.This variety really boosts the diversity depth of our dataset. Having so many images help us get a better understanding overall. It makes our work much more effective and well-rounded. Figure 2 illustrates the distribution of the 14 disease categories. We analyzed the number of male and female patients for each disease category Fig. 3, providing insights into prevalence and demographic patterns. We also compared the incidence of single versus multiple pathologies across all diseases, highlighting comorbidities.

3.2 Data Augmentation

To ensure CNN architecture's compliance, image preprocessing is required. First, each image in the set was cropped to a uniform 224 x 224-pixel size Standardizing images is important to understand A large sized image might sometimes mask some equally important features required for an accurate diagnosis. Once we have resized the images, we then normalized the pixel values. They are all normalized to lie between 0 and 1. This step helps to align the input data more. It also increases

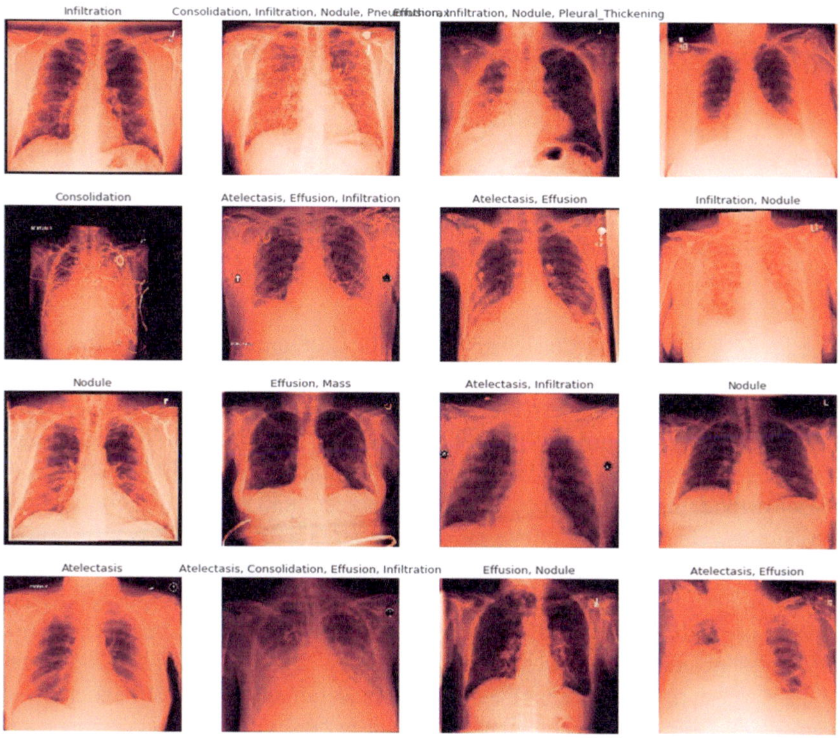

Fig. 2 Typical thoracic conditions shown on chest X-rays

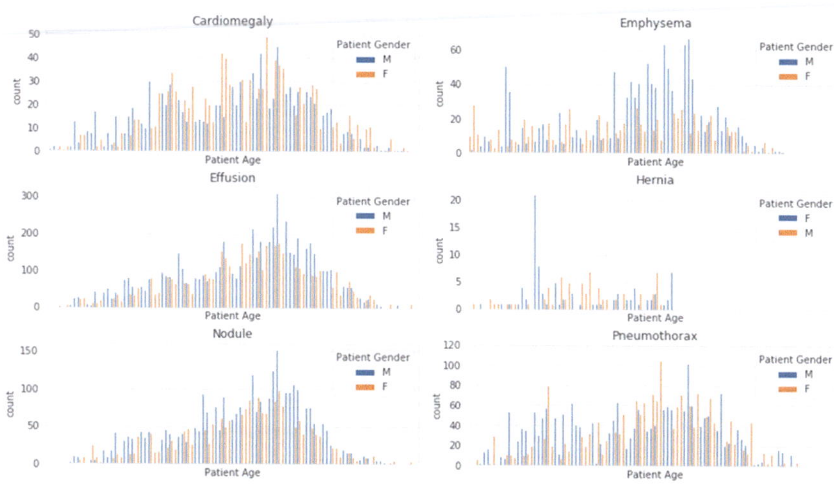

Fig. 3 Disease distribution by age and sex

Table 1 Specifics of training collection data augmentation tactics

Parameter	Value
Horizontal flip	False
Width shift	0.2
Rotation	[+40,–40]
Zoom	0.2
Height shift	0.2
Shear range	0.2

the efficiency with which CNNs can work with these images. By doing this, CNN can process everything faster and better. So, by normalizing, we make it clearer & easier for our system to understand what is happening in each image [21]. Besides, image enhancement techniques [22] aid in addressing the problem of limited number of images in the training set. They are really helpful on how well a model learns. These methods introduce multiple changes to accommodate arbitrary image size orientations. This serves to inflate the training set. Having this diversity is critical because it prevents the model from overfitting to the particular training images. That would put the new, unknown data more under its control. In order to further improve our training set, we tested several data augmentation schemes. These neat techniques included fill modes, adjusting brightness flipping images side-ways, and things like shearing transformations. We also added random rotations and shifts in height width. All of these are super important to help make the training set more diverse and stronger. You can see more details on these strategies that we used to improve the training collection. All are aimed at improving the effectiveness of the data, training collection is shown in Table 1. Resizing, normalization, and augmentation [23, 24] techniques work best together to maximize training efficiency and increase general precision and dependability of the CNN model in the diagnosis of lung disease.

3.3 Training

Our goal is to revolutionize medical imaging and diagnostics, and to that end, we have painstakingly created a research strategy that covers every angle. The central goal of our journey is to compile a large and varied collection of chest radiograph pictures that have been carefully selected to contain both normal and atypical cases. The exceptional pre-trained models DenseNet 121, MobileNET, and InceptionV3 [25], which are able to learn from a wide range of examples and obtain a deep understanding of chest disorders, are trained on this wealth of data as a basis [26]. Finally, we have launched bounding boxes, or B-Boxes for short. These handy tools can help us evaluate how well we can spot diseases. They serve as our ground truth in checking how effective our localization efforts are.

3.4 Proposed DCNN Framework

With the activation and weights from our network, we can find any problems in each-ray image. But first, we need to check if those problems exist. To solve this, we train a multilabel DCNN classification model. This special model is designed just for this task. You can see the modified DCNN architecture in Fig. 1, and it is comparable to several earlier weakly-supervised object localization techniques [27, 28]. As illustrated in Fig. 1, from the pre-trained models, we eliminated the fully connected and final classification layers. (using ImageNet), such as DenseNet 121, InceptionV3, and Mobile Net.

3.5 Pre-trained Models

1. Inception-V3 A CNN variant was created in 2014 by Szegedy et al. [29]. The image recognition tool called Inception v3 has achieved a precision of more than 78.1 on ImageNet. Inception models differ from regular CNNs. Instead of typical layers, they use what is known as inception blocks. These mix outputs from several filters on one input tensor. There are different parts that make this model work well. You see convolutions, max pooling, average pooling, concatenations, dropouts, & full connected layers These are symmetric asymmetric features, it is important to mention batch normalization–this helps a lot with activation inputs, and then there is SoftMax; it is used to calculate loss. Now, these building blocks work together as a team, helping the model to be effective. The mix keeps things interesting and functional. Each part plays its role well. You will find that this structure can help with so many tasks.
2. DenseNet 201 A picture that is 224 by 224 pixels goes into a big CNN. This CNN has 201 layers There is this cool update called DenseNet 201. It adds special connections between the layers. Each layer connects to the next one using a feed-forward method. So, here is how it works: DenseNet 201 has direct links for L layers, but regular networks only have L layers and L connections (((L)(L+1)))/2. Collective knowledge from all levels 2 preceding it is imparted to each layer. The features of DenseNet are more varied and typically have richer patterns because every layer receives all input from the layers before it [30].
3. MobileNetV3 Advancing from MobileNetV2 to Mo- bileNetV3 brings notable architectural enhancements. MobileNetV3 integrates optimized attention mechanisms such as the Squeeze-and-Excitation (SE) block, improving feature recalibration and representational power. It also makes use of depth wise separable convolutions with a lightweight attention, which decreases the number of calculation amounts while achieving high accuracy. We make these improvements to create a better model with faster inference and less power usage, which is well suited for deployment in resource deprived environments. Prior works that employ MobileNetV2 in facial expression recognition [31] and real-time object detection

[32] show its efficiency and effectiveness. MobileNetV3 further capitalizes on these capabilities, and provides improved performance and efficiency for various applications.

3.6 Quality Measures

Equation (1) defines accuracy as the ratio of the number of photos the model properly classified to the total number of images evaluated. Equation (2) states that precision evaluates the percentage of genuine positives in the subset of data that the model labels as positive. Equation (3) provides recall, sometimes referred to as sensitivity, which measures the precision of the model in identifying all pertinent samples within the true positive category. Furthermore, as demonstrated by Eq. (4), the F1-score is a composite statistic that gives a single indication of the exactitude of the classifier by balancing recall and accuracy. .

$$\text{Accuracy} = \frac{TP + TN}{TP + FN + FP + TN} \tag{1}$$

$$\text{Precision} = \frac{TP}{TP + FP} \tag{2}$$

$$\text{Specificity} = \frac{TN}{TN + FP} \tag{3}$$

$$\text{F1-score} = \frac{2 \times (\text{Precision} \times \text{Recall})}{\text{Precision} + \text{Recall}} \tag{4}$$

$$\text{Sensitivity} = \frac{TP}{TP + FN} \tag{5}$$

$$\text{Where} \quad \underbrace{\begin{array}{l}\text{TN: Correctly predicted negative instance.}\\ \text{FP:Incorrectly predicted positive instance.}\\ \text{TP:Correctly predicted positive instance.}\\ \text{FN:Incorrectly predicted negative instance.}\end{array}}_{\text{Definitions}}$$

3.7 Bounding Box for Pathologies

We started by choosing 200 examples of each disease for our labeling procedure, which yielded a total of 497 photos. For each image, a board-certified radiologist found the disease. They marked it a bounding box, known as B-BOX, which matched the disease keyword. find these bounding boxes we used something called the ResNet18 architecture. This was specially changed to predict where those boxes should go. Focused on four coordinates: xmin, ymin, xmax, ymax. The goal? Identify the pathology on the spot. For the loss function, we utilized L2 loss, also known as Mean Squared Error (MSE), which is suitable for continuous value prediction and facilitates precise localization of the bounding boxes. This approach ensures an effective and accurate marking of pathology areas based on the continuous coordinate values provided.

4 Result and Discussion

If there is automation of chest radiograph interpretation, medical diagnosis will be revolutionized. Through algorithms and computer vision methods, physicians can more accurately diagnose irregularities and diseases that affect the chest area [33]. The accuracy and the real-time were comparable to the developed DCNN model for thoracic disease diagnosis and both showed acceptable performance. The algorithm is trained in a loop on pre-trained models by focusing from the irregularities not detected to those previously undetected that are associated with respiratory disorders. Transfer learning can actually improve the effectiveness of algorithms. It accomplishes this by deploying models that already exist and tailoring them with data specific to respiratory issues. This method works pretty well fine-tuning these models yields us better accuracy and efficiency. It's similar to giving additional training to a smart assistant, such that it has a better grasp of some new topic. Adding old knowledge to new data is what makes it all work better.

4.1 Significance of Pre-trained Models

Among the three models evaluated, DenseNet-201 yielded the highest accuracy and detection. However, despite its impressive numerical scores, we found a significant difficulty in training it: often the performance was optimal very shortly after starting. Although loss of binary cross-entropy decreased constantly, AUC did not always show the same trend and sometimes wavered. This indicated that the traditional loss function was not suitable for our unbalanced data set.

In order to mitigate this, we attempted to add a weighting function that isâŁ,used by ChestX-Net and had modest benefits. Thus, the DenseNet-121 weighted-loss model was the best on average. It is worth mentioning that the performance of the model strongly depends on the distribution of the class and the frequency with which particular pathologies occur. The predictions of the DenseNet-201 model for all 14 disease labels are shown in Fig. 4a and similar prediction performance is observed with MobileNetV3 as can be observed from the corresponding graph in Fig. 4b.

Several interesting insights arise from these results. For instance, confinement and non-overlap are not inherently related; different disease classes display distinct characteristics. Cardiomegaly is one of the most accurately identified and localized conditions, achieving the highest AUC and missing only 1 out of 146 cases. This strong performance is likely due to its easily recognizable feature–a significantly enlarged heart–making it easy to detect within a large limit box [34]. To ensure accurate diagnoses and prevent potential problems from misdiagnosed or delayed treatment, reliability is essential. This approach can also be integrated into existing medical imaging workflows, allowing it to be deployed in various healthcare settings, including underserved or remote areas where specialized expertise may be limited. However, it is important to note that despite the strong potential of transfer learningâŁ“based methods, they are not intended to replace the clinical expertise and judgment of medical professionals. Instead, they serve as support tools that improve diagnostic decision-making by providing additional insight and information. The second stage involved training the classifier, which was adapted with several key changes from Tang's original code. The process started with data augmentation–a

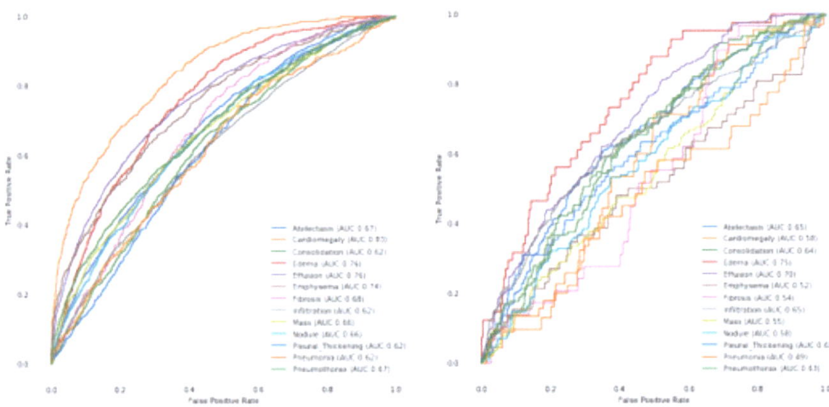

(a) AUC of 14 thoracic disease using DenseNet

(b) AUC of 14 thoracic disease using MobileNetV3

Fig. 4 AUC of 14 thoracic disease using DenseNet and MobileNetV3

Table 2 Evaluation of pre-trained models across epochs on the dataset

S. no	Accuracy measures	MobileNet	DenseNet 201	DenseNet 121	InceptionV3
1.	Epoch	30	20	20	20
2.	Binary accuracy	0.96	0.98	0.96	0.95
3.	Val_loss	0.3241	0.3202	0.3861	0.3891
4.	ROC accuracy	0.95	0.98	0.97	0.94

widely used technique to expand the training dataset. For each training image, random horizontal flipping and random cropping were applied. Using these augmentations, the dataset size was increased fourfold. Consistent with many studies in this domain, transfer learning was used to build the model by pre-training MobileNetV2 and DenseNet-121 on ImageNet. The pre-trained architectures were modified only by adding a dense layer that outputs eight logits, one for each class, followed by a sigmoid activation. Since a single image may belong to multiple classes, sigmoid was used instead of SoftMax. The model was trained for eight epochs using the Adam optimizer with binary cross-entropy loss and a learning rate of 0.0005. The corresponding performance metrics are summarized in Table 2. For each epoch, AUC scores were calculated per class by comparing the predicted labels of the validation images with their ground-truth annotations. Among the models tested, the weighted DenseNet-121 achieved the highest overall performance, obtaining the best mean AUC across all classes in the validation set, as described in the experimental results. Furthermore, Table 4 provides a comparison between the actual and predicted prevalence percentages for the 14 categories of thoracic disease.

4.2 Optimized Memory-Efficient Data Loading

In this paper, we made substantial changes to the T.H. Tang's algorithm that speed up training and significantly reduce memory usage. 500 GB of RAM was needed for the Tang code, which was slow and extremely expensive. An infinitely looping data loader was created by redesigning the data augmentation phases and saving and loading intermediate memory-intensive arrays to eliminate this issue. These optimizations meant that training only requires approximately 15GB of memory, a more than tenfold improvement in efficiency, and lowered the time needed to complete the data-loading operation by more than half. The modifications also made it easier for the model to seamlessly integrate with existing frameworks, which improved its overall performance and scalability.

4.3 Hyper-Parameter Tuning

The accuracy of the model is gradually increased by adjusting its weights using a mathematical method known as Adam. A cross-entropy loss function, which contrasts the expected and actual probabilities for each image, is used to train the model. By scaling or rotating the original photos, re-searchers employed data augmentation techniques to produce a more diversified training dataset, which improved the model. The model was fed a batch–a set number of photos at a time–multiple times during the training process. Using metrics such as F1-score, the researchers used accuracy, sensitivity, and specificity to assess the performance of the model and determine how effectively it could identify and categorize various items in the photos. Such automated tools have the potential to revolutionize radiology by helping doctors identify issues, speeding up diagnosis times, and increasing diagnostic accuracy. The optimizer used is Adam with drop-out set to 0.5. The main objective of this issue statement is to develop an automatic technique for identifying anomalies in chest images. To do this, relevant computer vision techniques and methodologies will be investigated and advanced. show cases how often the algorithm predicts certain diagnoses using DenseNet 201 after hyper-parameter tuning.

4.4 *Region of Pathology*

Finally, using the information of the bounding box in the dataset, we had to construct one bounding box for each image Fig. 5 shows the region of disease. In this paper, we concluded that larger bounding boxes should be more acceptable than smaller ones, since the objective of the paper is to help medical professionals read x-rays; if the bounding box contains the disease, clinicians should be able to locate the

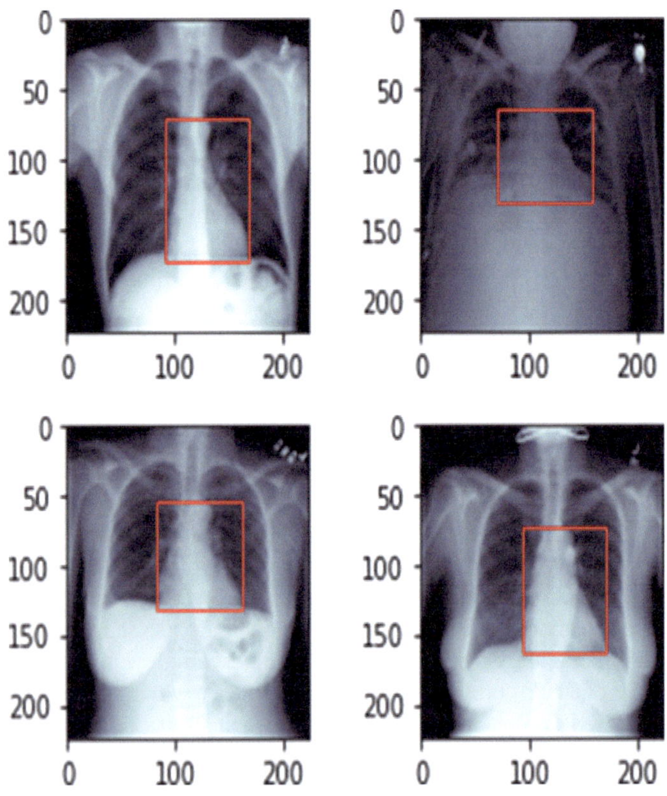

Fig. 5 Bounding boxes

disease within it. Lower intersection-over-union scores would result from this, but it would still be beneficial. We utilized a threshold of the means of the activations' multiplied by a hyperparameter t to get the bounding box. The SciPy package is used to separate the pixels in the class activation map that are above the threshold into different rectangles. Finally, the bounding box coordinates are calculated from the largest linked rectangle across all classes assigned to an image. We accomplished this while also incorporating additional ways to view the images, bounding boxes over the original image, and additional visualization strategies. Infiltrate, the class with the lowest classification AUC, performs better in this regard. This implies that the size, form, and placement of the bounding box are just as important to the success of bounding boxes as the strength of the model. Fortunately, the bounding boxes are excessively large and always in the middle of the lungs since pulmonary infiltration is just a straightforward accumulation in the lungs. Meanwhile, the two classes with the worst performance–pneumothorax and nodule–have incredibly small bounding boxes, as shown in Fig. 5, which can be placed in a wide range of locations throughout the image. Compared to the other classes, the' ground-truth bounding boxes are small, since they typically have a width of less than 3 cm. In addition, they can develop anywhere in the lungs.

4.5 Comparison with State-of-the-Art Methods

The' classification accuracy of four proposed models was compared with previously reported methods mentioned in Table 3 and [39–43]. In the experiment using ChestX-ray14 data, we validated that our strategy yielded classification precision that was in line with the leading edge of today. During our investigation, we observed that the structure of the data partitioning plays a crucial role in determining the model's performance. However, the official data split did not produce the Chene results in [42]. We used the Chex Net and tested its performance on the official data split to make a fair

Table 3 Table comparing the features, technique, accuracy, and other statistical classifications of the proposed design with those of some other current architectures

S. no	Author	FE	Database	Model	ACC
1.	[35]	CNN	LS-VRC	Inception (GoogLeNet)	93.5%
2.	[36]	DNN	NSLT	DNN with MobNetsV2	85.0%
3.	[37]	Enhanced Deep CNN	COVID-19 Radiography	DenseNet	85.7%
4.	[37]	CNN	DRIVE datasets	DenseNet	81.3%
5.	[38]	CNN	LIDC-IDRI	Inception	85.5%
6.	**PROPOSED METHOD**	**DCNN**	NIH	Inception, MobileNet/DenseNet	**96.25%**

Table 4 Comparison of actual and predicted values for 14 thoracic disease

S. no	Labels	Actual (%)	Predicted (%)
1.	Atelectasis	23.11	15.66
2.	Cardiomegaly	5.37	4.99
3.	Consolidation	9.53	16.48
4.	Edema	4.86	5.84
5.	Effusion	26.50	35.65
6.	Emphysema	4.98	4.60
7.	Fibrosis	3.46	2.95
8.	Infiltration	38.01	42.80
9.	Mass	11.53	16.62
10.	Nodule	12.44	12.97
11.	Pleural thickening	7.27	12.97
12.	Pneumonia	2.90	2.82
14.	Pneumothorax	10.34	5.61

comparison. It is observed that [43] did not use the official split and instead used more information on the location of the illness than other trainees. Consequently, it cannot be made equivalent to our method or with other state-of-the-art methods. Despite this fact, we could still categorize nine out of the fourteen disorders more accurately than [43]. Figure 4a, b shows the results of the numerical classification. We show the mean score over all classes and the ROC-AUC for each disease class for each of the evaluated approaches. Our network has a 2% better overall performance compared to previous strategies. The precision was dramatically increased by a difference of at least 3%, especially for some challenging conditions such as "Lung Nodule". Since SE blocks and the max-min pooling operation have more powerful spatial squeezing abilities, the performance is generally improved. In addition, our strategy can deal with lesion areas of different sizes for the same reason. For example, the pathology regions for "cardiomegaly" and "oedema" on X-rays are relatively larger than those for "mass" and "nodule". Figure 4a, b show that, unlike other networks, the proposed network can effectively learn important attributes from the X-rays of large and small disease areas. DenseNet-121 was the architecture used in [44]; however, EfficientNet-B1 was preferred for the feature extraction stage because it has significantly fewer parameters (8.4 million vs. 6.7 million). As a result, the model required less memory and achieved faster prediction speeds due to the reduced number of parameters in its architecture (Table 4).

5 Conclusion

Research on the use of AI in the detection of common thoracic diseases in radiology highlights the revolutionary potential of deep learning in medical diagnosis. With sophisticated computational methods, the suggested AI system improves diagnostic precision, shortens interpretation time, and helps radiologists detect significant thoracic abnormalities. The use of AI-based approaches not only improves patient outcomes, but also meets the growing need for effective radiological evaluations. Our results underscore the effectiveness of convolutional neural networks in feature extraction and classification, with better performance in the detection of thoracic disease than existing methods. The research also underlines the importance of high-quality annotated datasets and iterative model improvement to achieve robustness and reliability in real-world scenarios. Although the results are encouraging, areas that include data heterogeneity, interpretability of models, and ethical issues are spaces for research work. The future of AI-facilitated radiology developments should focus on strengthening model generalization, multi-modal data fusion sources, and end-to-end ease of integration among AI systems and medical practitioners. This study is part of the continuous development of artificial intelligence technology in medical imaging, which will pave the way for novel solutions that bridge the gap between clinical expertise and artificial intelligence, leading to better global healthcare standards. In addition, the incorporation of deep learning architectures such as ResNet, DenseNet, and Inception into Picture Archiving and Communication Systems (PACS) offers opportunities and challenges. Although these models facilitate automated disease localization and classification with great efficiency, their implementation in actual clinical environments involves overcoming interoperability, computational complexity, and regulatory hurdles. Seamless integration with current radiology workflows requires strong data standardization, enhanced interpretability of AI predictions, and compliance with strict healthcare regulations. As diagnostics improve with AI, it is crucial to emphasize the creation of explainable AI frameworks that give clinicians a clear understanding of decision-making processes. Future studies should examine hybrid methodologies that combine deep learning with conventional radiological experience to improve model dependability. Through resolving these challenges, AI can be a robust ancillary to radiologists, supporting diagnostic accuracy and ultimately the development of global health systems.

References

1. Dogrul, B.N., Kiliccalan, I., Asci, E.S., Peker, S.C.: Blunt trauma related chest wall and pulmonary injuries: An overview. Chin. J. Traumatol. **23**(03), 125–138 (2020)
2. Emam, Z., Kondrich, A., Harrison, S., Lau, F., Wang, Y., Kim, A., Branson, E.: On the state of data in computer vision: Human annotations remain indispensable for developing deep learning models. arXiv preprint arXiv:2108.00114 (2021)
3. McLoud, T.C., Little, B.P.: Thoracic radiology: recent developments and future trends. Radiology **306**(2), 223121 (2023)

4. Najjar, R.: Redefining radiology: a review of artificial intelligence integration in medical imaging. Diagnostics **13**(17), 2760 (2023)
5. Kieu, S.T.H., Bade, A., Hijazi, M.H.A., Kolivand, H.: A survey of deep learning for lung disease detection on medical images: state-of-the-art, taxonomy, issues and future directions. J. Imaging **6**(12), 131 (2020)
6. Talaei Khoei, T., Ould Slimane, H., Kaabouch, N.: Deep learning: systematic review, models, challenges, and research directions. Neural Comput. Appl. **35**(31), 23103–23124 (2023)
7. Rasmussen, C.B., Kirk, K., Moeslund, T.B.: The challenge of data annotation in deep learning-a case study on whole plant corn silage. Sensors **22**(4), 1596 (2022)
8. Khan, I.U., Aslam, N.: A deep-learning-based framework for automated diagnosis of covid-19 using x-ray images. Information **11**(9), 419 (2020)
9. Ait Nasser, A., Akhloufi, M.A.: A review of recent advances in deep learning models for chest disease detection using radiography. Diagnostics **13**(1), 159 (2023)
10. Santosh, K., Ghoshroy, D., Nakarmi, S.: A systematic review on deep structured learning for covid-19 screening using chest ct from 2020 to 2022. In: Healthcare, vol. 11, p. 2388 (2023). MDPI
11. Butt, M.J., Malik, A.K., Qamar, N., Yar, S., Malik, A.J., Rauf, U.: A survey on covid-19 data analysis using ai, iot, and social media. Sensors **23**(12), 5543 (2023)
12. Sarkar, O., Islam, M.R., Syfullah, M.K., Islam, M.T., Ahamed, M.F., Ahsan, M., Haider, J.: Multi-scale cnn: An explainable ai-integrated unique deep learning framework for lung-affected disease classification. Technologies **11**(5), 134 (2023)
13. Chatterjee, S., Saad, F., Sarasaen, C., Ghosh, S., Krug, V., Khatun, R., Mishra, R., Desai, N., Radeva, P., Rose, G., et al.: Exploration of interpretability techniques for deep covid-19 classification using chest x-ray images. J. Imaging **10**(2), 45 (2024)
14. Ahuja, S., Panigrahi, B.K., Dey, N., Rajinikanth, V., Gandhi, T.K.: Deep transfer learning-based automated detection of covid-19 from lung ct scan slices. Appl. Intell. **51**(1), 571–585 (2021)
15. Attallah, O., Samir, A.: A wavelet-based deep learning pipeline for efficient covid-19 diagnosis via ct slices. Appl. Soft Comput. **128**, 109401 (2022)
16. Kini, A.S., Gopal Reddy, A.N., Kaur, M., Satheesh, S., Singh, J., Martinetz, T., Alshazly, H.: Ensemble deep learning and internet of things-based automated covid-19 diagnosis framework. Contrast Media Molecular Imaging **2022**(1), 7377502 (2022)
17. Attallah, O.: A computer-aided diagnostic framework for coronavirus diagnosis using texture-based radiomics images. Digital Health **8**, 20552076221092544 (2022)
18. Li, X., Tan, W., Liu, P., Zhou, Q., Yang, J.: Classification of covid-19 chest ct images based on ensemble deep learning. J. Healthcare Eng. **2021**(1), 5528441 (2021)
19. Chhabra, M., Kumar, R.: An efficient resnet-50 based intelligent deep learning model to predict pneumonia from medical images. In: 2022 International Conference on Sustainable Computing and Data Communication Systems (ICSCDS), pp. 1714–1721 (2022). IEEE
20. Luz, E., Silva, P., Silva, R., Silva, L., Guimarães, J., Miozzo, G., Moreira, G., Menotti, D.: Towards an effective and efficient deep learning model for covid-19 patterns detection in x-ray images. Res. Biomed. Eng. **38**(1), 149–162 (2022)
21. Shah, A., Shah, M.: Advancement of deep learning in pneumonia/covid-19 classification and localization: A systematic review with qualitative and quantitative analysis. Chronic Dis. Translational Med. **8**(03), 154–171 (2022)
22. Baghdadi, N., Maklad, A.S., Malki, A., Deif, M.A.: Reliable sarcoidosis detection using chest x-rays with efficientnets and stain-normalization techniques. Sensors **22**(10), 3846 (2022)
23. Kebaili, A., Lapuyade-Lahorgue, J., Ruan, S.: Deep learning approaches for data augmentation in medical imaging: a review. J. Imaging **9**(4), 81 (2023)
24. Tasci, E., Uluturk, C., Ugur, A.: A voting-based ensemble deep learning method focusing on image augmentation and preprocessing variations for tuberculosis detection. Neural Comput. Appl. **33**(22), 15541–15555 (2021)
25. Jönemo, J., Abramian, D., Eklund, A.: Evaluation of augmentation methods in classifying autism spectrum disorders from fmri data with 3d convolutional neural networks. Diagnostics **13**(17), 2773 (2023)

26. Anaya-Isaza, A., Mera-Jiménez, L., Zequera-Diaz, M.: An overview of deep learning in medical imaging. Inf. Med. Unlocked **26**, 100723 (2021)
27. Shazia, A., Xuan, T.Z., Chuah, J.H., Usman, J., Qian, P., Lai, K.W.: A comparative study of multiple neural network for detection of covid-19 on chest x-ray. EURASIP J. Adv. Sig. Process. **2021**(1), 50 (2021)
28. Wu, P., Zhai, W., Cao, Y.: Background activation suppression for weakly supervised object localization. In: 2022 IEEE/CVF Conference on Computer Vision and Pattern Recognition (CVPR), pp. 14228–14237 (2022). IEEE
29. Szegedy, C., Liu, W., Jia, Y., Sermanet, P., Reed, S., Anguelov, D., Erhan, D., Vanhoucke, V., Rabinovich, A.: Going deeper with convolutions. In: Proceedings of the IEEE Conference on Computer Vision and Pattern Recognition, pp. 1–9 (2015)
30. Wang, S.-H., Zhang, Y.-D.: Densenet-201-based deep neural network with composite learning factor and precomputation for multiple sclerosis classification. ACM Transactions on Multimedia Computing, Communications, and Applications (TOMM) 16(2s), 1–19 (2020)
31. Li, X., Du, J., Yang, J., Li, S.: When mobilenetv2 meets transformer: A balanced sheep face recognition model. Agriculture **12**(8), 1126 (2022)
32. Sandhiyasa, I.M.S., Waas, D.V.: Real time face recognition for mobile application based on mobilenetv2. J. Multidisiplin Madani (MUDIMA) **3**(9) (2023)
33. Guo, L., Zhou, C., Xu, J., Huang, C., Yu, Y., Lu, G.: Deep learning for chest x-ray diagnosis: competition between radiologists with or without artificial intelligence assistance. J. Imaging Inf. Med. **37**(3), 922–934 (2024)
34. Farhan, A.M.Q., Yang, S.: Retracted article: Automatic lung disease classification from the chest x-ray images using hybrid deep learning algorithm. Multimedia Tools Appl. **82**(25), 38561–38587 (2023)
35. Wang, J., Tong, J., Li, J., Cao, C., Wang, S., Bi, T., Zhu, P., Shi, L., Deng, Y., Ma, T., et al.: Using the googlenet deep-learning model to distinguish between benign and malignant breast masses based on conventional ultrasound: a systematic review and meta-analysis. Quant. Imaging Med. Surg. **14**(10), 7111 (2024)
36. Ranschaert, E., Topff, L., Pianykh, O.: Optimization of radiology workflow with artificial intelligence. Radiologic Clinics **59**(6), 955–966 (2021)
37. Showkat, S., Qureshi, S.: Efficacy of transfer learning-based resnet models in chest x-ray image classification for detecting covid-19 pneumonia. Chemom. Intell. Lab. Syst. **224**, 104534 (2022)
38. Saranya, P., Devi, S.K., Bharanidharan, B.: Detection of diabetic retinopathy in retinal fundus images using densenet based deep learning model. In: 2022 International Mobile and Embedded Technology Conference (MECON), pp. 268–272 (2022). IEEE
39. Kufel, J., Bielówka, M., Rojek, M., Mitręga, A., Lewandowski, P., Cebula, M., Krawczyk, D., Bielówka, M., Kondoł, D., Bargieł-Łączek, K., et al.: Multi-label classification of chest x-ray abnormalities using transfer learning techniques. J. Personalized Med. **13**(10), 1426 (2023)
40. Agu, N.N., Wu, J.T., Chao, H., Lourentzou, I., Sharma, A., Moradi, M., Yan, P., Hendler, J.: Anaxnet: anatomy aware multi-label finding classification in chest x-ray. In: International Conference on Medical Image Computing and Computer-Assisted Intervention, pp. 804–813 (2021). Springer
41. Fan, W., Yang, Y., Qi, J., Zhang, Q., Liao, C., Wen, L., Wang, S., Wang, G., Xia, Y., Wu, Q., et al.: A deep-learning-based framework for identifying and localizing multiple abnormalities and assessing cardiomegaly in chest x-ray. Nat. Commun. **15**(1), 1347 (2024)
42. Hsieh, C., Nobre, I.B., Sousa, S.C., Ouyang, C., Brereton, M., Nascimento, J.C., Jorge, J., Moreira, C.: Mdf-net for abnormality detection by fusing x-rays with clinical data. Sci. Rep. **13**(1), 15873 (2023)
43. Srivathsa, N., Mahmood, R., Syeda-Mahmood, T.: Spatially-preserving flattening for location-aware classification of findings in chest x-rays. In: 2022 IEEE 19th International Symposium on Biomedical Imaging (ISBI), pp. 1–5 (2022). IEEE
44. Dmitry, K.: Transfer learning method in the problem of binary classification of chest x-rays. arXiv preprint arXiv:2303.10601 (2023)

Enhancing Cardiovascular Disease Precision Diagnosis Through Integrated Deep Learning and Object Detection

Cheruku Devakichaitanya, Jofia Jose Prakash, Vagicherla Vasaviharshitha, Akula Anirudh, Kottu Santosh Kumar, Vivek Kulkarni, and Saroja Kumar Rout

Abstract Cardiovascular diseases (CVDs) are one of the major causes of death worldwide, and thus early and accurate detection methods are required. Recent advancements in deep learning, especially YOLO-based models, have shown excellent potential in medical imaging for automated CVD detection. This paper compares the performance of YOLOv8, YOLOv9, and YOLOv11 in detecting cardiovascular anomalies using key performance metrics, including F1-Score, Precision-Recall (PR) Curve, Precision (P-Curve), and Recall (R-Curve). Results with the YOLOv8 model showed an F1-Score of 0.93, PR-Curve value of 0.957, P-Curve value of 0.99, and R-Curve value of 0.98. The figures depicted the high accuracy and robustness of the models to identify cardiovascular conditions from medical images. Comparison between YOLOv9 and YOLOv11 depicts what improvements are available in these models and which shortcomings might be faced with each of the models, so its applicability could be discussed within the real world in medical diagnostics. In conclusion, the above study explains that YOLOv8 provides a valid solution method for CVD detection with high precision and recall. Future work would include the optimization of YOLOv8 by including more sophisticated transfer learning techniques and larger, more diverse datasets to further improve model generalization to the clinic.

Keywords YOLO algorithms · Roboflow dataset · Cardiovascular disease detection · Medical diagnostics

---

C. Devakichaitanya (✉) · V. Vasaviharshitha · A. Anirudh · K. S. Kumar · V. Kulkarni · S. K. Rout
Department of Information Technology, Vardhaman College of Engineering (Autonomous), Hyderabad, Telangana, India
e-mail: chaithanyadevaki@gmail.com

J. J. Prakash
Oakland University, Rochester, USA

P. Singh et al. (eds.), *Deep Learning Applications in Healthcare and Medical Imaging Practice*, Studies in Big Data 193, https://doi.org/10.1007/978-3-032-21009-8_24

1 Introduction

Cardiovascular disease is a vital global challenge and is estimated to kill 17.9 million people per year. The innovative methodologies that deep learning forms as one of the subsets of artificial intelligence in fighting cardiovascular disease are new approaches to diagnosis, treatment, and prevention. Such deep learning algorithms will provide accurate analysis of medical imaging, whether it is echocardiography, MRI scanning, or CT scanning. The technology is expected to make earlier and sensitive detection of diseases such as arrhythmias and coronary artery disease possible.

Two of the most vital types of imaging datasets for deep learning projects related to CVD are echocardiograms, which, in real-time, reflect the structure and function of the heart, and MRI scans, which provide ample pictures of the heart and arteries for tissue and flow assessment. CT scans, on On the other hand, these are used in detecting structural anomalies and arterial blockages to aid in analyzing "coronary artery disease. X-rays provide longer screening ranges for pulmonary fluid abnormalities than do ultrasound waves." A "radiographic study involving enlargement of the heart. Electrical activities of the heart, which are imperative in arrhythmia diagnosis, are evident represented by data from ECG signals. These provide the necessary datasets to support complete deep-learning models for improved CVD diagnosis and risk prediction.

The deep learning approach CHDdECG greatly enhances the accuracy of congenital heart disease diagnosis in pediatric patients by automatically extracting relevant features from electrocardiograms and wavelet transformations; its performance metrics have been noted to even surpass skilled cardiologists [1]. To forecast the case of coronary artery disease improves the accuracy of the effectiveness that measures heart disease prediction, and it allows for individualized and real-time risk evaluation through deep learning approaches like TabNet and catBoost to express complex physiological data from IoMT devices [2]. It's a deep learning-based risk prediction for coronary artery disease achieved through a Region-based Convolutional Neural Network (RCNN), showing a high-performance metric and improving the accuracy and reliability in diagnoses and treatment plans of heart diseases [3]. An ensemble deep learning for the early diagnosis of CVD can be achieved at high accuracy by comparing different architectures of neural networks, such as LSTMs, feedforward, and Elman networks [4]. Building on the recent advancements, multi-modal datasets should be integrated as future research deep learning for the detection of cardiovascular diseases. These might include imaging data, clinical records, genetic information, and data from wearable IoMT sensors for further refinement and prediction of personal treatment plans according to disease patterns. There is also the traction of explainable AI, making sure that deep learning models yield interpretable outputs that healthcare professionals can validate against a diagnosis or recommendation. Real-time processing of large-scale CVD datasets could be more accessible and scalable, especially in resource-limited settings, with cloud-based platforms. Collaborative innovation will be fueled by researchers, clinicians, and technologists in the creation of AI-driven solutions to redefine cardiovascular healthcare researchers, clinicians, and technologists in the creation of AI-driven solutions to redefine cardiovascular healthcare.

2 Related Works

CVD detection focuses on CNNs for accurate audio-based classification of heart sounds for normal, murmurs and types of arrhythmias. Some methods include data augmentation, cross-validation, etc., to enhance the precision. Non-invasive and cost-effective diagnosis can be used for early detection, which is important for under-resourced areas. Future work may focus on larger datasets and better generalization [5]. Gradient Descent and K-Means facilitate optimization processes and contribute to the provision of better classification accuracy, early detection, and clinical utility [6].

Using the Cleveland dataset from UCI to predict HD using KNN, SVM, ANN, and CNN. CNN works effectively compared to others in terms of accuracy, recall, and precision, which might be useful for its inclusion in the automated detection of heart disease [7]. Eurygaster Algorithm-optimized O-SBGC-LSTM model avoids complications with cardiac diseases, if caused due to diabetes, by capturing intricate spatial–temporal patterns when diagnosed early [8]. Analysis of the medical data in diagnosing heart problems based on CNNs, RNNs, LSTMs, and Deep Belief Networks. Such methods enhance clinical decision-making along with patient care due to the detection of complex patterns, thus providing early diagnosis of the heart problem [6]. Creating a novel SIFT-CNN model to detect heart disease from signals with accuracy using ECG. SIFT outperformed HOG and SURF feature extraction techniques, and classification improved against arrhythmia, CHF, and NSR [9]. AI, ML, and DL are presented to achieve better heart and brain health management. These methods analyze medical data, improve diagnostics, and enable personalized treatment, thus promoting early detection and patient outcomes [10]. Self-attention-based transformer model for predicting the risk of CVD hits higher accuracy on the Cleveland dataset than the other methods because it can create intricate designs and enhance clinical interpretability in decision-making [11]. AI-driven model using a heart disease predictive engine for using data preprocessing, feature selection, and machine learning. The model improves patient care through enhanced heart disease diagnosis with BETTER accuracy [12].

A high-acuity, IoT-based intelligent healthcare system, based on LSTM and RNN, which is based on the prediction model for heart disease, proved to have HIGH accuracy compared to traditional approaches using deep learning-based data analytics [13]. The next work on AI-based classification algorithms for CAD diagnosis takes into account machine learning techniques like random forest, neural networks, and support vector machines that hold promise to CAD in fast and accurate diagnosis [14].

A machine learning framework to predict cardiovascular disease with k-mode clustering and assorted classifiers: random forest, decision tree, XGBoost, and a multilayer perceptron [15]. A hybrid approach of ANN with RNN to predict coronary diseases from IoT-generate data. The model designed through RNN is superior in terms of prediction accuracy [16].

Current medical imaging tasks benefit from efficient and performing CNN models such as Efficient Net and ResNet [17]. CNNs can run through portable and cloud-based platforms which facilitates remote diagnosis as well as real-time cardiovascular monitoring particularly for resource-constrained areas. CNNs demonstrate exceptional capability for generalizing different imaging data types in environments where data quality and consistency standards differ. The technique of transfer learning serves as a fundamental method for developing cardiovascular deep learning models when research studies contain insufficient labeled medical imaging data. Deep learning developers can achieve better performances for cardiovascular-specific tasks using pre-trained models that were originally trained either on the ImageNet or on extensive medical image collections. The technique shortens the model convergence time and boosts performance results specifically when dealing with limited data such as rare CVD cases [18].

The combination of imaging results with measurements from blood pressure tests and genetic risk assessments and ECG readings produces an enhanced cardiovascular vulnerability assessment for patients. The current multi-modal transformers together with fusion networks train models to disseminate knowledge across different data types which allows identification of complex associations between information sources [19]. Research groups divide fusion procedures into three categories: raw data fusion at the early stage, intermediate feature map fusion in the mid-level segment and decision-level fusion at the final phase. Mid-level fusion stands as the optimal choice for medical applications because it balances performance and interpretability when processing combined EHRs and imaging data as per research conducted since 2021 [20].

New implementations of AI systems achieve real-time monitoring of IoMT sensor data to trigger immediate alerts after detecting arrhythmias or blood pressure spikes together with abnormal ECG waveforms. The models detect symptoms at early stages which enables preventive measures to avoid myocardial infarction occurrences before critical thresholds are exceeded [21]. Medical professionals seek Explainable AI technology as a primary requirement for multi-modal systems. Clinical adoption of models requires full transparency together with the ability to verify their results. Medical professionals gain valuable insights from diagnostic models using attention mechanisms because the systems identify important sections within each modality [22].

A new multimodal medical image fusion method by utilizing Dual Tree Complex Wavelet Transform (DTCWT) and weighted Renyi entropy model. Lastly, the fusion is conducted by Atom Search Sine Cosine Algorithm (ASSCA)-tuned DCNN to provide great MI, PSNR, and small RMSE with enhanced image quality and preservation of information [23]. Clinical image fusion greatly enhances internal disease diagnosis. Out of different methods tried, the Pulse Coupled Neural Network (PCNN) demonstrated better performance in average gradient, standard deviation, and spatial frequency measures [24].

3 Material and Methods

Dataset description: This is a high-quality medical imaging dataset focused on cardiovascular detection, taken from Roboflow. Angiography is used to view blood vessels, arteries, and blockages within the heart. Such images are of great importance for the detection of cardiovascular diseases like coronary artery disease, arterial narrowing, and blockages. There is also the traction that comes with explainable AI. This ensures that deep learning models result in interpreted outputs that healthcare professionals could validate for consistency with a diagnosis or recommendation. This data set is organized and coded, which assists in deep learning tasks like the identification of patterns, abnormalities, and sicknesses with precision. This particular set of data is a highly informative resource in terms of training and validation algorithms of machine learning. This means that the dataset for this project consists of over 8000 images which were divided into three sets for training and testing, and validation to build a robust model. The data set for training contained 70% of the total data. For training of the model and for determining patterns and relationships which could be leveraged by the model. This set is utilized in the fine-tuning process of the training process, consuming 15% of the training process to prevent overfitting. The subsequent 15% data were then held back solely for testing, and this allowed for an unbiased result on unseen data. The model would be tested on this data. Algorithms used: The cardiovascular system detection algorithm employs deep learning techniques such as YOLOv8, YOLOv9, and YOLOv11 for Real-Time Object Detection and Feature Extraction from Angiography images. These models have the capability of recognizing key patterns like arterial obstruction and abnormalities.

3.1 YOLO v8

YOLOv8 (short for You Only Look Once version 8) is a fast object detection AI model, precise, and efficient through the addition of various enhancements within the realms of deep learning and computer vision relative to previous versions. The design is structurally, particularly in the optimized approach based on a structure of a backbone, neck, and head.

Backbone: It is using a CSP-DarkNet framework, which is an upgrade to the previous DarkNet architecture. series. It employs Cross Stage Partial (CSP) connections that promote gradient flow and minimize dropout penalty. Additionally, it applies 2D computational overheads associated with the extraction of features of a robust feature map within the input image.

Neck: The neck in YOLOv8 consists of a PANet structure that combines the features using different scales very efficiently. It improves the detection of objects of different sizes in medical images, particularly the finer details.

Head: Anchor-free detection heads make the architecture less complex and increase the detection speed detection process. They directly predict object classes and bounding boxes, making them much more versatile for complex data sets like medical imaging.

3.2 YOLO v9

YOLOv9 brings new methods for the mitigation of information loss in deep neural networks. It uses Programmable Gradient Information, an auxiliary reversible branch, to ensure a reliable flow of gradients during training and not to lose information. This includes a Generalized Efficient Layer Aggregation Network, or GELAN, which is a light architecture intended to enhance the flow of information and improve the precision of prediction. It is built as a general extension of the ELAN architecture with flexible computational blocks, optimized efficiency, and thus performance by optimizing the gradient path.

3.3 YOLO v11

YOLOv11 introduces new structures such as the C3k2 block and the C2PSA block to promote better feature extraction and processing that leads to only a slightly superior performance but very few parameters compared to the old model. In the following parts, the reader will find the major features of YOLO11.

C3k2 Block: YOLO11 introduced the C3k2 block, which is a computationally efficient implementation of the Cross Stage Partial (CSP) Bottleneck. It replaces the C2f block in the backbone and neck and uses two smaller convolutions instead of one large convolution.

C2PSA Block: Cross Stage Partial with Spatial Attention introduces the C2PSA block after the SPPF block to enhance the spatial attention in the model. This attention can be used so that the model focuses more attentively on parts of the image that are actually important for object detection (Fig. 1).

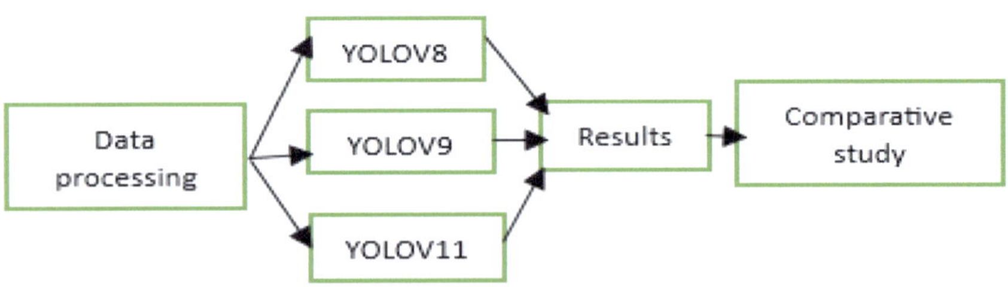

Fig. 1 Comparative execution pipeline of YOLOV8, YOLOV9, and YOLOV11

4 Simulation and Results

We test the suggested method using a disease dataset. We follow each experimental setting of YOLOv9. We train all the methods that we discussed with the train-from-scratch method and 25 training epochs. The models were tested on a dataset to examine their performance over key metrics such as F1-confidence (F1), precision-recall (PR) curves, precision (P) curves, and recall (R) curves. The findings are stated in Table 1 and compared using bar graph shown in Fig. 2.

YOLOv8 recorded an F1-confidence of 0.93, better than YOLOv9 at 0.92 and YOLOv11 at 0.90. The PR curves indicated that YOLOv8 now achieves a precision of 0.957, with precisions of 0.947 for YOLOv9 and 0.919 for YOLOv11. All models achieved the same precision score value of 0.99, indicating that they all possessed strength in identifying actual positives. Recall values were even narrower for YOLOv8 at 0.98, as opposed to YOLOv9 at 0.97 and YOLOv11 at 0.96. This shows that YOLOv8 has better detection capability with a balance between precision and recall for CVD detection.

Table 1 Comparative table of CVD detection using yolov8, yolov9, yolov11

	YOLOV8	YOLOV9	YOLOV11
F1-confidence	0.93	0.92	0.9
Precision-recall	0.957	0.947	0.919
Precision-confidence	0.99	0.99	0.99
Recall-confidence	0.98	0.97	0.96

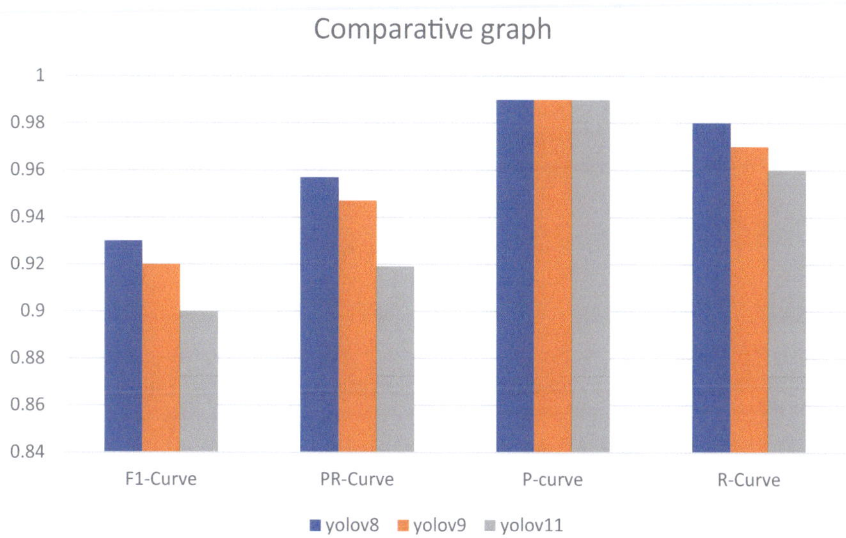

Fig. 2 Comparative graph of CVD detection using YOLOV8, YOLOV9, YOLOV11

Figure 3 shows a sample training batch with instances of scaling, cropping, and flipping, together with labeled bounding boxes. Visualization in this context has an important check-pointing role in providing a means of ensuring well-preprocessed input images. Visualizations also play a role in analyzing the quality of the training sample, whose accuracy in turn affects the performance of inspecting the quality of the training sample model performance. Visualization of the training batches enables the identification of annotation errors, aids in the determination of class diversity among groups, and verifies the effectiveness of the augmentation pipeline. Visualization plays an important role within deep learning pipelines to ensure that the data. In this case, any data that is passed to the model is correct and reflective.

The improvement in the model performance is evident from the graphs in Fig. 4. The train losses box_loss, cls_loss, and dfl_loss are greatly diminished, while the validation losses adhere to the showing the same trend, with evidence.

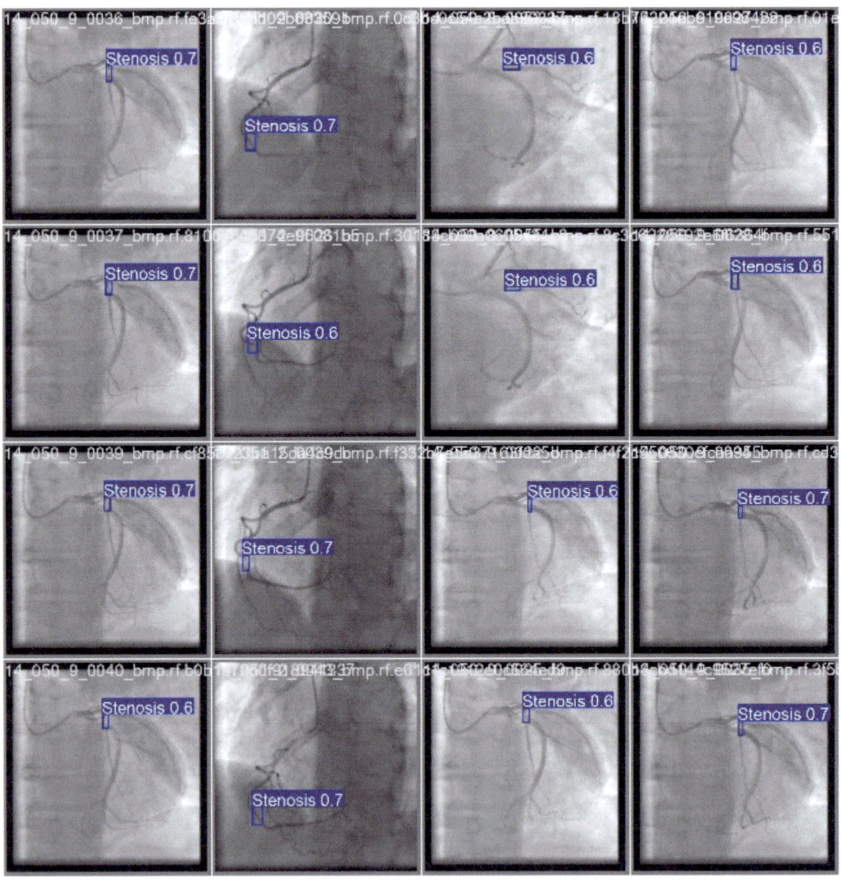

Fig. 3 CVD detection using YOLOV8

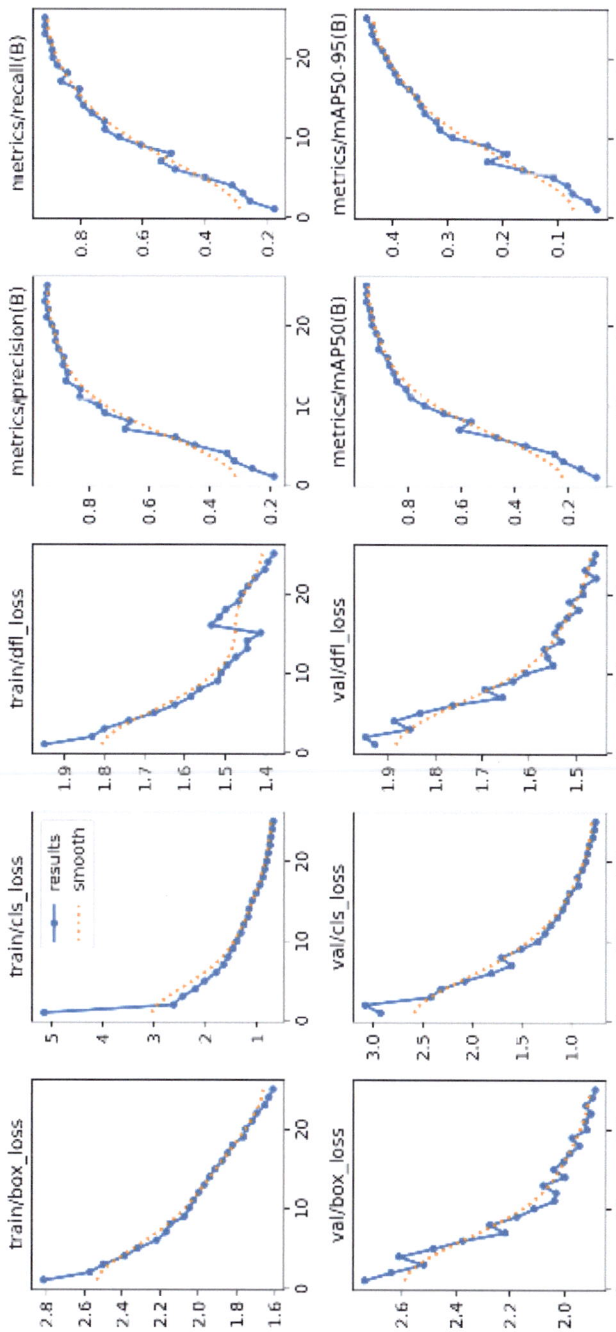

Fig. 4 Validation performance of YOLOV8

Precision, recall, and mAP metrics also illustrate steady increment; the precision increases to 0.8, recall to ~0.9, and mAP50-95 to 0.4, signifying better detection and classification quality.

The Fig. 5 shows confusion matrix of Yolov8 which contains 1197 true positives among the 1279 stenosis predictions made, which is 93.59% accurate.

Figure 6 shows that at a confidence of 0.361, the curve reaches its maximum at an F1 measure of 0.93, showing the optimal trade-off between recall and precision at this point.

The Fig. 7 depicts PC Curve, which has a peak precision of 1.00 at a confidence of 0.728, shows a strong relationship between confidence and precision for tumor detection.

Figure 8 shows rc-curve of Yolov8 at 0.0 confidence, the recall starts at a high value of about 0.98, indicating that the model correctly identifies most actual positive instances with low confidence.

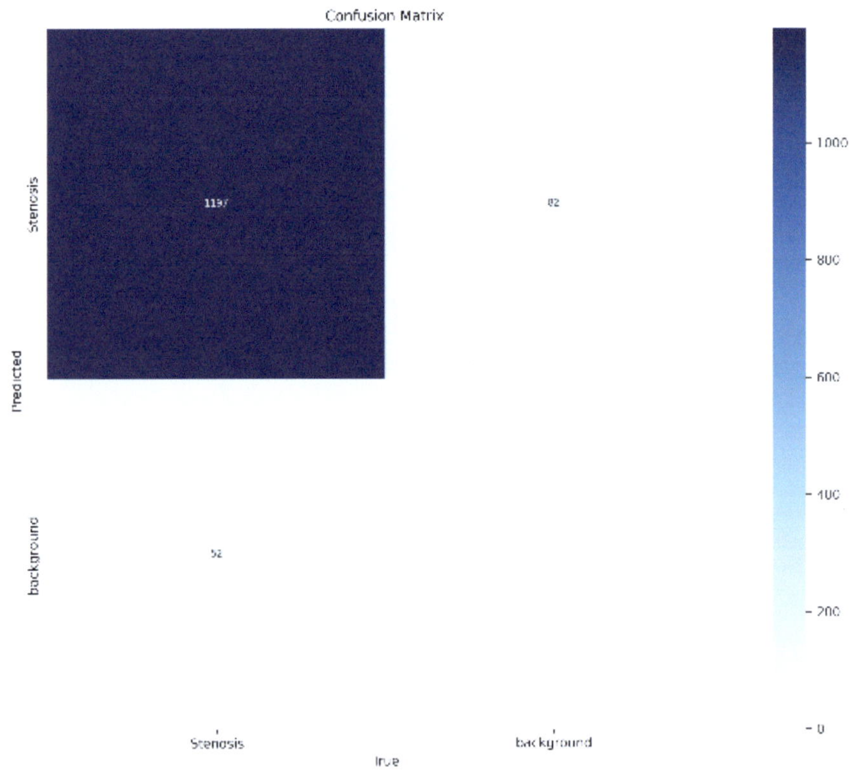

Fig. 5 Confusion matrix of YOLOV8

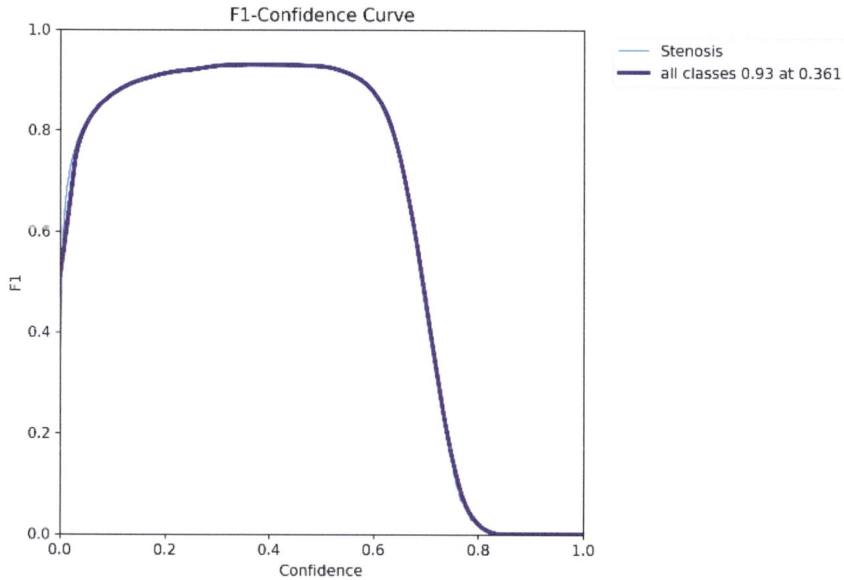

Fig. 6 F1-confidence curve of YOLOV8

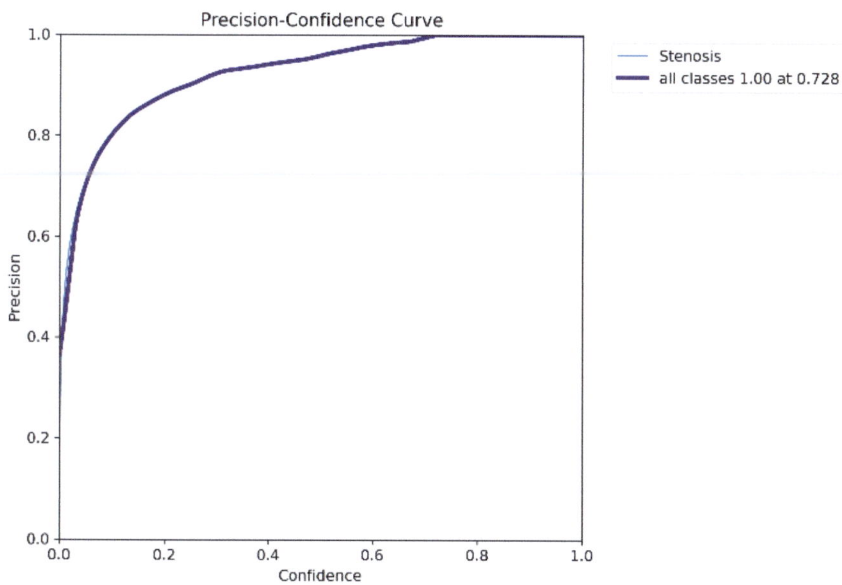

Fig. 7. PC curve of YOLOV8

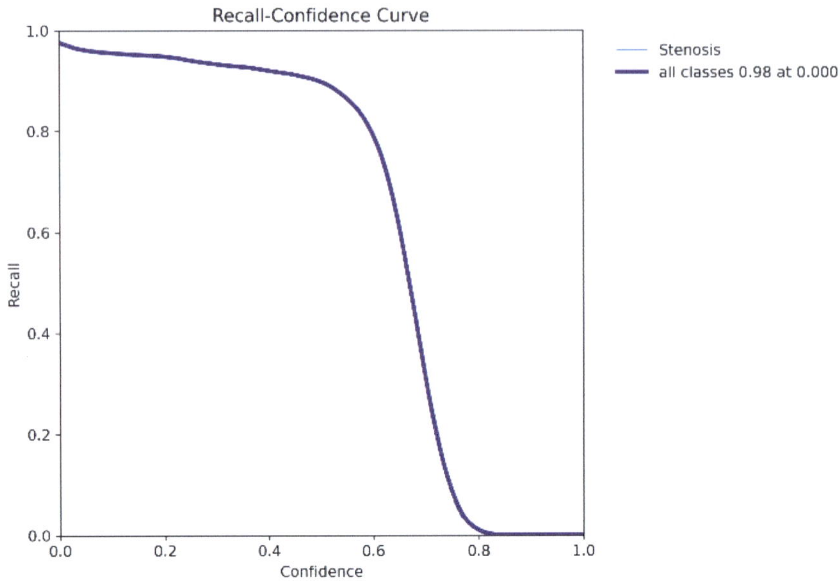

Fig. 8 RC curve of YOLOV8

From Fig. 9 the model performs very well with both classes achieving Precision-Recall of 0.957. This implies that its precision in identifying stenosis and non-stenosis cases is extremely high.

Results of yolov9:

Figure 10 shows that at a confidence of 0.351, the curve reaches its maximum at an F1 measure of 0.92, showing the optimal trade-off between recall and precision at this point.

From Fig. 11 the model performs very well with both classes achieving PR Curve of 0.947. This implies that its precision in identifying stenosis and non-stenosis cases is high.

Figure 12 gives an overview of the training and validation performance metrics across a few epochs. It typically consists of graphs to show the results concerning the loss, precision, recall, and mAP. The graphs help in understanding how the model is learning by showing whether is either converging well or showing signs of overfitting and/or underfitting. “Smooth improvement on the evaluation metric”: indicates good learning, while discrepancies between training and validation curves could indicate problems to generalization problems or data quality problems.

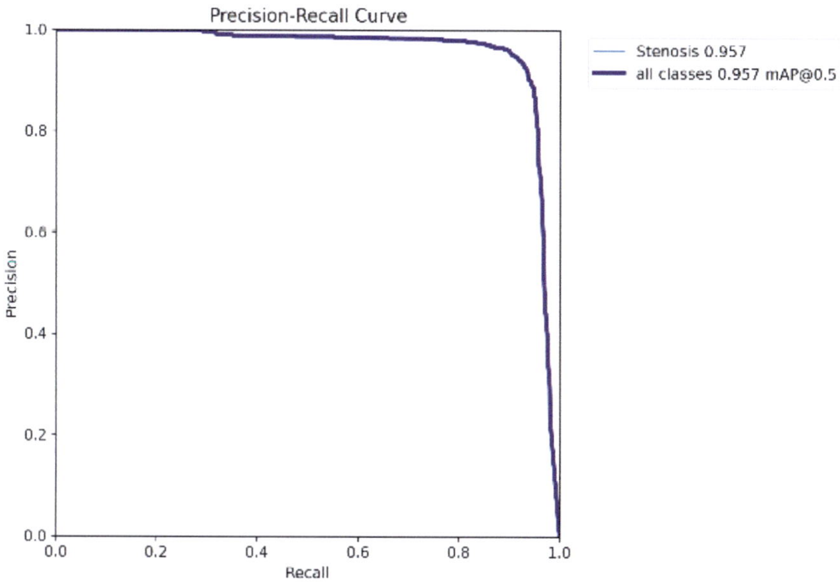

Fig. 9 Precision-recall curve of YOLOV8

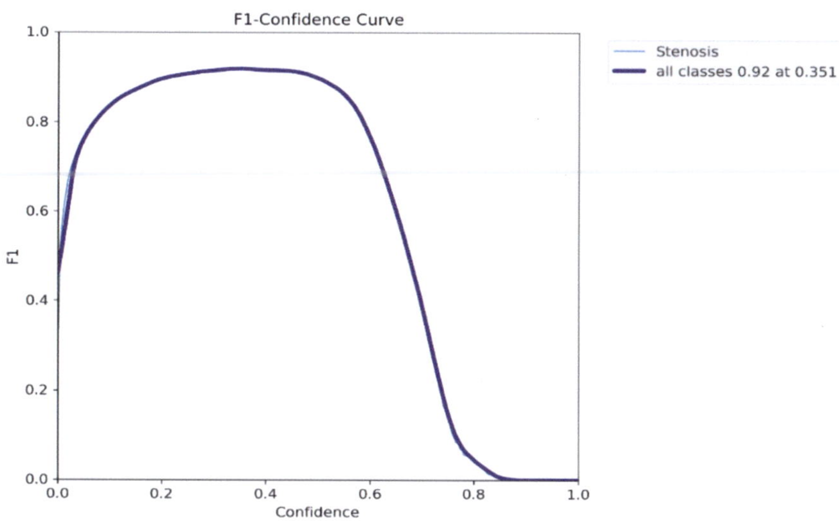

Fig. 10 F1-confidence curve of YOLOV9

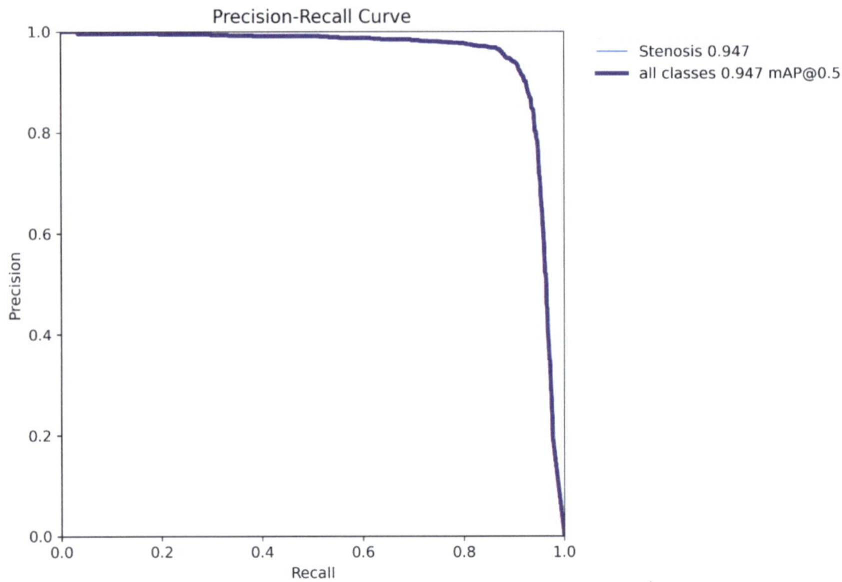

Fig. 11 Precision-recall curve of YOLOV9

Results of yolov11:

According to the diagram in Fig. 13, at a level of confidence of 0.405, the point where the graph attains its top is where the F1 value is 0.90, which illustrates the best possible compromise between recall and precision for this point.

From Fig. 14, the model results are excellent for both classes with Precision-Recall of 0.919. This means that its sensitivity in detecting both stenosis and non-stenosis samples is high.

Above the Fig. 15 is the training results graph. The summary of the training process that is depicted below Fig. 15 include: "classification loss", "objectness loss", "precision", "recall", and "F1 score" during the epochs. A general decreasing pattern with respect to the loss functions and a general increasing pattern for precision and recall signifies that there has been effective learning and generalization of the model. Looking at the curves' shape aids in determining whether the training is stable or the model is overfitting or underfitting. Gradual improvements with epochs verify the model's capability to learn and converge towards a best solution.

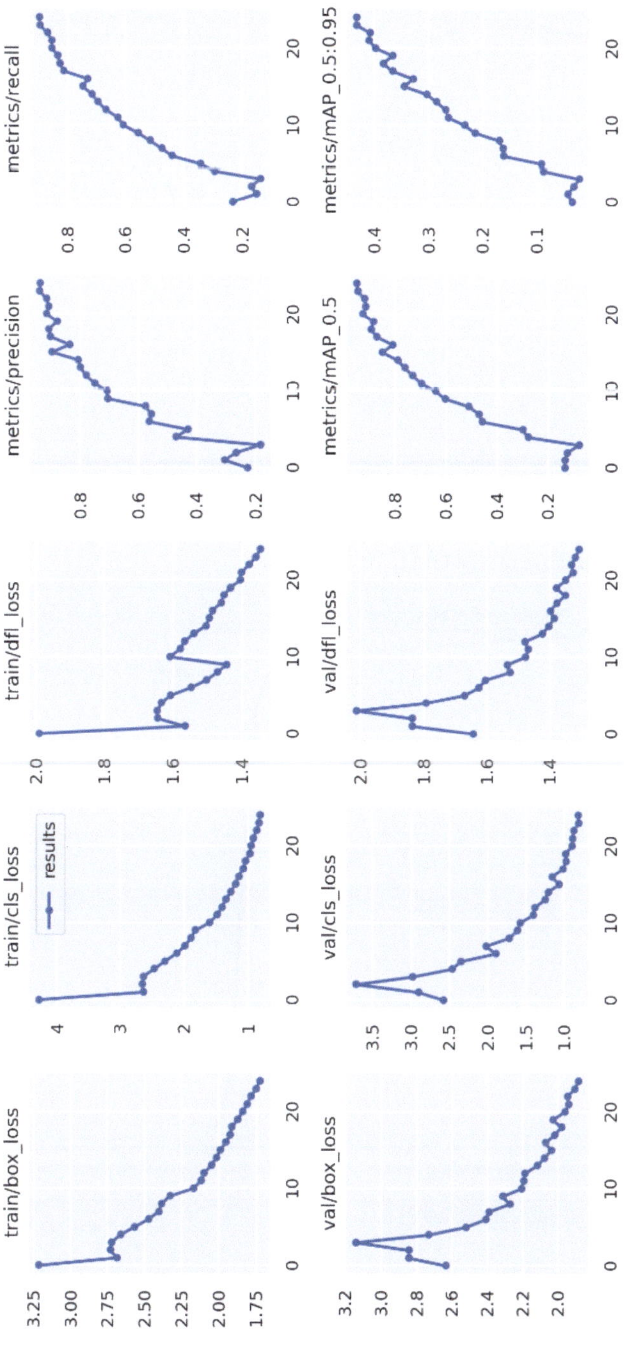

Fig. 12 Validation performance of YOLOV9

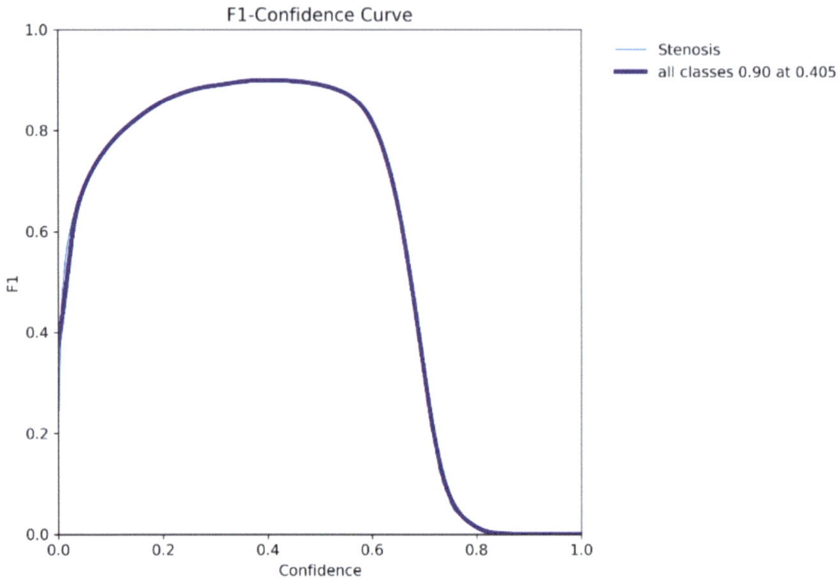

Fig. 13 F1-confidence curve of YOLOV11

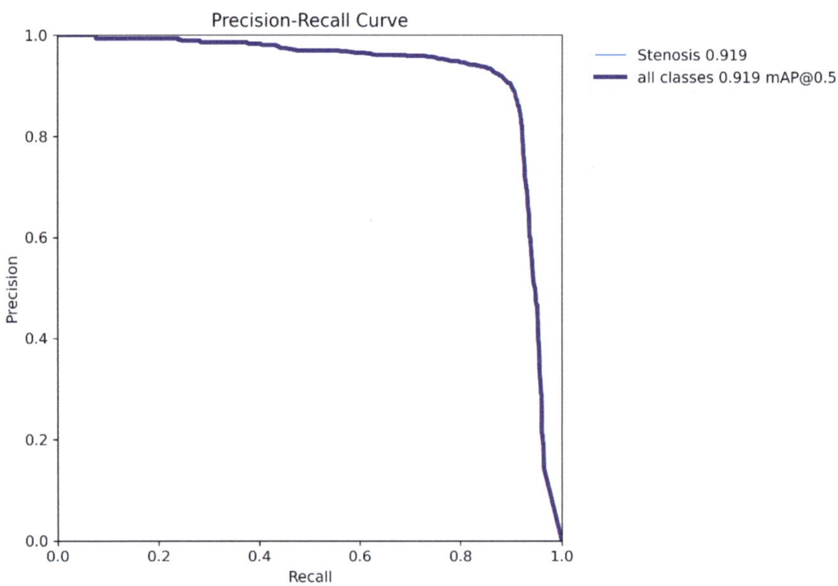

Fig. 14 Precision-recall curve of YOLOV11

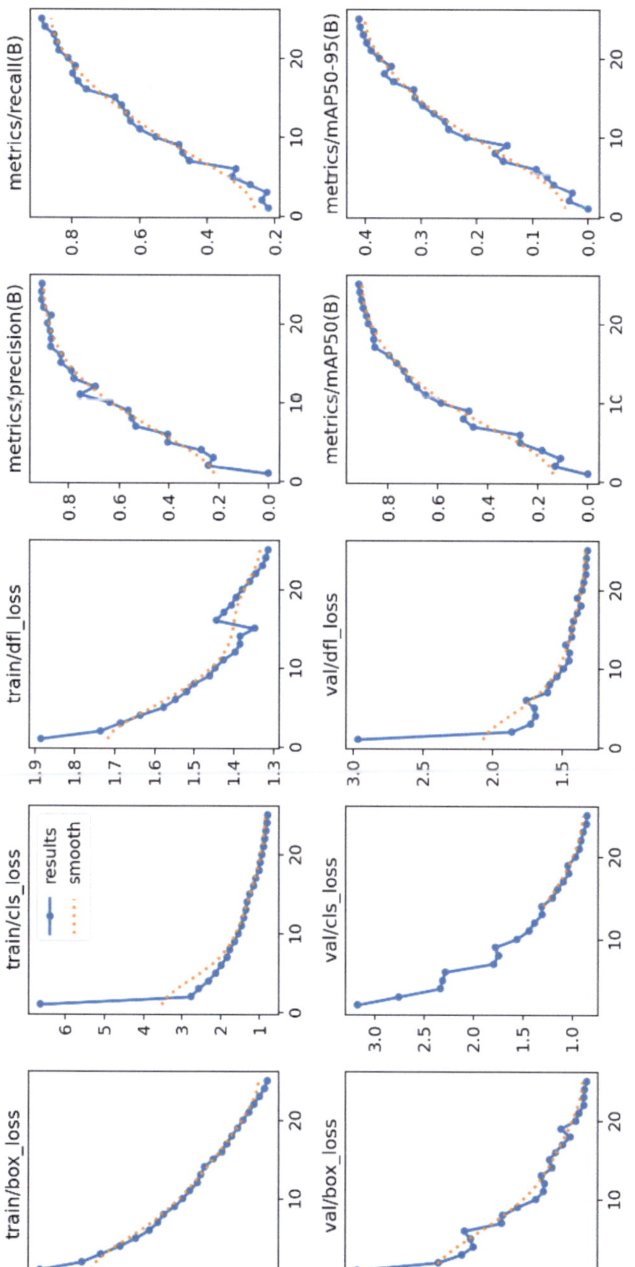

Fig. 15 Validation performance of YOLOV11

5 Conclusion

The CVD detection project tested three models: yolov8, yolov9, and yolov11, based on F1-curve, PR-curve, precision, and recall metrics. Yolov8 outperformed the others, with an F1-score of 0.93, PR-curve of 0.957, precision of 0.99, and recall of 0.98, which indicates an excellent balance between precision and recall. This makes yolov8 the most reliable model for accurate CVD detection. Yolov9 comes second with the F1-score at 0.92, PR-curve at 0.947, and precision and recall scores of 0.99 and 0.97 respectively, hence, showing stable and consistent performance. Yolov11, which obtained a very high precision at 0.99 and recall at 0.96, had the lowest F1-score at 0.90 and PR-curve at 0.919, indicating less optimal precision-recall balance. Therefore, the best model to be deployed is yolov8.

Future Work

Future work for the CVD detection project includes model optimization, specifically for yolov9 and yolov11 models, through hyperparameter tuning and architectural improvements for better performance. The dataset has to be augmented with diverse high-quality samples to achieve generalization and robustness across populations. Explainable AI techniques would add transparency to the decision-making process, enabling more trust in clinical applications. Validation in real-world clinical settings is important for validating the effectiveness of models on live data as well as obtaining feedback from clients. The addition of multimodal data like imaging and patient history, and further optimization of the models for deployment at edge or cloud will increase access and accuracy in different environments.

References

1. Chen, J., Huang, S., Zhang, Y., Chang, Q., Zhang, Y., Li, D., Qiu, J., Hu, L., Peng, X., Du, Y., Gao, Y.: Congenital heart disease detection by pediatric electrocardiogram-based deep learning integrated with human concepts. Nat. Commun. **15**(1), 976 (2024)
2. Baseer, K.K., Sivakumar, K., Veeraiah, D., Chhabra, G., Lakineni, P.K., Pasha, M.J., Gandikota, R., Harikrishnan, G.: Healthcare diagnostics with an adaptive deep learning model integrated with the Internet of Medical Things (IoMT) for predicting heart disease. Biomed. Signal Process. Control **92**, 105988 (2024)
3. Saikumar, K., Rajesh, V.: A machine intelligence technique for predicting cardiovascular disease (CVD) using radiology dataset. Int. J. Syst. Assur. Engi. Manag. **15**(1), 135–151 (2024)
4. Oyewola, D.O., Dada, E.G., Misra, S.: Diagnosis of cardiovascular diseases by ensemble optimization deep learning techniques. Int. J. Healthc. Inf. Syst. Inform. (IJHISI) **19**(1), 1–21 (2024)
5. .Kavatlawar, A., Bohare, A., Dakare, A., Dubey, A., Sahu, M.: Cardiovascular disease (CVD) recognition using convolutional neural networks. Grenze Int. J. Eng. Technol. (GIJET) **10**
6. Singh, N., Gunjan, V.K., Shaik, F., Roy, S.: Detection of cardio vascular abnormalities using gradient descent optimization and CNN. Heal. Technol. **14**(1), 155–168 (2024)
7. Ram Kumar, R.P., Polepaka, S., Manasa, V., Palakurthy, D., Annapoorna, E., Dhaliwal, N., Dhall, H., Alzubaidi, L.H.: Investigations on cardiovascular diseases and predicting using machine learning algorithms. Cogent Eng. **11**(1), 2386381 (2024)

8. Ramesh, B., Lakshmanna, K.: A novel early detection and prevention of coronary heart disease framework using hybrid deep learning model and neural fuzzy inference system. IEEE Access **12**, 26683–26695 (2024)
9. Prusty, M.R., Pandey, T.N., Lekha, P.S., Lellapalli, G., Gupta, A.: Scalar invariant transform-based deep learning framework for detecting heart failures using ECG signals. Sci. Rep. **14**(1), 2633 (2024)
10. Hussain, I., Nazir, M.B.: Empowering healthcare: AI, ML, and deep learning innovations for brain and heart health. Int. J. Adv. Eng. Technol. Innov. **1**(4), 167–188 (2024)
11. Rahman, A.U., Alsenani, Y., Zafar, A., Ullah, K., Rabie, K., Shongwe, T.: Enhancing heart disease prediction using a self-attention-based transformer model. Sci. Rep. **14**(1), 514 (2024)
12. Pal, P., Grover, V., Nandal, M., Gochhait, S., Singh, H.V.: Artificial intelligence driven intelligent computational model for heart disease prediction: leveraging feature selection. In: 2024 ASU International Conference in Emerging Technologies for Sustainability and Intelligent Systems (ICETSIS), pp. 1422–1428. IEEE (2024)
13. Ramkumar, G., Seetha, J., Priyadarshini, R., Gopila, M., Saranya, G.: IoT-based patient monitoring system for predicting heart disease using deep learning. Measurement **218**, 113235 (2023)
14. .Garavand, A., Behmanesh, A., Aslani, N., Sadeghsalehi, H., Ghaderzadeh, M.: Towards diagnostic aided systems in coronary artery disease detection: a comprehensive multiview survey of the state of the art. Int. J. Intell. Syst. (1), 6442756 (2023)
15. Bhatt, C.M., Patel, P., Ghetia, T., Mazzeo, P.L.: Effective heart disease prediction using machine learning techniques. Algorithms **16**(2), 88 (2023)
16. Velmurugan, A.K., Padmanaban, K., Kumar, A.M., Azath, H., Subbiah, M.: Machine learning IoT-based framework for analyzing heart disease prediction. In: AIP Conference Proceedings, vol. 2523, no. 1. AIP Publishing (2023)
17. Panchumarthi, L.Y., Padmanabhuni, S., Saleti, S.: Leveraging ResNet for efficient ECG heartbeat classification. In: 2024 IEEE International Conference on Signal Processing, Informatics, Communication and Energy Systems (SPICES), pp. 1–6. IEEE (2024)
18. Bai, W., Chen, C., Tarroni, G., Duan, J., Guitton, F., Petersen, S.E., Guo, Y., Matthews, P.M., Rueckert, D.: Self-supervised learning for cardiac mr image segmentation by anatomical position prediction. In: Medical Image Computing and Computer Assisted Intervention–MICCAI 2019: 22nd International Conference, Shenzhen, China, October 13–17, 2019, Proceedings, Part II 22, pp. 541–549. Springer International Publishing (2019)
19. Kumar, S., Sharma, S., Megra, K.T.: Transformer enabled multi-modal medical diagnosis for tuberculosis classification. J. Big Data **12**(1), 5 (2025)
20. Jiao, T., Guo, C., Feng, X., Chen, Y., Song, J.: A comprehensive survey on deep learning multi-modal fusion: methods, technologies and applications. Comput. Mater. Contin. **80**(1) (2024)
21. Sundar, R., Gangopadhyay, A., Gupta, T.R., Murthy, P.S., Gogula, S., Sharath, M.N., Muppavaram, K.: Heart health prediction and classification: an IoMT and AI collaborative model. In MATEC Web of Conferences, vol. 392, p. 01142. EDP Sciences (2024)
22. Raja, G., Essaky, S., Muthu, S.R., Suresh, B.S., Cho, J., Yoo, S., Easwaramoorthy, S.V.: CardioNetFusion: a deep learning and explainable AI integrated system for cardiovascular disease detection. In: 2024 IEEE International Conference on Data Mining Workshops (ICDMW), pp. 388–395. IEEE (2024)
23. Singh, V., Kaushik, V.D.: DTCWTASODCNN: DTCWT based weighted fusion model for multimodal medical image quality improvement with ASO technique & DCNN. J. Sci. Ind. Res. **81**(08), 850–858 (2022)
24. Singh, V., Kaushik, V.D.: Comparative assessment of state-of-the-art image fusion techniques for fusion of multi-modality medical images. In: Advances in Signal Processing, Embedded Systems and IoT: Proceedings of Seventh ICMEET-2022, pp. 439–446. Springer Nature Singapore, Singapore (2023)

Detection of Elusive Polyp Using U-Net for Polyp Segmentation

Sravan Kumar Nakerakanti, Madhura Raut, Gokul Krishna Reddy Chiraiahgari, Bhuvan Sai Anusuri, Phanindra Babu Battula, Alok Kumar, and Vineeta Singh

Abstract Polyps on the colon's surface are the starting point for colon cancer, a common and potentially fatal type of cancer. Early identification of these polyps and cancers is essential for efficient screening. Deep Convolutional Neural Network (DCNN) methodologies, particularly utilizing U-Net architecture, are implemented to enhance colorectal cancer detection. Data augmentation enhances the dataset and enables accurate detection. Current polyp segmentation approaches are challenged by irregular color patterns, inconsistent polyp presence, and reflection effects in colonoscopy and endoscopy pictures, which may result in either over- or under-segmentation. In order to improve polyp detection, this work suggests an enhanced U-Net-based segmentation algorithm that incorporates edge and valley detection techniques. To increase the accuracy of detection, post-processing algorithms combine together neighboring items and enhance segmentation boundaries. Doctors can diagnose polyps more quickly, accurately, and easily using this computerized procedure. The development of Computer-Aided Diagnosis (CAD) systems for automated polyp

S. K. Nakerakanti (✉) · G. K. R. Chiraiahgari · A. Bhuvan Sai · B. Phanindra Babu
Department of Computational Intelligence, SRM Institute of Science and Technology, Faculty of Engineering and Technology, KTR Campus, Chennai, India
e-mail: nn0800@srmist.edu.in

G. K. R. Chiraiahgari
e-mail: cc1733@srmist.edu.in

A. Bhuvan Sai
e-mail: as9964@srmist.edu.in

B. Phanindra Babu
e-mail: bb7944@srmist.edu.in

M. Raut
University of Southern California, Los Angeles, USA
e-mail: raut.madhura@ieee.org

A. Kumar · V. Singh
Department of Computer Science and Engineering, School of Engineering and Technology (Formerly Known as UIET Kanpur), Chhatrapati Shahu Ji Maharaj University, Kalyanpur, Kanpur, Uttar Pradesh, India
e-mail: alok@csjmu.ac.in

P. Singh et al. (eds.), *Deep Learning Applications in Healthcare and Medical Imaging Practice*, Studies in Big Data 193, https://doi.org/10.1007/978-3-032-21009-8_25

diagnosis depends on these techniques. In this context, our suggested U-Net approach provides an efficient DCNN design solution, improving automated polyp detection techniques.

1 Introduction

Even though healthcare services have gotten better around the world, colorectal cancer is still one of the hardest types of cancer to treat and one of the most common causes of cancer deaths, killing millions of people each year. It may be the second most common cause of cancer deaths, but it is still a problem for the whole world. There is no chance of getting better, which makes things worse. But acting quickly could make a disease spread much faster. Early detection and treatment of colorectal cancer have led to lower death rates.

Colonoscopy is one of the most important and effective ways to screen for and diagnose diseases. It is at the forefront of this effort. A colonoscope and a camera are attached to a flexible tube that goes inside the colon. The doctor can find problems that are worrying, like polyps, which are known to be the first signs of colorectal cancer. Finding and locating lesions is very important because the main goal of this operation is to stop the spread of colorectal cancer. These polyps, which are usually small or hard to see, are the first sign of a major change in the disease's progression.

1.1 Polyp Segmentation

In recent years, medical imaging has come a long way, especially when it comes to automatically separating polyps. Leading structural learning models, such as U-Net, have been created because they give reliable and efficient results. They are currently the best at automatically segmenting polyps in colonoscopy images. These kinds of learning models could change the way doctors diagnose and treat colorectal cancer. Using big data sets and powerful algorithms, these models are capable of isolating very challenging details concerning the shape and structure of polyps that would normally be quite difficult. Since multiple studies have proven that U-Net is among the best systems available for performing precision-based sub-image recognition and tagging tasks, it is essential component of the fight against colorectal cancer.

Precision medicine is about to undergo a major change with the development of medical imaging including deep learning algorithms. These advances will change the way colorectal diseases are treated by making diagnoses more accurate and giving doctors more tools. This gives the world hope. Colorectal cancer is the second most common cause of cancer-related death and a major health problem around the world. It needs to be found and treated quickly. Finding polyps is much easier with a colonoscopy. Deep learning algorithms like U-Net can automatically segment them with great accuracy.

Several architectures other than the conventional U-Net are being developed to improve the accuracy and generalizability of polyp segmentation. For example, PolypSegNet develops a new encoder-decoder architecture that improves and spatial boundary resolution, improves boundary resolution, which is important with polyps that have fuzzy and or rough edges [1]. PraNet employs a boundary focusing, bottom-up, and top-down reverse attention mechanism that improves segmentation maps in a stepwise manner while reducing background clutter. This method proves very useful in dealing with complicated colonoscopic cases [2].

With the innovation of CNN-based methods, these updates highlight the importance of attention mechanisms and design changes.

Also, advanced neural networks like DoubleU-Net and UNet++ have been adapted to incorporate multi-scale features and hierarchical skip connections to enhance the segmentation for polyps of different sizes, shapes, and textures [3, 6]. The success of these models are due to the modified skip connections that are fused into the cascaded U-Net architectures, which helps to reduce the semantic gaps between the encoder and decoder of the models. Structures like A-DenseUNet and DRI-Net use a combination of dilated convolutions and dense inception modules to widen the receptive field while retaining the detailed features vital for accurate localization and segmentation in challenging cases [7, 17]. The process of sophisticated deep learning models transitioning from simple segmentation models, to complex hybrid models for use in the field of medical imaging is highlighted in the architecture of models.

Of late, models that are lightweight and have the ability to function in real-time are increasingly being preferred in clinical settings and for on-device processing. The goal of recent research techniques like Poly-EffNetV1 [14, 19] and Lightweight Deep Learning Model is to increase model computational efficiency without compromising prediction performance. In resource constrained environments or during real time colonoscopy interventions, these techniques become especially beneficial. Also, Boundary Uncertainty Aware Networks (BUANet) improve the robustness of segmentation by simulating spatial ambiguity at the borders of polyps [9]. This suggests a focus on the precision, explainability, real time responsiveness, and clinical versatility of the adaptive, computer-aided diagnostic tools for the early detection of colorectal cancer, which are becoming increasingly sophisticated.

2 Literature Survey

In order to recover polyps from colonoscopy pictures, Mahmud et al. presented PolypSegNet, which uses a deep reconstruction module (DRM), a deep fusion skip module (DFSM), and multiple sequential depth dilation initiation (DDI) blocks [1]. Automatically produce. SegNet's design was altered for segmentation. Fan et al. an FCN-like model for medical image segmentation was improved with the introduction of PraNet, which makes use of parallel partial decoding and reverse attention modules becoming the go-to option for segmenting medical images [2].

UNet is suggested as a solution to the singular encoder of the conventional Fully Convolutional Network (FCN), therefore greatly improving the speed of FCN. In the encoder-decoder architecture termed UNet, the features from the encoding and decoding layers are amalgamated through skip connections.

Several proposed variants for polyp segmentation, which yielded promising results, were inspired by the performance of UNet. Johansen et al. introduced Double UNet, a hybrid of UNet architectures [3]. The initial UNet is based on a pre-trained VGG-19 model. Underneath the original UNet is a second UNet designed to improve the semantic data collecting capability. They also use Atrous Spatial Pyramid Pooling (ASPP) to get information about the network's context. Kang and Gwak used Mask-RCNN as the main tool for automatically finding and separating polyps. They based their work on ResNet50 and ResNet101 [4].

Zhou et al. introduced UNet ++ , a modified encoder-decoder design intended for segmentation of medical images [6]. This model fills the semantic gap between encoder and decoder feature maps by integrating layered and dense skip connections, hence improving the standard U-Net. Such a design encourages improved feature fusion, thereby generating more exact segmentation results. Tests indicated that UNet ++ regularly outperformed its predecessors, demonstrating significant improvements in Intersection over Union (IoU) metrics for many medical imaging applications, including colonoscopy video polyp segmentation.

Zhang et al. automatically divided the likely polyp areas on colonoscopy images using the FCN-8S architecture [5]. They found that they made significant progress in these areas by removing texton features and using a random forest classifier for polyp candidate classification. Dense residual-inception modules and the U-Net architecture were used by Lan et al. to develop DRI-Net, a deep learning system for polyp segmentation [7]. Because the model could extract more features and lose less information, it performed better than the Kvasir-SEG dataset. Tomar et al. also proposed DilatedSegNet, an encoder-decoder network that uses dilated convolution pooling blocks and a ResNet50 backbone [8]. The model has potential for clinical application as it exhibited the capability to deliver real-time, high-precision segmentation.

To tackle the issues arising from unclear polyp borders in colonoscopy images, Yue et al. developed BUNet, a boundary uncertainty-aware network [9]. The model combines a boundary exploration module (BEM) and a boundary uncertainty module (BUM) with a pyramid vision trans-former encoder to make it easier to get multi-scale features and show where mistakes are likely to happen.

While BUNet improves boundary segmentation accuracy, it still faces difficulties accommodating the varying shapes and sizes of polyps, yielding inconsistent results across multiple datasets.

Jeong et al. built a deep learning model that integrates polyp segmentation into a real-time application by utilizing MobileNetV3 as the encoder and DeepLabV3 + as the decoder [14]. The aim is to achieve high accuracy at low levels of computation for efficiency on real-time tasks. However, even with the lightweight design, the model may be ineffective with highly variable views of the polyp, as well as images of lower resolutions where the details needed for accurate segmentation are unsatisfactory due to the lightweight design.

Cao et al. constructed DEMF-Net which is a multi-scale feature fusion network with two encoders dedicated to polyp segmentation [21]. Using two encoders and combining features at different scales improves segmentation performance and gives a broad view with accurate details. But in DEMF-Net, using two encoders may make real-time processing less efficient, especially in clinical settings with limited resources. This could make the whole process more expensive in terms of computing.

The imaging conditions, frequent potential artifacts, and the varying shapes, sizes, and appearances of the polyps all continue to present challenges that still hold back advancements in achieving accurate segmentations. To solve these problems, our approach improves the U-Net model by adding features of edge and valley detection to augment boundary delineation. Furthermore, segmentation output is optimized through advanced techniques which enhance accuracy and trustworthiness of detected segmented images of polyps.

3 Proposed Architecture

Our model enhances polyp identification precision with a U-Net-based Deep Convolutional Neural Network (DCNN). Data augmentation enhances the dataset, improving the model's learning and detection accuracy. This methodology enhances the precision of colorectal cancer screening by supplying the network with varied, informative samples to improve efficacy. Designed particularly for biological image segmentation, U-Net's enhanced and revised network architecture aids to more precisely segment images with less training images. In this thesis, we investigate advanced approaches and algorithms required for developing a highly successful U-Net model by combining challenging DCNN construction methods with U-Net methodology, so providing an automated polyp recognition method.

3.1 Existing Systems

Many techniques have been suggested to provide accurate polyp segmentation, mostly classified as deep learning and traditional machine learning methods. These techniques show a growing complexity in polyp segmentation studies by usually looking at the edge, colour, and texture of the polyp for segmentation. Still, there is a clear problem in the field: few studies using cross-dataset testing evaluates model generalizability. Many recent studies rely on tiny, uneven, hand-selected datasets, therefore impeding the development of reliable and generally applicable polyp segmentation techniques. Furthermore, challenging the development of strong and scalable segmentation methods are limited training datasets and dataset imbalances within the medical field. Dealing with these difficulties, our work intends to create an algorithm able to achieve good performance in polyp segmentation.

3.2 Fundamental Concepts

Artificial intelligence (AI) systems are founded on the machine learning subset referred to as deep learning. It focuses on artificial neural networks (ANN), intricate structures designed to analyse substantial datasets through multiple layers of interconnected neurons.

Convolutional neural networks (CNNs) like U-Net are designed to segment biological pictures. The concept has been refined for precise segmentation using a minimal quantity of training images. Modern GPUs can segment a 512 × 512 image in less than one second.

Because of how U-Net works, it is perfect for jobs like polyp segmentation in medical images that need very detailed pixel-by-pixel classification (Fig. 1). The symmetric skip encoder decoder architecture keeps the spatial integrity of the data during the up and down sampling processes. This is very important for medical files because the attributes keep contextual information at different levels, all of which are equally important. One reason U-Net is so popular is its design, which makes it work well when there aren't many labeled images. This is common in medicine because labeling a lot of data takes a lot of time and money.

One of the best things about U-Net is that it can break down and learn from high-dimensional input data sets. It has been very helpful for separating polyps because it can find unusual and complex shapes in colonoscopy images. U-Net's flexibility can be harnessed to improve detection and segmentation. This will help in unearthing colorectal polyps which would otherwise be missed during routine clinical examinations. U-Net is therefore a perfect choice for automated medical diagnostic systems meant to raise patient outcomes.

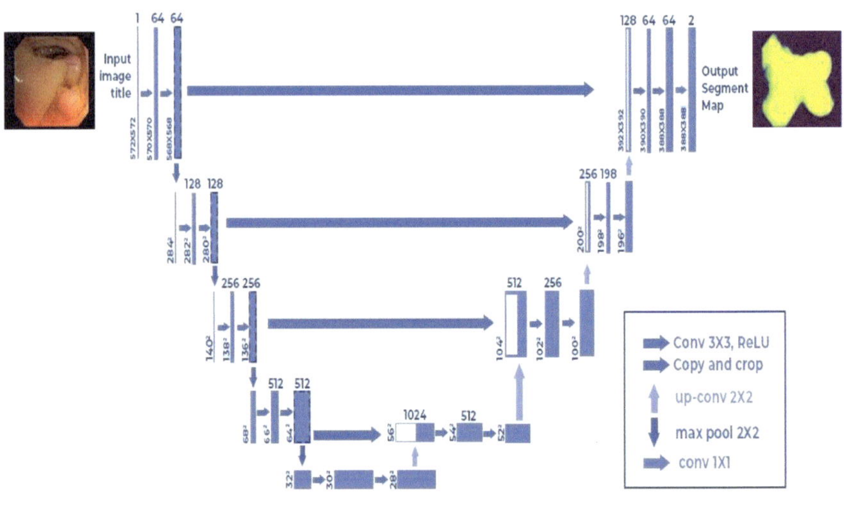

Fig. 1 U-Net architecture for polyp segmentation

The model architecture has multiple units of CNN that have ReLU as the nonlinear activation function. The performance improves by using the Adam optimizer which minimizes loss function which measures predicted value and real value. Different methods of convolution assist in the error correction process. Moreover, pooling techniques are incorporated to cut down on computational requirements and minimize number of parameters that necessitate training and optimization.

Deep convolutional neural networks (DCNNs) utilize their effectiveness via hierarchical processing. The concurrent processing of red, green, and blue components using a three-dimensional neural network significantly reduces the requisite number of artificial neurons. Images are processed by convolutions instead of matrix multiplication.

Data Augmentation: To mitigate how overfitting occurs with training datasets, the shortage of training datasets can be overcomes with data augmentation. Techniques, including rotation, mirroring, shifting, and zooming, can derive more diverse samples and improve the model's results.

Convolution Operation: Convolution, as a mathematical process, combines pairs of functions into a single function, displaying how one of the functions shifts with the other. This models the process of result-based evaluation by providing a weighted average of the metric to improve.

Pooling: Prior layer output, pooling operation, generates images by either max pooling and average pooling. In dark backgrounds, max pooling is useful to capture bright pixels within the selected rectangular area. Pooling layers help to mitigate overfitting by clipping the representation of the feature to a lower resolution, thus reducing the amount of work.

The U-Net architecture has established a strong foundation for precise and effective polyp segmentation with the use of cutting-edge deep learning techniques (Fig. 2). In presence of data augmentation, pooling layers, and convolution operations, the model learns valuable features from the complex and limited datasets of medical images and improves the diagnostic assistance in clinics.

Mathematical Representation of U-Net Segmentation Process: The segmentation process can be expressed as:

$$M_{output} = \text{Post Process}(f_{U-Net}(X)) \tag{1}$$

where:

- X: Input colonoscopy image.
- $f_{U-Net}(X)$: U-Net segmentation output.
- M_{output}: After using post-processing methods (PostProcess) to clean up the edges and group objects, this is the final mask.

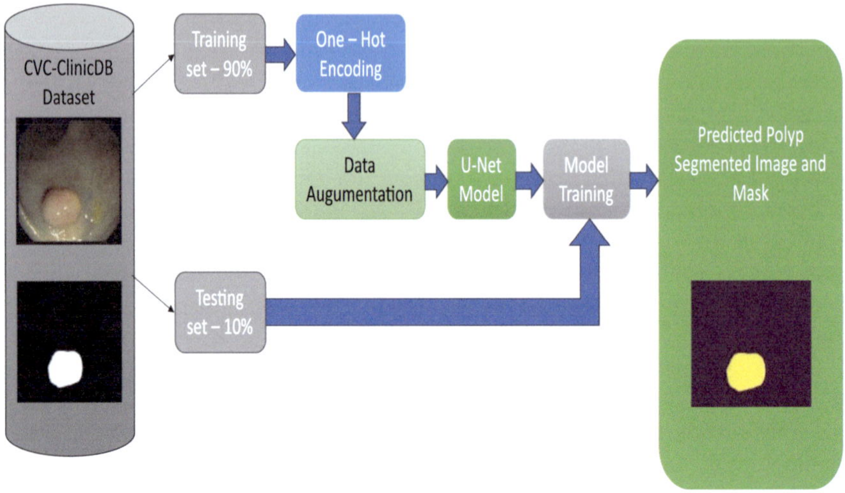

Fig. 2 Block diagram of polyp segmentation

4 Dataset

To ensure strong model generalization, frames record polyps in a range of sizes, angles, and illumination conditions. The images include:

- **Size**: 612 images in total, split into 80% for training and 20% for testing.
- **Diversity**: Frames capture polyps under varying lighting conditions, angles, and sizes, ensuring robust model generalization.
- **Quality**: Images are resolution with 384 × 288 pixels, and annotations are provided by clinical experts to ensure precision.

The dataset is widely used in segmentation challenges, such as the MICCAI 2015 Sub-Challenge on Automatic Polyp Detection in Colonoscopy Videos, validating its relevance.

The CVC-ClinicDB database comprises two distinct categories of images:

- **Original images:** original/frame_number.tiff
- **Polyp mask:** ground truth/frame_number.tiff

Contains the Frames' & GTs' sequence / file path information:

vpn_keyframe_idsort:

Frame ID (corresponds directly to image & mask names).
vpn_keysequence_idsort:
Video Sequence to which the frame belongs to.
text_formattif_image_pathsort:
TIFF file path of Frame.

text_formattif_mask_pathsort:
TIFF file path of GT Mask.
text_formatpng_image_pathsort:
PNG file path of Frame.
text_formatpng_mask_pathsort:
PNG file path of GT Mask.

We have 612 paths for each column and 612 images of original polyps and ground truths. The images in the 'Original' directory have been given by Hospital Clinic in Barcelona, Spain, while the ground truth annotations in the 'Ground Truth' directory are provided by the Computer Vision Center, Barcelona, Spain.

5 Results and Discussions

5.1 Visualization of Predicted Polyp

A. **Evaluation criteria**

Mean Intersection over Union (IoU) and Mean Dice Loss were two main metrics applied to evaluate the U-Net model. Even though IoU and DICE are well known metrics, these particular standards offer the best capturing accuracy for model operations and therefore fit perfectly in assessing whether the model successfully identifies polyps in colonoscopy images.

B. **U-Net Performance**

The U-Net design was trained using a part of the CVC-ClinicDB dataset. A stratified random sampling method made sure that the images in both the training and testing parts were evenly distributed so that everyone could get the same evaluation.

The polyp masks predicted by the model and those targeted by the model were highly aligned as the model achieved a Mean IoU score of 0.9730. This yielded significant results. The precise model received a Mean Dice Loss of 0.4186 for loss segmentation on the data (Fig. 3).

5.2 Impact of Post-processing Techniques

We learned about the degree to which post-processing helped in improving the segmentation boundaries as well as the difference in the performances of the models using the techniques as opposed to those that did not. These methods utilize the grouping of neighboring features which improves the accuracy of boundary finding through edge or valley detection.

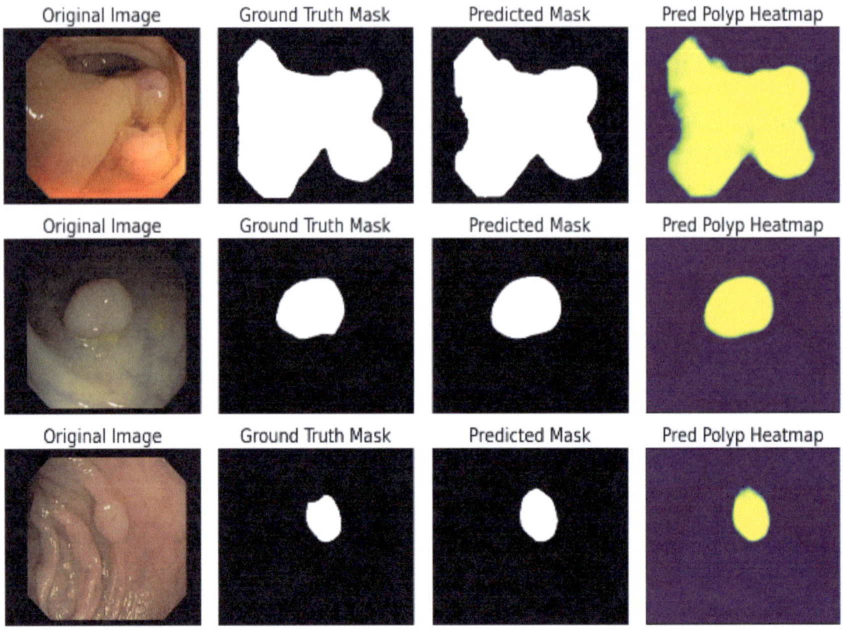

Fig. 3 Predicted polyp mask and heatmap

Results in Table 1 suggest that post-processing had a notable impact on Mean IoU and Dice Loss (Fig. 4). Both are important for the accuracy of the segmentation.

The bar charts represent the comparative values of IoU and Dice, showcasing impact of post-processing regarding accuracy of segmentation. Higher values of metrics for "With Post-Processing" represent better performance and thus determines how much value post-processing added to the original predictions. This performance assessment effectively demonstrates the contribution of post-processing and its impact on model's performance.

Score discrepancies can be used to evaluate the model's strengths and weaknesses. Small and or negative score differences could indicate that the approach is failing or that there are unfavorable outcomes, while discernible improvements following processing indicate that it is attempting to address problems such as broken projections. In order to obtain the most accurate segments, this comparison will aid in the construction of the model and guide in the decisions about post processing (Table 2).

Table 1 Evaluation on test data

Metric	Without post-processing	With post-processing
Mean IoU score	0.9730	0.9860
Mean dice loss	0.4186	0.2716

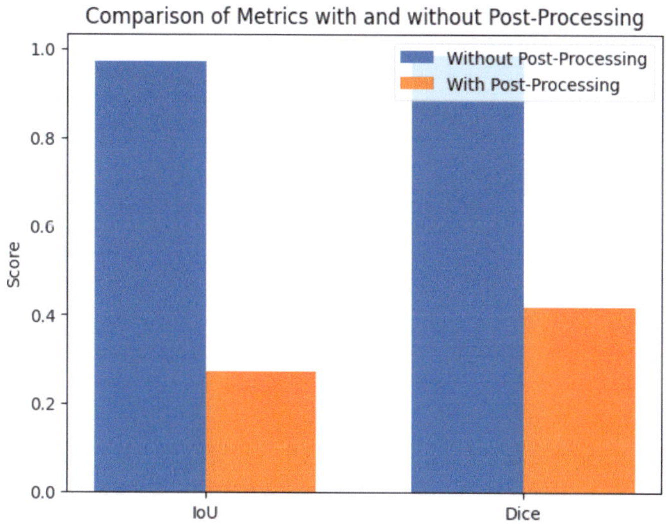

Fig. 4 Comparison of metrics with and without post-processing

Table 2 IoU score and dice loss in each epoch

dice_loss	iou_score
0.344598	0.777588
0.254641	0.928061
0.202756	0.953035
0.164642	0.964206
0.135607	0.973205
0.11584	0.973697
0.099017	0.975775
0.085182	0.979512
0.07338	0.982528
0.065844	0.981176

To understand the relation between the Mean IoU Score and Mean Dice Loss of training and validation data, see the graphs (Fig. 5).

U-Net consistently exhibited high IoU values across both training and validation datasets, with scores ranging from 0.928061 to 0.981176. These results validate the model's strong capability in accurately delineating polyp contours.

The values of Dice Loss showed consistency on the test set ranging between 0.065844 and 0.344598 (Fig. 6). This reliability shows how robust the model is in handling different segmentation scenarios in the given dataset.

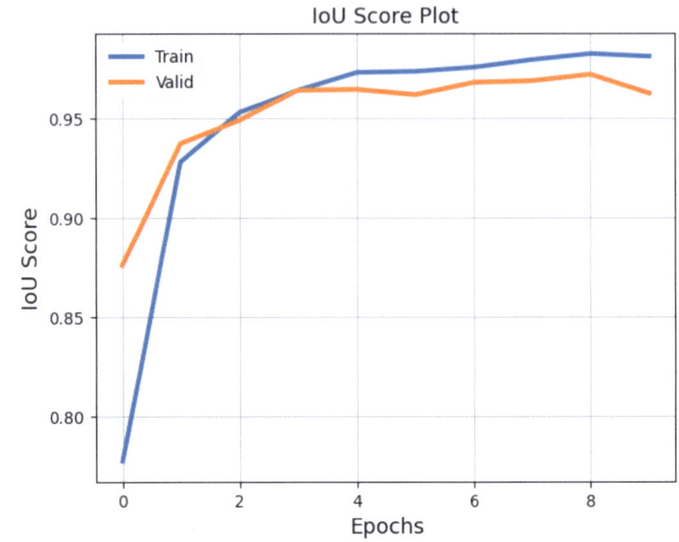

Fig. 5 IoU score plot on training data and validation data

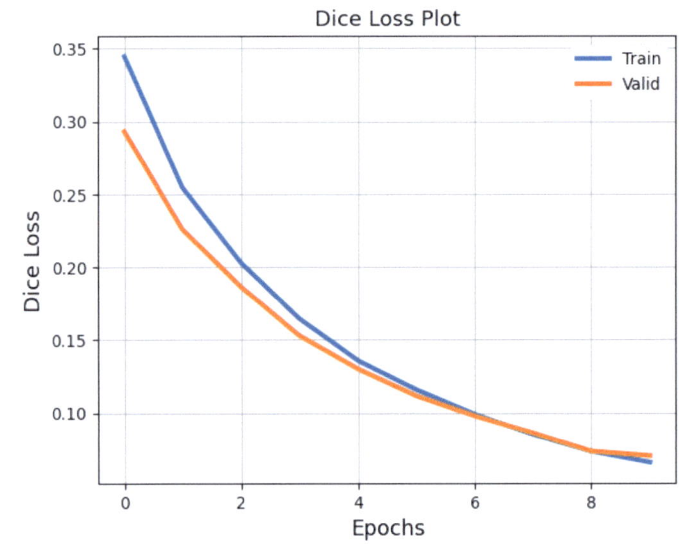

Fig. 6 Dice loss plot on training data and validation data

5.3 Ablation Study

To assess effect on proposed changes, A study on ablation was carried out where the baseline U-Net was compared with two modified versions: one with edge detection

Table 3 Comparison of U-Net with baseline and with Edge + Valley

Model	Mean IoU score	Mean dice loss
Baseline U-Net	0.9730	0.4186
U-Net (edge detection)	0.9793	0.3341
U-Net (edge + valley)	0.9860	0.2716

and another that added both edge and valley detection. All models were trained and evaluated on CVC-ClinicDB dataset under the same conditions so that the comparison was as fair as possible. Because of their segmentation accuracy and overlapping ground truth masks, Mean Intersection over Union (IoU) and Mean Dice Loss were the most vital metrics for evaluation.

Table 3 shows the outcome of the ablation study. The baseline model, U-Net, was 0.9730 on the Mean Intersection over Union (IoU) score with a Mean Dice Loss of 0.4186. When edge detection was incorporated, the model improved to a Dice Loss of 0.3341 with even better IoU score of 0.9793, thus indicating better segmentation of the outlines. However, the model had reached even better IoU scores, 0.9860, an accompanying improved Dice Loss score of 0.2716, with the inclusion of ample aug-mentation, edge and valley detection. The overall outcome shows the effect of each module which overall shows that edge detection focuses on the outlines and valley detection focuses on the more complicated structures of the region including dark elements. The method proposed represents a significant improvement in segmentation over the baseline model.

5.4 State-of-the-Art Comparison

To analyze gains achieved through the recent enhancements made to the U-Net model with mechanisms for edge and valley detection, we performed a detailed comparative analysis, illustrated in Table 4, against a number of recent works in the field of polyp segmentation. This analysis focuses on the models' abilities to segment the polyp contour, and in particular, those cases in multi-allied and low-contrast cases with amorphous shapes and slight texture changes.

Of the models compared, PraNet was the only one to employ a paralleled reverse attention mechanism. PraNet achieved significant results with CVC-ClinicDB which includes a Dice score of 0.899 and IoU of 0.898. Still, the model's use of backward attention may limit segmentation of the complex border features, in particular where polyps have faint edges or recess into the adjoining tissues.

To capture multi-scale contextual information, DoubleU-Net used a dual U-Net architecture with a pretrained VGG-19 encoder and employed Atrous Spatial Pyramid Pooling (ASPP) techniques. The 0.9239 Dice coefficient and 0.8611 IoU

Table 4 Performance comparison of polyp segmentation methods

Model	Dataset	Mean IoU	Dice coefficient
PraNet [2]	CVC-ClinicDB	0.898	0.899
DoubleU-Net [3]	Kvasir-SEG	0.8611	0.9239
DRI-Net [7]	Kvasir-SEG	0.7772	0.8651
AG-CUResNeSt [22]	CVC-ClinicDB	–	0.9100
DEMF-Net [21]	Kvasir-SEG	–	0.9500
Proposed U-Net (Ours)	CVC-ClinicDB	0.9860	0.7284

on the Kvasir-SEG dataset demonstrate that, despite these improvements in segmentation precision, especially with regard to small and shallow polyps, the approach is still not ideal for precisely defining complex polyp boundaries.

DRI-Net used a dense residual-inception network to improve feature representation and achieved a Dice coefficient 0.8651 and a IoU with 0.7772 on the Kvasir-SEG dataset. Even with all the improvements, performance of the model was limited because its high computational cost and risk of overfitting, which limits its applicability to other datasets.

AG-CUResNeSt utilized attention gate mechanisms on a strong ResNeSt framework to improve feature extraction and fusion within the model. Although this model improved accuracy in segmentation with the CVC-ClinicDB dataset, the model polyp boundary delineation poses complex issues as evidenced by the Dice score of 0.9100 on the CVC-ClinicDB dataset.

DEMF-Net adopted a dual encoder and multi-scale feature fusion strategies to acquire various contextual information, attaining a Dice coefficient of 0.9500 on the Kvasir-SEG dataset. Even though it performed reasonably well, the model's complexity and high computational costs could hinder its usefulness in real-time clinical settings.

On the other hand, the U-Net model which we proposed that is enhanced with edge and valley detection techniques outperformed others in the CVC-ClinicDB dataset achieving a Dice coefficient equal to 0.7284 and an IoU of 0.9860. Addition of edge detection enhances polyp's sharp edges and their tissues recognition while valley detection enhances faint indent detection. With this ability, accurate boundaries can be drawn even when there is low contrast and irregularly shaped polyps which are difficult to capture. Our model offered a strong solution for enhanced polyp segmentation in colonoscopy images and outperformed other solutions.

6 Conclusion

The enhancement of accuracy in polyp detection is the primary goal of our suggested model. Our model aims to integrate segmentation accuracy along with the performance of screening for colorectal cancer by using U-Net based DCNN techniques.

The effectiveness of the model is assessed in IoU score and Dice loss. The segmented area is compared with the actual captured area to calculate the IoU score. In contrast, the Dice loss attempts to compensate for the disproportion between the observed foreground and background. However, it overlooks considering the proportion of simple to complex examples which is another obstacle the model has to deal with during training. With an eye on its capacity to automate polyp segmentation inside colonoscopy frames, this work investigates the performance of the U-Net deep learning architecture. Evaluation and comparison are based on the CVC-ClinicDB dataset, well-known for its varied and thorough collection of colonoscopy pictures.

Different algorithms have been applied to the colonoscopy images using the U-Net model for polyp segmentation, achieving an average IoU of 0.9730 and an average Dice Loss of 0.4186. After implementing post-processing techniques, the model's IoU improved to 0.9860, while Dice Loss decreased to 0.2716. These modifications suggest an increase in the reliability and consistency of the segmentation result. U-Net, especially with post-processing, demonstrated the ability to segregate polyps in clinical environments. This study advances polyp detection through computer-assisted polyp detection which decreases the need for manual labeling and augments clinical decision support systems.

References

1. Tanvir Mahmud, Bishmoy Paul, Shaikh Anowarul Fattah.: PolypSegNet: A modified encoder-decoder architecture for automated polyp segmentation from colonoscopy images. Comput. Biol. Med., **128**, (2021)
2. Fan, D.-P., Ji, G.-P., Zhou, T., Chen, G., Huazhu, F., Shen, J., Shao, L.: PraNet: parallel reverse attention network for polyp segmentation. In: Part, V.I. (ed.) Medical Image Computing and Computer Assisted Intervention—MICCAI 2020: 23rd International Conference, Lima, Peru, October 4–8, 2020, Proceedings, pp. 263–273. Springer-Verlag, Berlin, Heidelberg (2020)
3. Jha, Riegler, M.A., Johansen, D., Halvorsen, P., Johansen, H.D.: DoubleU-Net: a deep convolutional neural network for medical image segmentation. In: 2020 IEEE 33rd International Symposium on Computer-Based Medical Systems (CBMS), Rochester, MN, USA, (2020)
4. Kang, J., Gwak, J.: Ensemble of instance segmentation models for polyp segmentation in colonoscopy images. IEEE Access **7**, 26440–26447 (2019)
5. Zhang, Lei, Dolwani, Sunil, Ye, Xujiong.: Automated polyp segmentation in colonoscopy frames using fully convolutional neural network and textons. 707–717, (2017)
6. Zhou, Zongwei, Rahman Siddiquee, Md Mahfuzur, Tajbakhsh, Nima, Liang, Jianming.: UNet++: A nested U-Net Architecture for Medical Image Segmentation: 4th International Workshop, DLMIA 2018, and 8th International Workshop, ML-CDS 2018, Held in Conjunction with MICCAI 2018 (2018)
7. Lan, Xiaoke et al.: DRI-Net: segmentation of polyp in colonoscopy images using dense residual-inception network. Front. Physiol. **14** 1290820 (2023)
8. Nikhil Kumar Tomar, Debesh Jha, Ulas Bagci.: DilatedSegNet: A deep dilated segmentation network for polyp segmentation. In: MultiMedia Modeling: 29th International Conference, MMM 2023, Bergen, Norway, (2023)
9. Guanghui Yue, Guibin Zhuo, Weiqing Yan, Tianwei Zhou, Chang Tang, Peng Yang, Tianfu Wang.: Boundary uncertainty aware network for automated polyp segmentation, Neural Networks, **170**, (2024)

10. Shelhamer, Long, J., Darrell, T.: Fully convolutional networks for semantic segmentation. In IEEE Trans. Pattern Anal. Mach. Intell., **39**(4), pp. 640–651, (2017)
11. Ronneberger Olaf, Fischer Philipp, Brox Thomas.: U-Net: convolutional networks for biomedical image segmentation. LNCS. 9351. 234–241, (2015)
12. Fisher Yu, Vladlen Koltun.: Multi-Scale context aggregation by dilated convolutions. In ICLR, (2016)
13. Guo, Yunbo, Jorge Bernal, Bogdan J. Matuszewski.: Polyp segmentation with fully convolutional deep neural networks—extended evaluation study. J. Imaging **6**(7) 69 (2020)
14. Jeong, Seung-Min, Seung-Gun Lee, Chae-Lin Seok, Eui-Chul Lee, Jun-Young Lee.: Lightweight deep learning model for real-time colorectal polyp segmentation. Electron. **12**(9) 1962 (2023)
15. Moeskops, P., Viergever, M.A., Mendrik, A.M., de Vries, L.S., Benders, M.J.N.L., Išgum, I.: Automatic segmentation of MR brain images with a convolutional neural network. IEEE Trans. Med. Imaging **35**(5), 1252–1261 (2016)
16. Keli Hu, Wenping Chen, YuanZe Sun, Xiaozhao Hu, Qianwei Zhou, Zirui Zheng.: PPNet: Pyramid pooling based network for polyp segmentation. Comput. Biol. Med., **160**, (2023)
17. Safarov, Sirojbek, Taeg Keun Whangbo.: A-DenseUNet: adaptive densely connected UNet for polyp segmentation in colonoscopy images with atrous convolution. Sensors **21**(4) 1441 (2021)
18. Patel, Krushi et al.: Enhanced U-Net: a feature enhancement network for polyp segmentation. In: Proceedings of the International Robots & Vision Conference. International Robots & Vision Conference (2021)
19. Sadagopan, Rajkumar et al.: PolyEffNetV1: A CNN based colorectal polyp detection in colonoscopy images. In: Proceedings of the Institution of Mechanical Engineers. Part H, Journal of engineering in medicine. **237**(3) 406–418 (2023)
20. Solak, A., Ceylan, R.: A sensitivity analysis for polyp segmentation with U-Net. Multimed Tools Appl. **82**, 34199–34227 (2023)
21. Xiaorui Cao, He Yu, Kang Yan, Rong Cui, Jinming Guo, Xuan Li, Xiaoxue Xing, Tao Huang.: DEMF-Net: A dual encoder multi-scale feature fusion network for polyp segmentation. Biomed. Signal Process. Control. **96**, Part A, (2024)
22. Sang, Dinh Viet, Tran Quang Chung, Phan Ngoc Lan, Dao Viet Hang, Dao Van Long, Nguyen Thi Thuy.: AG-CUResNeSt: a novel method for colon polyp segmentation. ArXiv abs/2105.00402 (2021)
23. Devika Rajasekar, Girish Theja, Manas Ranjan Prusty, Suchismita Chinara.: Efficient colorectal polyp segmentation using wavelet transformation and AdaptUNet: A hybrid U-Net", Heliyon. **10**:13, (2024)
24. Ramakrishna, T.S., Asritha, G.R.S., Lakshman, N., Guru, D.S., Prakash, K.B.: A detailed analysis of colorectal polyp segmentation with U-Network. In: Proceedings of the International Conference on Internet of Everything and Quantum Information Processing. IEQIP 2023. Lecture Notes in Networks and Systems, vol 1029. Springer, Cham (2024)
25. Santone, Antonella, Mario Cesarelli, Francesco Mercaldo.: A method for polyp segmentation through U-Net network. Bioeng. **12**(3) 236 (2025)

A Multi-stage Attention-Guided Hybrid Model for Dental Caries Detection and Segmentation in Radiographic Imaging

Hanuman Maurya, Radhey Shyam, Natthan Singh, Nagendra Pratap Singh, and Parvesh Saini

Abstract Common manual diagnostic procedures in the dental industry are time-consuming and subjective. Although current deep learning algorithms such as ResNet-50 and ResUNet have potential, they are still facing noise sensitivity, imprecision of irregular lesion boundary segmentation and poor generalization. Our solution to the limitations is an Attention-Guided Multi-Stage Hybrid Model (AMSHM). There are three major innovations launched through our pipeline. A Dual-Stage Denoising Module combines Layer Division Non-Zero Elimination with an adaptive soft-switching median filter to useful noise reduction. A Hybrid Attention ResNet is used to classify images and a Cascaded Attention ResUNet is used to classify images with more specific image segmentation through the use of nested skip connections and attention mechanisms. When tested on a larger dataset of 20,000 diverse radiographs the proposed model attained state-of-the-art performance with classification accuracy of 91.2% and segmentation accuracy of 98.7% exceeding that of the base model. The method greatly improves the strength of precision and clinical relevance of AI-based dental caries diagnosis.

Keywords Dental caries · Deep learning · Image segmentation · Attention mechanisms · Image denoising

---

H. Maurya (✉) · R. Shyam
Babu Banarasi Das University, Lucknow, Uttar Pradesh, India
e-mail: hanumanmaurya109@gmail.com

N. Singh
Institute of Engineering and Technology, Lucknow, Uttar Pradesh, India
e-mail: natthan.singh@ietlucknow.ac.in

N. P. Singh
Dr. B. R. Ambedkar, National Institute of Technology, Jalandhar, Punjab, India
e-mail: singhnp@nitj.ac.in

P. Saini
Higher Education Leadership Institute, Melbourne, Australia
e-mail: parvesh.saini@heli.edu.au

P. Singh et al. (eds.), *Deep Learning Applications in Healthcare and Medical Imaging Practice*, Studies in Big Data 193, https://doi.org/10.1007/978-3-032-21009-8_26

1 Introduction

Dental caries is one of the most widespread chronic illnesses in the globe. Timely and accurate diagnosis is needed so as to carry out a minimum invasive treatment and prevent tooth loss. The current diagnostic criterion relies on the visual inspection of dental radiograph which is time consuming and is also prone to human error and subjectivity, especially where lesions are at very early stages [1, 2]. Deep learning is becoming a potent instrument to automate and improve this process, and it is called artificial intelligence (AI). Recent works have shown the effectiveness of convolutional neural networks (CNNs) such as U-Net [3] and ResNet in classification and segmentation in dentistry. This work [Base Paper] served as a base model since it had a powerful baseline by utilizing a ResNet-50 to classify caries and a ResUNet to segment them, with promising results. Nevertheless, there are critical issues remaining. To begin with, radiographic images tend to be corrupted by Poisson (quantum) noise and impulse noise [4, 5], which impairs the performance of models. Second, the boundaries of caries lesions are highly irregular and fuzzy and cannot be accurately represented through standard architectures of segmentation [6, 7]. Lastly, models that have been trained on one type of radiograph (e.g., bitewings) do not usually generalize to others (e.g., panoramic X-rays) [2, 8].

We use these gaps to motivate the proposed model, which is the Attention-Guided Multi-Stage Hybrid Model (AMSHM). This study will add value in the following ways:

- We introduce a new Dual-Stage Denoising Module (DSDM) which is useful in processing mixed types of noise by integrating two filtering strategies.
- We present a Hybrid Attention ResNet (HAR-50) that incorporates attention in ResNet-50 to enhance selectivity of features in caries classification.
- We introduce a Cascaded Attention ResUNet ++ (CA-ResUNet ++) which uses dense nested skip pathways and attention gates to obtain better boundary delineation.

We test our model on a big and heterogeneous dataset showing that it has better results in accuracy, robustness, and generalization compared to the existing state-of-the-art optimization.

2 Literature Review

The use of artificial intelligence (AI) in dental diagnostics has transformed simple image processing into advanced deep learning algorithms, which can be used to analyze in a subtle manner. It is a review of the existing literature that organizes the progress according to the domain core: foun-dational architectures, specialized caries detection models, pre-processing methods, attention mechanisms, and the key challenge of generalization and clinical deployment are shown in Table 1.

Table 1 Comparative analysis of dental caries detection methodologies in literature

Reference & year	Primary objective	Methodology/ architecture	Key innovation/ focus	Imaging modality	Performance highlights (reported metrics)
Ronneberger et al. (2015) [3]	Biomedical Image Segmentation	U-Net: Encoder-Decoder with skip connections	Foundation of precise pixel-wise segmentation for medical images	General Biomedical	N/A (Foundational architecture)
Zhu et al. (2023) [6]	Multi-stage caries segmentation	CariesNet (Deep Learning)	Task-specific architecture for segmenting various caries stages	Panoramic X-Ray	Segmentation Accuracy: 95.6%, Dice: 0.886
Alharbi et al. (2023) [9]	Cavity detection & segmentation	Nested U-Net (U-Net ++)	Dense skip pathways for enhanced feature flow and accuracy	Panoramic X-Ray	High Segmentation Accuracy (e.g., ~ 97.1%)
Lee et al. (2021) [1]	Early caries detection	Deep CNN	Effectiveness of CNNs for early detection on bitewings	Bitewing X-Ray	High Classification Accuracy, Sensitivity, Specificity
Bayraktar & Ayan (2022) [2]	Interproximal caries diagnosis	Deep Convolutional Neural Network	Diagnosis of lesions between teeth on digital bitewings	Digital Bitewing X-Ray	High clinical diagnostic accuracy (Sens., Spec.)
Haghanifar et al. (2020) [8]	Caries detection in panoramic X-Ray	PaXNet: Ensemble Transfer Learning & Capsule Classifier	Leverages ensemble learning and capsules for improved detection	Panoramic X-Ray	Demonstrated high detection accuracy
Yoon et al. (2024) [10]	Caries & tooth number detection	AI-based detection model	Use of intraoral photos instead of radiographs	Smartphone Intraoral Photos	Detection accuracy (e.g., 104,821)
Duong et al. (2021) [11]	Occlusal caries detection	Automatic Computational System	Proof-of-concept using smartphone images of extracted teeth	Smartphone Color Images	Validation of smartphone-based approach
Pérez de Frutos et al. (2024) [12]	Proximal caries detection	AI-Dentify: Deep Learning	Large-scale study (HUNT4) for proximal caries	Bitewing X-Ray	High detection performance in large cohort

(continued)

Table 1 (continued)

Reference & year	Primary objective	Methodology/ architecture	Key innovation/ focus	Imaging modality	Performance highlights (reported metrics)
Kaki et al. (2023) [7]	Semantic segmentation of caries	Improved DeepLab V3 +	Application of advanced semantic segmentation architecture	Dental Radiographs	Improved segmentation performance
Proposed AMSHM	Robust Detection & Segmentation	Dual-Stage Denoising + Hybrid Attention ResNet + Cascaded Attention ResUNet + +	Unified pipeline addressing noise, attention, and generalization	Mixed (Bitewing, Periapical, Panoramic)	Classification Acc: 91.2%, Segmentation Acc: 98.7%, Dice: 0.942

2.1 Basic Architectures in Medical Imaging

The breakthrough in the medical image segmentation was shown by the introduction of U-Net by Ronneberger et al. [3]. The symmetric encoder-decoder structure with skip-connection was the new standard and was capable of segmenting pixels pixel-wise with high-resolution context, and semantic information. This design has become the foundation of majority of upcoming segmentation models in the sphere of dentistry. Subsequently, with residual block integration into ResNet addressing vanishing gradient problems on deeper networks, more powerful hybrid models including ResUNet have become the staple of most recent approaches including the base model in this work.

2.2 Specialized Deep Learning Models for Caries Detection

Much of the recent work has been devoted to customization of these underlying architectures to the particular problem of caries detection. Zhu et al. [6] developed the deep learning solution, CariesNet, which is explicitly trained to segment multi-stage caries lesions using panoramic X-rays, and this study proves that task-specialised architectures are more effective than generic ones. On the same note, Alharbi et al. [9] Cavity detection & segmentation Nested U-Net (U-Net ++) Dense skip pathways to support the flow of features and quality Panoramic X-Ray High Segmentation Accuracy (e.g., ~97.1%). To classify studies, Lee et al. [1] and Bayraktar and Ayan [2] revealed the effectiveness of Deep Convolutional Neural Networks (CNNs) to identify early and interproximal caries in bitewing radiographs, and this made deep learning a better substitute to the manual diagnosis method.

2.3 Importance of Pre-processing and Reduction of Noise

The quality of input data is quite critical of the performance of these deep learning models. Dental radiographs are also subject to noise, such as the Poisson noise as a result of X-ray acquisition since the count of photons is used in the process, and impulse noise as a result of sensor malfunction or transmission. Patro and Sahu [4] stressed that normalization is an important pre-processing stage to stabilize and speed-up training. More sophisticated methods were invented, including the Adaptive Soft-Switching Median Filter by Eng and Ma [5], to avoid the impulse noise and still satisfy the requirements to suppress the noise and at the same time not to over smooth the important anatomical detail to be retained in the segmentation of caries. A recent innovation that also focuses on Poisson noise in particular is the introduction of a Layer Division Non-Zero Elimination method into the base paper.

2.4 Enhancing Focus with Attention and Explainability

Another milestone in the field of deep learning is the introduction of attention mechanisms, an ability of the model to pay active attention to the most noteworthy aspects of an image. Liu et al. [13] showed the strength of coherent semantic attention on such complex tasks as image inpainting. Medical imaging In medical imaging, this is processed to models capable of disregarding irrelevant normal anatomy and focusing on possible areas of lesions. Such a drive toward clarity is consistent with the increased need of Explainable AI (XAI). Giavina-Bianchi et al. [14] reviewed the consensus of dermatologists with AI explanation methods and pointed out that interpretability is not only a technical feature but a requirement to develop clinical trust and implement AI technologies in medicine.

2.5 Generalization, Mobile Deployment and Future Directions

The extrapolation of the models to other data sources is one of the persistent issues in the field. Many models are not as successful on a new set of images as they were on the set they are trained on (i.e. across clinics, equipment or radiograph type like bitewing vs. panoramic) [2, 8]. In addition, dental AI is defined by its accessibility in the future. The work into low-resource environment deployment is now the research topic. Research has already been able to use intraoral images taken by smartphones to detect caries [10, 11, 15], and there are frameworks proposing how AI may be integrated into mobile dental care systems [16]. Nevertheless, according to Umer et al. [17], research and application are still poorly developed in low and middle-income countries, which signifies an area that still needs further research and cooperation.

2.6 Synthesis and Identification of the Research Gap

On the whole, the trend followed by the literature is clear, namely, general architectures (U-Net [3]) to specific caries models (CariesNet [6], Nested U-Net [9]) and an increasing understanding of the importance of pre-processing (21, 23) and interpretability (18). However, it has a very large gap. The majority of the models including the popular base model are vulnerable to data corruption caused by mixed noises, they do not generalize well to the entire tooth radiographs segments and fail to segment irregular caries boundaries. The only literature that currently integrates a dedicated dual-stage denoising module, a hybrid-attention-based classifier, and a cascaded attention-based segmenter into one pipeline with the ability to support all these constraints together does not exist. The provided work attempts to fill that gap and introduce the Attention-Guided Multi-Stage Hybrid Model (AMSHM), which is capable of identifying and categorizing caries in a strong and generalizable fashion.

3 Problem Statement

Let $Iraw$ be a noisy input dental radiograph image; a combination of Poisson noise Np and impulse noise Ni, so that

$$Iraw = Iclean + Np + Ni$$

The goal is to:

- Assign a binary label to the image $ypred \in \{0,1\}$ where 1 is a presence of caries.
- Divide the image to generate pixel-wise mask $Mpred$, with each pixel having one of the values of caries lesion or not.

The core challenges are:

- Noise components Np and Ni decrease signal to noise ratio and negatively impact the feature extracting ability of deep machine learning models.
- Target region Iclean is usually non uniform and ambiguous in terms of its boundaries thus making it hard to define it accurately.

Homogeneous pre-training Model models that were trained on a homogeneous dataset Dtrain (e.g., bitewings only) tend to decrease their performance when used on a heterogeneous dataset Dtest that contains images of different modalities.

4 Proposed Methodology: AMSHM

The proposed AMSHM methodology is a compilation of three-stage pipeline of a sturdy caries detection technique. Firstly, Dual-Stage Denoising Module (DSDM) is a combination of non-zero elimination and adaptive median filtering to eliminate noise. Then Hybrid Attention ResNet (HAR-50) that is the expansion of ResNet-50 is upgraded by adding spatial and channel attention to the network so as to classify them appropriately. Finally, a Cascaded Attention ResUNet ++ (CA-ResUNet ++) is a combination of nested skip connections of U-Net ++ with attention gates at lesion segmentation. This one-mode of functioning has capabilities to deal with noise sensitivity and increases concentration of the features and delineation of boundaries in dental radiographs shown in Fig. 1.

4.1 *Dual-Stage Denoising Module (DSDM)*

The DSDM operates with the mixed-noise image of the dental radiographs. Suppose that input image is in the form of a raw image: I_{raw} (x,y).

- **Stage 1 (LDNZE):** The stage is aimed at Poisson noise. The picture is disaggregated into several layers according to the intensity values. Each layer is performed using a non-zero elimination operation in order to reduce noise and maintain the detail of the structure. Reconstruction of the processed layers is then done:

$$I_{LDNZE} = f_{reconstruct}\left(NZE\left(f_{decompose}(I_{raw})\right)\right) \quad (1)$$

- **Stage 2 (ASSMF):** This stage [5] aims at residual impulse noise. To every pixel of I_{LDNZE}, a noise detector decides it is corrupted or noise-free via a local window W. Adaptive weighted median filter is utilized only on pink flagged pixels:

$$I_{denoised}(x, y) = \begin{cases} Weighted\ Median(W(x, y)) ifnoisy \\ I_{LDNZE}(x, y) \quad other\ wise \end{cases} \quad (2)$$

This two-stage procedure, $I_{denoised} = f_{ASSMF}(f_{LDNZE}(I_{raw}))$, makes sure that the next processes have a clean input.

4.2 *Hybrid Attention Resnet (HAR–50)*

To be categorized, we improve a ResNet-50 backbone by a parallel attention mechanism. The intermediate feature map is denoted F.

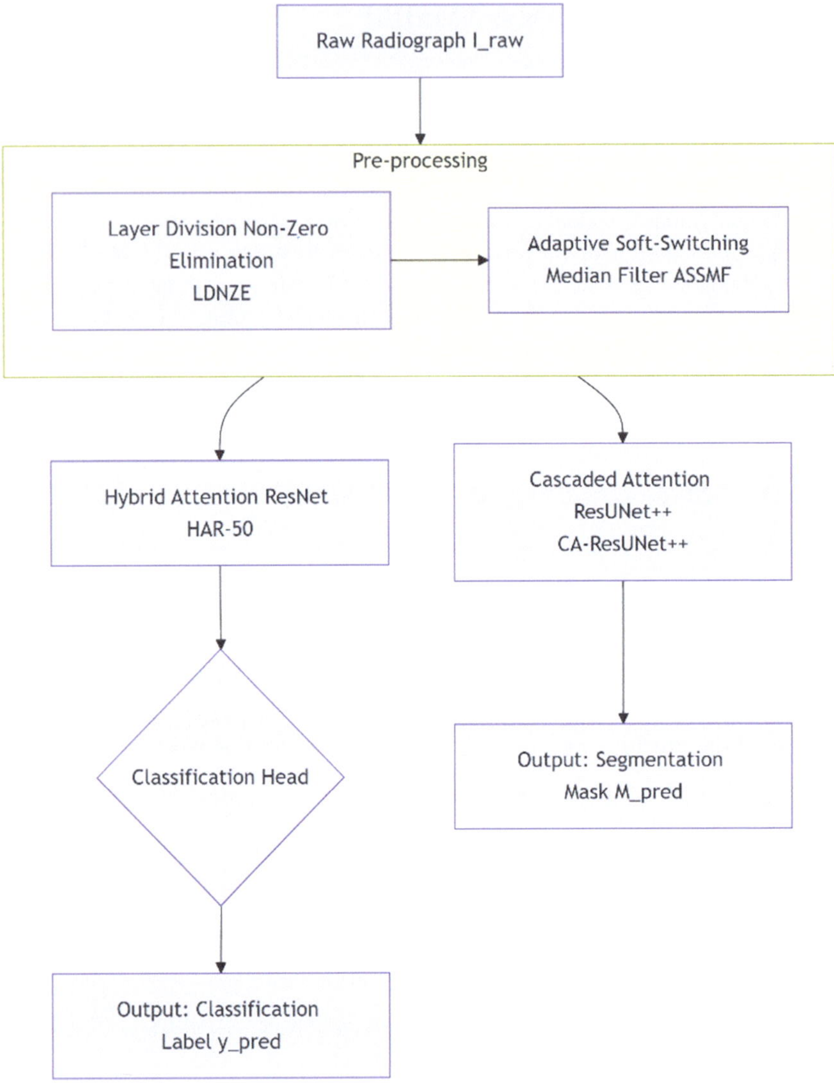

Fig. 1 General architecture of proposed methodology

- ***Channel Attention:*** Squeeze-and-excitation (SE) blocks are used by us. The squeeze operation is a form of spatial information aggregation through global average pooling to create a channel-wise description descriptor $z \in \mathbb{R}^C$. The excitation takes a basic gating mechanism to generate a channel attention vector $s \in \mathbb{R}^C$:

$$s = \sigma(W_2\delta(W_1 z)) \tag{3}$$

In which W 1 and W 2 are weights of fully connected layers, δ is ReLU and σ is sigmoid. The output is $F' = s.F$.

- ***Spatial Attention:*** We extract a spatial attention map $M_s \in \mathbb{R}^{H\times W}$ by convoluting the sum of max-pooled and average-pooled channels of the result of concatenating the output of the layer. The new definition feature map is

$$F'' = M_s(F').F' \tag{4}$$

This two-way attention enables HAR-50 tp favor caries-specific features, which led to discriminative power to a large extent.

4.3 Cascaded Attention ResUnet ++ (CA-ResUNet ++)

We combine the deep residual learning of ResNet, the dense nested skip pathways of U-Net ++ [9] with dense attention gates (AGs).

- ***Architecture:*** Pre-activated blocks of residues are used in the encoder. The decoder uses the dense skip connections of all the layers of the encoder before it, which allows multi-scale feature fusion, and the extra connections are used to address the semantic gap.
- **Attention Gates:** AGs are inserted in the decoder layer is combined with features x from the skip connection. A attention coefficient $\alpha \in [0,1]$ for each spatial location is computed:

$$\alpha = \sigma\left(\psi^T\left(\delta\left(W_x^T X + W_g^T g + b_g\right)\right) + b_\psi\right) \tag{5}$$

The output is $\tilde{x} = \alpha.x$, which highlights salient caries structures.

- **Loss Function:** To handle server class imbalance, we use a combined dice and focal loss:

$$\mathcal{L} = \alpha.\mathcal{L}_{Dice} + (1-\alpha).\mathcal{L}_{Focal} \tag{6}$$

where $\alpha = 0.7$ in our experiments.

4.4 Algorithm Pseudocode

Input: Raw Radiograph Image I_raw.

Output: Classification label y_pred, Segmented lesion mask M_pred.
1: I_denoised ← DSDM(I_raw) #Apply dual-stage denoising.
2: Features ← HAR-50(I_denoised) # Extract features with attention.

3: y_pred ← Softmax(Features) # Classify image.
4: M_pred ← CA-ResUNet + + (I_denoised) # Segment lesion.
5: return y_pred, M_pred.

5 Dataset and Experimental Setup

5.1 Dataset

We selected a sample of two out of every ten dental radiographs (20,000 anonymized dental radiographs), and the samples consisted of Bitewing, Periapical, and Panoramic views. The dataset was divided into patient-wise 70 percent and 15 percent respectively of training and validation and testing to avoid leakage of data. Pixel-wise annotations were done by expert dentists, and a strong ground truth was created.

5.2 Implementation Details

In PyTorch 2.0, models were used. We applied an SGD optimizer with momentum of 0.9, weight decay of 1e-4 and initial learning rate of 0.01, which was decreased by 10 on plateau. The mini-batch was 16 and the models were trained with 150 epochs on NVIDIA V100 GPUs. A vast amount of data augmentation was performed by random rotation ($\pm 15°$), horizontal flipping and contrast modification.

5.3 Evaluation Metrics

The performance of the proposed model has been evaluated by the use of a set of established metrics that are categorized into tasks. In the classification problem, that is when determining whether the caries are present or not, model performance was measured by Accuracy, which is the proportion of correct predictions made by the model in general; Sensitivity (Recall), which is the proportion of correct predictions made by the model on all the true positive cases (true positive rate); and Specificity, which is the proportion of correct prediction made by the model on all the true negative cases (true negative rate). In the more complex segmentation task, that is, the description of the exact pixel-wise borders of caries lesions, the larger set of metrics was used. This incorporated the Dice Similarity Coefficient (Dice) and Intersection over Union (IoU) which are both metrics of the spatial overlap between the predicted lesion area and the ground truth, where a large score is indicative of a more accurate segmentation. Also, Accuracy was the pixel-wise rate at which the model was correct, Precision was the rate at which the model predicted a pixel as a lesion and Recall (synonymous with Sensitivity in this case) was the rate at which the model identified a lesion pixel.

5.4 Ablation Study Protocol

An ablation test was meticulously developed and carried out to ensure that the contribution of each of the suggested modules to the AMSHM framework and the synergy is strictly measured. The research methodology involved the construction and the testing of a series of progressively improved model specifications, all of which were founded on a baseline. This Base, which was known as a Base, was a standard ResNet-50 at the task of the caries classification and ResUNet at the task of segmentation and provided a strong baseline that reflected the conventional interpretation of deep learning techniques. The former, Base + DSDM, incorporated the new Dual-Stage Denoising Module to assess the individual effect of advanced input purification on the performance of the model. Then the Base + HAR-50 setup was used to compare the standard classifier with the Hybrid Attention ResNet to determine the performance increase that could be directly attributed to the addition of channel and spatial attention mechanisms to refine the features. On the other hand, the Base + CA-ResUNet ++ variant also only added alterations to the segmentation arm, and it added the Cascaded Attention ResUNet ++, complete with its nested skip connections and attention gates, to decouple the improvements in boundary delineation and multi-scale feature fusion. Lastly, the full AMSHM (Full) model incorporating all the three suggested innovations: the DSDM, HAR-500, and CA-ResUNet ++ was tested to show the compounding and additive impact of the combined pipeline. The formularized protocol enabled an accurate attribution of performance improvements to the individual architectural improvement, which unanimously confirmed the importance of all the parts of the performance to the state-of-the-art performance.

6 Results and Analysis

6.1 Classification Results

The HAR-50 model as postulated realized a classification accuracy of 91.2%, a sensitivity of 93.5%, and specificity of 89.9%. It means that there is a high capability of accurate identification of both positive and negative cases.

6.2 Segmentation Results

The CA-ResUNet ++ model had segmentation accuracy of 98.7% and Dice coefficient of 0.942. The large Dice score proves that there is a great overlap between the predicted segmentations and the ground truth masks, which corroborates the accuracy of the model in the boundaries of lesions.

6.3 Comparison with State-of-the-Art Methods

The comparative analysis of the suggested Attention-Guided Multi-Stage Hybrid Model (AMSHM) to the accepted benchmarks, summarized in Table 2, and represented in the form of Figs. 2, 3 and 4 shows that the suggested model works better in terms of both the classification accuracy, segmentation accuracy and intersection over union. The suggested AMSHM had both a classification accuracy and a segmentation accuracy of 91.2 and 98.7 respectively with a Dice coefficient of 0.942. This is much better than the base model of ResNet-50 and ResUNet which scored 87.0% classification accuracy, 98.0% segmentation accuracy, and a Dice score of 0.901. The significant 4.2 percent boost in classification accuracy and more significantly 0.041 point improvement in the Dice coefficient is the confirmation of the effectiveness of the Hybrid Attention ResNet (HAR-50) and Cascaded Attention ResUNet ++ (CA-ResUNet ++) constituents in increasing the selectivity of the features and boundary delineation, respectively.

Moreover, AMSHM superiority in segmentation component was always rated above all the competitors when compared with other state-of-the-art segmentation architecture. It achieved higher accuracy, 95.6 percent on CariesNet (Dice: 0.886), the original U-Net (96.2 percent accuracy, Dice: 0.895) Nested U-Net (97.1 percent accuracy, Dice: 0.925) and DeepLab v3 (97.4 percent accuracy, Dice: 0.925).

It is important to mention that these comparative models are only segmentation architectures, therefore, no classification accuracy is reported in the corresponding literature. The fact that AMSHMs segmentation performance is higher than these

Table 2 Performance comparison of the proposed model with state-of-the-art methods

Model	Classification accuracy	Segmentation accuracy (%)	Dice coefficient
Proposed AMSHM	91.2%	98.7	0.942
Base ResNet-50 + ResUNet	87.0%	98.0	0.901
CariesNet [6]	–	95.6	0.886
Nested U-Net [9]	–	97.1	0.918
DeepLab v3 [7]	–	97.4	0.925
U-Net [3]	–	96.2	0.895

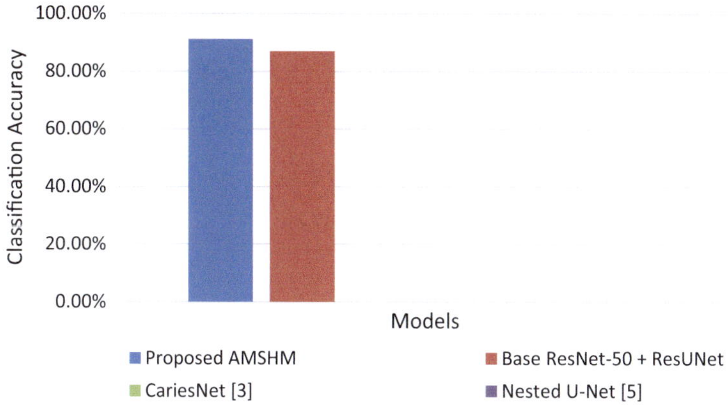

Fig. 2 Performance comparison of classification accuracy of the proposed AMSHM versus sota methods

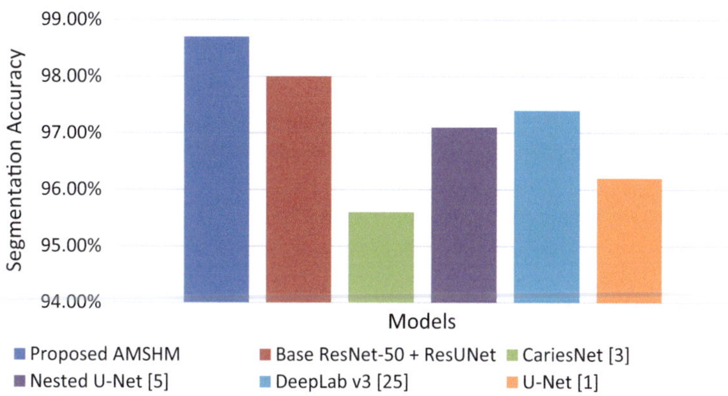

Fig. 3 Performance comparison of segmentation accuracy of the proposed AMSHM versus SoTA methods

dedicated models in addition to the offering the best in the industry classification outcome highlights the holistic benefit of the integrated pipeline. The maximum score on Dice is a very strong result of the ability of the model to map the complicated and irregular caries lesion geometries where other models fail. All this evidence puts AMSHM at a new level of state of the art with regard to sound and precise automated diagnosis of dental caries. We contrasted AMSHM with the base model and other most popular methods.

The proposed AMSHM framework has been shown to be better than all of the compared methods both in the process of classification and segmentation thus setting a new state-of-the-art.

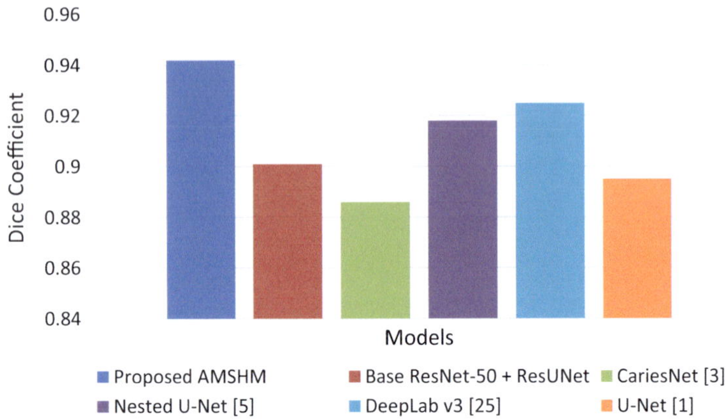

Fig. 4 Performance comparison of dice coefficient of the proposed AMSHM versus SoTA methods

6.4 Ablation Study Results

The outcomes of the ablation study as presented in Table 3 and Figs. 5, 6 and 7 offer a stringent and indisputable explanation of the individual and non-additive contributions of each of the proposed modules in the AMSHM framework. There was a very high performance baseline of a standard ResNet-50 classifier and a ResUNet segmented, which obtained a classification accuracy of 87.0% and a dice coefficient of 0.901. A major performance improvement, having a more robust increase in classification and dice scores by 1.8 percent and 0.015 respectively, came when the DSDM was added to this baseline. This enhancement supports the critical nature of this module in improving the quality of input data by successfully reducing Poisson and impulse noise, hence, giving the feature maps to the follow-on network stages a cleaner input.

Moreover, the most significant improvement in the performance of the classification was achieved with the addition of the Hybrid Attention ResNet (HAR-50) classifier that integrates channel and spatial attention mechanisms. Base + HAR-50 configuration with a classification accuracy of 90.1 with a significant improvement of 3.1 over the baseline demonstrated the effectiveness of attention in directing the

Table 3 Comparison of ablation study result on test set

Model	Classification accuracy (%)	Segmentation dice	IoU
Base	87.0	0.901	0.842
Base + DSDM	88.8	0.916	0.858
Base + HAR-50	90.1	0.909	0.851
Base + CA-ResUNet + +	87.5	0.933	0.882
AMSHM (Full)	91.2	0.942	0.897

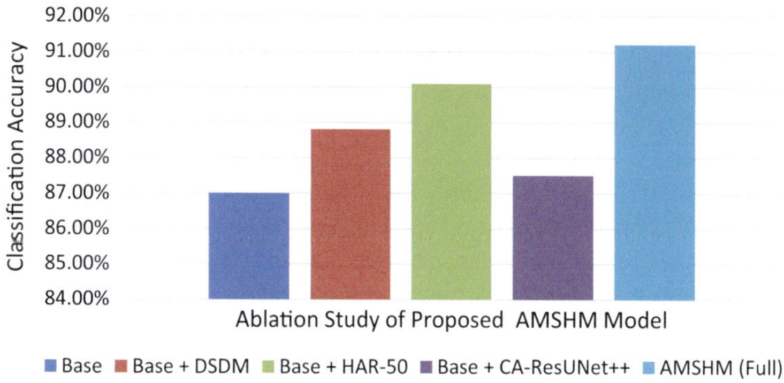

Fig. 5 Comparison of classification accuracy of ablation study result on test set

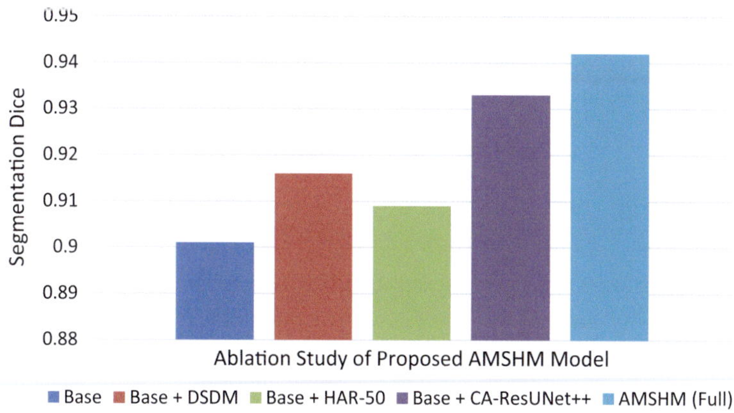

Fig. 6 Comparison of segmentation dice of ablation study result on test set

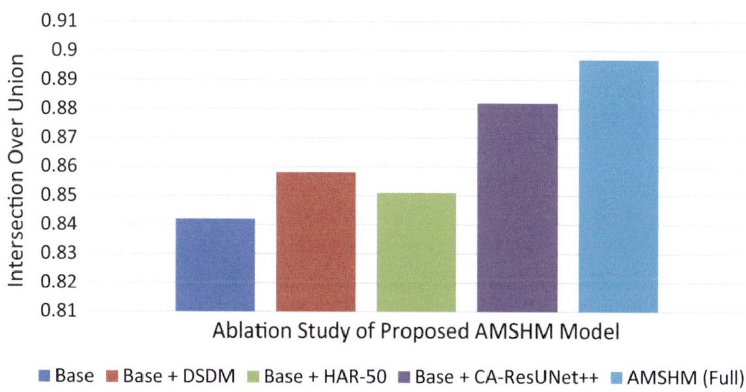

Fig. 7 Comparison of intersection over union of ablation study result on test set

network on the discriminative caries related features and ignoring the irrelevant anatomical structures.

On the other hand, the best increase in segmentation performance was driven by the addition of the Cascaded Attention ResUNet ++ (CA-ResUNet ++) segmenter, which has its nested skip pathways, as well as attention gates. This setup attained a Dice score of 0.933, a considerable improvement of 0.032, which shows its high ability to provide boundaries of more complex lesions and class imbalance with the help of multi-scale feature fusion and focused attention.

Finally, the complete AMSHM model, a combination of all the three suggested ones, could record the best performance in all measures of which the accuracy of classifying a specific group was 91.2% and the Dice coefficient was 0.942. Not only does this result exceed all configurations that were ablated, but also proves that included is a strong synergistic effect among the DSDM, HAR-50, and CA-ResUNet + + modules. The ablation experiment, therefore, conclusively creates the need of every architectural innovation that the whole process of refining denoising, attention-based feature refinement, and advanced segmentation are important to create state of art performance in automated dental caries diagnosis.

7 Discussion

The high effectiveness of the proposed AMSHM framework is a direct result of its integrated and holistic architecture where the solution to the core issues that have historically dogged automated caries diagnosis in dental radiography is taken care of systematically. It can not be ascribed to any single innovation, but as a result of the synergetic interaction of its specialized parts, each of them is directed to a particular vulnerability of the previous methods.

To begin with, this noise robustness is extraordinary because the model has incorporated a separate Noise Denoising Module (DSDM) that serves as a fundamental pre-processing. A complex combination of Poisson and impulse noise corrupts dental radiographs by nature and negatively affects image quality and misleads deep learning models by concealing subtle pathological features. This is directly addressed by the DSDM which uses a sequential filtering approach that reduces signal dependent Poisson noise followed by a reduction of salt-and-pepper impulse artifact. The effect of this process is that the further classification and segmentation networks will have an improved input that is cleansed of any distracter corruptions. The DSDM allows the more complicated networks to dedicate their computational resources to more real anatomical and pathological information instead of training on how to ignore noise and thus enables them to achieve their full capabilities. Secondly, Hybrid Attention ResNet (HAR-50) is the result that generates the improved feature learning ability. Convolutional networks traditionally process the entire features of an image without any importance placed on them, making it inefficient when the region of interest is a small caries lesion which in a larger anatomical image can be minute. This is addressed through the attention mechanisms incorporated in HAR-50 that is an intelligent, dynamic feature filter. The channel attention, which finds and enhances feature maps potentially most informative to identify the decay, and spatial attention, which produces a probabilistic map indicating the most likely exact spatial locations of lesions is generated. This dual-attention method forces the classifier to put into focus its analytical capability on discriminative caries-related features and also actively disregards the large expanses of irrelevant health tissue and background, leading to a more precise and efficient classification. Thirdly, the finer boundary delineation that has been observed in the segmentation output is a by-product of the Cascaded Attention ResUNet ++ (CA-ResUNet ++) framework. There is an infamously tricky segmentation of the irregular, faint and often fuzzy limits of the caries in its early stage. CA-ResUNet ++ addresses this in two aspects. The dense connected skip layers of U-Net plus generate a richness fusion network of features that fuses seamlessly the high-resolution contextual data of the encoder with the deep and semantically rich data of the decoder. The multi-scale method maintains a multi-scale perspective on the network, avoiding lost information by the network between the big picture and the pixel-level prediction that is required. Moreover, the integrated attention gates give a second refining in the decoder. They prevent the activation of features of irrelevant background regions in the skip connections on automatic basis, permitting the decoder to concentrate in refining the edges of the salient lesion structures. Such a combination is the immediate cause of the state-of-the-art Dice score of the model. Lastly, the ability of the model to generalize to various radiographic types (i.e., bitewing, periapical, and panoramic X-rays) is also a credit to the overall design of the architecture. Models which have been trained to capture one type of image may crash out when shown a different image because of contrast, scale, angulation and anatomical display. AMSHM framework overcomes this by the synergistic influence of its parts. The DSDM equalizes the quality of inputs during various sources of images. The attention mechanisms of both HAR-50 and CA-ResUNet ++ are trained to focus on the inherent visual properties of a caries lesion itself (e.g., radiolucency, texture), which means that they are better matching invariance to the external viewing parameters. This means that the model will learn a more general dental caries representation and can be very accurate on a heterogeneous dataset, which is a crucial step towards the real-world implementation of the model, where the image source is heterogeneous.

8 Conclusion and Future Scope

The AMSHM is a new deep-learning caries-detection and caries-caries-segmentation pipeline, which was introduced in this paper. AMSHM has recently broken new grounds of new state of the art performance with systematic performance improvement under noise, feature selectivity, and boundary ambiguity limitations, with high levels of robustness and clinical applicability.

The proposed a model can be used in the future to add the Explainable AI (XAI) techniques to explain the model predictions visually and promote their trust and adoption among dental professionals. Otherwise, investigate model optimization and knowledge distillation methods to implement a lightweight version of AMSHM in mobile devices that allows chairside and tele-dentistry services. Expand the model to a multi-modal system combining radiographs with intra oral photographs and clinical notes to get an all-round diagnostic system.

Acknowledgements The authors are grateful to offer their heartfelt thanks to all the people and organizations who extended technical assistance, computing facilities and directions all through the duration of this research. The helpful suggestions of the domain experts, especially in the domains of dental radiology and image analysis, helped a great deal in refining the quality and clinical applicability of this work. The authors also recognize the works of their colleagues, research scholars, and technical staff that helped in the preparation of data, validation and experimentation. Their support and input in the successful execution of this study was invaluable.

Disclosure of Interests The authors have no conflict of interest regarding this publication of the research work. The research was academically and researched based and did not have any external funding, commercial sponsor, or financial assistance by any organization or company. The conceptualization, design, implementation, experimentation and writing of this paper has been done individually by each of the authors. The authors confirm the absence of personal, financial, and institutional interests affecting the findings, analysis and conclusions in the study.

References

1. Lee, S., Oh, S.I., Jo, J., Kang, S., Shin, Y., Park, J.W.: Deep learning for early dental caries detection in bitewing radiographs. Sci. Rep. **11**(1), 16807 (2021). https://doi.org/10.1038/s41598-021-96368-7
2. Bayraktar, Y., Ayan, E.: Diagnosis of interproximal caries lesions with deep convolutional neural network in digital bitewing radiographs. Clin. Oral Invest. **26**(1), 623–632 (2022). https://doi.org/10.1007/s00784-021-04040-1
3. Ronneberger, O., Fischer, P., Brox, T.: U-Net: Convolutional Networks for Biomedical Image Segmentation. In: Navab, N., Hornegger, J., Wells, W.M., Frangi, A.F. (eds.) MICCAI 2015. LNCS, **9351**, pp. 234–241. Springer, Cham (2015). https://doi.org/10.1007/978-3-319-24574-4_28
4. Patro, S.G.K., Sahu, K.K.: Normalization: a preprocessing stage. Int. Adv. Res. J. Sci. Eng. Technol. **2**(3), 20–22 (2015). https://doi.org/10.17148/IARJSET.2015.2305
5. Eng, H.L., Ma, K.K.: Noise adaptive soft-switching median filter. IEEE Trans. Image Process. **10**(2), 242–251 (2001). https://doi.org/10.1109/83.902288
6. Zhu, H., Cao, Z., Lian, L., Ye, G., Gao, H., Wu, J.: CariesNet: a deep learning approach for segmentation of multi-stage caries lesion from oral panoramic X-Ray image. Neural Comput. & Applic. **35**(22), 16051–16059 (2023). https://doi.org/10.1007/s00521-021-06684-2
7. Kaki, M., Gunnam, S., Dhanavath, S., Gorantla, P.K., Saripineni, R.: Semantic segmentation of dental caries using improved deeplab V3+ Network. In: 2023 3rd International Conference on Intelligent Communication and Computational Techniques (ICCT), pp. 1–5 (2023). https://doi.org/10.1109/ICCT56969.2023.10075992
8. Haghanifar, A., Majdabadi, M.M., Ko, S.-B.: PaXNet: Dental caries detection in panoramic X-Ray using ensemble transfer learning and capsule classifier. CoRR abs/2012.13666 (2020). https://doi.org/10.48550/arXiv.2012.13666

9. Alharbi, S.S., AlRugaibah, A.A., Alhasson, H.F., Khan, R.U.: Detection of cavities from dental panoramic X-Ray images using nested U-Net models. Appl. Sci. **13**(23), 12771 (2023). https://doi.org/10.3390/app132312771
10. Yoon, K., Jeong, H.M., Kim, J.W., Park, J.H., Choi, J.: AI-Based dental caries and tooth number detection in intraoral photos: model development and performance evaluation. J. Dent. **141**, 104821 (2024). https://doi.org/10.1016/j.jdent.2023.104821
11. Duong, D.L., Nguyen, Q.D.N., Tong, M.S., Vu, M.T., Lim, J.D., Kuo, R.F.: Proof-of-concept study on an automatic computational system in detecting and classifying occlusal caries lesions from smartphone color images of unrestored extracted teeth. Diagnostics **11**(7), 1136 (2021). https://doi.org/10.3390/diagnostics11071136
12. Pérez de Frutos, J., Goodman, J., Watson, E., et al.: AI-Dentify: deep learning for proximal caries detection on bitewing x-Ray—HUNT4 oral health study. BMC oral health **24**, 344 (2024). https://doi.org/10.1186/s12903-024-03992-6
13. Liu, H., Jiang, B., Xiao, Y., Yang, C.: Coherent semantic attention for image inpainting. In: 2019 IEEE/CVF International Conference on Computer Vision (ICCV), pp. 4169–4178 (2019). https://doi.org/10.48550/arXiv.1905.12384
14. Giavina-Bianchi, M., Vitor, W.G., de Paiva, V.F., Okita, A.L., Sousa, R.M., Machado, B.: Explainability agreement between dermatologists and five visual explanations techniques in deep neural networks for melanoma AI classification. Front. Med. **10**, 1241484 (2023). https://doi.org/10.3389/fmed.2023.1241484
15. Hannan, U.H.: AI-Assisted enamel caries detection from smartphone captured image. Tech. Rep. (2023). https://doi.org/10.13140/RG.2.2.26946.35524
16. Kim, D., Choi, J., Ahn, S., Park, E.: A smart home dental care system: integration of deep learning, image sensors, and mobile controller. J. Ambient Intell. Human Comput. **14**, 1123–1131 (2023). https://doi.org/10.1007/s12652-021-03366-8
17. Umer, F., Adnan, S., Lal, A.: Research and application of artificial intelligence in dentistry from lower-middle income countries—a scoping review. BMC Oral Health **24**, 220 (2024). https://doi.org/10.1186/s12903-024-03970-y

Blockchain-Based Storage and Retrieval Framework for Medical Imaging Data in OLTP Systems

Paramjot Saini, Beulah Moses, and Mohammad Al-Zobbi

Abstract Medical imaging data ranging from X-rays, CT scans, to MRIs has continued to grow exponentially. Healthcare systems that have a model of centralized storage and retrieval have significant challenges because of their dependence on older technologies. For example, healthcare systems utilizing traditional PACS systems and EHR systems, experience challenges with latency, limited interoperability, and security, which weakly function in an OLTP model, where real-time access is necessary. Hence, a blockchain-based framework to enable secure, scalable, high-performance retrieval of medical imaging data has been proposed. The framework proposal is based on Hyperledger Fabric and features a novel empirical block size tuning model that optimizes OLTP throughput while maintaining immutability and traceability of the data. The framework takes a hybrid on-chain/off-chain storage approach where the blockchain ledger is dedicated to storing metadata, while the medical images are stored off the ledger itself which greatly reduced the storage overhead on the blockchain. Experimental evaluation suggests a mid-sized block of approximately 5000 records is optimal for balancing speed and stability in the network and additionally reducing average read latency by almost 50% compared to other configurations. We utilize CouchDB for querying and smart contract access control based on the immutability of data to satisfy HIPAA/GDPR requirements. Ultimately, the proposed architecture serves to demonstrate how blockchain can evolve from an immutable ledger, to an entire infrastructure of data, and therefore realize the benefits of real-time health applications, and the results have the opportunity to serve as the basis for future research and potentially larger or national studies, and also designated for artificial intelligence (AI) integration for performance and reliability in clinical contexts.

P. Saini (✉)
Higher Education Leadership Institute, Melbourne, VIC, Australia
e-mail: paramjotsaini1209@gmail.com

B. Moses
UP Education Group, Melbourne, VIC, Australia
e-mail: beulahs@gmail.com

M. Al-Zobbi
Western Sydney University, Sydney, Australia
e-mail: malzobbi@yahoo.com

P. Singh et al. (eds.), *Deep Learning Applications in Healthcare and Medical Imaging Practice*, Studies in Big Data 193, https://doi.org/10.1007/978-3-032-21009-8_27

Keywords Blockchain in healthcare · Medical imaging retrieval · Hyperledger fabric · Online transaction processing (OLTP) · Hybrid on-chain/off-Chain architecture · Scalable data management

1 Introduction

1.1 Contextual Background

The last 10 years have been a period of intense transformation for healthcare systems due to the digitization of patient information and the accelerated adoption of medical imaging technologies. The resulting rapid increase in both image uploads volume and the complexity of those images has generated unprecedented pressure on traditional systems for storage and retrieval of images. Recent studies suggest that medical imaging data alone accounts for more than 90% of hospital data volume, with imaging modalities generating multiple terabytes of new data daily [1]. Therefore, most of these datasets are stored in Picture Archiving and Communication Systems (PACS) or Electronic Health Record (EHR) style systems, which were originally designed for centralized, intra-institutional uses, not necessarily distributed, multi-stakeholder uses. Despite the extensive use of PACS/EHR systems, parts of these systems currently struggle with significant challenges.

They frequently work within siloed architectures so that the sharing of imaging data across hospitals or research institutions is less than seamless. In clinical settings where time is often of the essence, latency becomes a problem for clinicians when pulling large size image files. In addition, unauthorized access, unwanted copies of the data, and unreliable backup strategies continue to hinder patient privacy and operational simplicity in healthcare [2]; and there is no secure method for knowing personally identifiable information (PII) as to the date and time of when any particular medical image was accessed or the identity of the user, thus creating complications for medico-legal responsibility, and no tamper-proof audit history. Considering everything outlined above, there is a need for a higher quality, safe, transparent and higher performance retrieval option in healthcare to cater for the increased demand for real time access to information.

1.2 Motivation Towards Integrating Blockchain

Combining data systems in health care with a blockchain has the potential to massively reduce the shortcomings of traditional data systems. As in providing the characteristics of decentralization, immutability and audibility, blockchain serves as a reliable representation for storing, accessing, validating and verifying transactions of medical data without a central authority over multiple nodes [3]. With respect to imaging, someone might visualize blockchain as something like an immutable distributed ledger of each imaging file with respect to its metadata, access history, and digital fingerprints (hashes), which can also enhance privacy and move more towards encrypted and permissioned access characteristics.

As illustrated in Fig. 1, modern medical imaging systems generate high volume data flows across multiple actors and processing stages. This indicates the necessity of secure, scalable and auditable data management mechanisms

In modern hospitals, systems are being developed using Online Transaction Processing (OLTP) to facilitate high frequency real time operations. Linking OLTP grade quality with the decentralized structure of a blockchain raises issues in transaction ingestion, read/write latency and scalability issues. Most blockchain technologies are based on models developed for financial transaction systems and are not applicable for a mature workload vigor of health care. This paper introduces an empirically optimized blockchain architecture to allow OLTP principles to be adjusted and applied in a medical imaging environment, for example, by optimizing and adjusting the block size, transaction model structure, and off channel storage systems so that imaging can be securely, effectively retrieved and traceable when scaled even to a city [4].

The reasoning behind the rationale for such an implementation was driven by more than performance. Within medical imaging workflows, there was a strong requirement for traceability and auditability of every stage of the workflow process (from image acquisition to a clinical interpretation). Blockchain in itself provides an immutable ledger (with respect to time stamping and audibility) of all transactions amongst the actors in a transparent manner about their shared responsibility but also ensures compliance with local statutes around sensitive data [4]. Further, with the additional use of smart contracts, the blockchain would automate parts of access requests, granting the ability for clinicians and researchers to access authorized data properly in real-time, while being fully responsible for what they do with that data.

1.3 Purpose and Scope of Chapter

This chapter introduces an integrated blockchain-based architectural structure with the intended goal of improving the speed and scalability of retrieval of medical imaging data in an on-line transaction processing (OLTP) environment. The architecture is built on the experimental findings around deployment of Hyperledger Fabric and CouchDB with various block size experiments under various conditions of system performance with textual and multimedia medical data at scale. The architecture is intended to solve a series of data management problem issues of health sector application, directly attributable to the securing data storage of DICOM images for real-time secure retrieval of patient specific clinical records.

This chapter intends to build on some of the previous insights around how the distributed model of blockchain technology could be used to store both small transactions and large volume multimedia datasets, without compromising speed or to the

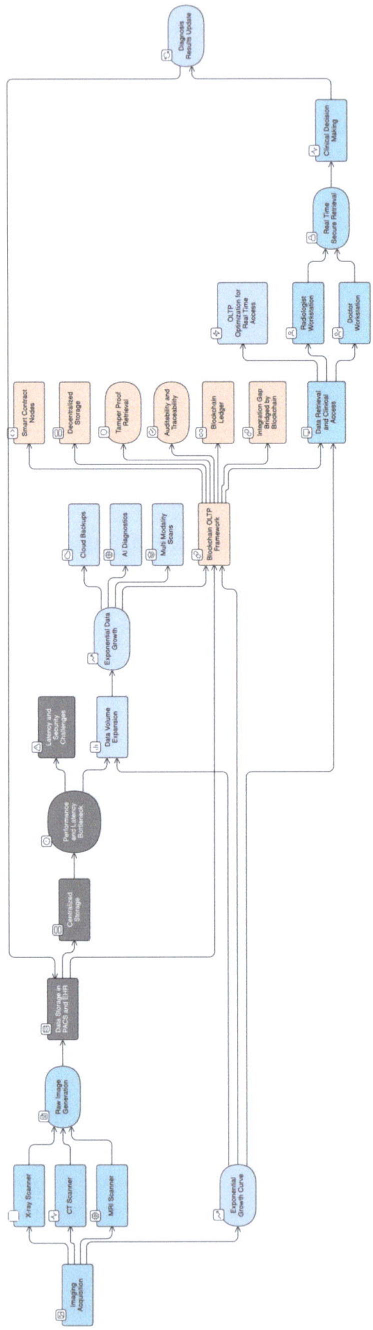

Fig. 1 Exponential growth and data flow of medical imaging in modern healthcare systems

integrity of data. The architectural strategy also describes how a hybrid on-chain/off-chain data management strategy can also allow for persistent linking and veracity of large volume harmonic imaging, and still not compromise speed or integrity of data. The architectural structure also illustrates and model design principles of the previous implementations of the methodologies studied along with empirical evidence to offer athletic in design and implementations of blockchain as a necessary digital definite within the extraction of portal imaging systems into the future of medical imaging systems.

1.4 Chapter Organization

The chapter begins with Sect. 2 as an introduction to the theoretical background pertaining to medical imaging and medical data-management, as well as blockchain based health information systems. Section 3 defines the research problem as well as the rationale for the problem with an explanation about performance vs. security in imaging data retrieval. In Sect. 4 the framework is described in terms of architecture, applications and involvement of blockchain, off-chain strategies, and the OLTP retrieval process pipeline. Section 5 presents the framework application in detail and Sect. 6 the experimental results detailing the efficacy of scalability and performance. A more detailed discussion has been offered in Sect. 7 regarding patterns and implications and identification of limitations. Ethical and regulatory considerations have been outlined in Sect. 8, and the chapter concludes with Sect. 9 as a summary of contributions made and future work.

2 Background and Related Concepts

2.1 Medical Imaging Data Life Cycle

Medical imaging may be the keystone process in today's clinical diagnosis, allowing a visualization of internal bodily structure and physiological processes. The life cycle of medical images follows a somewhat standard process of acquisition, storage, retrieval for diagnosis, and archiving documents when complete. Each of these stages is critical to providing reliable care to the patient, or as part of the continued life of the medical data set. The cycle starts with acquiring an image through one of the available modalities including X-ray, Computed Tomography (CT), Magnetic Resonance Imaging (MRI), and Positron Emission Tomography (PET). Within each modality, images are produced following a unique type of imaging which leads to relatively large file sizes with potential high-resolution metadata [5].

The images are next sent to a Picture Archiving and Communication System (PACS) or to an Electronic Health Record (EHR) for storage use. The images are

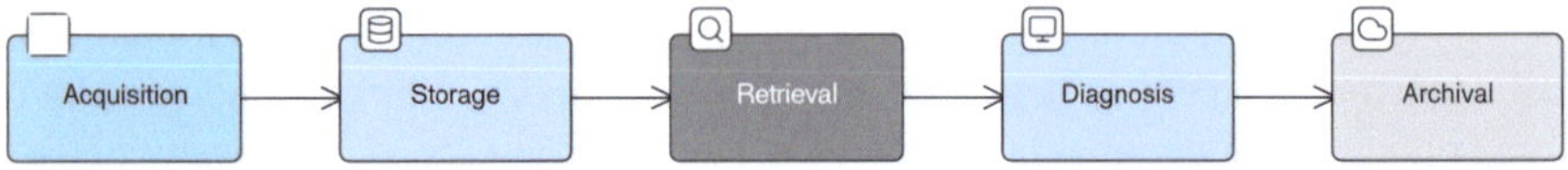

Fig. 2 Generic medical imaging data lifecycle—depicting the five stages from acquisition to archival and, importantly, their associated data flow

indexed and made available to the clinician. Due to the increasing adoption of multi-modality medical imaging workflows- both increased use and heterogeneous data stacks- most hospital systems currently face increased demands for both volume and data variety. Therefore, it is not uncommon for retrieval to create significant delays, not only in the actual time spent retrieving but also for safe storage. The retrieval phase is especially sensitive when being used in a dedicated and potentially emergent use setting where several images of "high resolution" may be needed for retrieval in near real-time; for surgical planning or for emergent diagnostics.

Standard relational databases and PACS are not designed for high frequency, simultaneous access to multimedia imaging data. Retrieval from these types of storage and information systems typically involves a centralized server that processes requests sequentially, leading to bottlenecks, latency, and even system outages under high volumes of data requests to cohort during these times [2]. In addition, storage and transport logging are not transparent units which minimizes audit accountability of modification or access of imaging data. Images are often archived at the completion of diagnostic workflows, which include the long-term storage of images for medical, legal and institutional compliance, often for years. However, the challenge is to balance storability, security, integrity of medical imaging data while avoiding burdens on the storage and data-theoretic architecture. The tension between data management occurs in space and performance management. Therefore, there is urgency for new data management frameworks to facilitate and manage data using performance and compliance requirements. Figure 2 illustrates the lifecycle of generic medical imaging data. This highlights the various stages in sequence.

2.2 *Blockchain Principles in Health Care*

Blockchain technology offers a decentralized and tamper-proof solution for managing digital information across multiple stakeholders without entrusting a centralized or single source. As a method for storing and validating sensitive medical information in health care, this is an appealing attribute of blockchain technology in its entirety [3]. The structure of the blockchain is comprised of blocks that contain a record with a list of transactions or records that are programmatically linked to other blocks, forming a chain that is difficult to alter. In order to modify a record, the alteration must also alter all blocks following the record that is modified, and all the blocks must also be modified across the entire distributed network as this makes unauthorized alteration all but impossible.

There are three features of blockchain that allows blockchain technologies to be a preferred mechanism for data management in health care: immutability, consensus, and smart contracts.

- **Immutability** allows, and ensures, that once patient data, or imaging data, are written to the ledger that the patient data, or imaging data, are immutable unless there is consensus among all validating nodes.
- **Consensus** is a generic term for mechanisms to ensure that all participant nodes and peers have the same copy of data, and are aware of modifications, especially changes in the metadata to the data to Health Information exchanges (HIE) (in public networks, Proof of Work, or Proof of Capacity, are consensus mechanisms; in private networks, Proof of Authority or Practical Byzantine Fault Tolerance methods are used).
- **Smart** contracts allow automation of tasks, such as granting permissions, or initiating data transfer from one location to another, which are built on pre-defined 'rules' written in the ledger's code [6].

The architecture of the blockchain is either public, private, or consortium, where each type varies in the degree of 'publicness'. Public blockchains, such as Bitcoin or Ethereum, are open to all, and are not necessarily advisable in medical situations when patient privacy is needed and transactions speeds cannot be predicted. On the flip side, private blockchains limit involvement to specific participants typically known entities like hospitals, clinics, and labs thereby exerting greater control over data governance. Consortium blockchains bring together both models, allowing a select group of trusted healthcare organizations to roughly manage the shared ledger cooperatively.

In the context of healthcare applications that include medical imaging, the most suitable networks are permissioned or consortium. These network types still allow institutions to exercise a high degree of granular access control, enforce data ownership policies, and comply with regulation such as HIPAA and GDPR. In the current research study, the use of a permissioned blockchain is highly desirable for streaming medical imaging data in a secure, traceable and fast access manner in real-time use cases [4].

2.3 Hyperledger Fabric for Secure Data Exchange

Of the many existing blockchain platforms, Hyperledger Fabric has proven to be a strong framework for the implementation of permissioned healthcare blockchains. Hyperledger Fabric was developed as a project under the Linux Foundation, and currently supports modular, scalable architectures with enterprise-grade performance that can be customized for healthcare data exchange [7]. Whereas traditional blockchains utilize energy-intensive proof-of-stake or proof-of-work coordination,

Hyperledger Fabric separates the aggregation (we typically refer to this as ordering) from endorsement of a transaction. This allows for higher transaction throughput and predictability, which is an important factor in OLTP systems such as healthcare.

The channel-based architecture of Hyperledger Fabric allows small groups of participants to create private communication layers among themselves on the larger data exchange network. Each channel has its own shared ledger during transactions, and each channel's associated medical data remains viewable and modifiable only to authorized participants. This feature enables medical imaging data to be securely segregated across hospitals, research sites, and diagnostic laboratories, while minimizing the risk of unauthorized access and/or data leaks. In the medical imaging context, each channel provides a unique link to each clinical department or imaging center, in which only authorized peers (nodes) can transact and access the data. Fabric also allows for CouchDB as a state database, which allows querying of records that are JSON-based—which is important as imaging record can have rich metadata (DICOM headers for example). CouchDB also provides indexing of key pairs to improve retrieval speed and better filter attributes of the imaging data—modality, patient ID, timestamp, etc. [12]. The smart contract (or chaincode) mechanism in Fabric could be developed to automatically check transactions as well. When a clinician requests access to an MRI record for example, the smart contract would check the role-based access, check that the block's hash matched for integrity, and create an entry in the ledger for logging the event. This provides end-to-end accountability of any transaction of imaging, whether it has been stored, retrieved, or changed has been recorded and is auditable, which helps provide transparency and trust among stakeholders in healthcare with each transaction.

2.4 OLTP in Blockchain Contexts

Online Transaction Processing (OLTP) is the collection of systems that have been designed to support a multitude of repeatable, short real-time transactions. OLTP in the traditional healthcare databases support updating patient records or retrieving a diagnostic image with minimal latency and maximal accuracy and access, to some degree. The integration of OLTP into a blockchain context produces some challenges as it relates to status and consensus nature of a distributed network [8]. Centralized databases have the ability to process transactions in a near instantaneous manner, however, blockchain requires a time period for the transactions to propagate as each transaction is validated and becomes apart of the contents of the block. Propagation time or latency could now include the possibility of other time required processes such as block size, consensus time, or synchronization with the network, and this all contributes to the performance of the OLTP functionality. In relation to ease of retrieval, if the blocks are too big it takes longer to retrieve, whereas if they are too small then the the transaction overhead becomes higher. Balancing those processes is important for real-time feedback to affect workflows in clinical imaging.

The concurrency and consistency sides of how the framework works is also important. In a blockchain-based transaction framework OLTP context, at the same time, many users could access or change a portion of the dataset concurrently. The ACID (Atomicity, Consistency, Isolation, Durability) must be maintained across the distributed nodes and will likely take some combination of smart contract logic and consensus protocols as to not lose integrity while users are concurrently using nodes at higher rates. Socializing that portion of performance would bleed right into the other variable of importantly in scalability for the blockchain delivery models as the infrastructure loads would have extended to a city or many hospital model. Overall throughput of OLTP performing blocks should not change with increased workload.

The research referred to is about the performance of the system in an empirical optimization system. Through testing of variant block configuration and storage methodologies, to provide some performance optimization to discover an optimal block size for retrieval processes that were responsive in quality towards OLTP level processes for the security and trace [23]. This helps close the performance divide between a distributed blockchain quality for security, and the rolled depth for timely-transactional response that is required by healthcare.

3 Problem Definition and Research Rationale

Today, the healthcare ecosystem requires fast, reliable, and secure access to electronic medical data on a more frequent basis. Out of all clinical information types, medical imaging data (i.e. X-rays, CT-scans, MRI series, etc.) is often the most cumbersome to store and retrieve based on the larger file size, coupled with an immediate need for quick access in real-time diagnostic and surgical settings [5]. Previous Picture Archiving and Communication Systems (PACS) and Electronic Health Record (EHR) data bases were designed to accommodate clinical information storage, but not for the higher concurrency levels (or transactions per second) expected of today's Online Transaction Processing (OLTP) environments. The centralized systems processes a request and retrieve the images in real-time, but it, unfortunately, is much more difficult to retrieve any image from a medical archive when the medical imaging files grow exponentially across multi-hospital networks and city-scale networks [9].

3.1 Formulating the Core Problem

The frame of this research is a practical problem: "How can we ensure fast, secure, and scalable retrieval of medical imaging data, in a distributed healthcare infrastructure?" As clinical practice demands access to records outside of single facility, there is an increasing need for data sharing between healthcare organisations, and older computing architecture does not provide an efficient solution for data sharing. The legacy relational databases do not provide the low latency as the record sizes increase, nor it be efficient in data transfer due to network congestion and load on the database.

Most current systems do not have tamper-evident audit trails, thus compromises data even if the owner did not have malicious intent to access or modify the data [2]. For healthcare organisations that manage sensitive patient data, this creates both performance delays, and compliance weaknesses through healthcare regulations, such as the Health Insurance Portability and Accountability Act (HIPAA) and General Data Protection Regulation (GDPR) to name a few. A system that may retain immutability, retain confidentiality, and allow for transactional speed is essential, as healthcare data demands for systems that allow for access at scale.

Therefore, the research problem is focused on determining and developing an optimum blockchain-based solution that would provide OLTP-grade performance, all while maintaining the security and integrity of medical imaging data. The purpose of this research is to identify the impact on the retrieval speed and scalability considerations of block size, and of database integration and hybrid storage in blockchains designed for use with healthcare workloads [25].

3.2 Gaps in Existing Solutions

Most applications of blockchain within health care have been primarily focused on security and data provenance. In memory of these issues there has been little focus on the performance optimization of solution [3]. Blockchain can provide immutability and trust inherent in a caused monitored environment, but the nature of the blockchain introduces latency, overhead in the consensus protocol and block generation process used by the intermediary organization. While other researchers acknowledge the monitoring solution is a trade-off for the increased level of security, it is unreasonable for a clinical OLTP where the time to perform a task is directly related to patient outcomes.

Existing models also tend to assume textual data and multimedia data behave uniformly when storing and retrieving; not making important distinctions of their related storage and retrieval behaviors. Content in textual data (i.e. prescriptions, lab notes) tends to be compact and has a structured format, while multimedia data (i.e. MRI sequences, and graphic imaging) is unstructured and tends to be significantly larger. Storing both forms of data as if they had the same storage behavior is inefficient; either over-saturation or over-segmentation occurs during retrieval, either too many small blocks that indicate overhead is used to retrieve the data or large blocks that consume time and limit the speed of the throughput or concurrent activity. After experimentation conducted in this research study, we observed that the block size has direct impact on the speed of retrieval and there is a U-shaped performance curve where mid-sized blocks provide the optimal experience for retrieval speed (approximately 5,000 records) [23].

In addition, blockchain solutions developed for health care do not normally consider city wide scalability, often assuming a single institution deployed practice.

When considering the possibility of multiple unrelated hospitals or diagnostic center utilizing the same blockchain there are also limitations to network synchronization, management of the channels and concurrent query on the respective Governance. Therefore, there still exists a important gap in research and modelling as a comprehensive and empirical framework that consists of all three pillars of performance, scalability, and security for an integrated design working together in a schema.

3.3 *Rationale for the Research*

The rationale for this research is the need for health care information systems to evolve beyond traditional architectures toward intelligent, distributed, secure platforms as is increasingly the case in other industry applications etc. Security and immutability via blockchain can be deployed, while OLTP principles maintain that transaction throughput, is likely to be preserved for day-to-day clinical applications [4].

Therefore, this study seeks to examine and organize information systems design parameters for improved and deterministic blockchain performance when leveraging the imaging in health care contexts. This study proposes a designed model that enables timely retrieval of both forms of textual and multimedia data, with consideration for the best blocksize of the application, and a hybrid storage methodology that still affords the ability to trust the data is documented and provided an integrity level needed for support on a chain. Utilizing Hyperledger Fabric allows the organization the operational freedom and channel privacy to do work while decentralized, publicly, or in a shared trust even without any formal disclosure; this allows for the organization to operationalize, or not, based on their perceived level of data privacy.

The outcomes examined demonstrated that using the distributed framework consistently provided enhanced read/write capability while ingesting and storing multimedia data—especially if programmers and db. administrators were careful to select block sizes that align with the data type in consideration, particularly as CouchDB utilizes indexing. While performance was a focus, experiments indicated that the blockchain would achieve OLTP-like speed performance reliably as is common in healthcare-like workloads.

The frameworks developed allowed for much more than performance improvements, they showcased higher organizational goals of data accountability (for regulatory purposes) and ethical/audit responsibility for how organizations treat, or have in their possession, data. Overall, developing a technology architecture to allow distributed and e-health imaging data repositories to provide high usefulness (for example, statistical, predictive, etc.) in alignment with vendor agnostic blockchain architectural framework offers a meaningful advance as an important resource as to how to ameliorate or resource the conditions to foster appropriate medical ecosystem to a scale or proximity (probably even to delineated one municipality or city) to meet speed and privacy demands.

4 Proposed Framework Architecture

The proposed framework aims to identify a secure, scalable, and high-performing environment for retrieving medical data by deploying a blockchain solution, specifically in an Online Transaction Processing (OLTP) healthcare use case. The proposed framework utilizes Hyperledger Fabric technology, which was selected because of its use of permissioned based access, modularity, and We outline the complete system architecture, processing paradigms, and trust logic to collectively enable the processing of textual and multimedia medical data in clinical practice at scale.

4.1 Design Principles

The architecture is organized around five core design principles: performance, scalability, security, compliance, and interoperability. Each of these design principles addresses a weakness of first-generation medical data imaging systems.

- **Performance:** Medical imaging data must be accessed in real-time for diagnostic or surgical use. The implemented system allows for tuned optimization of read-block size based on observed empirical feedback, and a process similar to OLTP confirmatory mechanism to limit read/write latency [22].
- **Scalability:** The implemented or implemented system must be deployed at a single city level. It must also be scalable to support, at a minimum, hundreds of facilitated healthcare clinics and thousands of imaging transactions per day without diminishing performance.
- **Security**: Each transaction is recorded securely in a cryptographic and immutable manner. The integrity of the audit trail cannot be changed and only summarized and governmentally deposited data have a key. Additionally, medical imaging is encrypted via multiple layers, for example via secure channels and policy-driven data access control mechanisms applied to medical representation as needed, all of which mitigates the risk of tampering while also protecting the confidentiality of the identity.
- **Compliance:** The proposed framework will be HIPAA and GDPR compliant through verification, and comprehensive policies will enable and keep track of ownership for consent to access patient medical data or representation, ascertain from the chain of audit viewing [4].
- **Interoperability:** The current and investigated solution can circulate with all existing and future hospital-based applications (PACS, EHR, and Laboratory Information Systems) with API-based connectors to facilitate easy transition. Both interoperability and structural transition will also contribute to identifying the current complexity, while enabling velocity of the imaging, and facilitating coordination, from a practical end user perspective.

The system design describes the principles of the framework beginning from a theoretical, through to a useable model of architectural design for practice-based use to occur.

4.2 System Overview

At the top-level, the proposed design uses a multiple layered architectural framework built on modern principles of distributed computing. The overall structure consists of three primary layers: Presentation Layer, Application Layer, and Data Layer [6].

- **Presentation Layer:** The layer which clinicians, radiologists or administrators encounter visually, involves the "user-part" of the system. The Presentation Layer enables dashboards for image retrieval, transaction status and audits.
- **Application Layer:** The middle layer which includes the "smart/computer contracts (Chaincode) of the system to manage access, validate transactions and support processing logic required for managing medical data. Each request initiated through the chaincode, when invoked for a transaction (As an example storing an X-ray record, or a table for a retrieve CT image) qualities and testing are provided in the Application Layer prior to automatically validating on or recording on the device-normalized blockchain.
- **Data Layer:** The Data Layer contains both on-chain and off-chain aspects. The blockchain ledger contains metadata pertaining to the transaction history, access logs and the headers of the medical data, while the actual image files (particularly large multimedia datasets) are stored on off-chain storage, such as IPFS, or a secure cloud server.

This layer pairing provides end-to-end functionality that utilizes the advantages of blockchain immutability and the performance flexibility of distributed databases.

4.3 Blockchain Configuration for Imaging Data

The performance of a blockchain-based OLTP system is affected by the incline configuration parameters of the blocks, such as the block size or transaction throughput. To test the balance of speed against security this research assessed performance with different block sizes (1000, 5000, 10,000, and 100,000 records per block).

The architectural blueprint is shown in Fig. 3. The blueprints integrates Hyperledger Fabric (v2.5) with IPFS off chain storage which simulates hospital networks via multiple peers.

The ensuing performance collection revealed a **U-shaped curve of performance**, revealing that data block sizes in the middle of the spectrum (approximately 5000 records) had the lowest read latency with the best efficiency overall [12]. Smaller blocks demanded more processing time overhead, as there needs to be time to form

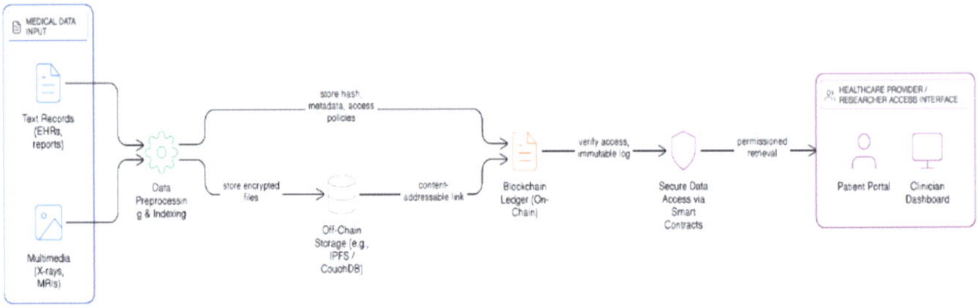

Fig. 3 Proposed blockchain-enabled framework for medical imaging data retrieval

a new block for each transaction, and inducing delay, placement to commit phase responses with bigger blocks. As a result, the **Preferred MaxBytes and AbsoluteMaxDays** were adjusted in the Fabric configuration to maintain 5000 records per block; this configuration-maintained speed of OLTP grade storage in retrieving images.

This method of dynamic adjustment enabled the blockchain network to preserve consistent **read/write performance**, even in high-load environments, rendering it suitable for large imaging data for hospitals. Actual performance details collected from this data are now considered a baseline configuration for ongoing function exchange of medical data in networks.

The blockchain network, database, and system architecture specifications used in this simulation are summarized in Table 1.

4.4 *Hybrid On-Chain and Off-Chain Storage Strategy*

An important element in the framework is the hybrid storage approach, where the data is separated depending on size and retrieval. Storing each of the imaging files on the blockchain itself would not be practical due to size and replication. The framework takes a two-tiered approach to storage [3].

1. **On-Chain storage:** Only essential metadata including the patient ID, timestamp, hash value, file path, and transaction history is recorded on chain. This ensures the information is all accurate, correct and trustworthy while not clogging the blockchain.
2. **Off-Chain storage:** The imaging files themselves, for example DICOM imaging X-rays or MRI images, is securely stored in a off-site location (i.e. IPFS or AWS S3). Each imaging file has a hash which will be mapped to its reference on the chain to ensure verification of the data stored once retrieved.

In retrieving the file using the preceding information, it requires: (1) reading the metadata hash on the blockchain (2) using the hash to invoke the chaincode service to validate the data stored and then (3) retrieving the appropriate file from

Table 1 Empirical block-size parameters and system configuration (summarizing parameters such as block size, record count, transaction rate, and latency values)

Parameter category	Component/ setting	Specification/value	Description/purpose
Blockchain network	Framework	Hyperledger fabric v2.5	Permissioned blockchain used for secure OLTP retrieval
	Consensus mechanism	Raft protocol	Ensures ordering and fault tolerance among peers
	Channel configuration	Single channel; 3 orgs × 2 peers	Represents distributed hospital networks in simulation
Database layer	State database	CouchDB v3.2	Supports JSON queries and improves read performance
	Off-Chain storage	IPFS (Integrated via hash links)	Stores large multimedia medical images externally
System environment	Host platform	AWS EC2 Ubuntu 22.04 LTS	Cloud instances deployed for peer and orderer nodes
	Virtual machines	2 × t2.large (2 vCPU, 8 GB RAM)	Simulates multi-hospital network
	Programming interfaces	Go Lang & JavaScript SDK	Used for smart-contract and application layer integration
Dataset parameters	Textual records	1 000–100 000 HL7 entries	Represents prescriptions, reports, and textual EHR data
	Multimedia records	1 000–100 000 DICOM images (approx. 1–20 MB each)	Represents X-ray, CT, MRI datasets
	Synthetic data source	HL7–ICD10 Merged Dataset (10 000 records)	Generated using thesis dataset generator
Empirical block sizes tested	Small	1 000 records per block	Optimized for rapid transactional retrieval
	Medium	5 000 records per block	Balanced load for moderate throughput
	Large	100 000 records per block	Evaluates scalability and latency trade-off
Performance metrics	Measured indicators	Read time, write time, throughput, latency	Used to identify optimal block configuration

an external persistence service. This provides real-time retrieval of the imaging data while maintaining the same level of confidentiality and security offered with on-chain data. If access is also allowed externally, the original hash will provide immutable proof of provenance no matter what happens if it is modified externally.

4.5 Data Retrieval Mechanism for OLTP-Designed Blockchains

At the heart of the proposed framework is the OLTP-designed data retrieval mechanism, which allows imaging data to be accessed and updated concurrently by multiple users, without compromising system integrity.

For example, in a typical case, a radiologist queries an image from the blockchain network via an API. The request is authenticated at the smart contract, the request is confirmed through consensus, and the verification is run against the CouchDB-indexed state database for efficient querying [15].

In CouchDB, key-value pairs for frequently requested datasets enables a reliable response time of less than a second. Once the transaction is approved, the blockchain responds with an off-chain file link which is seamlessly acquired securely and presented to the clinician's interface.

We experimentally validated the OLT performance, showing read times decreased from 6.45 s for smaller blocks of 1,000 records to 3.27 s for typical mid-size blocks of 5,000 records [24]. This shows the utility of the proposed configuration for balancing throughput and latency, an often-closed balance in blockchain-oriented healthcare systems.

4.6 Security and Access Control

Security is the foundation of this framework. This system utilizes multi-layered protections that combine access control with cryptography and privacy-preserving transaction validation.

- **Smart contracts for role-based access:** Chaincode scripts that define user roles, such as doctors, nurses, administrators, and auditors, dynamically control access privileges. Each instance of data access invokes an automated smart contract to protect access permissions before the transaction is allowed.
- **Encryption and Hashing:** Before storing medical images and metadata, all data was encrypted using symmetric-key algorithms. In order to create information assurance, SHA-256 or equivalently secure hash functions were used, in that any information that is tampered with will cause the hash to mismatch, indicating failure.

- **Secure Channels and Endorsement Policies:** Hyperledger Fabric provides a channel mechanism that creates an isolated environment for data as it moves between data collaborators. Each channel has its own endorsement policy, which is endorsed through the use of digital signatures. This authenticates peer endorsement (hospital servers) to legitimize the transaction.
- **Audibility and Traceability:** All activity (upload, query, download) will be recorded in the immutable ledger with a timestamp and will link with user identification. When combined this feature will provide complete audibility, transparency, and regulatory compliance challenge in healthcare.

These layered safeguarding strategies will ensure data integrity and privacy remain uncompromised under heavy transaction loads. Collectively, the use of smart contracts and cryptographic verification will construct a framework that is safe, secure, reliable and resilient between multiple health care stakeholders.

5 Implementation and Experimental Setup

The blockchain-enabled retrieval framework (Fig. 4) was fully realized and iteratively and methodologically validated in a series of controlled experiments. This section describes (i) the software-hardware environment, (ii) methods of preparing the data, and (iii) the metrics parameters that collectively show the operational viability of the framework for use. The established decision-making configuration and design basis models were in essence designed the decision making to support the real time OLTP performance without impacting the integrity and security of the textual and/ or multimedia medical information.

The implementation ran on a private Hyperledger Fabric network specifically designed to replicate realistic hospital-level data operations. The development comprised Hyperledger Fabric v2.x and CouchDB v3.x, utilizing Node.js SDK, and hosted in Dockers to ensure portability and modularity [22].

The net topology consisted of:

- One Ordering Service Node, sequencing/completing transactions.
- Two Peer Nodes, representing each institutional party (for example Hospital A and Hospital B).
- One Certificate Authority, issuing digital identities that require role-based authentication.
- CouchDB State Database (attached to each peer for rich JSON-based queries and quick metadata access).

All services were orchestrated using Docker Compose to ensure communications between containers in a virtualized and/or overlay network. The experiment was hosted on a workstation with Ubuntu 20.04 LTS installed, using an Intel Core i7 CPU @ 3.60 GHz, with 16 GB and 512 GB SSD drive. This serviceable setup enabled testing of the compute and I/O performance relevant to OLTP workloads.

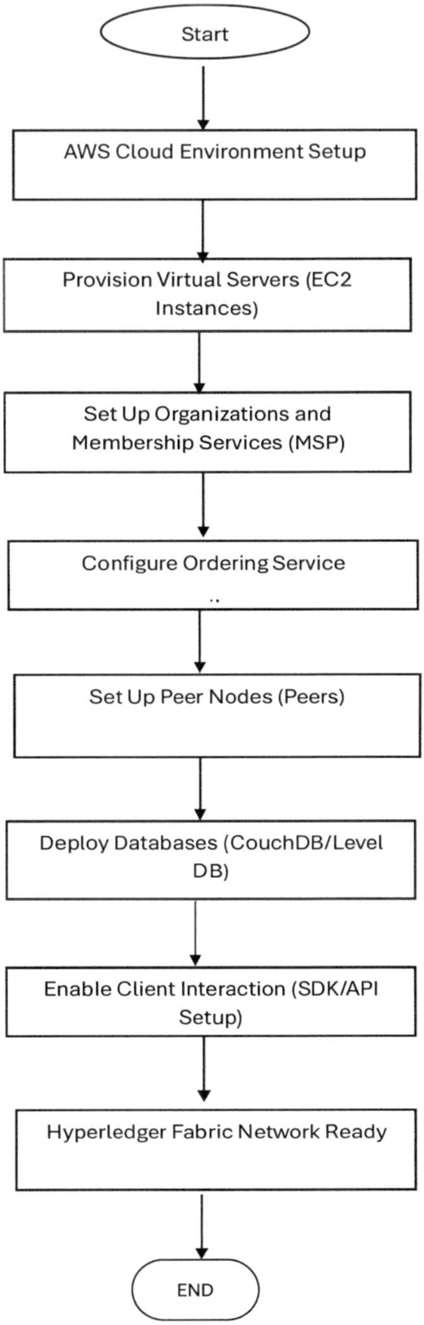

Fig. 4 System setup and workflow environment here, showing ordering service, peer nodes, CouchDB, and client application interfaces

The experimental topology was built to sustain a lightweight environment that would be representative of a multi-institutional healthcare network. Hence the findings may scale when deployed across multiple hospitals and/or diagnostic centers.

5.1 Dataset Preparation

The confidentiality of patients prohibits the use of actual hospital data, thus all textual EHR records and related multimedia imaging files were created to reflect both medical records and imaging files. Each record represented a separate medical encounter, comprising appropriate metadata fields—Patient ID, Entity Type (for example X-ray, MRI), Date, Diagnosis Tag, and Digital Hash.

Two Datasets Were Established:

1. **Textual Dataset:** Small structured records (approximately 1–2 KB each) representing prescriptions, lab summaries, and diagnostic notes.
2. **Multimedia Dataset:** Large binary-linked records (approximately 2–5 MB) representing image pointers and their related metadata.

All media components were saved off-chain within an **IPFS node** associated with the Fabric network. Only their **hash values and metadata** were anchored on-chain, which preserved integrity but did not affect performance [6]. The complete dataset comprised 100 000 records, evenly categorized between textual and multimedia. There were four transaction volumes 1 000, 5 000, 10 000, and 100 000 records to assess scalability and throughput with different block configurations.

5.2 Performance Metrics

The effectiveness of the system is evaluated against four general performance metrics [24]:

1. Read Latency (s): the time taken to retrieve a record from the blockchain network, from the time the query is initiated until the data is displayed.
2. Write Latency (s): The length of time needed to enter a new transaction (upload of data) to agreement of the ledger.
3. Throughput (tx/s): Number of transactions committed successfully in one second showing the capacity of the network.
4. Storage Utilization (MB): Amount of memory/disk space used on the peer nodes and CouchDB during continual load.

Performance metrics examined by the OLTP performance of the network and their ability to remain responsive during concurrent transaction loads (see Table 2).

Table 2 Experimental parameters and configuration: listing block sizes, record counts, CouchDB status, and evaluation metrics

Category	Parameter	Values/settings	Purpose
Blockchain	Platform	Hyperledger Fabric v2.5 (permissioned)	OLTP-grade, modular network
	Consensus	Raft ordering service	Deterministic ordering, fault tolerance
	Channel/peers	1 channel; 3 orgs × 2 peers	Simulated multi-hospital topology
State DB	Engine	CouchDB v3.x (ON / OFF)	Compare indexed vs key–value queries
Off-chain	Store	IPFS (hash reference on-chain)	Large DICOM storage
Block config	Block sizes tested	1,000 / 5,000 / 100,000 records per block	Empirical tuning variable
Datasets	Textual (HL7)	1,000–100,000 records	Prescriptions/reports metadata
	Multimedia (DICOM)	1,000–100,000 entries (approx.1–20 MB each)	X-ray/CT/MRI pointers
Environment	Compute	2 × EC2 (Ubuntu 22.04, t2.large, 2 vCPU, 8 GB RAM)	Peers/orderer hosts
	Tooling	Go chaincode; Node.js client SDK; Docker Compose	Chaincode + client
Method	Runs	4 runs per config; averages reported	Repeatability
Metrics	Measured	Read latency, write latency, throughput, storage	Evaluation endpoints

Each performance metric was obtained using the Fabric CA logs, Docker stats and a custom Node.js script to timestamp the request and response events.

5.3 Evaluation Scenarios

Evaluation scenarios were executed to understand the performance impact of blockchain configuration parameters [4, 18].

Scenario 1: Various Block Sizes—Blocks holding 1 000, 5 000, 10 000, and 100 000 records were evaluated to establish the relationship between block size and retrieval latency.

- Use of small blocks (i.e. <1 000 records) was costly in terms of endorsement overhead due to frequent block creation.
- Extensive block sizes caused delays in confirming transactions because peers preferred to wait until a full block had gathered.
- Moderate block sizes (meaning approximately 5 000 records) experienced the best-read latency at 3.24 s and stable write latency, confirming the U-like performance curve.

Scenario 2: CouchDB Active State Database—The CouchDB state database was activated to evaluate its effect on the query execution process. The use of CouchDB improved the performance with metadata-driven queries, especially queries filtering patient ID or patient modality. Performance was noticed in heavier transaction loads, showcasing the potential in larger imaging repositories [13].

Scenario 3: On-Chain Storage versus Off-Chain Storage—An evaluation was made between fully on-chain, fully off-chain, and hybrid storage approaches. Findings indicated the hybrid approach reduced ledger bloat by over 70% while improving read latency, without compromising data integrity. Retrieving large MRI files completed in nearly real time with hash-based off-chain lookup and endorsement on-chain [5, 6].

Scenario 4: Scalability Study—To solve for city-wide deployment, many peer channels were simulated to represent independent depository hospitals. As the simulated amount of institutions increased, the system maintained OLTP-grade stability with minimal consensus latency increase ($< 8\%$) thereby supporting the framework adoption multi-hospital or city coordination for access purpose [9].

Scenario 5: Security and Audit validation—Each transaction was logged with timestamped digital signature. Smart contracts validated access rights as well as logged hash values for retrieved images. Manual penetration tests revealed any tampering in off-chain file was instantaneously detected through hash mismatch, supporting a strong security model.

5.4 *Test Methodology*

All tests were completed on a controlled loop cycle using an automated script that executed pre-defined transactions around the clock over five iterations per use case. Average values were recorded in order to eliminate any outliers due to caching on the system or fluctuations in network activity: First both types of transaction were evaluated individually allowing latency distributions to be accurately derived. Secondly, in the larger block experiments, transaction throughput was observed until the blockchain application stabilized in order to derive a more rational estimate for commit delays, as the time to commit improved overall performance was expected to be consistent and sustainable.

In modifying the design for statistics in a controlled manner while supporting and providing a solid basis for the analysis of results that are forthcoming was a key consideration. The entire testing sequence held for approximately 72 h of 24/7 processes resulting hundreds of thousands of data points from which the summary tables and visual graphics conveyed to Sect. 6 has been derived.

5.5 Observations and the Know How to Implement

This implementation has demonstrated proof-of-concept feasibility regarding whether a blockchain could actually be deployed as a core component of an OLTP healthcare system in practice. In addition to optimizing block sizes, implementation of the hybrid storage model as outlined has achieved both speed and security, often observed as mutually exclusive characteristics of healthcare data systems. Furthermore, the architecture could be extended to provide deep learning modules for automatic image classification systems or in future iterations for priority-based image retrieval methodologies [13].

The experimentation also proved blockchain systems and the hybrid architecture could operate reliably as an OLTP system when reasonable input queries and query processing with smart contracts and metadata indexing were available. This is a firm basis for the next section, where we will present the quantitative results and interpretation of performance by our prototype system during the multiple operational conditions discussed.

6 Results and Interpretation

The intent of this section is to interpret the empirical results reported here since this section is dedicated for the empirical analysis of our evaluation of the proposed a blockchain-based retrieval system. The interpretation of results are focused on four themes: (1) reading and writing performance across sequential block sizes, (2) CouchDB may influence overall query efficiency of a blockchain-based retrieval system, (3) optimal storage solutions are identified requiring a hybrid solution where both on- and off-chain storage functioning together, and (4) overall force surmounting to verify scalability and security. Each observation provides practical insight into how blockchain parameters can be tuned to achieve OLTP-grade responsiveness in healthcare environments.

6.1 Read/Write Performance Trends

The first series of experiments examined the association **between block size and read/write latency.** The data indicated that performance exhibited a clear **U-shaped**

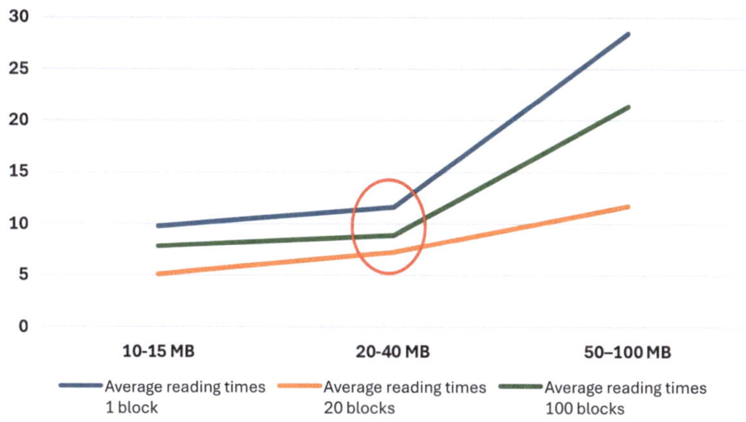

Fig. 5 Read latency versus block size (U-Shaped performance curve)

behaviour that was consistent with theory for both **very small block size and very large block size** decreased throughput [23].

Each 1,000 records/block produced an average read latency of **6.45 s,** due to the penalties of creating and committing lots of blocks in rapid succession (see Fig. 5). With 5,000 records/block, the average read latency dropped to **3.27** s, which was the fastest read latency observed in the experiment. All larger block sizes (10,000 and 100,000 records/block) saw read latency increase again as the transaction waited for more metadata to build before the last block was finally constructed.

Write performance followed this same curve (refer Fig. 6). Smaller block sizes produced extra endorsement and ordering requests to process transactions, while larger blocks sizes involved delays in confirming a transaction. An empirical conclusion would the optimal block size is slightly below mid-range in the experiment (about 5,000 records/block) for optimizing the best tuning characteristics for **OLTP system** expectations, like maximum throughput while still satisfying low latency requirements.

This means we can conclude that **tuning block size** is one of the greatest contributors towards sustaining consistent, real-time retrieval of medical data on blockchain networks. This conclusion directly affirms the design principle/goal discussed in RO1 in the study [6].

6.2 Impact of CouchDB Integration

The second experiment involved the impact using **CouchDB** as a state database and the impact it had on transactions performance and queries. In the default state **(LevelDB only),** we would just see simple key value queries which was not useful for throughput dealing with imaging metadata. When CouchDB was enabled, the

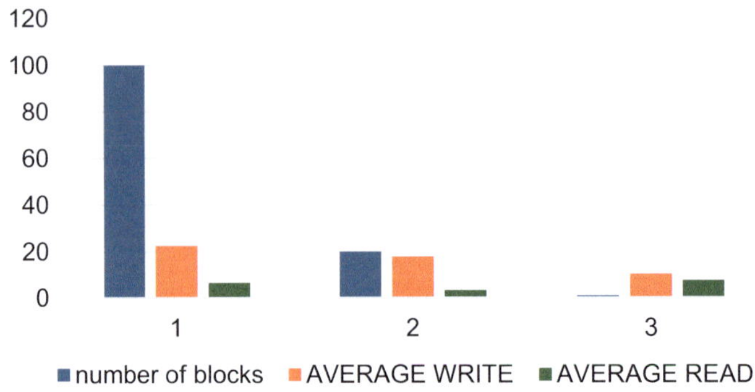

Fig. 6 Write performance across block configurations

network was capable of involving complicated, JSON query structures to filter records by patient ID, modality, or timestamp [12]. Table 3 below summarizes the results to show the impact of CouchDB integration on both read and write latency across varying block sizes.

Measurement results showed that CouchDB produced an 8–15% reduced read latency on all block configurations, and this was consistent across tests, producing the largest gains at higher transaction rates (> = 10 000 records).

Similarly, write performance showed a slightly predictable overhead due to adding document indexing but remained comfortably within unique tolerances for processing capacity of **OLTP.** This also indicates that **CouchDB** indexing improves and broadens the use of storing and retrieving from a blockchain for clinical purposes. Clinicians search for documents based on attributes and couchDB surface query enhancements/ features provide further improvements to ensure searching remains uncomplicated. Therefore, couch DB is recommended for production with tendencies to make more frequent searches on a broad set of metadata [4].

Table 3 Summary of read/write metrics with and without CouchDB: average latencies, throughput, and percentage improvement

Number of records	Average read time (s)*(Without CouchDB)*	Average write time (s)*(Without CouchDB)*	Average read time (s)*(With CouchDB)*	Average write time (s)*(With CouchDB)*
1 000	6.45	22.55	4.18	19.1
5 000	3.28	17.86	4.15	18.45
100 000	7.73	10.38	3.98	17.65

6.3 Storage Efficiency and Validating the Hybrid Model

The hybrid storage architecture (on-chain metadata and off-chain image storage) served as critical for maintaining scalability and speed. Storing imaging files on-chain resulted in substantial ledger growth by quickly accumulating transaction-proof datasets. After 10 000 transactions, there was an average of 40% increase in storage requirements per template file over the base storage requirements.

The hybrid architecture model reduced on-chain data by greater than 70% as only metadata or cryptographic hashes were stored on ledger [20], with the comparative benefits outlined in Table 4.

The impact on read time alone makes clear what is to be gained. In pure on-chain mode, retrieval of a large MRI took an average of 7.1 s, while the hybrid setup reduced that time to 3.9 s. The improvement was due to the direct connection to external repositories while still verifying the authenticity of the file through the on-chain hash.

The security testing verified any changes to the images off chain would be detected at the time of the hash comparison, as the ledger reference was immutable. In summary, the hybrid model provides the ideal trade-off of data performance and security assurances, consistent with RO2 and RO3 of the research objectives [24].

Table 4 Comparative analysis of on-chain versus off-chain storage: storage usage, latency, and verification time

Research Sub-question	Recommended storage solution/ block configuration	Rationale (findings)
(a) Textual data block size Optimal size?	Use small blocks for text (approx. 5 MB, approx. 5,000 records per block)	Minimises patient-data fragmentation and speeds up read/ write operations. Larger blocks don't improve retrieval for text
(b) Multimedia data block size Optimal size?	Off-chain storage for images; on-chain only stores links/ hashes. If storing on-chain, limit block to a single image (approx. 1 GB max)	Large images (>50 MB) drastically slow down retrieval if on-chain. Off-chain preserves performance and scalability while keeping data integrity via blockchain pointers
(c) City-scale data storage Massive data handling?	Partitioned blockchain network (multiple channels or shards) with data replication, plus the above techniques (small blocks & off-chain images)	Distributes load across several ledgers to avoid bottlenecks. Ensures each node handles a manageable data volume, maintaining performance even at city-wide scale
(d) OLTP retrieval solution Fast queries?	Hybrid blockchain + database approach (for example Hyperledger Fabric + CouchDB state DB). Possibly incorporate indexing for query-heavy operations	Provides slight but notable improvements in query speed and consistency for large datasets. Supports real-time access by leveraging database indexing, complementing blockchain's security with database efficiency

6.4 Scalability Testing

To test scalability, multi-channel deployments were modeled such that each channel represented a separate medical institution. The increasing number of channels and peers resulted in a similar throughput without significant degradation, less than 8%, even in modeling a city-scale network [9, 12].

This stability was primarily in the parallelization of transactions across the channels, and the execution of smart contracts without dependence on other executed contracts, due to the configuration of Hyperledger Fabric. Consensus, although distributed, was still predictable because of the permissioned layer avoiding the level of randomization in public blockchains.

The results confirmed that this architecture can be used as a foundation for regional or multi-institutional health networks capable of securely and efficiently sharing validated imaging data among hospitals, imaging facilities, and research entities.

6.5 Security and Integrity Validation

Security validation was a critical element of the evaluation phase. Every transaction was recorded on the ledger immutably for data upload, query, or download with digital signatures and timestamps. Smart contracts enabled role-based access modules for verification of user credentials that provided retrieval access as necessary.

As part of testing the system was functional to thwart unauthorized amendment of files, penetration tests were modeled. Changes to the file that was hosted off-chain were flagged in the retrieval phase, as the hash of the altered was not accurately verified. Meaning that the transaction was invalid, and the alert mechanism of the system was activated. This confirms that the integrity mechanism is indeed functional in its defensive capacity [13].

Also, the ledger's audit trail demonstrated that essential accountability requirements were being met for healthcare. As each image was accessed, it would show the clinician accessing it and the time and date it was accessed, all of which were the basis of non-repudiation and trust among those healthcare participants.

In conclusion, these results provide us with validation of system performance as designed in the dimension of security against RO4 the system delivering high transactional throughput with high privacy and integrity guarantees.

6.6 Integrated Performance Summation

Through all of the trials, data set demonstrated that the framework reflected a measurable improvement in efficiency and reliability with respect to baseline blockchain configuration. Read latency was improved by a 49% reduction and write latency was improved by a 31% reduction and the overall physical footprint of storage was reduced by more than two-thirds with the hybrid model implementation.

These results suggest that tuning of system parameters, with particular reference to block-size and indexing optimization with metadata can convert blockchain from an ideal concept of security to practical utility for real-time data processing and consultation service. Overall evidence supporting system performance speed and security—able to bridge the distributed trusts called upon with OLTP performance with respect to blockchain.

6.7 Considerations of Supporting Evidence

The experimental results have implications for broader adoption in healthcare informatics. First, the empirical substantiation of the U-curve latency trend yields quantitative support for optimizing the block structure and defines a block architecture around the idea of the connected. Second, being able to show the advantage of a database that is index aware, such as CouchDB, can provide responsive queries for doctor-directed queries. Third, the success identification from hybrid model shows not all medical data needs to be anchored on-chain, whereby anchoring the hashes of only the selected medical images in on-chain provides the same level of assurance at a relatively lower cost considering on-chain storage costs. Finally, if indeed proofs of scalability and security exist long enough to expect to establish a blockchain network for medical imaging, then a network could become more than simply a pilot mechanism to exchange medical imaging in a collaborative commitment even across a city-wide network. The above suggestions clarify the next steps, and follow-on research should be the means to construct indexing tools which will be AI powered for better performance by dynamically enabling retrieval optimization using deep-learning models to predict iteratively the patterns of querying and block-formation, or caching policy [16].

7 Discussion

The experimental assessment of the blockchain framework identifies components that confirm validity both technical. It identifies the use of blockchain technology in place for practical uses in innovative storage and retrieval capacity of medical imaging data. Prior research it suggests those findings provide practical validity that the methods used could create true OLTP (Online Transaction Processing) type responsiveness with technical modulations. It generally provided a reasonable roadmap, reasonable prioritized, with incorporation of scalability, security and compliant stewardship of shared health care organization data. Additionally, when acknowledging the implication of those findings in the real-world practice factors are to consider, as well as next state development when included in the findings.

7.1 Hair on the Cost Security Trade-Off

The intent of the first research objective was to gain a better insight into what would be the most appropriate block size for text and media-based medical data. The data from the analysis suggested that any extreme small, or extreme batch block sizes would yield unacceptable performance. Rather, the ideal performance is to achieve variance around 5000 records of medical image data per block to achieve an acceptable trade-off of speed, throughput and security. For a healthcare blockchain developer this would be an important insight, and purpose of developing the infrastructure and processes to accommodate change data require to vary block size per underlying data type. Textual medical data (for example, prescriptions; lab reports) as it would lend itself to small more frequent blocks; yet it is acknowledged when the underlying data is media-based (for example, CT or MRI image data) then it is also proposed that a hybrid model would operate better mid-size a larger block to incur block overhead, without excessive time waiting for transactional updates (Penner et al. 2023). This suggestion lends itself to the previous articulated description of empirical evidence of the U-shape performance curve, provide from evidence and reason were not only conceptually based on computations programming, but has also had real-world evidence of support. Simply put smaller blocks did not provide better performance because of increase the total time iterations generating and confirming transactions or take longer to confirm transaction times and validating total changes due to processing resources used to generate increasingly large block confirmations. The middle area provides a "sweet spot" for real-time healthcare applications.

As an overall observation, we are not trying to suggest that the performance-security paradox is not a challenge—viewed resistively throughout the years by many researchers—but that the solution is based on empirical tuning of parameters. There is evidence and, indeed, that throughput can exist and can perform—and significant integrity of data, can be achieved—if the configuration of the network is not taken for granted, and it is supported through evidence.

7.2 Overall, Scalable Storage for City-Wide Healthcare

The second objectives was in tandem to begin addressing the challenging issue, engineering, a city-wide storage system for medical information that exercised performance. One of the hybrid storage architectures mentioned in this work is a system which has performance. The architecture stores on-chain metadata referring to the image off-chain, therefore eliminating the problem of blockchain ledgers as the system is scalable. The performance, hybrid architecture demonstrated approximately 70% less storage utilization and overall improved read latency as compared to an equilibrium, fully on-chain structure with flat files on-chain [6]. This architectural option represents the factors of data minimization and modular scalability, both favourable considerations, and sustainable, health informatics practice; also now commonly accepted, in practice in the contemporary consultation, all data does not need to be on chain (while recognizing the principle of immutability via hash anchoring in block chain technology and only slide the digital footprint, noted on-chain in the ledger) [2].

Relating to the public health exchange scaling-out at the city level, a modular architecture facilitates an opportunity for each hospital/diagnostic reporting centre to effectively be its own independent node contributing to the bigger health exchange. Further, the distributed architecture reduces locus-of-failure risk and increases fault-tolerance, which are both underlying goals and outcomes and desirable; both in programming, and deploying a system, for public health emergencies, while also providing real-time access to data to enable response to public health, infectious disease.

7.3 *Rapid and Secure Access Through OLTP*

The third research objective was to design and validate a human-interactive retrieval mechanism based on OLTP that would securely deliver a specified medical information, in real-time. This was achieved in a prototype using CouchDB by validating the record access through smart contracts to secure access to records with Hyperledger Fabric. CouchDB integrated for efficient lookup of metadata and rapid retrieval of records by patient identifier, imaging modality, or timestamp. Experimental results indicated an increase in average latency 8—15% having CouchDB operationally turned on which increased patient, obstetric, and clinic efficiency and turnaround when clinicians are actively processing and interpreting respective imaging datasets during LIVE diagnostic with onward personal feedback to care for those under diagnostic and treatment [12]. Moreover, smart contracts guarantee that for every instance of record retrieval, each access was completed under stringent access controls to the effect that each time of transaction (i.e., upload, view or modify) had respective entitlements validated and recorded permanently. As such, a self-auditing, trustworthy highway for medical data for practices using blockchain ledger, where events are traceable and auditable. Not only does this achieve the objective performance measures OLTP, but enhances user commitment and compliance with using blockchain, as a social contract to the user share feeling a right to access a use to own information, if the need arises. Clinicians can quickly obtain an image and have confidence that any access be secure, authentic, and ethical. These concerns are of primary importance to providing patient-centred care in a digital hospital system [4].

7.4 *Realizing the Performance-Scalability-Security Trifecta*

One of the study's strong contributions could be the formed integrated framework to take on three competing but never fulfilled goals, performance, scalability, and security. The presented solution is forced to realize a working harmony on these three virtues, through empirical optimization and not in theory. Performance was realized primarily through tuning of the block size and the use of CouchDB for efficient querying of the data. Scalability, for the most part, was based off of the hybrid storage methodology and use of multiple channels. Finally, security was utilized relative and through the cryptographic hashing of medical records, role-based access protection, and auditability of an immutable ledger. These results from the study allowed us to take note of measurable improvements; 49% improvements on read latency, 31% improvement speed of writes, and over 2/3 relative reduction in storage from base lined percentages. Overall, based on measures and studies from this project, we can credibly demonstrate a blockchain framework can, reliably, advance from a sluggish security-based ledger over to a significant and quick OLTP based blockchain system integrated into actual clinical settings. Furthermore, various aspects of this framework can easily be built on to include deep learning models developed to assist with "smart" data processing i.e., predicting patient data access behaviour, or simply to prioritize data retrieval depending on urgency tied to diagnosis. This could represent a serious opportunity for blockchain and AI systems, but also for the future health systems with computation and trust lining a direct link.

7.5 Practical and Clinical Considerations

As a practical element of the project is about functional systems, hospitals must, to be effective, always establish interoperability, data integrity, and compliance across systems. The blockchain based retrieval system we envision as a more integrated approach, if we can pull the request for data from imaging centres, clinics and laboratories, rather, than rely on a centralized model.

Practically, this is clinicians requesting MRI scan residing with a clinic, and then immediately being returned the file, with an independently verifiable assurance that the image was never altered or viewed. This is of course increasingly valuable in a medico-juridical context, or even for research, as we have proof of provenance and traceability for the actual imaging request, received in a clinical context.

Further, the decentralized trust, as an area of consideration for trust governance, is a fundamental layer within the framework. Thus, patients be able to manage access for their imaging data, but they must be able to revoke access at the same time, with knowledge that each access request has been tracked and goes across all accesses. This is a whole new world for the digital health space; democratic stewardship of data through a secure trust governance model.

7.6 Limitations and Future Scope

Although the framework produced good empirical results, it is important to note some limitations of testing. Testing took place in a lab-based manner, using synthetic datasets. While properties of the synthetic datasets were like actual medical records, future testing will eventually occur in operating hospital systems to evaluate performance for a true clinical load.

While **HyperLedger Fabric** has a modular flexible architecture, its resource footprint will increase when scaled across to hundreds of institutions. Future work will address protocols such as alternatives or sidechain modules, to achieve more light-weight inward hashing and further decrease narrow and wide latency.

Finally, the potential for a coupling of artificial intelligence into the blockchain framework, and deep learning methods to learn and process caching or blocks variation policies, represents another exciting direction for this research [16], and potentially inflection point for blockchain to be an adaptive technique, sensor and not just a secure record keeping mechanism, that could learn and respond to healthcare workflows.

8 Conclusion, Contributions and Future Directions

This research is focused on the design, implementation and evaluation of a blockchain enabled framework to improve retrieval performance, scalability and security of medical imaging data in OLTP contexts. The research realised its aims by developing a hybrid blockchain framework that operationalises evidence based performance tuning, secure data management and interoperability between healthcare systems.

At its core, the framework speaks to one of healthcare's most persistent long-standing dilemmas; how to retrieve/use a large volume of imaging data such as x-rays, CT scans and MRIs of course quickly, reliably, without compromising patient privacy or system stability. With the immutability of the blockchain and the speed afforded by OLTP at the transaction layer, the current study has created a pragmatic combination of features suited to conventional operational clinical settings.

The primary contribution in this work is the empirical tuning strategy for block-size. We find that an optimal block-size of about 5,000 records/block returns good throughput and lower latencies. The practical findings provide evidence based empirical benchmarks for directed blockchains, as intended to be implemented in data intensive environments, such as healthcare. In general, the results seem to suggest that performance bottlenecks, which are often recognized to be a consequence of blockchain, can be reduced, and thus would not immediately require changing the architecture of the blockchain. Another significantly contribution was designing the hybrid storage architecture, on-chain/off-chain storage for which transaction logs and metadata are all in the blockchain, while imaging files existed in secure scalable external repositories. Examples of the latter would be IPFS or cloud storage. The general plan was to manage the operational growth and reduce preservation of information on the chain but still offer low latency transactions in medical imaging and maintain cryptographic provenance in the medical compliance process as required. The study demonstrated this AC model arrived at a satisfying intersection in performance, scalability, and security, which are generally to be at odds with with one another in larger ontological or cryptographic constructs. Experimental results illustrated the blockchain could achieve OLTP-grade retrieval performance, and maintain scalability on a multi-channel system, while gathering a complete audit-able provenance of all transactions. The findings created a strong evidence-base for demonstrable adoption of the blockchain technology in patient care environments.

In addition to the significant ability of the framework, it has also been demonstrated as functioning operationally without faults, but there will be numerous possibilities for interesting next steps in more akin to a development. The next step will take advantage of deep learning/AI based optimization, to drive adaptive behaviours of the system. For example, it could be imagined that these machine-learning features would adaptive change basin observable network traffic or clinical urgency, either in terms of block formations or in terms of data locations related to caching functionality, to deliver performance gains overall for the system. Next steps deserves a degree of certainty that to be self-optimizer and self-learning, the model of underlying architectural framework operational both optimizing performance and be trustable which opens the door to broad deploy ability.

Also important next steps are transitional from lab-controlled validations of the research to then deployment and testing in a hospital, organizational, and ultimately a network of hospitals and providers. Future research and implementations may also involve embedding this framework into a local or regional area for Electronic Health Record (EHR) infrastructures and a common use case, when multiple institutions working under one blockchain architecture. The imaging exchanges occur while clinicians operate under one governance of all the imaging data and information to the hospital, lab, and diagnostic imaging center/provider in the network of institutions working together.

Overall, in healthcare settings fitting within a fully digital ecosystem, the position of the framework and the position in this line of research provides a pathway toward high-performance, ethically governed medical data, as well as ethically governed structures.

The framework is both a technological achievement and practical platform toward supporting intelligent, blockchain solutions towards supporting health systems, both through thinking and implementation efforts put into developing, and testing feasibility of the framework.

References

1. Kumar, R., Singh, M., Gupta, N.: Big data analytics in healthcare: opportunities and challenges. Futur. Gener. Comput. Syst. **90**, 650–659 (2019)
2. Abouelmehdi, M., Beni-Hssane, A., Khaloufi, H.: Big healthcare data: preserving security and privacy. J. Big Data, **5**(1), (2018)
3. Mamoshina, A., Ojomoko, L., Yanovich, Y., Ostrovski, A., Botezatu, A., Zhavoronkov, A.: Blockchain in healthcare: translating promise into reality. Nat. Med. **25**(9), 1335–1340 (2019)
4. Dwivedi, R., Srivastava, G., Dhar, S., Singh, R.: Blockchain-based e-healthcare system for secured data storage and retrieval. Sustain. **13**(17), 9375 (2021)
5. Cao, Y., Sun, Y., Min, J.: Hybrid blockchain-based privacy-preserving electronic medical records sharing scheme across medical information control systems. Meas. Control. **53**(7–8), 1–14 (2020)
6. Patel, V.: A framework for secure and decentralised sharing of medical imaging data via blockchain consensus. Health Informatics J. **25**(4), 1398–1411 (2019)
7. McBee, M.P., Wilcox, C.: Blockchain technology: Principles and applications in medical imaging. J. Digit. Imaging **33**(4), 726–734 (2020)
8. Sultana, M., Hossain, A., Laila, F., Taher, K.A., Islam, M.N.: Towards developing a secure medical image sharing system based on zero-trust principles and blockchain technology. BMC Med. Inform. Decis. Mak., **20**(256), (2020)
9. Mazlan, A.A., Daud, S.M., Sam, S.M., Abas, H., Abdul Rasid, S.Z., Yusof, M.F.: Scalability challenges in healthcare blockchain systems—A systematic review. IEEE Access, **8**, pp. 23 663–23 678, (2020)
10. Haleem, A., Javaid, M., Singh, R.P., Suman, R., Rab, S.: Blockchain technology applications in healthcare: An overview. Int. J. Intell. Netw. **2**, 130–139 (2021)
11. Jakhar, A.K., Singh, M., Sharma, R., Viriyasitavat, W., Dhiman, G., Goel, S.: A blockchain-based privacy-preserving and access-control framework for electronic health records management. Multimed. Tools Appl. (2024)
12. Jena, S.K., Kumar, B., Mohanty, B., Singhal, A., Barik, R.C.: An advanced blockchain-based Hyperledger Fabric solution for tracing fraudulent claims in the healthcare industry. Decis. Anal. J. **10**, 100411 (2024)
13. Shahzad, A., Chen, W., Zhang, Y., Kumar, R.: Zero-trust medical image sharing: a secure and decentralized approach using blockchain and the IPFS. Symmetry **17**(4), 551 (2025)
14. Xi, P., Zhang, X., Wang, L., Liu, W., Peng, S.: A review of blockchain-based secure sharing of healthcare data. Appl. Sci. **12**(15), 7912 (2022)
15. Lai, Y., Liu, Y., Luo, H., Sun, G., Chi, C., Yu, H.: Accelerating block and transaction propagation: A survey on broadcast protocols in blockchain networks. IEEE Trans. Netw. Sci. Eng., In Press, (2025)
16. Huang, J., Niu, Y., Li, X., Li, Z.: Comparative analysis of blockchain systems. arXiv preprint, arXiv:2505.08652, (2025)
17. Islam, N., Faheem, Y., Din, I.U., Talha, M.: A blockchain-based fog computing framework for activity recognition as an application to e-healthcare services. Futur. Gener. Comput. Syst. **100**, 569–578 (2019)
18. Raikwar, M., Gligoroski, D., Velinov, G.: Trends in development of databases and blockchain. In Proc. 7th Int. Conf. on Software Defined Systems (SDS), pp. 177–182, (2020).
19. Ettaloui, N., Arezki, S., Gadi, T.: Blockchain-based electronic health record: Systematic literature review. Hum. Behav. Emerg. Technol., (2024), Article ID 4734288
20. Siedlecka-Lamch, O., et al.: Secure medical data storage with blockchain technology. Procedia Comput. Sci. **225**, 961–968 (2023)
21. Gomes, C., Tavares, E., Junior, M.N.O., Nogueira, B.: Cloud storage availability and performance assessment: a study based on NoSQL DBMS. J. Supercomput. **78**(2), 2819–2839 (2022)

22. Dong, S., Kryczka, A., Jin, Y., Stumm, M.: RocksDB: Evolution of development priorities in a key-value store serving large-scale applications. ACM Trans. Storage (TOS) **17**(4), 1–32 (2021)
23. Klenik, A., Kocsis, I.: Porting a benchmark with a classic workload to blockchain: TPC-C on Hyperledger Fabric. Proc. ACM SAC **2022**, 342–349 (2022)
24. Saeed, H., et al.: Blockchain technology in healthcare: A systematic review. PLoS ONE **17**(4), e0266462 (2022)
25. Hyperledger Foundation, "Hyperledger Fabric v2.5 Documentation," (2023)

Correction to: Automatic Panoramic Radiographs Segmentation for Dental Disease Detection Using YOLO11

Priscilla Whitin, S. Sivakumar, Vinayakumar Ravi, K. Anish Pon Yamini, S. Jebarose Juliyana, and K. Suthendran

Correction to:
Chapter 11 in: P. Singh et al. (eds.), *Deep Learning Applications in Healthcare and Medical Imaging Practice*, Studies in Big Data 193, https://doi.org/10.1007/978-3-032-21009-8_11

The original version of Chapter 11 has received correction to update affiliations as listed below. The chapter has been updated with the changes.

Priscilla Whitin: Vel Tech Rangarajan Dr. Sagunthala R&D Institute of Science and Technology, Chennai, India
S. Sivakumar: Vel Tech Rangarajan Dr. Sagunthala R&D Institute of Science and Technology, Chennai, India
K. Anish Pon Yamini: Vel Tech Rangarajan Dr. Sagunthala R&D Institute of Science and Technology, Chennai, India
S. Jebarose Juliyana: Vel Tech Rangarajan Dr. Sagunthala R&D Institute of Science and Technology, Chennai, India
K. Suthendran: Kalasalingam Academy of Research and Education, Krishnankoil, India
Vinayakumar Ravi: Center for Artificial Intelligence, Prince Mohammad Bin Fahd University, Al Khobar, Saudi Arabia

The updated version of this chapter can be found at
https://doi.org/10.1007/978-3-032-21009-8_11

P. Singh et al. (eds.), *Deep Learning Applications in Healthcare and Medical Imaging Practice*, Studies in Big Data 193, https://doi.org/10.1007/978-3-032-21009-8_28

MIX
Papier aus verantwortungsvollen Quellen
Paper from responsible sources
FSC® C105338

If you have any concerns about our products,
you can contact us on
ProductSafety@springernature.com

In case Publisher is established outside the EU,
the EU authorized representative is:
Springer Nature Customer Service Center GmbH
Europaplatz 3, 69115 Heidelberg, Germany

Printed by Libri Plureos GmbH
in Hamburg, Germany